FIFTH EDITION

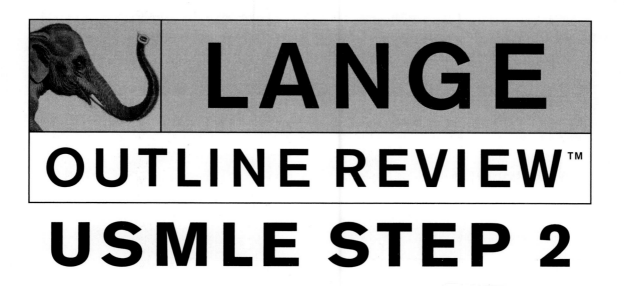

LANGE
OUTLINE REVIEW™
USMLE STEP 2

D1501197

Joel S. Goldberg, DO
Assistant Professor of Medicine
Department of Medicine
Drexel University College of Medicine
Philadelphia, Pennsylvania

McGraw-Hill
Medical Publishing Division

New York   Chicago   San Francisco   Lisbon   London   Madrid   Mexico City   Milan
New Delhi   San Juan   Seoul   Singapore   Sydney   Toronto

Lange Outline Review: USMLE Step 2, Fifth Edition

2 3 4 5 6 7 8 9 0   QPD/QPD   0 9 8 7 6

ISBN 0-07-145192-7

Notice

Medicine is an ever-changing science. As new research and clinical experience broaden our knowledge, changes in treatment and drug therapy are required. The authors and the publisher of this work have checked with sources believed to be reliable in their efforts to provide information that is complete and generally in accord with the standards accepted at the time of publication. However, in view of the possibility of human error or changes in medical sciences, neither the authors nor the publisher nor any other party who has been involved in the preparation or publication of this work warrants that the information contained herein is in every respect accurate or complete, and they disclaim all responsibility for any errors or omissions or for the results obtained from use of the information contained in this work. Readers are encouraged to confirm the information contained herein with other sources. For example and in particular, readers are advised to check the product information sheet included in the package of each drug they plan to administer to be certain that the information contained in this work is accurate and that changes have not been made in the recommended dose or in the contraindications for administration. This recommendation is of particular importance in connection with new or infrequently used drugs.

This book was set in Palatino by Rainbow Graphics.
The editor was Marsha Loeb.
The production supervisor was Sherri Souffrance.
Project management was provided by Rainbow Graphics.
The cover designer was Aimee Nordin.
Quebecor World Dubuque was the printer and binder.

This book is printed on acid-free paper.

Library of Congress Cataloging-in-Publication Data

Goldberg, Joel S.
   Lange outline review. USMLE step 2 / Joel S. Goldberg.— 5th ed.
      p. ; cm
   Rev. ed. of: Appleton & Lange outline review for the USMLE step 2. 4th ed. c2004.
   Includes bibliographical references and index.
   ISBN 0-07-145192-7
   1. Medicine—Examinations, questions, etc. 2. Medicine—Outlines, syllabi, etc. I. Title: USMLE step 2. II. Goldberg, Joel S. Appleton & Lange outline review for the USMLE step 2. III. Title.
   [DNLM: 1. Medicine—Examination Questions. WB 18.2 G618La 2006]
R834.5.G6467 2006
610'.76—dc22
                                                                                        2005054664

For Mickey, Daniel, and Kasey

Contents

Contributors

Reviewed and revised by:

Jennifer C. Bellino, MD
The William W. Backus Hospital
Norwich, Connecticut

Contributors to the previous edition:

Bharat Awsare, MD
Clinical Assistant Professor of Medicine
Division of Critical Care, Pulmonary, Allergic and
    Immunologic Diseases
Department of Medicine
Jefferson Medical College of Thomas Jefferson
    University
Philadelphia, Pennsylvania
Chapter 16, "Pulmonary Medicine"

Arthur K. Balin, MD, PhD, FACP
Clinical Senior Investigator
Lankenau Institute for Medical Research
Jefferson Health System
Wynnewood, Pennsylvania

Attending Physician
Division of Dermatology
Department of Internal Medicine
Riddle Memorial Hospital
Media, Pennsylvania
Chapter 2, "Disorders of the Skin and Subcutaneous Tissue"

Siamak Barkhordarian, MD
Vascular Fellow
Section of Vascular Surgery Department of Surgery
Yale University School of Medicine
New Haven, Connecticut
Chapter 18, "Surgical Principles"

Evan Bash, MD
Clinical Assistant Professor
Department of Orthopedic Surgery
MCP–Hahnemann School of Medicine and
    Temple University School of Medicine
Philadelphia, Pennsylvania
Attending Orthopedic Surgeon
Division of Orthopedic Surgery, Department
    of Surgery
Crozer–Chester Medical Center
Upland, Pennsylvania
*Chapter 10, "Musculoskeletal and Connective Tissue
    Disease"*

Vikas Batra, MD
Fellow
Division of Critical Care, Pulmonary, Allergic and
    Immunologic Diseases
Department of Medicine
Jefferson Medical College of Thomas Jefferson
    University
Philadelphia, Pennsylvania
Chapter 16, "Pulmonary Medicine"

Jennifer C. Bellino, MD
Senior Medical Resident
Department of Internal Medicine
Thomas Jefferson University Hospital
Philadelphia, Pennsylvania
Chapter 19, "Symptoms, Signs, and Ill-Defined Conditions"

Amy C. Brodkey, MD
Clinical Associate Professor
Department of Psychiatry
University of Pennsylvania School of Medicine
Philadelphia, Pennsylvania
Chapter 15, "Psychiatry"

Maria Childers, MD
Instructor
Department of Pediatrics
Jefferson Medical College of Thomas Jefferson
    University
Philadelphia, Pennsylvania
*Chapter 12, "Normal Growth and Development and General
    Principles of Care"*
*Chapter 14, "Congenital Anomalies and Perinatal
    Medicine"*

Christina M. Clay, MD
Clinical Instructor
Department of Medicine
Jefferson Medical College of Thomas Jefferson
    University
Philadelphia, Pennsylvania
Chapter 5, "Hematology"
Chapter 6, "Oncology"

Thomas Fekete, MD
Professor of Medicine
Section of Infectious Diseases
Departments of Internal Medicine and Microbiology
Temple University School of Medicine
Philadelphia, Pennsylvania
Chapter 9, "Infectious and Parasitic Diseases"

Jeffrey Freeman, DO, FACOI
Professor and Chairman
Division of Endocrinology and Metabolism
Department of Medicine
Philadelphia College of Osteopathic Medicine
Philadelphia, Pennsylvania
Chapter 3, "Endocrine and Metabolic Disorders"

Vivian Gahtan, MD
Associate Professor
Section of Vascular Surgery
Department of Surgery
Yale University School of Medicine
New Haven, Connecticut
Chapter 18, "Surgical Principles"

Richard Goldman, MD
Clinical Assistant Professor
Department of Internal Medicine
MCP–Hahnemann University School of Medicine
Philadelphia, Pennsylvania
Attending Physician
Division of Internal Medicine
Department of Hematology/Oncology
Crozer–Chester Medical Center
Upland, Pennsylvania
Chapter 5, "Hematology"
Chapter 6, "Oncology"

Jeffrey I. Greenstein, MD
Chairman
Department of Neurology
Graduate Hospital
Philadelphia, Pennsylvania
Chapter 11, "Neurology"

Victor A. Heresniak, DO
Chairman
Department of Emergency Medicine
Crozer–Chester Medical Center
Upland, Pennsylvania
Chapter 8, "Injury and Toxicology"

Samuel L. Jacobs, MD
Associate Professor, Clinical Obstetrics and
    Gynecology
Division of Reproductive Endocrinology and
    Infertility
Cooper Hospital/University Medical Center
UMDNJ–Robert Wood Johnson School of Medicine
Camden, New Jersey
Chapter 13, "Obstetrics and Gynecology"

Ancil A. Jones, MD
Adjunct Clinical Assistant Professor
Department of Medicine
MCP–Hahnemann University School of Medicine
Philadelphia, Pennsylvania
Clinical Associate Professor
Department of Medicine
Temple University School of Medicine
Philadelphia, Pennsylvania
Invasive/Interventional and Clinical Cardiologist
Department of Medicine
Taylor Hospital
Ridley Park, Pennsylvania
Medical Director
Cardiac Catheterization Laboratory
Crozer–Chester Medical Center
Upland, Pennsylvania
Chapter 1, "Cardiovascular Medicine"

Morris D. Kerstein, MD
Professor and Vice Chairman
Division of General and Vascular Surgery
Department of Surgery
Mount Sinai Hospital and Medical Center
New York, New York
Chapter 18, "Surgical Principles"

Thomas Klein, MD
Chief
Division of Allergy and Immunology
Delaware County Memorial Hospital
Drexel Hill, Pennsylvania
Chapter 7, "Immunology and Allergy"

S. Bruce Malkowicz, MD
Associate Professor
Co-Director, Urology–Oncology Program
Division of Urology
University of Pennsylvania School of Medicine
Philadelphia, Pennsylvania
Chapter 17, "Renal System and Urology"

Charles A. Pohl, MD, FAAP
Clinical Associate Professor and Associate Dean
Department of Pediatrics
Jefferson Medical College of Thomas Jefferson
    University
Philadelphia, Pennsylvania
*Chapter 12, "Normal Growth and Development and General
    Principles of Care"*
*Chapter 14, "Congenital Anomalies and Perinatal
    Medicine"*

Arthur F. Tuch, MD
Clinical Assistant Professor
Department of Medicine
Drexel University College of Medicine
Philadelphia, Pennsylvania
Attending Physician
Division of Gastroenterology
Department of Medicine
Crozer–Chester Medical Center
Upland, Pennsylvania
and
Riddle Memorial Hospital
Media, Pennsylvania
Chapter 4, "Gastroenterology"

Preface

In 1993, I developed a book for medical students specifically designed to allow a rapid and effective review for the USMLE Step 2. *The Instant Exam Review for the USMLE Step 2* was a comprehensive compendium of general medical knowledge in a revolutionary format designed to directly and completely cover the "high impact" fact list of the United States Medical Licensing Exam.

After extensive student feedback, student group discussions, and analysis of current test questions and material, a new text was created and subsequently revised, now known as the *Lange Outline Review: USMLE Step 2,* Fifth Edition. This review book shares the same goals as my original work as a rapid, effective exam review tool. It is up to date, concise, accurate, and highly reflective of current testing material and conditions.

Each and every chapter of *Lange Outline Review: USMLE Step 2,* Fifth Edition has been prepared with the assistance of renowned physicians and specialists. This review book will provide a valuable resource in preparation for the Step 2 examination. As always, the material presented is comprised only of the essential core exam facts necessary for exam success. This book will not waste your valuable time with irrelevant material.

Therefore, remember that this text was not designed to teach general medicine, nor to be a substitute for accepted methods of student education. Its sole purpose is to help ensure exam success.

Joel S. Goldberg, DO
Philadelphia, Pennsylvania

Acknowledgments

I wish to extend my appreciation to Ms. Marsha Loeb and the other publishing staff of McGraw-Hill. They have been a tremendous help and continual valuable resource in the development and production of this text.

I wish to thank all my coauthors for their help with this revision. This group of dedicated physicians was willing to participate in this endeavor despite their busy professional schedules.

How to Use This Book

This book is a practical and easy-to-read study guide designed to be used in both the initial phase of USMLE Step 2 exam preparation as a comprehensive study outline and in the final few days and hours before the exam as a quick review manual.

USING THE BOOK AS A STUDY OUTLINE

When you begin to study, turn to the contents to obtain an overview of this text. At this time, *do not* omit any chapters, but instead start at the beginning and read the book in its entirety. Notice that the outline format is streamlined to allow the rapid assimilation of facts in a minimal amount of reading time. Extraneous and time-consuming information and phrasing have been omitted so you will learn more from this review book than any other text in a comparable amount of time. Since the text is concise, your mind should be clear and focused on the material without distractions. It is important to be both well rested and in a comfortable and quiet study area in order to obtain maximal benefit from *Lange Outline Review: USMLE Step 2,* Fifth Edition.

USING THE BOOK AS A QUICK REVIEW

In the final several weeks and days prior to your examination, *Lange Outline Review: USMLE Step 2* will serve as a rapid review tool. For this type of review, be sure to scan all the pictures, cram facts, and differential diagnosis boxes. Also, it would be a good idea to review the first few words of the diagnosis and treatment steps sections for each disorder. This type of review will provide a good last-minute review.

Cardiovascular Medicine

1

I. ISCHEMIC HEART DISEASE

A. Stable Angina Pectoris

► Description

Disagreeable **chest discomfort,** commonly **substernal** and often described as **heaviness** or squeezing. Can be felt anywhere from epigastrium to jaw, arm(s), neck, or back. **Dyspnea** may accompany chest discomfort or occur alone. **Provoked by exertion or emotional upset, relieved within minutes by rest.**

► Symptoms

The **relationship of symptoms to effort,** and **relief by cessation of activity,** is characteristic. Asymptomatic at rest.

► Diagnosis

Typical symptoms, especially in presence of one or more risk factors (see section I.D). Exam often normal. Electrocardiogram (ECG) can be normal in absence of prior myocardial infarction. **Cardiac stress testing** (exercise or pharmacologic), with or without adjunctive nuclear imaging or echocardiography. In selected cases, **coronary angiography.** Cardiac enzymes (creatine kinase [CK], troponin) will show laboratory evidence of severe ischemia/myocardial infarction (MI) (see following sections).

► Pathology

Increase in myocardial demand for oxygen and nutrient substrate that **exceeds available supply.** Coronary blood supply restricted by arterial narrowing due to **atherosclerotic plaque.** In some cases, excessive myocardial demand (e.g., left ventricular hypertrophy due to aortic stenosis, thyrotoxicosis) can outpace blood supply through normal coronary arteries, or anemia can impair oxygen delivery.

► Treatment Steps
1. **Nitrates, β-blockers, aspirin, empiric anticoagulation** may be used (heparin, low-molecular-weight heparin).
2. Reduction of cardiovascular risk factors.
3. Treatment of MI if present (see section I.C).
4. Revascularization if indicated (see section I.C).

B. Unstable Angina Pectoris

► Description

Disagreeable **chest discomfort,** commonly **substernal** and often described as **heaviness** or squeezing. Can be felt anywhere from the epigastrium to pharynx, arm(s), neck, or back. Occurs unpredictably **at rest** or in a sharply and **abruptly worsening pattern compared to previous stable angina. Dyspnea** may accompany chest discomfort or occur alone. Duration of unstable angina attacks generally 20 minutes or less (an attack lasting hours suggests myocardial infarction).

► Symptoms

Discomfort identical to stable angina pectoris, except usually more severe, and occurs under conditions of **rest** or **minimal activity.** Unstable angina may occur de novo or in patient with known stable angina pectoris. **Commonly occurs at night or in early morning** and may wake patient. May progress to acute myocardial infarction.

► **differential diagnosis**

CARDIOVASCULAR CAUSES OF DYSPNEA

- Cardiomyopathy (dilated, hypertrophic, or restrictive)
- Myocarditis
- Ischemic heart disease (stable or unstable angina, acute MI, acute pulmonary edema)
- Valvular heart disease (especially aortic stenosis, aortic regurgitation, mitral stenosis, mitral regurgitation)
- Pulmonary embolism
- Primary pulmonary hypertension
- Pericardial effusion/tamponade
- Congenital heart disease (depending on form and severity)
- Arrhythmia

ISCHEMIC HEART DISEASE SYNDROMES

Stable Angina Pectoris
- Central chest discomfort, can be felt in back, arm(s), jaw, upper abdomen
- Predictable with physical activity or emotional upset, relief with rest
- Cardiac stress test usually abnormal, cardiac catheterization shows CAD
- Medical therapy with nitrates, β-blockers, calcium channel blockers, aspirin, risk factor modification (long term)
- Revascularization with coronary artery bypass graft (CABG) or PCI

Unstable Angina Pectoris
- Central chest discomfort, can be felt in back, arm(s), jaw, upper abdomen
- Unpredictable at rest or abruptly worsening pattern of angina, prolonged duration (20 minutes or more)
- Cardiac catheterization shows CAD, often with ruptured plaque and/or thrombus
- ECG often abnormal (ST depression or T inversion) but no myocardial necrosis by serum cardiac markers
- Medical therapy with nitrates, β-blockers, aspirin, heparin (unfractionated or low molecular weight), glycoprotein IIbIIIa platelet receptor blockers, risk factor modification (long term)
- Revascularization with CABG or PCI

Acute Myocardial Infarction
- Central chest discomfort, can be felt in back, arm(s), jaw, upper abdomen
- Onset without warning, duration prolonged (often hours)
- ECG usually abnormal, often diagnostic (ST elevation) or suggestive (ST depression)
- Myocardial necrosis by serum cardiac markers
- Medical treatment with aspirin, heparin (unfractionated or low molecular weight), glycoprotein IIbIIIa platelet receptor blockers, β-blockers, nitrates, risk factor modification (long term)
- Urgent reperfusion with thrombolytic drug or PCI
- Cardiac catheterization shows CAD with ruptured plaque and/or thrombus
- Possible complications: mitral regurgitation, ventricular septal defect, cardiac rupture, left ventricular aneurysm

► Diagnosis
Typical symptoms, especially in presence of one or more risk factors. Exam may be normal. The **ECG** may show ischemic ST-T abnormalities, especially if recorded during an attack. Exercise stress testing contraindicated until patieent is asymptomatic and stable. **Coronary angiography** in selected cases.

► Pathology
Decrease in supply of coronary blood flow and oxygen to a level **below that required for baseline metabolic needs of myocardium.** Coronary blood flow is interrupted by **fibrin and platelet plug** developing on a **fissured or ruptured atherosclerotic plaque.** Coronary vasospasm plays role in some patients.

► Treatment Steps
1. **Nitrates, β-blockers, aspirin, empiric anticoagulation** may be used (heparin, low-molecular-weight heparin).
2. Reduction of cardiovascular risk factors.
3. Treatment of MI if present (see section I.C).
4. Revascularization if indicated (see section I.C).

C. Acute Myocardial Infarction (AMI)

► Description

Clinical syndrome of ischemic myocardial necrosis. Amount of necrosis variable depending on quantity of myocardium affected by ischemia, duration of ischemia, collateral blood supply, and treatment administered within the first few hours.

► Symptoms

Prolonged chest discomfort, most commonly **substernal,** but may be felt in arm(s), jaw, back, pharynx, epigastrium. **Dyspnea, diaphoresis** common. **Syncope** may occur. Pain is sometimes "atypical," particularly in females and diabetics (see Clinical Pearl).

► Diagnosis

Typical history, especially in patient with one or more risk factors for coronary artery disease. Exam may disclose **bradycardia, tachycardia, hypotension, hypertension, cardiac gallop(s), cardiac murmur, congestive heart failure (CHF).** The ECG is **usually suggestive or diagnostic** (ST elevation) of acute myocardial ischemia. Serial **serum cardiac marker** testing (creatine phosphokinase [CPK] with myocardial isoenzyme, troponin I or T) confirmatory. Look for **evolution of infarction pattern on serial ECGs.**

► Pathology

Caused by an **abrupt decrease in coronary arterial blood flow** or, less commonly, by a severe and **prolonged increase in myocardial oxygen need** that cannot be met by available coronary arterial flow. Abrupt decrease in coronary artery flow usually due to **thrombus formation on fissured** or **ruptured atherosclerotic plaque** or hemorrhage into atherosclerotic plaque. Coronary vasoconstriction (spasm), coronary artery embolus, or spontaneous artery dissection rare causes. Tachycardia or sustained severe hypertension can cause prolonged increase in myocardial oxygen demand sufficient to cause myocardial necrosis. **Irreversible necrosis can develop within 1–6 (variable) hours after onset of persistent ischemia.**

► Treatment Steps

1. **Aspirin, nitrates, heparin (unfractionated or low molecular weight), glycoprotein IIbIIIa platelet receptor blockers, β-blockers, angiotensin-converting enzyme (ACE) inhibitors** (see Cram Facts).
2. **Urgent myocardial reperfusion** using **thrombolytic therapy** (alteplase [t-PA], reteplase [r-PA], streptokinase, anistreplase [APSAC], or emergency **percutaneous transluminal intervention** [PCI]) (Fig. 1–1).
3. **Treatment of arrhythmia** as required.
4. Cardiac catheterization followed by cardiac surgery or PCI may be required for complications of recurrent angina or infarction, mitral regurgitation (acquired) ventricular septal defect, cardial rupture, cardiogenic shock, ventricular aneurysm.

D. Risk Factors for Coronary Artery Disease (CAD)

► Description

Risk factors for CAD have a **strong epidemiologic correlation with likelihood of developing clinical CAD.** Multiple risk factors combine to significantly increase CAD risk compared to one factor alone.

- **Hyperlipidemia** (elevated low-density lipoprotein [LDL], low high-density lipoprotein [HDL], possibly elevated triglycerides).

► **clinical pearl**

ATYPICAL CHEST PAIN

Patients can have myocardial ischemia or infarction without classic symptoms of "chest pain." This is particularly common in females and diabetics. Clinicians need to keep cardiac ischemia in mind in patients with atypical presentations (e.g., abdominal pain, fatigue, neck pain).

► **cram facts**

BLOOD THINNERS USED IN AMI

HEPARIN

- Given as continuous intravenous infusion
- Advantage is it can be turned off and reversed quickly
- Disadvantage is it can be difficult to regulate, requiring frequent monitoring of the partial thromboplastin time (PTT)

LOW-MOLECULAR-WEIGHT HEPARIN (LMWH)

- Enoxaparin (Lovenox), dalteparin (Fragmin)
- Given subcutaneously once or twice a day
- No routine monitoring needed (unless patient is morbidly obese or in renal failure)
- Disadvantage is the inability to reverse the drug acutely

GLYCOPROTEIN IIb/IIIa INHIBITORS

- Eptifibatide (Integrilin)
- Acts to inhibit platelet aggregation
- Given intravenously with heparin or LMWH in acute coronary syndromes

ECG CHANGES

ST depression suggests myocardial ischemia.

ST elevation suggests myocardial infarction.

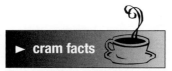

ACUTE MYOCARDIAL INFARCTION (AMI)

New terminology describes STEMI vs. NSTEMI. STEMI is an AMI with ST elevation seen on the ECG. NSTEMI is an AMI without ST elevation seen on the ECG.

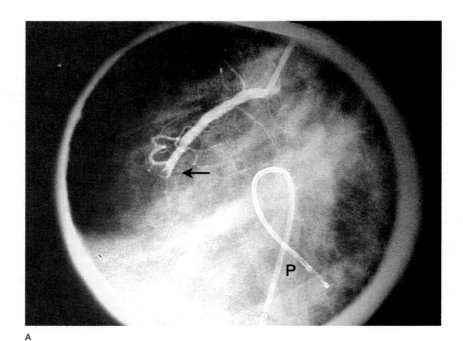

A

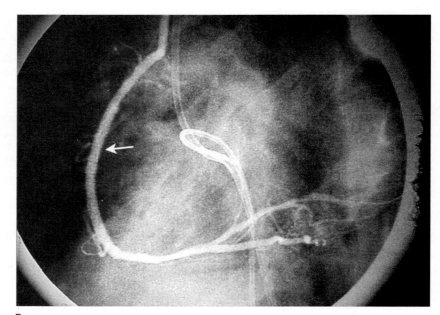

B

Figure 1–1. Right coronary angiogram of a patient with acute inferior myocardial associated with ST segment elevation of ECG. Note (A) total thrombotic occlusion (arrow) of mid-RCA and (B) successful reperfusion (arrow) with PCI and coronary artery stenting. Temporary right ventricular (P) pacing was required for infarct associated complete heart block.

- **Cigarette smoking.**
- **Systemic arterial hypertension.**
- **Diabetes mellitus.**
- **Family history of premature CAD** (< 55 yr of age).
- **Male sex** or **postmenopausal females.**
- An HDL level ≥ 60 mg/dL is actually a negative risk factor for CAD because high HDL levels correlate with a lower risk of CAD.

E. Prevention of Coronary Artery Disease

- **Primary prevention**—efforts to lower risk of CAD by risk-factor modification before clinical manifestations of CAD appear.
- **Secondary prevention**—efforts to lower risk of repeat CAD event in patient who has already developed clinical manifestations of CAD (e.g., angina, myocardial infarction).

Prevention efforts focus on modifiable risk factors:
- **Hyperglycemic control**
- **Cessation of cigarette smoking**
- **Control of systemic arterial hypertension**
- **Control of excess body weight**
- **Diet modification**
- **Behavior modification and stress reduction**
- **Exercise**
- **Lipid management**

► **cram facts**

CONGESTIVE HEART FAILURE (CHF)

Low-Output CHF

- Inability of heart to deliver blood adequate for metabolic needs without elevation of filling pressure. Depressed ejection fraction on echocardiogram.
- Systolic (depression of ventricular contractility) and diastolic dysfunction usually coexist; diastolic dysfunction alone less common.
- Multiple etiologies, including systemic hypertension, CAD, valvular disease, primary myocardial disease, rheumatic heart disease, congenital heart disease.
- Echocardiogram to assess cardiac function, valves.
- Neurohormonal pathophysiology (renin–angiotensin and sympathetic nervous systems).
- Dyspnea, orthopnea, fatigue, swelling, palpitations.
- Pulmonary rales, edema, cardiac gallop(s), ascites, cardiac enlargement.
- Salt restriction, diuretic, ACE inhibitor, digitalis, β-blocker, treat underlying cause.

High-Output CHF

- Inability of heart to deliver blood adequate for increased metabolic needs without elevation of filling pressure.
- Much less common than low-output CHF.
- Systolic and/or diastolic dysfunction.
- Etiologies include severe anemia, Paget's disease, beriberi, thyrotoxicosis, large arteriovenous fistula(e).
- Signs and symptoms similar to low-output CHF.
- Salt restriction, diuretic.
- Diagnose and treat underlying cause.

Cor Pulmonale

- Right ventricular failure secondary to pulmonary disease (multiple etiologies), parenchymal and/or vascular, causing significant pulmonary hypertension.
- Swelling, fatigue, palpitations, ascites, hepatosplenomegaly.
- Edema, neck vein distention, right ventricular (RV) enlargement, RV gallop(s), tricuspid regurgitation.
- ECG with RVH, echocardiogram with RV enlargement and signs of pulmonary hypertension.
- Salt restriction, diuretic, treat underlying cause.

NYHA CLASSES FOR HEART FAILURE

A useful and commonly used way to classify severity of heart failure is the New York Heart Association's classification:

- Class I—no symptoms with normal physical activity.
- Class II—ordinary physical activity results in fatigue, dyspnea, or other symptoms.
- Class III—marked limitation in normal physical activity.
- Class IV—symptoms at rest or with any physical activity.

"BNP"

- Brain natriuretic peptide, also known as B-type natriuretic peptide.
- Marked elevation of serum BNP can help differentiate CHF as a cause of dyspnea, rather than other conditions.
- May also help with prognosis of CHF exacerbation.

F. Cardiac Rehabilitation

► Description
Physician-supervised **program of exercise and risk-factor modification** for patients with angina pectoris, prior myocardial infarction, prior PCI, or prior coronary bypass surgery.

► Goals
Improvement in **exercise capacity, symptom level,** and **sense of well-being. Longer survival** through risk-factor modification.

II. HEART FAILURE

Heart failure is a clinical syndrome in which the heart is unable to pump blood at a rate adequate to meet metabolic needs at the tissue level. Heart failure is characterized by **abnormal cardiac muscle performance** (myocardial dysfunction), **pathophysiologic neurohumoral changes** (in both the renin–angiotensin system and sympathetic nervous system), and **peripheral circulation changes** (peripheral vasoconstriction).

A. Low-Output Heart Failure

► Description
Inability of the heart to deliver adequate blood to meet the metabolic needs of the body in the resting state or with day-to-day activities, or to do so only at the expense of elevated filling pressure (Frank–Starling relationship). **Most common form of heart failure.**

► Symptoms
See Table 1–1 for signs and symptoms of heart failure.

► Diagnosis
- **History** of **characteristic symptoms,** especially in patient with known heart disease.
- Workup includes chest x-ray, ECG, Doppler echocardiography, nuclear and cardiac imaging. New lab test is BNP (see Clinical Pearl).

► Pathology
Myocardial dysfunction can affect either **systolic** (contractile) or **diastolic** (relaxation) function. Often, systolic and diastolic dysfunction coexist, although in some cases (e.g., hypertrophic cardiomyopathy) diastolic dysfunction can dominate. **Systemic vascular resistance (SVR) usually increased.**

Left ventricle (LV) often affected alone early on, but in severe cases, both right ventricle (RV) and LV usually involved. Most common cause of RV failure is LV failure.

1-1

SIGNS AND SYMPTOMS OF HEART FAILURE

Symptoms of right- and left-sided heart failure often coexist. However, it is commonly taught to separate the two signs and symptoms.

LEFT-SIDED HEART FAILURE
- Symptoms: Dyspnea (at rest or with exertion), orthopnea, fatigue
- Signs: Pulmonary congestion (rales), cardiomegaly, left ventricular heave and/or gallop

RIGHT-SIDED HEART FAILURE
- Symptoms: "Swelling," fatigue
- Signs: JVD, cardiomegaly, RV heave or gallop, ascites, hepatosplenomegaly, lower extremity edema

Systemic hypertension and **coronary artery disease** are common causes of CHF. Other etiologies are numerous and include **rheumatic heart disease, valvular diseases,** and **myocardial diseases.**

► Treatment Steps
1. **Salt restriction, diuretic** as needed for fluid overload.
2. **Angiotensin-converting enzyme inhibitors (ACEIs), digitalis** for patients with impaired LV function.
3. **Angiotensin receptor blockers (ARBs)** or **hydralazine/nitrates** for patients intolerant of ACEIs.
4. **β-blockers** (carvedilol, metoprolol, bisoprolol) for patients with impaired LV function.
5. Treat arrhythmias as required.
6. Cardiac surgery for selected patients with severe valve dysfunction.

B. High-Output Heart Failure

► Description
Inability of the heart to pump adequate blood in face of a condition that requires an increased cardiac output to meet metabolic needs of the body.

► Symptoms
In contrast to patients with low-output CHF, patients with high-output CHF may have **bounding pulses** and **hyperdynamic circulation** with warm and flushed extremeties.

► Pathology
Arteriovenous shunting (peripheral circulation admixture) and persistent **increased cardiac output** (relative to low-output CHF) leads to **salt retention, increased blood volume,** and the CHF syndrome. **SVR is normal or reduced** (see Cram Facts).

► Treatment Steps
1. **Salt restriction, diuretic.**
2. **Treat underlying cause.**

C. Acute Pulmonary Edema

► Description
Abrupt **increase in pulmonary capillary pressure and vascular volume of lungs,** causing **impaired gas exchange** and constituting a medical emergency. **Most commonly occurs on cardiogenic basis,** but can occur as a result of noncardiac disease.

► Symptoms
Severe **dyspnea** and **orthopnea,** often of abrupt onset, with **diaphoresis.** See Table 1–1.

► Pathology
Cardiogenic pulmonary edema caused by **elevation of pulmonary venous pressure** (often precipitous).

► Treatment Steps
1. **Upright position** of head and thorax, supplemental oxygen.
2. **Intravenous loop diuretic, nitrates, morphine sulfate.**
3. **Mechanical ventilation** in severe cases.
4. Diagnose and correct contributing factors (see Clinical Pearl).

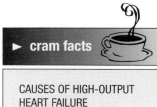

► **cram facts**

CAUSES OF HIGH-OUTPUT
HEART FAILURE

• Severe anemia
• Thyrotoxicosis
• Acute beriberi
• Paget's disease
• Large arteriovenous fistula(e)

► **clinical pearl**

When acute pulmonary edema occurs, the cause of the decompensation should be sought.

Causes include:
• Acute MI/ischemia
• Dietary indiscretion (high-sodium meal(s)
• Acute valvular dysfunction (i.e., rupture of mitral valve chordae leading to acute mitral regurgitation)
• Arrhythmia
• Severe anemia

D. Cor Pulmonale

▶ Description

Altered structure and function of the right ventricle due to primary pulmonary disease.

▶ Symptoms

Initial symptoms (fatigue, dyspnea) may be attributed to the pulmonary condition. Once RV failure is more advanced, passive hepatic congestion and lower extremity edema can occur. Exam findins include RV gallop or heave, jugular venous distention (JVD), ascites, and edema.

▶ Diagnosis

Clinical setting. The ECG may show **right atrial (RA) and right ventricular hypertrophy (RVH). Echocardiography** (RV enlargement/ hypertrophy, tricuspid regurgitation). Arterial blood gases and pulmonary function testing. Some patients may need **right heart catheterization** to confirm diagnosis and to assess response of pulmonary vasculature to vasodilators.

▶ Pathology

Lung disease can affect the heart through structural changes of pulmonary vasculature and/or severe hypoxia.

   Severe hypoxia can lead to moderate or severe **pulmonary hypertension** by causing pulmonary vasoconstriction.

   Obliteration of pulmonary vasculature sufficient to cause significant pulmonary hypertension can occur in pulmonary embolism, primary pulmonary hypertension, CREST syndrome (calcinosis, Raynaud's phenomenon, esophageal dysfunction, sclerodactyly, telangiectasia).

▶ Treatment Steps

Treatment of CHF (see section II.A) and treatment of the underlying condition.

III. CARDIAC ARRHYTHMIAS

A. Supraventricular Origin

1. Premature Beats

Premature Atrial Contraction (PAC)—An early (before the next expected sinus node depolarization) beat originating from an atrial focus outside of the sinus node (Fig. 1–2). Frequent PACs may portend atrial tachycardia, atrial fibrillation, or atrial flutter.

Premature Junctional Contraction (PJC)—An early beat originating from the atrioventricular junction (AV node).

2. Tachycardias

Paroxysmal Supraventricular Tachycardia (PSVT)—A regular tachycardia (usually 150–250/min) of atrial or atrioventricular junction origin. Most common mechanism is reentry within the atrioventricular junction, but may be due to automatic atrial focus or to reentry involving atria and ventricles utilizing a conduction tract bypassing to atrioventricular junction.

Nonparoxysmal Junctional Tachycardia—A regular tachycardia (usually < 130 per min) due to increased rate of automaticity of

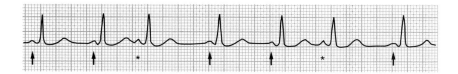

Figure 1–2. Premature atrial contraction (PAC). The P waves (*) of the PAC beats in this ECG lead II occur earlier than the next expected sinus beat and are of a different morphology compared to the sinus P wave (arrow).

the atrioventricular junction. Most commonly due to digitalis toxicity, acute myocardial infarction, or myocarditis.

Multifocal Atrial Tachycardia (MAT)—An irregular tachycardia (usually 120–200/min) due to rapid atrial depolarizations with varying nonsinus P wave morphologies (at least three different contours). Usually associated with severe and decompensated lung disease chronic obstructive pulmonary disease [COPD]).

Atrial Fibrillation—A grossly irregular supraventricular rhythm (may be slow but usually rapid in untreated state) with coarse or fine atrial fibrillation waves and no identifiable P waves (Fig. 1–3) (see Clinical Pearl).

Atrial Flutter—A supraventricular rhythm with identifiable ("sawtooth" ECG baseline) continuous atrial activity with atrial rate of 250–350 per minute (Fig. 1–4). Ventricular rate depends on degree of block at atrioventricular junction. Ventricular rate of 150 per minute (2:1 AV block) is common.

B. Ventricular Origin

1. Premature Beats

Premature Ventricular Contraction (PVC)—An early beat originating from any portion of either ventricle (Fig. 1–5). Found in a variety of diseases or in apparently normal individuals, **clinical significance depends on underlying cardiac diagnosis.**

2. Tachycardias

Ventricular Tachycardia (VT)—Consists of three or more consecutive ventricular beats originating from any portion of either ventricle. Usually paroxysmal and of abrupt onset and termination. May be sustained (≥ 30 beats), nonsustained (< 30 beats), monomorphic (each beat with similar or identical QRS morphology), or polymorphic (QRS morphology varies beat to beat). Can cause syncope, CHF, angina, or lead to ventricular fibrillation; P waves may or may not be identifiable.

▶ clinical pearl

ATRIAL FIBRILLATION

- Patients have an increased risk of stroke and are therefore given anticoagulation with Coumadin unless contraindications exist.
- No consensus on which is a primary goal of atrial fibrillation: rate control of atrial fibrillation versus conversion to normal sinus rhythm.

▶ clinical pearl

MEDICATIONS FOR ATRIAL FIBRILLATION

- β-Blockers (metoprolol) or calcium channel blockers (diltiazem) help with rate control.
- Digitalis slows conduction at the AV node and controls rate.
- Coumadin is used for anticoagulation unless contraindicated.
- Amiodarone is an antiarrhythmic with a multitude of side effects, including thyroid and liver dysfunction and hyperpigmentation of skin. Pulmonary toxicity (i.e., hypersensitivity pneumonitis) can be fatal.
- Other antiarrhythmics (sotalol, propafenone) are used but, because they can themselves be proarrhythmic with multiple side effects, are usually managed best with a cardiologist.

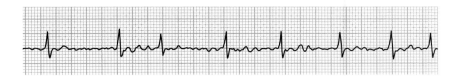

Figure 1–3. Atrial fibrillation. In this ECG lead II, note continuous, unorganized, chaotic atrial fibrillatory waves (of low amplitude in this example), best seen in the normally isoelectric segment between beats, and the irregularly irregular QRS cadence.

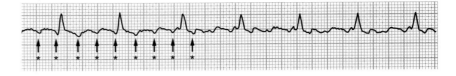

Figure 1–4. Atrial flutter. In this ECG lead II, note continuous sawtooth pattern of atrial activity. The atrial flutter waves (*) are slightly slower than the usual 300/min because of treatment with procainamide. QRS cadence (which may vary) is essentially regular due to repetitive atrial activity and near constant degree of block in the atrioventricular node.

Ventricular Fibrillation (VF)—A grossly chaotic ventricular tachyarrhythmia (ventricular rate > 250 per min or uncountable) without identifiable P waves. **Rapidly fatal if not treated immediately** by direct current countershock (defibrillation). Ventricular flutter, a ventricular tachyarrhythmia of 150–250 per minute without identifiable ST segments or T waves, has same clinical significance as VF.

3. Automatic Implantable Cardiac Defibrillator

Automatic implantable cardiac defibrillators (AICDs) are becoming more common. Patients often have an EPS (electrophysiology study). Whether their arrhythmias (usually ventricular tachycardia or fibrillation) are inducible, along with their baseline ejection fraction, will determine whether they are candidates for an AICD.

C. Bradyarrhythmias

1. Sinus

Sinus Arrest—Failure of impulse formation in the sinus node. Asystole will result unless an escape rhythm (ectopic atrial, junctional, ventricular) develops.

Sinus Bradycardia—An abnormally slow rate (< 50/min) due to a slowing of the rate of depolarization of the sinus node. May be found in healthy individuals, but may be associated with vasovagal reaction, MI, drug therapy, bradytachycardia syndrome, or aging. Usually asymptomatic, but can cause episodic weakness or syncope.

2. Heart Block

First-Degree AV Block—Prolongation of the PR interval > 0.20 seconds in adults due to slowing of conduction in the AV junction. May or may not be associated with bradycardia.

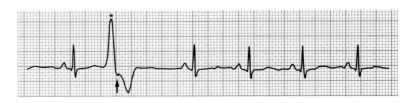

Figure 1–5. Premature ventricular contraction (PVC). In this ECG lead II, the PVC (*) occurs earlier than the next expected sinus beat, is wide (QRS ≥ 0.12 seconds due to intramyocardial conduction), and is not associated with a preceding atrial contraction. A compensatory pause follows the PVC. Note that intact ventriculoatrial conduction allows retrograde atrial depolarization, and the resulting P wave (∧) deforms the ST segment of the PVC.

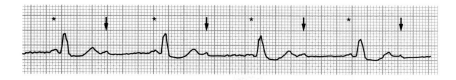

Figure 1–6. Mobitz II second-degree heart block. This ECG lead II shows a P wave conducted (*) to the ventricles followed by a nonconducted P wave (v) in alternating fashion (2:1 atrioventricular block). The wide QRS complex (0.13 second) is typical of infranodal block.

Second-Degree AV Block—Intermittent failure of the cardiac impulse originating in the atria to reach the ventricles, is of two types:

Mobitz Type I—Caused by block at the atrioventricular junction, is the most common type of second-degree heart block.

Mobitz Type II—Caused by block at site distal to the AV junction. Less common than type I, but often a precursor to complete infranodal AV block (see Fig. 1–6).

Third-Degree (Complete) AV Block—Due to complete block of cardiac impulse at the AV junction, His bundle, or both right and left bundle branches. Atrial and ventricular activities are independent. The resultant escape QRS complex is generally regular and will be normal (narrow, originating from the AV junction) or wide (idioventricular, originating from the ventricles), depending on the level of block. This bradyarrhythmia can cause weakness, angina, CHF, or syncope.

IV. MYOCARDIAL DISEASES

A. Congestive (Dilated) Cardiomyopathy

▶ Description
Congestive (dilated) cardiomyopathy is characterized by **dilated and poorly contractile ventricles.** Atria are often dilated as well. **Right and left ventricles are often affected together;** however, the right or left ventricle may be affected predominantly, depending on the specific cause or stage of the disease process.

▶ Symptoms
Symptoms of heart failure (see Table 1–1).

▶ Diagnosis
Clinical scenario. **Chest x-ray** with cardiomegaly, pulmonary congestion. **Echocardiography** shows cardiac dilatation with reduced ventricular ejection fraction. Laboratory studies may confirm specific etiologies.

▶ Pathology
Decreased ventricular contractility (systolic dysfunction) results in **reduced cardiac output** and/or **pulmonary congestion** (CHF). Basis for systolic dysfunction depends on etiology and, in some cases, is unknown. **Diastolic dysfunction** often coexists. Etiologies are numerous (see Cram Facts).

▶ Treatment Steps
1. Specific etiology of the cardiomyopathy should be determined to guide treatment and prognosis. Cardiac catheterization is usually indicated initially to rule out ischemic heart disease.
2. Treatment of CHF (see section II.A).

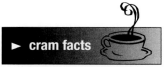
▶ **cram facts**

ETIOLOGIES OF DILATED CARDIOMYOPATHY

1. Ischemic CAD, prior MI
2. Systemic hypertension
3. Idiopathic (cause unknown)
4. Viral (including coxsackie, human immunodeficiency virus [HIV])
5. Familial (increasing evidence for genetic basis in many cases)
6. Postpartum/ peripartum
7. Alcoholic (toxic)
8. Chagas' heart disease (trypanosomiasis)
9. Radiation therapy
10. Beriberi (thiamine deficiency)
11. Drug induced (anthracyclines)
12. Cocaine abuse

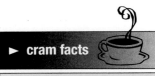

HYPERTROPHIC CARDIOMYOPATHY

- Important to diagnose due to an increased risk of sudden death, particularly in young people.
- The murmur of HOCM decreases with handgrip, increases with standing.

B. Hypertrophic Obstructive Cardiomyopathy (HOCM)

► Description

A form of cardiomyopathy characterized by a **hypertrophic and nondilated left ventricle** in the absence of a systemic or coexisting cardiac condition capable of producing left ventricular hypertrophy (LVH). Often **disproportionate hypertrophy of the ventricular septum,** which may produce variable amounts of obstruction in the left ventricular outflow tract. Right ventricle can be hypertrophied as well. May be **familial** or **sporadic.**

► Symptoms

Dyspnea, chest pain, near-syncope, or syncope, which can be caused by **arrhythmia** (ventricular tachycardia or atrial fibrillation) or LV outflow tract obstruction.

On exam, **systolic murmur** at lower left sternal border, **bifid carotid pulse** (in cases of LV outflow obstruction), **S4.** May have murmur of **mitral regurgitation.**

► Diagnosis

Patient history, family history, and exam. ECG shows LVH. **Echocardiography usually diagnostic.**

► Pathology

Clear evidence for genetically determined abnormalities of several contactile proteins in the cardiac myocyte. **Diastolic dysfunction** causes pulmonary congestion, restriction to adequate left ventricular filling. **Dynamic obstruction to left ventricular outflow common,** but does not always occur. Systolic dysfunction can occur in advanced cases.

► Treatment Steps

1. Avoid dehydration.
2. Strenuous activity prohibited.
3. **β-Blockers.**
4. **Calcium channel blockers.**
5. **Surgical myectomy** of hypertrophied ventricular septum in severely obstructed patients when medical therapy inadequate.
6. Permanent atrioventricular pacing beneficial in some refractory cases.
7. Alcohol ablation of a portion of the ventricular septum by PCI techniques.
8. Screening of family members.

C. Restrictive Cardiomyopathy

► Description

A form of cardiomyopathy characterized by **noncompliant, poorly distensible** ventricle(s) on basis of infiltrative process. Ventricular systolic function often normal, and heart may not be enlarged. **Least common** form of cardiomyopathy.

► Symptoms

Fatigue. Edema.

On exam, **neck vein distention, edema, ascites.** May mimic constrictive pericarditis.

► Diagnosis

Echocardiography may show endomyocardial fibroelastosis and/or restricive filling pattern. **Cardiac catheterization.** Endometrial biopsy sometimes used.

► Pathology

Any **infiltrative process** of myocardium that results in **interstitial fibrosis** or **thickening of heart wall** (not myocyte hypertrophy).
- **Amyloidosis**
- **Sarcoidosis**
- **Endomyocardial fibroelastosis** (may occur with or without idiopathic **hypereosinophilic syndrome**)
- **Glycogen storage disease**

► Treatment Steps
1. **Diuretic, salt restriction.**
2. **Treat underlying disease.**

D. Myocarditis

► Description

Inflammation of the myocardium with inflammatory cellular infiltrate and varying degrees of myocyte necrosis. Myocarditis may be difficult or impossible to distinguish clinically from cardiomyopathy (see preceding sections). Some forms of cardiomyopathy may evolve from myocarditis.

► Symptoms

Often **preceded by upper respiratory tract infection** (viral). Many cases mild and self-limited, may even be asymptomatic. In more severe cases, **fever, dyspnea, edema, chest pain.**

On exam, **tachycardia, pulmonary congestion, edema, gallops, cardiomegaly.**

► Diagnosis

History, exam. Chest x-ray with cardiomegaly, CHF. Elevated sedimentation rate. Viral cultures and titers useful in some cases. Blood cultures (bacterial). Right ventricular endomyocardial biopsy may have a role.

► Pathology

Viral—Very common; especially **coxsackie B,** but also influenza, varicella, echo virus, infectious mononucleosis, coxsackie A, measles, HIV-2 with the acquired immune deficiency syndrome (AIDS), and others. Bacterial fungal, rickettsial causes rare.

► Treatment Steps
1. **Treat congestive heart failure.**
2. **Treat underlying condition.**
3. **Immunosuppresive therapy** in selected cases.

V. PERICARDIAL DISEASES

A. Acute Pericarditis

► Description

Inflammatory process involving pericardium, by spread either from myoepicardium or from adjacent structure.

► Symptoms

Chest pain, often **sharp** and **knifelike,** central or left precordial, can radiate to shoulders or back. Often **positional** and with pleuritic component; however, may be asymptomatic. May evolve into chronic form.

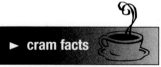

► cram facts

CAUSES OF PERICARDITIS

- Infectious—most commonly coxsackie B virus, other viral, bacterial, fungal, parasitic, or tuberculosis.
- Dressler syndrome (post cardiotomy and post myocardial infarct) likely autoimmune in nature.
- Malignancy.
- Idiopathic.
- Trauma.
- Radiation therapy.
- Uremia.
- Systemic lupus erythematosus.
- Rheumatic fever.
- Rheumatoid arthritis.
- Scleroderma.

► Diagnosis

History. On exam, hallmark is three-component **pericardial friction rub,** but only one or two components may be audible, or rub may not be present. Often leukocytosis, **elevated sedimentation rate.** Acute and convalescent viral titers. ECG with diffuse ST-T abnormality, typically with diffuse elevation of ST segment.

Echocardiography may show pericardial effusion. Important to establish etiologic diagnosis if possible.

► Treatment Steps

1. **Symptomatic** and **supportive.**
2. **Nonsteroidal anti-inflammatory drugs (NSAIDs)** or **aspirin.** Steroids occasionally required.
3. **Treat underlying disease.**

B. Pericardial Effusion

► Description

Accumulation of serous or serosanguinous **fluid in pericardial space.** Can be acute or chronic. Rapidity of fluid collection the major determinant of hemodynamic effect.

► Symptoms

May be **asymptomatic** or have **chest pain** of pericarditis. Cardiac tamponade with hemodynamic collapse can occur.

► Diagnosis

History, exam. May have **pericardial friction rub** or dullness at left lung base posteriorly due to compression of lung by pericardial sac **(Ewart's sign).** Chest x-ray with "cardiomegaly." The ECG may show pattern of pericarditis, also electrical alternans; **echocardiography** documents presence and size of effusion and may show signs of cardiac tamponade, if present. **Pericardiocentesis** and/or **pericardial biopsy** helpful in establishing etiology.

► Pathology

Most common causes are **viral, idiopathic, uremic, rheumatoid syndromes, thyroid disease,** and **malignant** pericarditis; however, **any cause of pericarditis** can cause pericardial effusion, and effusion may be the presenting sign of pericardial disease.

► Treatment Steps

1. **Treat underlying disorder.**
2. **Pericardial biopsy or pericardiocentesis** may be required.
3. **Treat pericarditis symptoms** (see above), if present.

C. Cardiac Tamponade (by Pericardial Effusion)

► Description

Marked reduction of cardiac output due to interference with normal cardiac filling by the **compressive effect of pericardial effusion.** Rate of accumulation of pericardial fluid important. Rapid accumulation of fluid can cause cardiac tamponade by relatively small volumes of pericardial fluid (as little as a few hundred milliliters).

► Symptoms

Acutely ill. Dyspnea and **hemodynamic collapse.** If tamponade develops slowly, can mimic CHF.

▶ Diagnosis

History, exam. **Neck vein distention** in setting of **hypotension and pulsus paradoxicus.** Heart sounds may be muffled, and pericardial friction rub may be heard.

▶ Pathology

Can occur with pericardial effusion of any cause, but most commonly associated with **trauma, cardiac surgery, malignancy.** Occasionally, cardiac tamponade is due to pericardial effusion from viral or idiopathic pericarditis or following radiation therapy.

▶ Treatment Steps
1. **Pericardiocentesis** or **surgical pericardiotomy** without delay can be lifesaving.
2. **Treat underlying disease** after relief of cardiac tamponade.

D. Constrictive Pericarditis

▶ Description

Chronic or subacute process of **thickening of pericardium** resulting in **cardiac encasement.**

▶ Symptoms

Edema, ascites, hepatic congestion, fatigue.

Exam shows signs of systemic venous congestion, especially **neck vein distention.** May have **Kussmaul's sign** and/or **pericardial knock.**

▶ Diagnosis

History, exam. The ECG is nonspecific, but often shows low QRS voltage. Chest x-ray often with cardiomegaly, may show **pericardial calcification.** Echocardiography may show thickened pericardium. **Cardiac catheterization** confirms diagnosis by demonstration of characteristic hemodynamics ("dip and plateau" contour of ventricular diastolic pressure).

▶ Pathology

Almost any cause of acute pericarditis can lead to pericardial constriction, but most commonly due to **radiation therapy, virus, idiopathic** process, **collagen vascular disease, uremia,** or **malignancy.**

Thickened **noncompliant pericardial sac** causes marked **limitation to cardiac filling** during ventricular diastole, resulting in **systemic venous congestion** and limitation of cardiac output reserve.

▶ Treatment Steps
1. **Diuretic, salt restriction.**
2. Definitive therapy requires **surgical pericardiectomy.**
3. **Treat underlying disease.**

VI. VALVULAR HEART DISEASES

A. Acute Rheumatic Fever

▶ Description

Inflammatory disease affecting skin, joints, heart, subcutaneous tissue, and central nervous system that develops following **group A streptococcal pharyngitis.** Common cause of **valvular heart disease,** but incidence declining in developed countries. Valvular sequelae include stenosis and/or regurgitation of aortic and/or mitral valves, less commonly affects right-sided heart valves.

► **cram facts**

VALVULAR HEART DISEASE

Aortic Stenosis (AS)

- Etiologies include degenerative process (calcific AS of the elderly), congenital malformation (e.g., bicuspid), and rheumatic heart disease (RHD)
- Symptoms of angina, dyspnea, syncope
- Harsh, mid- to late-peaking systolic murmur at base of heart radiating to neck; S4 gallop; LV heave; aortic regurgitation may coexist (see below)
- ECG with LVH, left atrial abnormality
- Confirm by Doppler echocardiography, cardiac catheterization
- Bacterial endocarditis prophylaxis
- Aortic valve replacement for symptomatic patients

Aortic Regurgitation (AR)

- Etiologies multiple, including congenital malformation, RHD, aortic root abnormality (e.g., Marfan syndrome, dissection), trauma, aortitis, endocarditis
- Symptoms of dyspnea, fatigue (angina, syncope rare)
- High-pitched, decrescendo diastolic murmur loudest at left sternal border or base, also heard at LV apex; S3 common; LV enlargement
- ECG with LVH, often left atrial abnormality
- Confirm by Doppler echocardiography, cardiac catheterization
- Bacterial endocarditis prophylaxis
- Aortic valve replacement in selected cases

Mitral Stenosis (MS)

- Usually due to rheumatic heart disease
- Symptoms of dyspnea, fatigue, or RV failure
- Low-pitched (rumble) diastolic murmur at LV apex; opening "snap" early in diastole; loud S1; MR (see below) may coexist
- ECG frequently with left atrial abnormality or atrial fibrillation, may have RVH
- Confirm with Doppler echocardiography, cardiac catheterization
- Bacterial endocarditis prophylaxis
- High risk of systemic thromboembolism, risk reduced with warfarin anticoagulation
- Mitral valve replacement/repair or percutaneous balloon valvuloplasty in selected cases

Mitral Regurgitation (MR)

- Etiologies multiple, including degenerative process (myxomatous change), ischemia, RHD, endocarditis, connective tissue disease (e.g., Marfan syndrome)
- Chronic or (less common) acute forms, depending on etiology
- Symptoms of dyspnea, fatigue
- High-pitched holosystolic (or crescendo systolic in case of MV prolapse) murmur at LV apex or left sternal border; S3 (chronic) or S4 (acute); LV enlargement (chronic)
- ECG with left atrial abnormality, LVH, may show atrial fibrillation
- Confirm with Doppler echocardiography, cardiac catheterization
- Bacterial endocarditis prophylaxis
- Mitral valve replacement/repair in selected cases

► **Symptoms**

Fever, malaise, polyarthritis, chorea, rash. Dyspnea from acute heart failure caused by valvular regurgitation and/or myocarditis. Acute pericarditis can occur. Many cases resolve without clinical sequelae. **Most common in children 5–15 years of age,** although can occur in any age group.

► Diagnosis

History, exam. Many of the signs, symptoms, and laboratory findings of acute rheumatic fever (ARF) are nonspecific, so the **modified Jones criteria** are often required for diagnosis: **two major criteria,** or **one major and two minor criteria,** and **evidence (usually serologic) of preceding streptococcal infection.**

1. Major Criteria
   - Carditis—most common and most reliable sign
   - Erythema marginatum
   - Polyarthritis
   - Chorea (Sydenham's)
   - Subcutaneous nodules

2. Minor Criteria
   - Fever
   - Arthralgia
   - Prior documented ARF or preexisting evidence of rheumatic heart disease
   - Prolonged PR interval on ECG
   - Elevated sedimentation rate or increased C-reactive protein

► Pathology

Invasive infection with **group A streptococcus** probably elicits an antibody response with **cross-reactivity with host tissues (autoimmune mechanism).**

► Treatment Steps

1. **Antibiotic treatment** (but treatment of established attack does not prevent subsequent heart involvement).
2. **Bed rest, salicylates.**
3. **Sedatives for chorea.**
4. **Corticosteroids** for moderate or severe **carditis.**
5. Diuretics, salt restriction if CHF. Cardiac surgery rarely required for severe valvular regurgitation during acute phase of illness.

► Prevention

Prevention of **initial attack** of ARF by adequate and prompt antibiotic therapy for streptococcal pharyngitis.

Prevention of **recurrent attack** of ARF by long-term prophylaxis against recurrent group A streptococcal infection.

B. Mitral Stenosis (MS)

► Description

Narrowing of the mitral valve orifice following inflammation of anterior and posterior mitral leaflets and variable degree of fusion and shortening of chordae tendineae. Causes obstruction to LV inflow from the left atrium. May coexist with mitral regurgitation.

► Symptoms

Dyspnea, often precipitated by **atrial fibrillation. Fatigue.** Left atrial thrombi can cause **systemic embolization.** In advanced cases, right heart failure with edema, hepatic congestion.

On exam, **loud S1, opening snap** in early diastole, **low-pitched diastolic murmur** ("rumble") at LV apex. May have **pulmonary congestion.** If RV failure, edema and neck vein distention.

► Diagnosis

History, exam. Acute pulmonary edema with new onset AF may be presenting symptom of previously clinically silent mitral stenosis (MS).

With left atrial enlargement or AF, ECG may have RVH. **Chest x-ray** with **left atrial enlargement, pulmonary venous hypertension. Doppler echocardiography** extremely helpful. **Cardiac catheterization.**

► Pathology

Almost always a **sequel of rheumatic fever** (years to decades after acute attack). Rarely, congenital or due to mitral annular calcification. Atrial myxoma can mimic hemodynamic abnormality of MS. **Increase in left atrial pressure** causes pulmonary congestion, left atrial enlargement, atrial arrhythmias.

► Treatment Steps
1. **Diuretic, salt restriction.**
2. **Control of atrial fibrillation,** if present.
3. **Anticoagulation** to lower risk of thromboembolism.
4. **Bacterial endocarditis prophylaxis.**
5. **Mitral valve surgery** or **percutaneous valvulotomy** in advanced cases.

C. Mitral Regurgitation (MR)

► Description

Reflux of blood from the left ventricle into the left atrium during ventricular systole through the mitral valve orifice. Severe regurgitation causes **left ventricular volume overload** and pulmonary congestion. May be acute or chronic, and may coexist with mitral stenosis.

► Symptoms

Will vary markedly from **asymptomatic to severely compromised due to CHF,** depending on degree and acuteness of MR, left ventricular function, and associated arrhythmias. Systemic embolization may occur in setting of atrial fibrillation.

On exam, **holosystolic or crescendo (mitral valve prolapse [MVP]) systolic murmur,** loudest at LV apex. May have **S3** (chronic MR) or S4 (acute MR). **Pulmonary congestion** in severe cases.

► Diagnosis

History, exam. Chest x-ray often shows cardiomegaly, and may show CHF. The ECG often shows LVH, left atrial abnormality. **Doppler echocardiography** very useful to assess mechanism and severity of MR. **Cardiac catheterization.**

► Pathology

Mechanism of MR can involve **dysfunction of any portion of the mitral valve apparatus:** annulus, leaflets, chordae tendineae, papillary muscles, or adjacent left ventricular wall. Pathologic processes with potential to affect one or more valve components are multiple and include **rheumatic fever, endocarditis, AMI, degenerative (MVP syndrome [Fig. 1–7]), Marfan's syndrome, congenital lesions, trauma, mitral annular dilatation, collagen vascular disease syndromes,** or **calcification.**

► Treatment Steps
1. **Salt restriction, diuretic** for CHF.
2. **Vasodilators** (ACE inhibitors, hydralazine, nitrates, sodium nitroprusside), especially in treatment of acute MR with CHF and/or low cardiac output.
3. **Treat arrhythmias** as required.
4. **Bacterial endocarditis prophylaxis.**
5. **Mitral valve surgery** (replacement or repair) for selected cases.

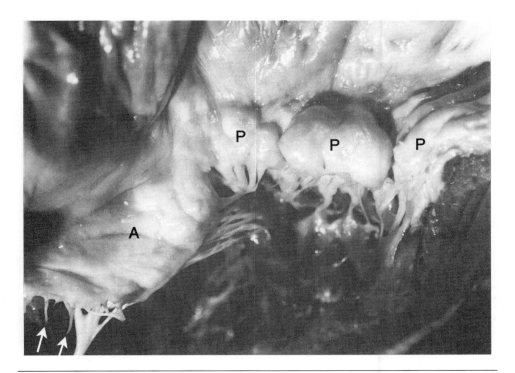

Figure 1–7. Degenerative mitral valve (mitral valve prolapse syndrome) obtained at necropsy in a 79-year-old woman who died in an automobile accident. Note that thickened posterior leaflet "scallops" (P) with marked hooding and reduncancy, and thickened anterior leaflet (A). Mitral valve cord rupture (arrows) is noted. LA = left atrium. LV = left ventricle.

D. Aortic Stenosis (AS)

▶ Description

Obstruction to blood flow from the left ventricle into the aorta at the level of the aortic valve. May coexist with aortic regurgitation.

▶ Symptoms

Angina pectoris, CHF, syncope.

On exam, **crescendo–decrescendo mid- or late-peaking harsh systolic murmur** in aortic area radiating to the neck. **Carotid upstroke diminished and delayed.** The S2 is absent or diminished.

▶ Diagnosis

History, exam. ECG with LVH. **Chest x-ray** with cardiomegaly, CHF in some cases. **Doppler echocardiography** very helpful. **Cardiac catheterization.**

▶ Pathology

Failure of the aortic valve orifice to open fully during ventricular systole may be caused by marked **thickening and calcification** of the aortic valve leaflets (as in degenerative calcific aortic stenosis [AS]), **commissural fusion from inflammation** (as in AS after rheumatic fever), or may be **congenital** in origin (as in AS developing on a bicuspid aortic valve [see Fig. 1–8]).

▶ Treatment Steps
1. **Surgical aortic valve replacement for symptomatic AS.**
2. **Bacterial endocarditis prophylaxis.**
3. **Diuretic, salt restriction for CHF.**

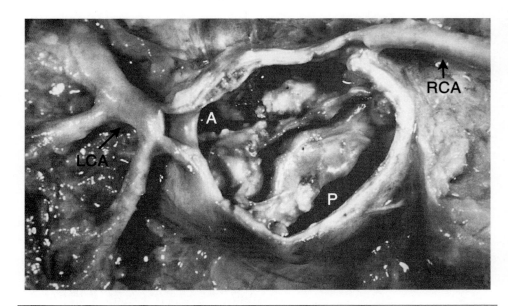

Figure 1–8. Congenitally bicuspid aortic valve obtained at necropsy in a 67-year-old man with NYHA Functional Class III angina pectoris and congestive heart failure who died suddenly. Viewed from superior aspect. Note narrow, slitlike valve orifice between anterior (A) and posterior (P) aortic valve cusps, which are markedly thickened, contain calcium nodules, and are not fused at the commissures. RCA = right coronary artery. LCA = left coronary artery.

E. Aortic Regurgitation (AR)

► Description

Reflux of blood from the aorta into the left ventricle during ventricular diastole due to **incompetent aortic valve.** Can take acute or chronic form. May coexist with aortic stenosis.

► Pathology

Loss of aortic valve competence can be caused by developmental abnormality, destruction of aortic leaflets, or by loss of support of aortic leaflets due to aortic root disease. Etiologic factors include **endocarditis, congenital** (including bicuspid aortic valve), **trauma, inflammation** (rheumatic fever), **dissection of the ascending aortic, aneurysm of the ascending aorta, aortitis** (ankylosing spondylitis, syphilis, Reiter's syndrome).

► Symptoms

Dyspnea. Fatigue. Palpitations. Syncope and angina uncommon. **CHF** in severe cases. Asymptomatic in mild cases.

On exam, **decrescendo diastolic murmur** loudest at left sternal border or aortic area, **cardiomegaly, S3 gallop.** In severe, acute aortic regurgitation, murmur may be inaudible.

► Diagnosis

History, exam. The ECG with LVH. Chest x-ray with cardiomegaly, possible CHF; aortic root dilatation often found. Doppler echocardiography. **Cardiac catheterization.**

► Treatment Steps
1. **Salt restriction, diuretics** for CHF.
2. **Vasodilators.**
3. **Bacterial endocarditis prophylaxis.**
4. **Surgical aortic valve replacement** in selected cases.

F. Endocarditis

▶ **Description**

Infection of endocardium, usually valvular but may involve mural endocardium or prosthetic heart valve. Subacute and acute forms, depending on organism involved and clinical setting. **Abnormal heart valves** and **congenital heart lesions** most often affected, but may occur in the normal heart.

▶ **Symptoms**

Fever. Malaise. Anemia, weight loss, emboli, renal failure, metastatic abscess, arthritis, CHF.

On exam, elevated temperature, evidence of systemic (left heart involvement) or pulmonary (right heart involvement) embolization, cardiac murmurs (any regurgitant lesion), signs of CHF.

▶ **Diagnosis**

History, exam. High index of suspicion if preexisting cardiac lesions or illicit intravenous drug use. **Blood cultures. Doppler echocardiography.** Elevated sedimentation rate, rheumatoid factor.

▶ **Pathology**

Most common causative organism of subacute bacterial endocarditis is *Streptococcus viridans.* Most common cause of acute bacterial endocarditis is *Staphylococcus aureus.* Other causes include *Staphylococcus epidermidis,* gram-negative bacteria, fungi, pneumococcus, gonococcus, and (rarely) spirochetes and rickettsiae. **Mitral valve most commonly involved,** followed by aortic and tricuspid. Pulmonic valve rarely affected by endocarditis.

▶ **Treatment Steps**

1. Early treatment (even while blood culture results pending) with **appropriate bacteriocidal or fungicidal antibiotics.**
2. **Cardiac surgery with replacement of affected valve** in selected cases. For CHF due to cardiac valve dysfunction, recurrent emboli on treatment, myocardial abscess.

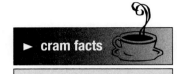

▶ **cram facts**

HACEK ORGANISMS

These are slow-growing gram-negative bacilli and are responsible for about 3% of all cases of endocarditis.

- *Haemophilus parainfluenza*
- *Haemophilus paraphrophilus*
- *Actinobacillus actinomycetemcomitans*
- *Cardiobacterium hominis*
- *Eikenella corrodens*
- *Kingella kingae*

G. Prosthetic Heart Valve

▶ **Description**

Artificial device designed to be **surgically implanted** as a functional **replacement for a cardiac valve** that is severely malfunctioning. Valve repair is sometimes an alternative to replacement.

1. Prosthetic Valve Types

Mechanical Prosthesis—Designs include ball-in-cage (Starr Edwards) and tilting disc (St. Jude, Hall Medtronic, Bjork Shiley) models, are considered durable, but require chronic anticoagulation.

Bioprosthesis—Designs (porcine, bovine pericardial, homograft) generally do not require long-term anticoagulation, but valve deterioration a problem especially in younger patients.

2. Complications of Prosthetic Heart Valves

Endocarditis—(Early or late after implantation), **embolization,** perivalvular **leak, mechanical failure, hemorrhagic complications** of anticoagulation.

VII. CONGENITAL HEART DISEASES

Present at birth, resulting from **abnormality of development.** Wide spectrum of clinical expression, depending on severity of defect. Cause unknown in most cases, but recognized contributing factors include chromosomal abnormalities (Down syndrome, Turner syndrome), older maternal age, maternal rubella infection in first trimester, maternal exposure to certain drugs. Prevention efforts involve adequate prenatal care, rubella immunization before conception, and genetic counseling in appropriate settings.

A. Ventricular Septal Defect (VSD)

▶ Description and Pathology

Most common congenital heart lesion, other than congenital abnormality of the aortic valve. Persistent **opening in the upper portion of the ventricular septum** (membranous septum) with resultant **left-to-right shunt** at the ventricular level.

▶ Symptoms

Harsh systolic murmur at left sternal border, radiates to right precordium. **Spontaneous closure 30–50% of cases.** If shunt small, may be asymptomatic. If shunt large, CHF and potential of pulmonary vascular disease with reversal of shunt and Eisenmenger syndrome.

▶ Diagnosis

History, exam. The ECG may show LVH. **Doppler echocardiography** should be diagnostic. **Chest x-ray** with cardiomegaly and increased pulmonary vasculature if shunt significant. **Cardiac catheterization.**

▶ Treatment Steps
1. For asymptomatic patient with **small VSD, observation.**
2. For patient with **large VSD and significant shunt flow, surgical repair.**
3. **Bacterial endocarditis prophylaxis.**

B. Atrial Septal Defect (ASD)

▶ Description and Pathology

Persistent **opening in atrial septum,** most commonly in region of fossa ovalis (ASD of secundum septum), but can also occur in lower portion of atrial septum (ASD of primum septum) or in sinus node region of the atrial septum (sinus venosus ASD). **Left-to-right shunt** at the atrial level. More common in females.

▶ Symptoms

Often asymptomatic as child or teenager. **Dyspnea, fatigue,** and **atrial arrhythmias** develop in early or middle adulthood, sometimes sooner. **Right heart failure** can occur. In advanced cases, severe pulmonary hypertension and Eisenmenger syndrome can develop.

On exam, **fixed splitting of second heart sound, systolic ejection murmur** at left upper sternal border, and **right ventricular enlargement.** If CHF has developed, neck vein distention and edema. Mitral regurgitation due to MVP (secundum ASD) or cleft in anterior mitral leaflet (primum ASD).

▶ Diagnosis

History, but note that patient may be asymptomatic. The ECG almost always with **incomplete or complete right bundle branch block**

(RBBB), and in addition usually has left axis deviation in cases of ASD of primum septum. **Chest x-ray** with cardiomegaly and **increased pulmonary vasculature. Doppler echocardiography** diagnostic in most cases. Cardiac catheterization.

► Treatment Steps
1. **Observation for small shunt** if asymptomatic.
2. **Surgical repair or percutaneous closure for significant shunt.**

C. Patent Ductus Arteriosus

► Description and Pathology
Arteriovenous fistula between aorta and left pulmonary artery due to failure of embryonic ductus to close after birth. **Left-to-right shunt** increases work on the left heart. Fistulous connection commonly inserts near origin of left subclavian artery. More common in births at high altitude, in births to mothers exposed to rubella in first trimester of pregnancy, in premature babies, and in females.

► Symptoms
Hallmark is **continuous "machinery" murmur** at upper left sternal border. S2 may be paradoxically split. **Wide systemic pulse pressure with abnormally low diastolic pressure.** Left ventricular volume overload can lead to CHF.

► Diagnosis
History, exam. The ECG with LVH. Chest x-ray with **cardiomegaly** and **increased pulmonary vasculature. Cardiac catheterization.**

► Treatment Steps
1. **Surgical closure,** optimal time 1–2 years of age.
2. **Bacterial endocarditis prophylaxis.**

D. Coarctation of Aorta

► Description and Pathology
Narrowing of aortic lumen, usually immediately **distal to origin of left subclavian artery** near insertion of ligamentum arteriosum. Associated with Turner syndrome. A cause of **secondary hypertension.** More common in males.

► Symptoms
Vary greatly from asymptomatic to severe **hypertension** resulting in **headache** or CHF, **intracranial hemorrhage,** lower extremity **claudication.** Aortic rupture a risk.

On exam, **upper extremity hypertension** with **reduced or absent lower extremity pulses, systolic ejection murmur** (may be continuous) anterior chest and upper back. May also have aortic regurgitation due to bicuspid aortic valve, which is associated with coarctation of aorta.

► Diagnosis
History, exam. The ECG often with LVH. Chest x-ray may show cardiomegaly, **rib notching, dilated aorta,** and left subclavian artery. Conventional **contrast aortography** or **magnetic resonance angiography (MRA).** Doppler echocardiography.

► Treatment Steps
1. **Surgical correction,** optimal time 4–8 years of age.
2. **Bacterial endocarditis prophylaxis.**

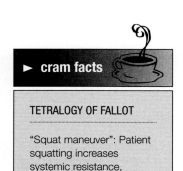

E. Tetralogy of Fallot

► Description and Pathology

Most common **cyanotic** congenital heart lesion in patients older than 1 year of age. Consists of:

1. **VSD** (usually large).
2. **Narrowing of right ventricular outflow tract** (usually infundibular, right ventricular airflow tract obstruction).
3. **Overriding of aorta above VSD** (aka dextroposition of aorta).
4. **Right ventricular hypertrophy.**

The result of this complex of abnormalities is a **right-to-left shunt** at the ventricular level and reduced blood flow to the lungs. About 25% of patients have a right-sided aortic arch.

► Symptoms

Polycythemia, retardation of growth, exercise intolerance. Characteristic **"squat maneuver"** after exercise.

On exam, **prominent right ventricular impulse, systolic ejection murmur** with **thrill** at left sternal border, single S2, **cyanosis, clubbing.**

► Diagnosis

History, exam. Chest x-ray with **decreased pulmonary vasculature, boot-shaped heart** ("coeur en sabot"). **Doppler echocardiography.** The ECG with RVH. **Cardiac catheterization** confirms diagnosis and defines level and severity of RV outflow obstruction.

► Treatment Steps

1. **Surgical corrections,** either palliative procedure followed by definitive operation at a later time or initial total surgical correction.
2. **Bacterial endocarditis prophylaxis.**
3. **Treat arrhythmias** (can occur before or after surgical correction) as required.

F. Endocardial Cushion Defect

► Description and Pathology

Persistent **opening in lower atrial and upper ventricular septa associated with developmental abnormalities of tricuspid and/or mitral valves,** caused by failure of the endocardial cushions to fuse properly during development. Spectrum of defect ranges from ostium primum ASD only (usually with some abnormality of mitral valve) to a complete atrioventricular canal defect with a common ASD/VSD and a common atrioventricular valve. The complete defect is associated with Down syndrome and mental retardation.

► Symptoms

Depends on severity and complexity of lesion. The complete endocardial cushion defect (common AV canal) usually presents in infancy with weight loss, CHF, recurrent pulmonary infections. Incomplete defects (e.g., ostium primum ASD) similar in presentation to more common ostium secundum ASD.

► Diagnosis

History, exam. Doppler echocardiography establishes diagnosis and extent of defect. The ECG with **first-degree AV block, left axis deviation. Chest x-ray** with cardiomegaly, **increased pulmonary vasculature** steps CHF in severe forms.

► Treatment Steps
1. **Depends on extent and complexity of defect.**
2. **Surgical repair** for "partial" or "incomplete" defect (ASD of primum septum) often occurs in childhood or young adulthood. Surgical repair for some patients with complete defect.
3. **Bacterial endocarditis prophylaxis.**

VIII. SYSTEMIC ARTERIAL HYPERTENSION

A. Primary (Essential, Idiopathic) Hypertension

► Description
Accounts for about **90% of cases of systemic hypertension,** usual onset 25–55 years of age. Many with family history of hypertension or atherosclerotic disease. Often found in patients with other cardiovascular risk factors. **More common in blacks** (20–30% of blacks) and patients with diabetes mellitus.

► Symptoms
Often asymptomatic. Headache.

► Diagnosis
The Seventh Report of the Joint National Committe on Prevention, Detection, Evaluation, and Treatment of High Blood Pressure (www.nhlbi.nih.gov) recommends the following classification of blood pressure (BP) for adults > 17 years:

Blood Pressure Category	SBP (mm Hg)	DBP (mm Hg)
Normal	< 120	≤ 80
Prehypertension	120–139	80–89
Hypertension Stage I	140–159	90–99
Hypertension Stage II	≥ 160	≥ 100

SBP = systolic blood pressure, DBP = diastolic blood pressure

Diagnostic workup should include: History and physical (assessing risk factors and comorbidities, revealing identifiable causes of hypertension, assessing presence of end-organ damage) (see below). Labs: urinalysis, blood glucose, hematocrit, lipid panel, potassium, calcium, creatinine. Urinary albumin/creatinine ratio is optional. ECG.

Identifiable causes of hypertension (see also section VIII.B): Sleep apnea, drugs/medications, chronic renal disease, primary hyperaldosteronism, renovascular disease, Cushing's syndrome or chronic steroid therapy, pheochromocytoma, coarcation of aorta, thyroid or parathyroid disease.

► Treatment Steps
1. Lifestyle modifications include weight reduction, DASH diet, sodium restriction, physical activity (aerobic), and moderation of alcohol intake.
2. Multiple medications exist, including thiazides, β-blockers, ACE inhibitors, calcium channel blockers, aldosterone antagonists, and angiotension receptor blockers. Select the drug(s) most appropriate for the patients (see Table 1–2).

B. Secondary Hypertension

► Description
Elevated blood pressure **associated with a documented condition known to cause hypertension.** Accounts for about **10% of all cases of**

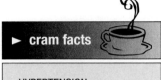

► **cram facts**

HYPERTENSION

- Known as silent disease because most patients are asymptomatic.
- Can cause LVH and CHF.
- Risk factor for MI, CVA, and renal failure.

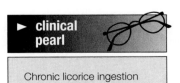

► **clinical pearl**

Chronic licorice ingestion can cause hypertension.

1-2

MEDICATIONS AND INDICATIONS

The following shows certain disease states (compelling indications) and which drugs are effective as initial therapy options (as per the JNCVII report):

Compelling Indications	Initial Therapy Options
CHF	THIAZ, BB, ACE, ARB, ALDO ANT
Post MI	BB, ACE, ALDO ANT
High cardiovascular risk	THIAZ, BB, ACE, CCB
Diabetes	THIAZ, BB, ACE, ARB, CCB
Chronic renal disease	ACE, ARB
Recurrent stroke prevention	THIAZ, ACE

THIAZ, thiazides; BB, β-blocker (BB); ACE, angiotensin-converting enzyme inhibitor; CCB, calcium channel blockers; ALDO ANT, aldosterone antagonists; ARB, angiotension receptor blockers.

hypertension. Can occur at any age, but suspect if patient < 25 years or > 60 years of age.

► Symptoms

Similar to essential hypertension, except may have signs and symptoms related to specific cause of secondary hypertension.

► Diagnosis

Pay close attention to symptoms and signs of secondary causes. Eliminate medications that can raise blood pressure, including oral contraceptives, illicit drugs, herbs, steroids, over-the-counter cold preparations with phenylephrine or pseudoephedrine, and all NSAIDs.

► Pathology

See Table 1–3.

► Treatment

1. **Eliminate secondary cause, if possible.** Surgical (e.g., surgery or stenting for renal artery stenosis, surgery for pheochromocytoma) possible in many cases.

1-3

CAUSES AND TESTS FOR SECONDARY HYPERTENSION

HYPERALDOSTERONISM
- Serum chemistries (hypoklemic metabolic alkalosis common)
- PRA ratio (random plasma aldosterone: plasma renin activity)
- Captopril-suppression test
- Serum aldosterone level
- 24-hour urinary aldosterone excretion
- Salt loading test

PHEOCHROMOCYTOMA
- 24-hour urine collection for creatinine, total catecholamines, vanillylmandelic acid (VMA), and metanephrines
- MRI to visualize adrenal tumors
- Scanning with iodine-131–labeled metaiodobenzylguanidine (MIBG) (reserved for cases when a pheochromocytoma is confirmed biochemically but computed tomography (CT) scan or magnetic resonance imaging (MRI) fail to visualize a tumor)

RENAL ARTERY STENOSIS
- Renal ultrasound with dopplers
- Radionuclide scanning with captopril
- CT or MR guided angiography

CUSHING'S SYNDROME OR DISEASE
- Overnight dexamethasone suppression test
- 24-hour urine for free cortisol
- See also Chapter 3

2. **Antihypertensive therapy** if specific approach to correct secondary cause impossible or not completely effective.

C. Accelerated (Malignant) Hypertension

▶ Description

Abrupt worsening of systemic arterial hypertension with **diastolic pressure** > 120 mm Hg associated with **neurologic dysfunction** (severe headache, cerebrovascular accident (CVA), visual disturbances, papilledema, convulsions), **acute renal failure** (with or without chronic renal insufficiency), or **cardiac dysfunction** (acute MI, pulmonary edema).

▶ Symptoms

Eyeground hemorrhages. May have **focal or nonfocal central nervous system (CNS) signs.** If CHF present, **pulmonary congestion** and cardiac gallops. **Cardiac ischemia (angina).**

▶ Diagnosis

Diastolic arterial pressure ≥ 120 mm Hg associated with acute and severe manifestations of cardiac, neurologic, or renal dysfunction.

ECG with LVH, may show acute cardiac ischemia.

Chest x-ray (CXR) may show cardiomegaly and/or CHF.

▶ Treatment Steps

1. **Prompt control of high blood pressure to moderate range with sodium nitroprusside, trimethaphan, nicardipine, hydralazine, labetalol.**
2. Adjunctive use of β-**blocker and/or diuretic.**
3. **Switch to oral antihypertensive agents** when stable.

D. Pre-eclampsia/Eclampsia

See Chapter 13, section II.A.

IX. SYSTEMIC ARTERIAL HYPOTENSION WITH SHOCK AND CYANOSIS

A. Systemic Hypotension with Shock

▶ Description

Hypotension is usually **defined as** < 90 mm Hg systolic in adults. Shock is said to exist when hypotension is accompanied by signs and symptoms of **poor tissue perfusion.** Shock can exist with systemic arterial pressure above 90 mm Hg systolic in some cases.

▶ Symptoms

Signs of poor tissue perfusion (altered mental status, cool extremities, oliguria, metabolic acidosis) associated with systemic arterial hypotension.

▶ Diagnosis

History, exam. Hypotension with symptoms and signs of poor tissue perfusion. History helps to distinguish hypovolemic from cardiogenic etiology. Neck vein distention and pulsus paradoxicus clues to possible cardiac tamponade.

▶ Pathology

Normal systemic arterial pressure is maintained by an **interplay between cardiac output and SVR.** A decline in one factor that cannot be compensated for by an increase in the other will cause systemic hypotension. Furthermore, at Cardiac Index under approximately 2.0 L/min per square meter of body surface area (BSA), peripheral perfusion will be inadequate, no matter how high the SVR.

Hypovolemia—Causes systemic hypotension by reducing venous return to the heart, thereby reducing cardiac output. Hypovolemia can be absolute (e.g., hemorrhage, dehydration) or can be relative (e.g., anaphylactoid reaction, sepsis).

Cardiogenic—Cause of systemic hypotension is due to an **inadequate output of the heart** under conditions of adequate venous return (i.e., hypovolemia not present). Inadequate cardiac output under these conditions can be due to severe mechanical (valvular or pericardial) or myocardial (e.g., cardiomyopathy, acute MI) dysfunction.

Severe pulmonary artery obstruction (e.g., severe pulmonary embolism, severe pulmonary vasculature disease) can uncommonly be a cause of hypotension by causing restriction of left heart filling.

▶ Treatment Steps

Hypovolemic Shock
1. **Intravenous fluids** (crystalloids, blood products if appropriate).
2. **Trendelenburg position** for optimal venous return to the central circulation.
3. If **pressors** (e.g., dopamine, norepinephrine, epinephrine) used, only temporary measure until intravascular volume is restored.
4. **Treat underlying cause.**

Cardiogenic Shock
1. **Inotropic agents** (dobutamine, dopamine, amrinone). **Vasodilator** if tolerated.
2. **Intra-aortic balloon counterpulsation.**
3. **Pericardiocentesis for cardiac tamponade.**
4. **Treat underlying cause.**

B. Cyanosis

▶ Description
Bluish, dusky discoloration of skin and mucous membranes.

▶ Symptoms
Central cyanosis is apparent on skin and warm mucous membranes.

Peripheral cyanosis is apparent on skin in exposed areas, where vasoconstriction may be present, and may not be visible on warm mucous membranes.

▶ Pathology
Due to an excess (> 4 g/dL) of reduced hemoglobin in capillary blood.

Central Cyanosis—Caused by abnormally high amount of reduced hemoglobin in arterial blood due to **right-to-left intracardiac shunt** (usually congenital heart disease) or patent Foramen ovale or to inability of **severely diseased lung parenchyma** to adequately oxygenate systemic venous blood. Methemoglobinemia.

Peripheral Cyanosis—Caused by excess removal of oxygen from normally saturated blood during **abnormally slow flow** through capillary bed during **shock** or **cold exposure.**

▶ Treatment Steps
Treat underlying condition.

X. ATHEROSCLEROSIS AND LIPOPROTEINS/ HYPERLIPIDEMIA

► Description

Although there are a number of different genetic diseases that cause abnormal lipid profiles, the majority of people have more of an acquired dyslipidemia from a poor diet. The two major concerns from a cardiovascular risk standpoint are an elevated LDL and a depressed HDL. In general, diet is recommended as a means to correct the LDL and HDL. Depending on the clinical scenario, however, drug therapy may also be initiated early (see Table 1–4).

The NCEP (National Cholesterol Education Program) has made recommendations on specific lipid (LDL) goals for patients in terms of the number of risk factors or the presence of coronary heart disease (CHD) they have.

Major cardiovascular risk factors (exclusive of LDL levels):

- Tobacco use.
- Hypertension (140/90 or patients taking blood pressure medications).
- Depressed HDL (< 40 mg/dL).
- Family history of premature CAD/CHD (in a male first-degree relative < 55 years old or female first-degree relative < 65 years old).
- Age: Males age ≥ 45 or females age ≥ 55.
- Note that an HDL ≥ 60 mg/dL counts as a negative risk factor. If present, a risk factor can be subtracted.

Atherosclerotic vascular disease (e.g., peripheral vascular disease, carotid stenosis, abdominal aortic aneurysm) and diabetes mellitus are regarded as CHD equivalents.

1-4

MEDICAL TREATMENT OF HYPERLIPIDEMIA

STATINS (hydroxymethylglutaryl coenzyme A [HMG CoA] reductase inhibitors)
- Atorvastatin (Lipitor), fluvastatin (Lescol), lovastatin (Mevacor), pravastatin (pravachol), rosuvastatin (Crestor), simvastatin (Zocor).
- Side effects (SE): elevated aspartate tramsaminase (AST) and alanine tramsaminase (ALT), myopathy, diarrhea.
- Monitor via baseline liver function tests (LFTs), repeat at 12 weeks, again every 6 weeks or with dose change. Check CK if patient has myopathy/myalgias.

BILE-ACID SEQUESTRANTS
- Cholestyramine (questran) colestipol, and colesevelam
- SE: Gastrointestinal (GI) distress, constipation, decreased absorption of drugs and vitamins, flatulence
- May have easy bruising due to decreased absorption of vitamin K

CHOLESTEROL ABSORPTION INHIBITOR
- The only drug in this class is ezetimibe (Zetia). It is used in patients who cannot take statins or who are on maximal therapy with statins and who are not at target cholesterol goals.
- SE: Diarrhea, myalgias, fatigue, cough
- Monitoring similar to that of statin

FIBRATES
- Gemfibrozil (Lopid), fenofibrate (Tricor)
- SE: Myopathy, hepatitis, cholelithiasis
- Monitor central venous catheter (CVC) and LFTs every 3 months during first year of therapy.

VITAMINS (Niacin)
- SE: Flushing, pruritus, diarrhea, decreased glucose tolerance at high doses
- Monitor LFTs, uric acid, and glucose periodically.

1-5

METABOLIC SYNDROME

With an increase in obesity, the metabolic syndrome is becoming increasingly common. Patients with the metabolic syndrome are at increased risk of cardiovascular disease and insulin resistance.

As defined by the NCEP (National Cholesterol Education Program), the metabolic syndrome is defined by three or more of the following:
- Central obesity (measured by waist circumference):
  Men ≥ 40 inches, women ≥ 35 inches
- Fasting triglycerides ≥ 150 mg/dL
- HDL cholesterol:
  Men < 40 mg/dL, women < 50 mg/dL
- Blood pressure ≥ 130/85 mm Hg
- Fasting glucose ≥ 110 mg/dL

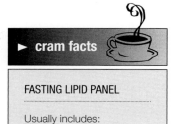

► **cram facts**

FASTING LIPID PANEL

Usually includes:
- Total cholesterol
- LDL
- HDL
- Triglycerides

A brief summary of the NCEP GUIDELINES:

High-risk (patients with CHD or a CHD equivalent):

- Goal LDL had been < 100 mg/dL. With newer published studies, it is deemed a "therapeutic option" to set the goal LDL at < 70 mg/dL for very high-risk patients—those with a recent MI, with either diabetes or severe or poorly controlled risk factors (i.e., continued tobacco use) or metabolic syndrome (see Table 1–5).

Moderately high risk (patients with two or more CHD risk factors):

- Goal LDL < 130 mg/dL

Low risk (patients with zero to one risk factor):

- Goal LDL < 160 mg/dL

XI. PERIPHERAL ARTERY VASCULAR DISEASES

A. Occlusive Arterial Disease

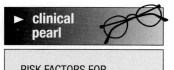

► **clinical pearl**

RISK FACTORS FOR PERIPHERAL ARTERY DISEASE

Occlusive vascular diseases have basically the same risk factors as coronary artery disease.

► Description
Narrowing or occlusion of **large- and medium-sized arteries** resulting in reduction or total disruption of flow of oxygenated blood. Associated with hypertension, hypercholesterolemia, cigarette smoking, male sex, diabetes mellitus.

► Symptoms
Claudication of lower (or, less commonly, upper) extremities distal to the point of occlusion. Pattern of claudication useful in predicting level of occlusion (buttock, thigh, sexual impotence in males [iliac]; calf [femoral, popliteal]). **Rest pain** and **ulceration** of skin can occur in advanced cases.

On exam, diminished arterial pulsations, vascular bruits, and consequence of poor arterial flow (sparse hair, ulceration) may be seen.

► Diagnosis
History, exam. Noninvasive evaluation includes measurement of ankle and brachial arterial pressures before and after exercise. **Angiography** confirms site of obstruction and evaluates distal arterial runoff.

► Pathology

Atherosclerosis is most common cause of occlusive peripheral artery disease; however, **inflammation** or **trauma** can also be a cause of arterial occlusive disease. Embolism or acute thrombosis can result in sudden total occlusion of an artery and is usually a medical emergency.

► Treatment Steps

1. **Medical therapy** (pentoxyfylline, cilastazol) may improve micro-circulation and peripheral oxygen delivery.
2. **Reconstructive arterial surgery** or **percutaneous angioplasty/stenting** for disabling symptoms or rest ischemia.
3. **Risk factor modification** (see above).
4. **Avoid vasoconstricting drugs.**

B. Giant Cell Arteritis (Temporal Arteritis)

► Description

Systemic disorder with involvement of **aorta and large branches (particularly carotid).** Usually in patients **older than 55 years of age.** Temporal arteritis is particularly worrisome because it can result in irreversible vision loss.

► Symptoms

Fever, malaise, myalgia. **Headache, scalp tenderness,** jaw claudication, **visual symptoms.**

► Diagnosis

Clinical scenario. Laboratory findings of **elevated sedimentation rate,** abnormal liver function tests, and anemia are nonspecific. **Biopsy** of involved artery (often **temporal artery**).

► Pathology

Segmental granulomatous inflammation of unknown cause, resulting in necrosis of media and occlusion of arterial lumen.

► Treatment Steps

Corticosteroids, usually for months.

C. Polyarteritis

► Description

Segmental **vasculitis of small- to medium-sized arteries,** causing dysfunction in **multiple organ systems.** Patients **usually middle aged.**

► Symptoms

Clinical pattern determined by which organ systems involved, but **systemic hypertension with kidney involvement in vast majority.** Acute MI may occur. Other symptoms may reflect involvement of **skin, gastrointestinal (GI) tract, spleen, CNS.**

► Diagnosis

Clinical picture. Multisystem involvement with **biopsy evidence of active arteritis.**

► Pathology

Small- to medium-sized arteries affected by **segmental necrotizing granulomatous inflammation** (varies from media only to full thickness) of **unknown cause.**

► Treatment Steps

Corticosteroids. Other therapy as indicated for specific organ dysfunction (e.g., acute MI).

D. Arteriovenous Fistula

► Description

Abnormal **communication between artery and vein.**

► Symptoms

Many asymptomatic, especially congenital AV fistulae, which tend to be smaller than acquired type. Venous and/or arterial insufficiency in extremity affected. CHF **due to high-output state.**

► Diagnosis

History, exam. Thrill and bruit over fistula. Prompt decrease in pulse rate (Nicoladoni Branham sign) when fistula is occluded. **Angiography** demonstrates location and size of fistula.

► Pathology

May be **acquired** as result of trauma (blunt or penetrating) or **congenital.** Sequelae of arteriovenous (AV) fistula can be local (increased venous pressure with swelling of extremity, or arterial insufficiency distal to the fistula) or systemic (high-output CHF, decreased diastolic BP), and will depend on size of fistula and site involved.

► Treatment Steps

Surgical excision or intra-arterial embolization in most acquired cases. Congenital forms are often followed conservatively.

XII. DISEASES OF VEINS AND PULMONARY EMBOLISM

A. Varicose Veins

► Description

Dilated and tortuous veins of lower extremities. Most common vascular disease of the lower extremities.

► Symptoms/Diagnosis

Many asymptomatic. May cause **pain** in legs, superficial skin **ulceration, increased pigmentation.**

► Pathology

Usually a secondary condition as a sequel to deep vein thrombosis (causing chronic deep venous insufficiency), or resulting from obesity, pregnancy, ascites, right heart failure, prolonged standing.

Less commonly, a **primary condition** as a result of hereditary weakness of valves and walls of veins.

► Treatment

Elastic support. May require sclerotherapy or **surgical treatment** (stripping).

B. Thrombophlebitis

► Description

Occlusion of a vein by thrombus with variable amount of **inflammation** of vein wall. Can occur in superficial veins (varicose or nonvaricose) or in deep venous system (iliofemoral, femoropopliteal, calf, axillary–subclavian). Predisposing factors include CHF, obesity, MI, trauma, postoperative state, malignancy, pregnancy, oral contraceptives.

▶ Symptoms

Superficial Thrombophlebitis—Pain and erythema in affected area. May cause fever and swelling. Embolism rare.

Deep Vein Thrombophlebitis (DVT)—Pain, swelling, fever. May cause increased superficial venous pattern around site of deep obstruction. **Pulmonary embolism** is common.

▶ Diagnosis

Superficial Thrombophlebitis—Exam, history.

Deep Vein Thrombophlebitis—Exam, history (especially regarding predisposing conditions). **Impedance plethysmography** and **Doppler flow studies** very helpful in documenting thrombosis proximal to calf veins. Contrast venography rarely needed.

▶ Treatment Steps

Superficial Thrombophlebitis
1. **Warm moist packs. Elevation of limb.**
2. **NSAIDs.**
3. In persistent or recurrent cases, **anticoagulation** and possible **surgery.**

Deep Vein Thrombophlebitis
1. **Full-dose anticoagulation with** heparin (unfractionated or low molecular weight) **followed by oral warfarin** for 3–6 months.
2. If anticoagulation cannot be used, consider inferior vena cava (IVC) filter device (commonly used Greenfield filter).
3. **Prevention with subcutaneous heparin** (unfractionated or low molecular weight), **warfarin,** or **calf compression devices** during periods of high risk for DVT.

C. Pulmonary Embolism and Infarction
See Chapter 16, section II.H.

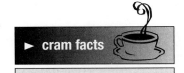

▶ cram facts

VIRCHOW'S TRIAD

Rudolf Virchow suggested three factors that predisposed a patient to developing a venous thrombosis:
- Stasis of blood flow
- Hypercoagulability
- Damage to the vascular endothelium

XIII. AORTIC ANEURYSMS

A. Dissecting Aneurysm of Aorta

▶ Description

Rupture of blood into the media of the aortic wall followed by dissection in circumferential and longitudinal fashion. **Severe clinical consequences.** Usually presents acutely (but may be chronic). Associated with **hypertension, Marfan's syndrome, pregnancy, coarctation of the aorta, trauma** (usually blunt). Men more commonly affected than women. **Peak incidence 35–70 years of age.**

▶ Symptoms

Sharp, knifelike chest pain of sudden onset, often felt initially substernally (ascending aortic dissection) but may then radiate to neck and interscapular area as dissection progresses distally. Pain of descending thoracic aorta dissection may be felt only in interscapular area. **Acute aortic regurgitation, acute myocardial infarction, hemopericardium with cardiac tamponade, paraplegia** (occlusion of spinal arteries); **CVA** can occur as a consequence of destruction by the plane of dissection.

Three anatomic patterns of aortic dissection have been described:

Type I—Dissection begins in proximal aorta and extends distally for variable distance.

Type II—Dissection limited to aortic arch.

Type III—Dissection begins distal to left subclavian artery and extends distally for variable distance.

► Diagnosis

History, exam. May have unequal blood pressure in upper or lower extremities, acute aortic regurgitation, cardiac tamponade, CHF. **Aortography** generally confirms diagnosis, but **transesophageal echocardiography (TEE), computed axial tomography (CT scan),** and **magnetic resonance imaging (MRI)** also highly accurate in detecting aortic dissection.

► Pathology

Separation of elements of media layer of aortic wall by an **intramural hematoma,** which gains access to the media through a **tear in aortic intima.** Occasionally, intramural hematoma may develop without intimal tear. Underlying condition in most cases appears to be cystic medial necrosis. The intramural hematoma may or may not exit into the true aortic lumen distally.

► Treatment Steps

1. **Severe clinical consequences** with grave outcome probable **if not detected and treated promptly.**
2. **Immediate control of BP, if hypertensive, with fast-acting parenteral agents** (e.g., sodium nitroprusside, trimethaphan, nicardipine).
3. **β-Blocker** (IV) to reduce shear forces in ascending aorta.
4. **Emergency surgical treatment of types I and II.**
5. **Medical therapy of type III** unless complications develop.

B. Aneurysm of the Thoracic Aorta (Nondissecting)

► Description

Significant **dilatation of one or more segments of thoracic aorta.** Most commonly involves ascending aorta from root to origin of innominate artery. May involve transverse arch segment alone. Aneurysm of the descending thoracic aorta may extend into the upper abdominal aorta (thoracoabdominal aortic aneurysm), and is often associated with significant hypertension.

► Symptoms

Depends on location and severity. May be asymptomatic. Dilatation of aortic root may lead to loss of aortic valve support and **aortic regurgitation** and CHF. **Compression** of adjacent structures can lead to symptoms of chest pain, hoarseness, dysphagia. With severely dilated aneurysms, **rupture** with fatal hemorrhage is a constant threat.

► Diagnosis

History, exam. Dilatation of the aorta will be apparent on **chest x-ray.** Conventional contrast or magnetic resonance **aortography** is required for anatomic localization of aneurysm if surgery is contemplated.

► Pathology

Atherosclerosis is the most common cause. **Cystic medial necrosis** may be seen in some aortic aneurysms, especially those of ascending aorta. Trauma, syphilis, aortitis less common causes. Marfan syndrome.

► Treatment Steps

Surgical resection with graft replacement for severe aneurysms, especially with significant aortic regurgitation (may need aortic valve replacement), rupture or impending rupture, local compression syndromes.

C. Aneurysm of the Abdominal Aorta

See Chapter 18.

XIV. HEART TRANSPLANTATION

► Description

Homograft cardiac orthotopic transplantation in carefully selected patients with life-threatening, severely symptomatic, and otherwise inoperable myocardial, valvular, coronary artery, or congenital heart disease. In some cardiac patients with severe pulmonary vascular disease (most commonly congenital heart patients), a heart–lung transplant is required.

A. Clinical Aspects of Posttransplantation Care

Infection with a variety of organisms and rejection are major causes of morbidity and mortality after cardiac transplantation, which requires chronic immunosuppressive therapy. Clinical signs of rejection (CHF, gallop rhythm, low QRS voltage on ECG) are insensitive, and the best method for evaluating acute rejection is **right ventricular endomyocardial biopsy.**

Graft coronary atherosclerosis, probably a form of chronic rejection, is a common problem. The transplanted cardiac patient will not experience angina because the transplanted heart is denervated.

XV. CARDIOPULMONARY ARREST

► Description

Cessation of effective cardiac and/or pulmonary function, resulting in **hemodynamic collapse** or severe cerebral dysfunction. Spontaneous cardiopulmonary arrest most often of **cardiac etiology in adults** (usually ventricular fibrillation due to CAD) and of **pulmonary etiology in children.**

► Symptoms

Loss of consciousness (usually abrupt) or **severe lethargy.** May be preceded by chest pain, palpitations, dyspnea. Must be distinguished from other causes of loss of consciousness or syncope (e.g., neurologic, hemorrhagic, metabolic, toxic).

► Diagnosis

Pulselessness (or ineffective very rapid or very slow pulse) in large artery of unresponsive victim, **absence of effective spontaneous respiration.**

► Treatment Steps

Basic Life Support (BLS)
- **Open airway.**
- **Ventilate effectively**—breathing.
- **Support circulation** with external cardiac compression.

Assess effectiveness of BLS with evaluation of pupillary reactivity and palpation of pulsation in large artery. Continue until advanced cardiac life support available.

Advanced Cardiac Life Support (ACLS)
- Maintain airway and adequate ventilation with adjunctive equipment (mask, endotracheal tube).
- Arrhythmia recognition (ECG) and appropriate treatment (electrical and pharmacologic).
- Intravenous access.

Often most important aspect of ACLS is **prompt defibrillation for ventricular fibrillation** (most common cause of cardiopulmonary arrest in adults). The use of portable automated external defibrillators (AEDs) has become much more common in schools, public venues.

BIBLIOGRAPHY

Braunwald E, Zipes D, Libby P. *Heart Disease*, 6th ed. Philadelphia: W.B. Saunders, 2004.

Fuster V, Alexander R, O'Rourke R. *The Heart*, 10th ed. New York: McGraw-Hill, 2001.

Fuster V, Ross R, Topol E. *Atherosclerosis and Coronary Artery Disease*. Philadelphia: Lippincott-Raven, 1996.

Julian DG, Campbell-Cowan J. *Cardiology*. Philadelphia: W.B. Saunders, 2005.

Disorders of the Skin and Subcutaneous Tissue

2

DISORDERS OF THE SKIN AND SUBCUTANEOUS TISSUE Health and Health Maintenance

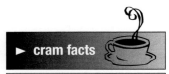

► cram facts

DERMATOLOGIC VOCABULARY

- **Bulla:** A vesicle with a diameter greater than 0.5 cm.
- **Crust:** Dry serum, blood or pus on the skin surface.
- **Erosion:** A defect in the epidermis with no change in the dermis.
- **Macule:** A change in skin color that is not palpable.
- **Nodule:** A palpable solid lesion > 1 cm.
- **Papule:** Palpable change in skin less than 1 cm in size.
- **Plaque:** A mesalike elevation that occupies a relatively large surface area in comparison with its height above the skin level.
- **Pustule:** A vesicle filled with pus.
- **Scale:** An accumulation of keratin.
- **Ulcer:** A tissue defect extending into the dermis.
- **Vesicle:** A circumscribed elevated lesion that contains fluid.
- **Wheal:** A rounded or flat-topped papule or plaque that disappears within a few hours.

I. HEALTH AND HEALTH MAINTENANCE

A. Economic/Social Impact of Skin Disorders

► Description

Consider ultimate cost in evaluation and treatment of skin-related disorders. Consider financial and social/psychological impact (i.e., acne). Skin conditions such as acne, psoriasis, nonmelanoma skin cancers, and occupational skin diseases create enormous financial impact.

B. Epidemiology and Prevention of Sun-Induced Skin Disorders

► Description

Sun exposure results in pathologic skin changes termed **actinic damage.** Skin damage depends on multiple factors including: (1) amount of sun exposure, (2) intrinsic sun protection ability (Fitzpatrick skin type), and (3) intrinsic ability to repair deoxyribonucleic acid (DNA) photodamage. Chronic sun exposure results in wrinkles and skin atrophy, as well as precancerous and cancerous lesions (basal cell carcinoma and squamous cell carcinoma). More than 1 million skin cancers diagnosed each year in the United States: approximately 800,000 basal cell carcinomas, 400,000 squamous cell carcinomas, and 50,000 melanomas. Photosensitive medication can make sun damage worse. Erythema, dyskeratotic cell potential high with **ultraviolet B (UVB)** (290–320 nm). **Ultraviolet C (UVC)** (1–290 nm) **absorbed by ozone layer. Black light (UVA)** (320–400 nm) **will go through glass, has longer wavelength, and causes aging and tanning; UVB will not go through glass, has shorter wavelength, and causes sunburn.** Prevention of sun-induced lesions involves education, avoiding sun exposure, and/or use of sun blockers, especially with higher SPF (sun protection factor; 15 or more is excellent). **Para-aminobenzoic acid (PABA) protects against UVB.** Parsol 1789 protects against UVA.

C. Epidemiology and Prevention of Contact Dermatitis and Drug Reactions

► Description

Contact dermatitis is **epidermal and dermal inflammation** secondary to chemical compounds. Two forms of contact dermatitis: irritant and allergic. Skin disease accounts for 24% of all reported cases of occupational disease. **Drug reactions** may present as multiple types of skin eruptions. History, physical with attention to drug allergies is important, as is early discontinuation of offending medication. **Common offending medications** include **penicillin, sulfa drugs, nonsteroidal anti-inflammatory drugs (NSAIDs),** and **anticonvulsants. Any medications ingested may cause skin reaction.**

D. Epidemiology and Prevention of Decubitus Ulcers

► Description

Decubitus ulcers involve **skin necrosis** resulting **from excessive pressure.** Disorder more common in individuals unable to move/react to this pressure (includes patients in coma, stroke/neurologic disorders). Seventy percent of patients with pressure sores are over 70

FUNCTION OF THE SKIN

1. Protection
   (A) Infection—The cutaneous lipid film is antimicrobial while the stratum corneum is a physical barrier against entry.
   (B) Trauma—Resistant to tearing, padded by subcutaneous fat.
   (C) Heat—Subcutaneous fat insulates to protect the body from temperature variations.
   (D) Light—Skin reflects and absorbs light.
   (E) Chemicals—Buffer capacity and mechanical protection against chemicals.
   (F) Prevents the interior of the body from drying out.

2. Sensation
   Pain, itch, light touch, heat, cold.

3. Metabolism

4. Communication
   (A) Antigen presentation through Langerhans' cells.
   (B) Medical condition—a jaundiced person's skin is yellow.
   (C) Emotional state and appearance.
   (D) Pheromones.

years of age. The mortality rate for this population is estimated at 8%. Key to **prevention** is **reduction** of **prolonged local pressure** via repositioning, therapy/ambulating if possible, or padding/pressure reduction via sheepskin, egg crate, air/waterflow beds.

II. INFECTIONS

A. Herpes Simplex

► Description
DNA virus of type 1 (nongenital) and type 2 (genital) variety.

► Symptoms
Fever and local tenderness. Primary infection of **type 1 most often presents as gingivostomatitis,** with erosions and adenopathy. Reactivated infection of type 1 mostly presents as cold sores. **Type 2 (fever blisters—herpes labialis)** has high incidence of **systemic symptoms,** fever, malaise; presents with genital papules, vesicles, erosions.

► Diagnosis
History, physical. Vesicle fluid virus culture, skin biopsy. **Tzanck preparation** demonstrates multinucleated giant cells.

► Pathology
A prevalent sexually transmitted disease, herpes simplex virus (HSV) is transmitted by direct contact, via mucosal surface to surface.

► Treatment Steps
Acyclovir, valacyclovir, famciclovir.

B. Herpes Zoster (Shingles)

► Description
Shingles is **recrudescence** of **latent infection** of **zoster/varicella virus.** Noted to be in boundary defined by a dermatome. Eruption is

GROUPED VESICLES

- **Herpes simplex**— Herpetiform grouping of vesicles on an erythematous base.
- **Herpes zoster**—Similar to herpes simplex but grouped vesicles confined to a dermatome.
- **Acute contact dermatitis**—Vesicles do not exhibit herpetiform grouping and may become confluent with large bullae.

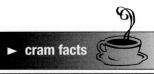

Herpetic whitlow is finger infection of HSV, a risk for physicians and dentists (wear gloves!).

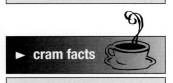

► cram facts

SHINGLES

- More common in people who are immuno-compromised (elderly, acquired immune deficiency syndrome [AIDS], cancer) but can occur in an otherwise healthy person under a great deal of stress.
- However, particularly in young patients, consider HIV testing.

most **often unilateral** and indicates partial immunity. Post-herpetic neuralgia may occur (see Clinical Pearl).

► **Symptoms**

Eruption of localized, painful, grouped vesicles, which is most often unilateral (Fig. 2–1). Burning and paresthesias in affected dermatome may be noted, as well as prodrome of fever and dermatome pain.

► **Diagnosis**

Typical presentation in individual dermatome. Viral culture may be performed along with serologic studies. **Tzanck** smear **positive for multinucleated giant cells.**

► **Pathology**

Dorsal nerve root latent virus reactivation.

► **Treatment Steps**

Acyclovir, valacyclovir, famciclovir.

C. Varicella (Chickenpox)

► **Description**

Varicella zoster virus infection. Chickenpox in children. More serious disease in adults.

► **Symptoms**

Classic presentation in children: Itchy rash, fever. Presents as crops of vesicles centered in pink papules.

► **Diagnosis**

Clinical picture is characteristic. Onset of papules, vesicles, and pustules located on thorax and face, prior to spread to extremities. Typical lesions have vesicle in center of an erythematous spot. **Lesions in all stages of development are noted.** Positive **Tzanck** smear not needed—diagnosed clinically.

► **Pathology**

Incubation of 2–3 weeks, with **transmission** possible **1 day prior to the rash to 6–7 days later.** Transmission via respiratory microdroplets as well as direct contact.

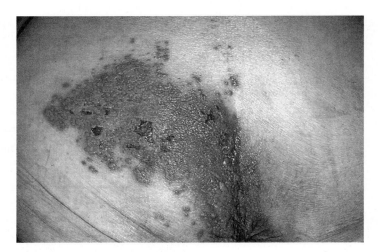

Figure 2–1. Herpes zoster. Grouped vesicles in S3 dermatologic distribution.

► Treatment Steps
1. Vaccine now offered to children.
2. Supportive care, benadryl for pruritus, acetaminophen for fever. **No aspirin in children.**

D. Cellulitis and Erysipelas

- An acute infection of dermal and subcutaneous tissues, most commonly due to *Staphylococcus aureus* or streptococci. (When cellulitis is due to group A streptococcus, it has a characteristic shiny reddish appearance, is warm and tender, and is referred to as erysipelas.)
- Diagnosis is clinical, and systemic antibiotic treatment is guided by the most likely organisms present. In simple cellulitis in a healthy person, gram-positive antibiotic coverage with medications such as cephalexin or clindamycin (see Clinical Pearl).

E. Erysipeloid

- An acute but slowly evolving cellulitis that occurs at sites of inoculation with the gram-positive rod *Erysipelothrix rhusiopathiae*. It occurs in those who handle fish, shellfish, meat, hides, bones, and poultry.
- Diagnosis is clinical. Almost never occurs in persons who do not handle dead animal matter in their work. Can include housewives, fishermen and fish handlers, butchers, farmers, veterinarians. Area usually well demarcated, painful, swollen, and reddish-purple, commonly occurring on finger or hand.
- Treatment: Prevention of infection with gloves. Penicillin or erythromycin.

F. Erythrasma

- A superficial bacterial skin infection caused by a gram-positive rod, *Corynebacterium minutissimum*. Usually affects intertriginous areas (toes, groin, axilla, beneath breasts) and mimics dermatophyte infections.
- Diagnosis: Wood's lamp shows a characteristic coral-red fluorescence, potassium hydroxide (KOH) is negative for fungi.
- Treatment: Erythromycin.

► **clinical pearl**

POSTHERPETIC NEURALGIA (PHN)

- PHN is persistent pain in the area of the healed zoster rash.
- Occurs in some patients after an outbreak of shingles.
- Various treatment options exist, including gabapentin (Neurontin), capsaicin cream (Zostrix), topical lidocaine patch.
- Early treatment of acute zoster (shingles) with antiviral agents (acyclovir) may decrease the risk of PHN.

► **cram facts**

Erysipelas in strep infection, more superficial than cellulitis (raised, sharply demarcated margin).

► **cram facts**

VARICELLA COMPLICATIONS

- Varicella can be a dangerous disease in pregnant women, neonates, adults, and immunocompromised patients.
- Pregnant women who were not previously immune to varicella (by prior infection or immunization): Contracting varicella during the first trimester can cause congenital varicella syndrome. Fetal defects can include microcephaly, chorioretinitis, intrauterine growth retardation (IUGR), and cataracts. Fetal risk of injury is not related to severity of disease in the mother.
- Neonatal varicella can result in life-threatening pneumonia or hepatitis. Treatment involves VZIG (varicella-zoster immune globulin) if the mother contracted varicella within 5 days of delivery, because there was not enough time to produce protective antibody.
- Adults and adolescents with varicella can have life-threatening pneumonia.
- Patients with underlying malignancy, particularly children with leukemia, have a very high risk of severe varicella. Care must be taken to prevent them from contact with other children with chickenpox.

ORGANISMS AND CELLULITIS

For certain clinical scenarios, specific organisms should be suspected of causing disease:

- *Vibrio vulnificus*—patient with underlying disorder (diabetes, cirrhosis, immunosuppression) who has ingested undercooked or raw seafood.
- *Aeromonas hydrophila*—patient with a preexisting wound, usually lower leg, exposed to fresh water.
- *Capnocytophaga canimorsus*—asplenic or immunosuppressed patient exposed to or bitten by a dog.
- *Pasteurella multocida*—following a cat bite

IMPETIGO

Highly communicable infection predominantly of preschool-age children; peak seasonal incidence late summer to early fall.

G. Impetigo

- A common superficial skin infection, most common in children. Usually caused by *S. aureus* or group A β-hemolytic strep.
- Diagnose clinically: Crusted, yellow lesions found on lips, nose, and cheek.
- Treatment: Usually responds to cleaning area well and using topical mupirocin ointment.

H. Folliculitis, Furuncle, and Carbuncle

- All are caused by *S. aureus* and represent a continuum of infection. A furuncle is an acute, deep, erythematous, hot, tender nodule that evolves from a staphylococcal folliculitis. A carbuncle is a deeper infection that results from interconnecting furuncles, usually arising in several contiguous hair follicles.
- Diagnose clinically. Culture of infected fluid can guide treatment.
- Treatment: Furuncles and carbuncles should be opened and drained, followed by systemic antibiotics effective against staphylococcus (i.e., dicloxacillin, cephalexin). (Simple folliculitis is often self-limited and treated with warm compresses.)

I. Abscess

- A localized collection of pus that can occur anywhere in the body, from small abscess near the nail (paronychia) to larger more complicated infection (intra-abdominal, spinal epidural).
- Diagnosis: Abscess can be obvious on skin but harder to find in other areas of the body. Clues include persistent pain, fever, elevated white blood cell (WBC) count. Often visualized on computed tomography (CT) or magnetic resonance imaging (MRI).
- Treatment: Almost always requires drainage of the abscess with systemic antibiotics. Antibiotics based on most likely organisms in the area of the abscess plus organisms found on culture.

J. Gas Gangrene/Necrotizing Soft Tissue Infection

- **A medical and surgical emergency.** Infection can be a necrotizing cellulitis, fasciitis, or myonecrosis. Infections need surgical debridement as well as systemic antibiotics and have a fairly high mortality rate.
- Diagnosis: Can mimic cellulitis but does not respond as well to systemic antibiotics. Skin may form bullae, blackened areas of necrosis. Sometimes severe pain is out of proportion to the physical findings.
- Treatment: Urgent consultation with a surgeon for exploration of the area and wide debridement. Broad-spectrum intravenous antibiotics needed. *Clostridium* species are a common cause.

K. Dermatophytoses, Tinea Pedis, Tinea Manuum, Tinea Cruris, Tinea Corporis, Tinea Capitis

► Description

Keratinized skin infection by fungi. Approximately 10% of the total population can be expected to have a dermatophytic foot infection at any given time.

► Symptoms

Tinea capitis may present as broken or hairless patch. **Tinea pedis** and **tinea manuum** may present as interdigital finger or toe-web scaling, cracking, or vesicles. **Tinea corporis** presents as annular plaques with raised edges (see Fig. 2–2 and Table 2–1).

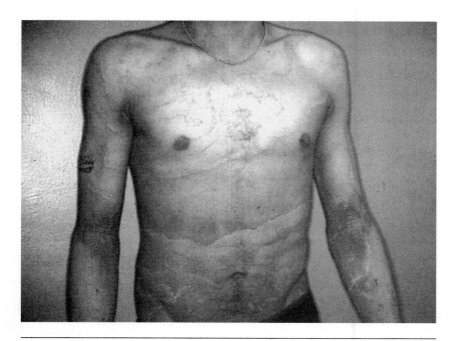

Figure 2–2. Tinea corporis. On the trunk are flat, erythematous lesions with sharp, raised, scaly, irregular borders. KOH positive for mycelia.

► Diagnosis

History, physical exam; fungal culture, KOH preparation.

► Pathology

Tinea capitis commonly due to *Trichophyton tonsurans* and *Microsporum audouinii.* **Tinea corporis, tinea cruris, tinea pedis,** and **tinea manuum** may be due to *T. rubrum, T. mentagrophytes,* or *Epidermophyton floccosum.*

► Treatment Steps

Tinea in hair or nails needs systemic (oral) therapy. All other can generally be treated topically:
• **Topical:** Ketoconazole (nizoral), clotrimazole (Lotrimin).
• **Oral:** Terbenafine (Lamisil), griseofulvin (mainl used in tinea capitis).

L. Onychomycosis

► Description

Infection of the nail caused by any fungus including nondermatophytes and yeasts. At least five subtypes exist and can coexist in the same patient.

2-1

TINEA INFECTIONS

Tinea infections are classified by region of the body:

• Tinea barbae—beard area and neck
• Tinea capitis—scalp hair
• Tinea corporis—trunk and extremities
• Tinea cruris—groin
• Tinea manuum and tinea pedis—palms, soles, interdigital webs

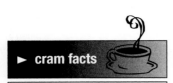

► cram facts

Monitoring of LFTs is usually needed with long-term use of azole therapy.

► clinical pearl

CONGENITAL RUBELLA SYNDROME

- If a pregnant woman contracts rubella in the early stage of gestation, the virus can be transmitted to the fetus via the placenta.
- Thankfully due to immunization, this is fairly rare.
- Classic triad in congenital rubella is hearing loss, visual defects (cataracts), and cardiac defects (patent ductus arteriosus), although multiple other complications can occur.

► Symptoms

Vary depending on etiology, but commonly thickened nail plate, yellow or white discoloration of nail plate, onycholysis.

► Diagnosis

Examination, KOH and fungal culture of debris under nail plate most common: *T. rubrum*, *T. mentagrophytes*, *E. floccosum* (dermatophytes), *Aspergillus* (molds), *Candida albicans*, *C. parapsilosis* (yeasts).

► Treatment Steps

Systemic therapy with either Lamisil (terbinafine), Sporanox (itraconazole), or ketoconazole. Often needs prolonged course of treatment (at least 8 weeks).

M. Rubella (German Measles)

► Symptoms

Spreading macules and papules, face downward to trunk **in 1 day,** fading by day 3. **Cervical, suboccipital, and postauricular node enlargement.**

► Diagnosis

History, physical exam. Serology to confirm if necessary. Incubation period is 14–21 days; spread by respiratory route.

► Pathology

Rubella virus infection.

► Treatment Steps

None. Prevention important as first trimester infection may cause fetal anomaly. Prevent by immunization.

N. Measles (Rubeola)

► Symptoms

Asymptomatic incubation period of 10–11 days; prodromal phase of fever, malaise, coryza, conjunctivitis, cough persists for 3–4 days; then rash lasts 5–6 days; Koplik's spots appear in mouth 24–48 hours before rash and remain 2–3 days.

► Diagnosis

Clinical picture. Photophobia, malaise, macules and papules may coalesce. May detect by serology. **Rash spreads over several days (rash behind ears and over forehead spreads over neck and trunk, then distally over extremities).**

► Pathology

Measles virus (paramyxovirus), causing hyaline necrosis of epidermal cells. Respiratory transmission. Highly contagious.

► Treatment Steps

Supportive therapy, rest, hydration. Prevent by immunization. Complications include pneumonia and encephalitis.

O. Roseola

► Description

An acute benign exanthem of childhood, with fever followed by rash.

► Symptoms

After a prodrome with high fever for 3–5 days, **rash then develops.** Occurs in first few weeks of life with incubation of 5 days to 2 weeks.

Rash of 1- to 5-mm macules or maculopapules, often tender, blanch on pressure and often surrounded by whitish halo, may be light pink in color. Diagnose clinically.

► **Pathology**
Caused by infection with human herpesvirus-6 infection (HHV-6).

► **Treatment Steps**
None. Most cases do not require treatment. Rarely, HHV-6 can cause hepatitis, meningitis, or encephalitis.

P. Erythema Infectiosum (Fifth Disease)

► **Symptoms**
"Slapped cheek" rash (confluent erythematous, edematous plaques on the malar eminences), reticulate pattern rash, mild fever. Rash lasts 5–9 days. Incubation period 4–14 days, spread by respiratory route. Infectious prior to onset of rash. Clinical diagnosis.

► **Pathology**
Parvovirus B19 (single-stranded DNA virus).

► **Treatment Steps**
None. Supportive therapy if aplastic crisis develops.

Q. Hand, Foot, and Mouth Disease

► **Symptoms**
Palatal erosions associated with vesicular lesions on the hands, feet, and buttocks (Fig. 2–3).

► **Diagnosis**
Ulcerative oral lesions, exanthema on hands and feet in association with mild febrile illness, usually caused by coxsackievirus A-16 and usually found in children < 10 years old.

► **Treatment Steps**
No specific treatment. Topical anesthetics for oral lesions.

R. Viral Warts
1. Common wart—cauliflower shaped (caused by papillomavirus).
2. Verrucae planae—flat wart (faces and hands of children).
3. Plantar wart—sole of feet.

► **Description**
Hyperkeratotic growths. The incidence of nongenital warts approaches 10% in children and young adults. Clinical diagnosis.

► **Symptoms**
One or more verrucae of typical appearance.

► **Pathology**
Human papillomavirus (HPV). At least 80 different genotypes of HPV have been identified: Type 1, plantar warts; Types 2, 4, 27, 29, common warts; Types 3, 10, 28, 49, flat warts.

► **Treatment Steps**
Multiple treatment approaches can be successful. Electrodesiccation and curettage are generally preferred, but depending on the patient, other modalities such as freezing, acid, surgical removal, immunotherapy, podophyllotoxin, imiquimod, intralesional bleomycin, interferon can be employed.

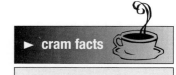

► **cram facts**

PARVOVIRUS B19

- Can cause an aplastic crisis, commonly in sickle cell disease patients.
- Can also cause self-limited polyarthritis/arthralgias.

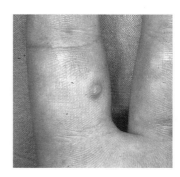

Figure 2–3. Hand, foot, and mouth disease. Vesicles and pustules on an erythematous base; often painful and are usually found on fingers and toes.

S. Rocky Mountain Spotted Fever

► Description
Rickettsial, febrile disorder.

► Symptoms
Fever, headache, myalgia, arthralgia. Rash develops about 4 days after constitutional symptoms. Pink, macular rash on wrists, ankles, forearms; then palms and soles; then centrally to arms, thighs, trunk, and face. The rash then becomes deeper red and petechial. Untreated fatality rate is 20–80%.

► Diagnosis
History, physical exam. Serologic testing, Weil–Felix test, acute and convalescent serum for confirmation (takes too long). Immunofluorescent staining of microorganisms in the walls of small blood vessels of skin biopsy. Cannot be done on paraffin-embedded sections.

► Pathology
Dermacentor andersoni **tick bite,** resulting in *Rickettsia rickettsii* transmission. Incubation 3–12 days, with mean of 7 days. Western U.S. vector is wood tick *D. andersoni;* Eastern U.S. vector is dog tick *D. variabilis.* Diffuse vasculitis, thrombosis of vascular lumen.

► Treatment Steps
Tetracycline. If pregnant, give chloramphenicol. Complications include disseminated intravascular coagulation (DIC), shock, and renal failure; **there may be no history of bite or rash in some cases.** Do not use sulfonamides; they enhance rickettsial infections.

T. Lyme Disease

► Description
Multisystem disorder caused by the spirochete *Borrelia burgdorferi.* Usually transmitted by the deer tick *Ixodes dammini.* A classic skin rash occurs early in infection. Other areas affected include cardiac, musculoskeletal, and neurologic.

► Symptoms
Dermatologic: Classic rash is **erythema chronicum migrans,** a flat to slightly raised erythematous rash with **central clearing.** In the early stage when the rash is present, patients may have flulike symptoms.

► Diagnosis
Clinical diagnosis. If the rash is noted in a patient who lives in or has visited an area with a high incidence of Lyme disease (particularly the Northeast United States), empiric treatment should be started. Serologic testing not needed as it may come back as a false negative early in the infection.

► Treatment Steps
First line: Doxycycline 100 mg BID for 14–21 days. Amoxicillin (used in pregnant women and children) for 14–21 days.

U. Dermatologic Manifestations of HIV (Human Immunodeficiency Virus)

1. **Oral thrush.** Presents as white patches in the oral cavity—tongue, buccal mucosa, oropharynx. Caused by *Candida albicans.* Treatment can include topical nystatin (swish and swallow) or oral fluconazole (Diflucan). Treatment is given only when thrush is present. Prophylaxis with long-term fluconazole is not

recommended due to issues with fluconazole-resistant *Candida* species.

2. **Molluscum contagiosum.** Firm, smooth, umbilicated papules, often flesh colored, sometimes white, yellow, or translucent. Caused by infection with a DNA poxvirus. Educate patients that it can be spread to others by direct contact. May be self-limited. Cryotherapy with liquid nitrogen can remove lesions. Other treatments exist.

3. **Kaposi's sarcoma.** A malignancy caused by human herpesvirus-8 (HHV-8). It presents as vascular, purplish-reddish lesions, often on the skin. However, lesions can exist in any area of the body, particularly the gastrointestinal or pulmonary systems. Treatment involves a multidisciplinary approach, including dermatologists, oncologists, and HIV specialists, and varies based on extent of disease.

III. ARTHROPODS

A. Scabies

▶ Description

Sarcoptes scabiei is an arthropod that spends its entire life cycle on human skin.

▶ Symptoms

Intense itching. Most common on hands, axillae, and genitalia (Fig. 2–4).

▶ Diagnosis

History of intense itching in several family members. Identify the mite by scraping on an intact tunnel. **Highly contagious.**

▶ Treatment Steps

Permethrin is the preferred treatment. It is applied topically to **the entire body.** Lindane is reserved for treatment failures because it can cause seizures.

IV. DERMATITIS

A. Atopic Dermatitis (Eczema)

▶ Description

Epidermal and dermal **inflammation;** defective cell-mediated immunity. There may be an increased risk of developing seasonal allergies or asthma.

▶ Symptoms

Itching and cutaneous reactivity; disturbances in vascular reactivity; dry, lackluster skin; lichenification.

▶ Diagnosis

History and physical exam. Family/personal history of atrophy. Chronic relapsing course, pruritus, flexural lichenification or linearity in adults, facial and extensor involvement in infants and children.

▶ **cram facts**

Nodular scabies: A localized allergic reaction; a cutaneous lymphocytic infiltrate occurs, even after the mites have been destroyed.

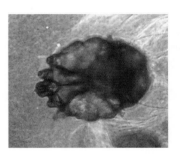

Figure 2–4. Scabies. The mite *Sarcoptes scabiei, var. hominis,* causes pruritic papules and vesicles with S-shaped or straight burrows.

▶ **cram facts**

ATOPIC DERMATITIS

• May have allergy/asthma history. **Positive association with cataracts** and keratoconus.
• Worse with itching and with stress.
• *Eczema* is a general term for several types of inflammation of the skin. Atopic dermatitis is the most common form of eczema.

Xerosis (dry skin) aggravated by decreased relative humidity, cold, and increased exposure to woolen clothing.

► Treatment Steps
1. Emollients.
2. Skin hydration.
3. Topical steroids.
4. Immunomodulators such as tacrolimus/pimecrolimus.
5. Phototherapy.
6. Avoid wool and polyester clothing.

B. Allergic Contact Dermatitis and Photodermatitis

► Description
Two forms of contact dermatitis: irritant and allergic. Dermal and epidermal inflammation secondary to chemical/foreign antigen exposure.

► Symptoms
In an allergic contact dermatitis caused by Rhus plant antigens, topical medications, and liquid antigens, the reaction is often acute vesicular dermatitis. For leather, rubber, or nickel antigens, the reaction is often low-grade chronic dermatitis. Commonly, an itchy area of erythema, in an exposed area (under watch, necklace, etc.). Irritant contact dermatitis occasionally occurs acutely with one exposure as a chemical burn; more commonly occurs slowly with chronic exposure to irritant or caustic substances. Dryness, scaling, fissuring, mild inflammation are manifestations.

► Pathology
Allergic contact dermatitis is a **type 4 delayed, cell-mediated, hypersensitivity reaction.** Irritant contact dermatitis is a direct toxic reaction.

► Treatment Steps
1. Remove cause.
2. Topical corticosteroids.
3. Systemic steroids if severe.

Photodermatitis is light induced, may show a clear border between light-exposed and light-protected areas.

C. Cutaneous Drug Reactions

► Description/Symptoms
Skin eruption resulting from medication (oral or topical). A drug reaction can develop up to 6 weeks after a drug is stopped. May present as almost any type of dermatitis.

► Pathology
Types 1, 2, 3, and 4 hypersensitivity reactions.

► Treatment Steps
1. Stop suspected medication.
2. Antihistamines.
3. Topical corticosteroids.
4. Systemic corticosteroids.

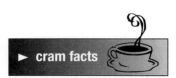

► cram facts

Exanthematous rash is most common drug rash. (Mono patient given amoxicillin). Fixed drug eruption will **present as lesion that will recur in same spot with same drug exposure.**

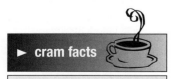

► cram facts

Psoriasis can be worsened by:
• Antimalarial drugs
• Lithium
• β-Blockers

V. PSORIASIS AND SEBORRHEIC DERMATITIS

A. Psoriasis

▶ Symptoms

Chronic scaling plaques, knees, elbows, nails. Red plaques and sil-ver-white scale. Guttate psoriasis: multiple small papules may be accompanied by psoriatic arthritis. Clinical diagnosis.

▶ Treatment Steps

1. Topical corticosteroids.
2. Calcipotriene.
3. Anthralin.
4. Tar products.
5. Phototherapy with UVB or psoralen plus ultraviolet A (PUVA).
6. Retinoids (for example, methotrexate).
7. Chemotherapy.

B. Seborrheic Dermatitis

▶ Description

Chronic scaling dermatitis. On the scalp, known as dandruff. On an infant's scalp, it is "cradle cap."

▶ Symptoms

Whitish scales with or without erythema common about nose, eyes, external ear canal, and central chest (active sebaceous gland areas).

▶ Pathology

Inflammatory reaction to the organism *Malassezia*.

▶ Treatment Steps

1. Ketoconazole shampoo or tar shampoo.
2. Topical corticosteroids.

VI. BULLOUS DISORDERS

A. Bullous Impetigo

▶ Description

Occurs in children < 2 years old; primary spontaneous infections of apparently normal skin.

▶ Symptoms

Vesicles and bullae on bland, noninflamed skin, although sometimes skin is erythematous. Can be pruritic. Vesicle is often filled with yellow fluid. Clinical diagnosis.

▶ Pathology

Exotoxin-producing *Staphylococcus aureus* that chemically splits the epidermis.

▶ Treatment Steps

1. Cleanse area.
2. Topical antibiotics can be curative (mupirocin).
3. Systemic antibiotics if extensive (cephalexin).
4. Inpatient care may be needed with widespread disease or in infants at risk for sepsis.

▶ **differential diagnosis**

- **Seborrheic dermatitis**—Ill-defined pink plaques with fine dandruff-like scale on scalp, eyebrows, beard, mesolabial and nasolabial creases, presternal skin.
- **Psoriasis vulgaris**—Less common on face. Scalp plaques, well-defined, often extending beyond hairline to forehead or neck.
- **Perioral dermatitis**—Papules in mesolabial folds, chin, upper lip.

▶ **cram facts**

Koebner's sign—Trauma resulting in eruption of psoriasis in the area of trauma.
Auspitz sign—Multiple bleeding points after scale removal.

▶ **cram facts**

Leiner's disease: generalized infantile seborrheic dermatitis, rule out histiocytosis X. Seborrheic dermatitis is most frequent cause of malar dermatitis. Seborrheic dermatitis on infant scalp is "cradle cap."

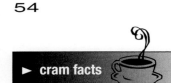

► cram facts

STAPHYLOCOCCAL
"SCALDED-SKIN"
SYNDROME

The toxin is blood-borne,
causing lysis and
denudation of large areas
of skin. Mortality rate
approaches 25% without
appropriate care.
Pyodermas are infections
of broken skin.

B. Bullous Pemphigoid

► **Description**

A subepidermal blistering skin disease usually occurring in the elderly. Thought to be a chronic, autoimmune, inflammatory disease.

► **Symptoms**

Bullous eruption in elderly. Large, tense blisters arising on normal skin or on erythematous base; often pruritus. Onset can be acute or subacute. Blisters; no Nikolsky sign.

► **Diagnosis**

Skin biopsy with immunofluorescence studies.

► **Pathology**

Autoimmune, immunoglobulin G (IgG) and C3 (complement) deposited at epidermal–dermal junction.

► **Treatment Steps**

1. Anti-inflammatories (prednisone, tetracycline, topical steroids of high potency).
2. Immunosuppressants may be used (azathioprine).

C. Dermatitis Herpetiformis

► **Description/Symptoms**

Itchy, chronic papulovesicular eruption. Symmetric vesicles on knees, elbows, shoulders, exterior surfaces, scalp. **No Nikolsky sign.** Intensely itchy.

► **Diagnosis**

Clnical scenario, skin biopsy.

► **Pathology**

Autoimmune vesicular disorder. IgA deposits in normal-appearing skin. **Commonly associated with celiac sprue.**

► **Treatment Steps**

1. **Gluten-free diet** will often control disease.
2. **Dapsone.** Other treatments include colchicine, cyclosporin, and prednisone.

D. Herpes Gestationis/Pemphigoid Gestationis

► **Description**

Pemphigoid gestationis is a rare autoimmune disease seen in pregnancy. (Originally named herpes gestationis on the basis of the morphology of the blisters, this is a misnomer because the disease is not related to any active or prior herpesvirus infection).

► **Symptoms**

During the second or third trimester of pregnancy, the abrupt onset of extremely pruritic papules and blisters, usually on the abdomen and trunk. Lesions can progress to tense vesicles.

► **Diagnosis**

Clinical picture, and skin biopsy with immunofluorescence (liner band of C3 deposition +/− IgG along the basement membrane).

► **Treatment Steps**

1. Management of pruritus can include bathing, moisurizers, emollients.

2. Topical steroids and topical or oral antihistamines can be effective if pruritus is mild.
3. If pruritus is severe, start prednisone, but taper as quickly as possible.

E. Pemphigus

► Description
Unusual, possibly fatal skin disorder.

► Symptoms
Multiple flaccid bullae, Nikolsky's sign (epidermal separation with pressure).

► Diagnosis
History and physical examination, immunofluorescence testing; skin/lesion **biopsy shows acantholysis.**

► Pathology
Unknown, but autoantibodies to epidermal antigen are present.

► Treatment Steps
1. Prednisone.
2. Fluids.
3. Antibiotics (tetracycline).
4. Immunosuppressives (mycophenolate, cyclophosphamide).
5. Gold.

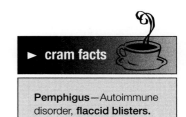

► cram facts

Pemphigus—Autoimmune disorder, **flaccid blisters.**

VII. PRURITIC DERMATOSES

A. Pruritus Ani

► Symptoms
Pruritus of anal area. May have minimal erythema or severe excoriations from itching. Clinical diagnosis.

► Pathology
Etiology in soaps, itching, diet(?), irritating toilet tissue, insufficient anal hygiene.

► Treatment Steps
1. Avoid etiologic factor and treat primary cause if evident (pinworms, psoriasis, etc.). Stop itch–scratch pattern.
2. Sitz bath.
3. Topical corticosteroids or tacrolimus/pimecrolimus.
4. Antihistamines.

B. Factitial Dermatitis

► Description
Self-inflicted dermatitis, therefore many types of dermatitis possible.

► Diagnosis
History, physical exam; may have bizarre pattern—patient denies causing rash but may have clear psychological problems. **No rash in nonreachable areas (midback, "butterfly sign").**

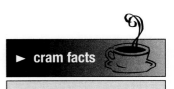

► cram facts

Rule out scabies, xerosis, uremia, Hodgkin's, and endocrine disorders in chronic itching.

► Treatment Steps

Psychiatric evaluation. **Neurotic excoriations: compulsive scratching. May also be termed** *lichen simplex chronicus.*

VIII. ACNEIFORM ERUPTIONS

A. Acne Vulgaris

► Symptoms/Diagnosis

Common acne, including comedones, nodules, papules, pustules, and cysts. Clinical diagnosis.

► Pathology

Follicle plugging and inflammation resulting from multiple factors including bacteria and androgenic influence. **Bacteria:** *Propionibacterium acne.*

► Treatment Steps
1. Benzoyl peroxide.
2. Topical and oral antibiotics.
3. Topical retinoids.
4. Isotretinoin (Accutane).

B. Rosacea

► Description

A common condition involving skin of the face.

► Symptoms/Diagnosis

Papules and papulopustules in the central face with red cheeks and telangiectasia. Recurrent flushing and blushing that becomes persistent. Leads to disfiguring hypertrophy of the sebaceous glands resulting in rhinophyma. Clinical diagnosis.

► Treatment Steps
1. Avoid irritants.
2. Avoid agents or situations that lead to facial flushing.
3. Topical metronidazole, clindamycin, or erythromycin.
4. Systemic tetracyline.
5. Intense pulse light (IPL) therapy for the telangiectasia and redness.

IX. DECUBITUS ULCERS

► Symptoms/Diagnosis

Erythema, skin breakdown, open sores, due to pressure necrosis. Decubitus ulcer commonly refers to a sacral ulcer, but any area that experiences pressure can develop a pressure sore. Examples include heels or elbows in bedbound patients. Clinical diagnosis.

► Pathology

Pressure-induced ischemia and tissue necrosis. Begins as blanchable erythema, then nonblanchable, then superficial to deep ulceration. Dry gangrene with tissue death may follow.

► Treatment Steps
1. **Prevent** by avoiding prolonged pressure in high-risk patients (special beds can be ordered; also various support modalities like ankle supports).

2. Avoid conditions promoting skin breakdown (excess moisture, particularly from urine or feces).
3. Occlusive dressing (Duoderm).
4. Surgical debridement if infected.

X. STASIS DERMATITIS

► **Description/Symptoms**

Chronic lower extremity dermatitis, with **hyperpigmentation, erythema,** and **edema.** Clinical diagnosis.

► **Pathology**

May result from phlebitis or venous insufficiency.

► **Treatment Steps**
1. Alleviate venous insufficiency.
2. Support stockings.
3. Elevate legs.
4. Treat infection.
5. Topical corticosteroids.

XI. URTICARIAL DISORDERS

► **Description**

Urticaria are hives. Angioedema is urticaria of deeper dermal depth.

► **Symptoms**

Fleeting, itchy papules and swellings (wheals). Hives last less than 24 hours.

► **Diagnosis**

History, physical exam.

► **Pathology**

Vast etiology including allergy (drugs, chemicals, bites, etc.), hereditary, heat/cold, solar and pressure. May include both type 1 hypersensitivity and type 3 reactions. Increased mast cells, dermal edema, and vascular fluid transudation.

► **Treatment Steps**
1. Eliminate offending agent.
2. Antihistamines.

XII. CYSTS

A. Pilonidal Cyst

► **Symptoms**

Swelling, tender, erythematous midline sacral mass. Clinical diagnosis.

► **Treatment Steps**
1. Antibiotics.
2. Surgical incision and drainage, or removal if severe.

B. Epidermoid Cyst

► **Description**

Keratin-containing cyst lined by surface epidermis.

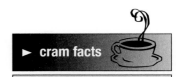

► **cram facts**

Stasis dermatitis may lead to stasis ulcer formation. Reduce edema and treat infection.

► **cram facts**

Hereditary angioedema: autosomal dominant, C1 esterase inhibitor deficiency, subcutaneous and submucosal edema. Dermagraphism: scratching results in urticaria due to histamine release.

► **Symptoms**
Slow-growing, asymptomatic. Some cysts get inflamed and secondarily infected.

► **Diagnosis**
Clinical diagnosis: An intradermal firm tumor, dome-shaped protuberance of the skin.

► **Treatment Steps**
If infected:
1. Drainage and culture.
2. Antiobiotic therapy.

Not infected cyst: enucleation or excision.

XIII. VASCULAR PROLIFERATIONS

A. Capillary Hemangioma (Strawberry Nevus)

► **Symptoms**
Red/purple hemangioma. Clinical diagnosis.

► **Treatment Steps**
1. Pulse dye laser therapy.
2. Elective cosmetic removal or cryosurgery. May regress.

B. Cavernous Hemangioma

► **Description/Symptoms**
Vascular anomaly, with swelling, may have purple color. Clinical diagnosis.

► **Treatment Steps**
1. Hope for regression.
2. Compression.
3. Systemic corticosteroids.
4. Embolization.
5. Surgical treatment.

XIV. BENIGN NEOPLASMS

A. Lentigo

► **Description**
Melanocytic and epidermal hyperplasia, increased melanin formation.

► **Symptoms**
Sharply circumscribed brown macule. Clinical diagnosis.

► **Pathology**
Intraepidermal melanocytic hyperplasia in the basal layer of elongated rete ridges without nest formation.

► **Treatment Steps**
None needed. Cryotherapy or Nd-YAG laser for cosmetic removal.

B. Seborrheic Keratoses

► **Description**
Benign skin tumors. Very common in elderly.

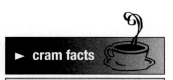
► **cram facts**

VASCULAR LESIONS

- **Kasabach–Merritt syndrome**—Hemangiomas and thrombocytopenia.
- **Senile angioma**—Cherry angioma, benign.
- **Venous lake**—Benign purple nodule in elderly, often on lip.
- **Spider angioma**—Found normally, also in pregnancy and liver disease.
- **Port-wine stain**—Congenital extensive purple lesion, will not regress.
- **Sturge–Weber syndrome**—Port-wine stain, brain calcifications and leptomeningeal angiomatosis, seizures.

► Symptoms

Flat, sharply demarcated brown macules that progress to poly-poidal, uneven warty surface (Fig. 2–5). Clinical diagnosis.

► Pathology

Proliferation of uniform basaloid cells, keratin cysts.

► Treatment Steps

1. Observation.
2. Shave excision.
3. Curettage.
4. Cryotherapy.

C. Nevomelanocytic Nevus

► Description

Proliferation of nevomelanocytes in the epidermis (junctional), dermis (intradermal), or both (compound). Usually asymptomatic.

► Diagnosis

Physical exam. Round or oval shape, well-demarcated and smooth borders.

► Treatment Steps

Excision and pathologic examination if suspicious for melanoma.

D. Dysplastic Nevus (Atypical Nevus)

► Description

Atypical-appearing melanocytic tumor with intraepidermal melanocytic dysplasia. Marker for increased melanoma risk. Usually asymptomatic.

► Diagnosis

Physical exam. Irregular, ill-defined, spreading borders with variation in color (Fig. 2–6).

► Pathology

Proliferation of intraepidermal melanocytes in irregular nests (architectural disarray) and cellular atypia.

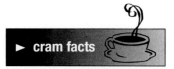

► cram facts

The eruptive appearance of multiple seborrheic keratoses in association with internal malignancies is called the sign of Leser–Trélat.

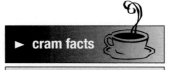

► cram facts

Risk factor for developing cutaneous melanoma:

- Dysplastic moles, prior melanomas, familial melanomas—500
- Dysplastic moles, no prior melanoma, familial melanoma—148
- Dysplastic mole, no prior melanoma, no familial melanoma—27

Figure 2–5. Seborrheic keratosis. Seborrheic keratosis showing "stuck-on" appearance and dull surface.

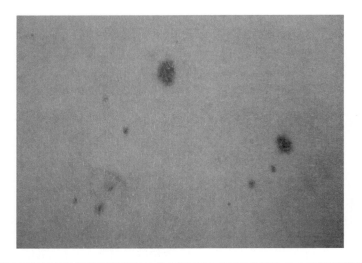

Figure 2–6. Dysplastic nevi. Dysplastic nevi showing variation in color and irregular ill-defined borders.

► Treatment Steps
1. Clinical photography.
2. Self examination every 4–6 weeks.
3. Excision of lesions with clinical suspicion of a high degree of cellular atypia or melanoma—new nevi or changing nevi.

XV. MALIGNANT NEOPLASMS

A. Actinic Keratosis

► Description
Also called **solar keratosis.** Precursors to squamous cell carcinomas.

► Symptoms/Diagnosis
Hyperkeratotic, coarse scale; hard to remove, erythematous.

► Pathology
Sun-induced keratinocyte damage. Malignant cells confined to the lower layers of the epidermis.

► Treatment Steps
1. Cryosurgery.
2. Chemosurgical destruction with phenol or trichloroacetic acid.
3. Fluorouracil (5-FU).
4. Excision.
5. Dermabrasion or laser surgery.

B. Squamous Cell Carcinoma

► Description
Skin and mucous membrane cancer. Two to four percent of the lesions metastasize. Sun (ultraviolet light) and radiation are risk factors.

► Symptoms
Indurated papule or nodule, may be in sun-exposed areas.

► Diagnosis
Clinical diagnosis, biopsy in certain cases.

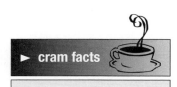

► cram facts

Most frequent premalignant skin lesion: actinic keratosis. On lips it is termed *actinic cheilitis.*

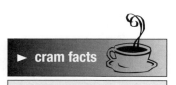

► cram facts

• Bowen's disease—Enlarging single lesion of carcinoma in situ. **May be arsenic induced.**
• Erythroplasia of Queyrat—Bowen's on the penis, also **carcinoma** in situ.

► Treatment Steps
1. Mohs' micrographic surgery provides the highest cure rate and spares the most normal tissue.
2. Surgical or radiation.

C. Basal Cell Carcinoma

► Description

Carcinoma of the skin arising from the basal cell layer. Related to one's lifetime cumulative exposure to ultraviolet light and irradiation. The most common cancer in people.

► Symptoms

Pearly nodule, rolled border (rodent ulcer). Nodular is most common type. May also be pigmented, morpheaform, superficial, and infiltrative (see Fig. 2–7). Lesions very rarely metastasize.

► Diagnosis

History, physical exam; biopsy.

► Treatment Steps
1. Mohs micrographic surgery provides the highest cure rate and spares the most normal tissue.
2. Other methods of removal include electrodesiccation and curettage, cryosurgery, radiation therapy, and scalpel excision.

D. Malignant Melanoma

► Description

Skin cancer arising from melanocytes. Some are sun related; others genetic predisposition (dysplastic nevus syndrome).

► Symptoms

May demonstrate **variegation of color, asymmetry,** and **irregular border.** Usually recognized when over 6 mm in size but can be smaller. May arise from dysplastic nevi.

► Diagnosis

See warning signs; also skin biopsy by **total excision.**

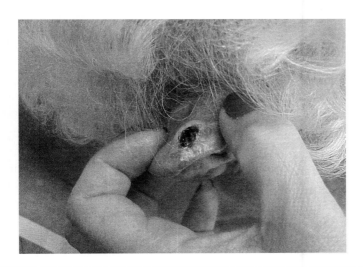

Figure 2–7. Basal cell carcinoma. Basal cell carcinoma showing ulceration and a "pearly" translucent border.

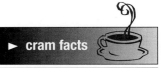

► cram facts

EARLY WARNING SIGNS OF MELANOMA

A. **Asymmetry:** One-half of the mole does not match the other half.
B. **Border:** Border or edge of the mole is ragged, blurred, irregular.
C. **Color:** Variation in the color of the mole—shades of tan, brown, black, red, white, or blue.
D. **Diameter:** Larger than 6 mm.

► cram facts

Most melanoma is superficial spreading type. Prognosis by Clark staging 1 to 5 and by Breslow thickness (depth of invasion < 0.75 mm, prognosis good; if > 4 mm, prognosis poor). Other types are nodular and lentigo maligna.

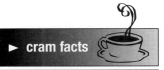

► cram facts

CLARK LEVEL STAGING OF MELANOMA

Level 1 Confined to epidermis
Level 2 Into the papillary dermis
Level 3 Fills the papillary dermis
Level 4 Into the reticular dermis
Level 5 Into the subcutaneous tissue

▶ Pathology

One-third of melanomas arise in a preexisting nevus. Metastasizes to the liver, brain, lymph nodes. The greater the depth of the melanoma, the higher the risk of metastases.

▶ Treatment Steps

Surgical. Mohs' micrographic surgery or wide excision. Metastatic workup and sentinal lymph node mapping for appropriate patients. Chemotherapy used for metastatic disease. If possible, resect isolated metastatic lesions.

XVI. CUTANEOUS MANIFESTATIONS OF SYSTEMIC DISEASE

A. Behçet's Syndrome

▶ Description

Syndrome of recurrent **aphthous ulcers, genital ulcers,** and **eye lesions (uveitis).**

▶ Symptoms

As described. **Painful ulcers, erythema nodosum.** Arthritis, inflammatory bowel disease.

▶ Diagnosis

History, physical exam. Pathergy lesions (cutaneous pustular vasculitis lesions induced by intradermal trauma).

▶ Pathology

Immune complex in blood with no known etiology. **Leukocytoclastic vasculitis.**

▶ Treatment Steps
1. Oral antibiotic suspensions.
2. Colchicine.
3. **Chlorambucil.**
4. Thalidomide.

B. Dermatomyositis

▶ Description

Multisystem disorder consisting of striated muscle inflammation.

▶ Symptoms

Progressive weakness, difficulty rising from low chairs, **proximal muscle weakness.** Maculopapular erythema on bony prominences, **heliotrope rash** (eyelid erythema), **Gottron's sign** (purple papules on knees, knuckles) (Fig. 2–8).

▶ Diagnosis

History, physical exam; elevated creatinine phosphokinase (CPK), skin/muscle biopsy, abnormal electromyogram (EMG), typical rash.

▶ Treatment Steps

Prednisone, rule out possible associated malignancy.

C. Erythema Multiforme

▶ Description

Self-limited syndrome of target-like skin lesions.

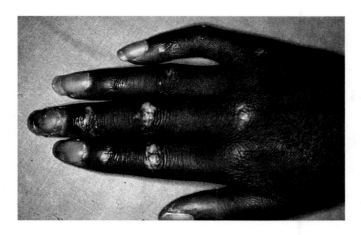

Figure 2–8. Dermatomyositis. On the dorsum of the hands over the metacarpophalangeal joints. Diffuse, erythematous papules (Gottron's papules) covered by fine scale and beginning atrophy.

► **Symptoms**

Fever, lethargy, **target lesions** affect palms and soles, mucous membranes. Clinical diagnosis.

► **Pathology**

Immune-mediated reaction. May be drug reaction (especially sulfa, phenylbutazone, phenytoin), from infection (HSV infection), toxins or other diseases. Perivascular infiltrate and dermal edema.

► **Treatment Steps**

1. Supportive therapy.
2. Identification of provocative agent.
3. Detect and prevent the most common fatal complications.

D. Erythema Nodosum

► **Description**

Inflammatory disorder of subcutaneous tissue. Immunologic.

► **Symptoms**

Lower extremity inflammatory nodules, often tender. Usually self-limited.

► **Diagnosis**

Clinical diagnosis, although skin biopsy may be needed.

► **Pathology**

Panniculitis inflammation.

► **Treatment Steps**

1. Supportive.
2. NSAIDs.
3. Corticosteroids.
4. Potassium iodide.

E. Livedo Reticularis

► **Description**

Mottled blue discoloration of the skin in a netlike pattern. Clinical diagnosis. Often asymptomatic.

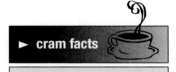

► **cram facts**

Erythema nodosum has been associated with:

- Inflammatory bowel disease
- Sarcoidosis
- Oral contraceptives
- Sulfa drugs
- Streptococcal infection
- Tuberculosis

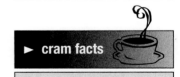

► **cram facts**

Lofgren syndrome—
Fever, erythema nodosum, possible sarcoid.

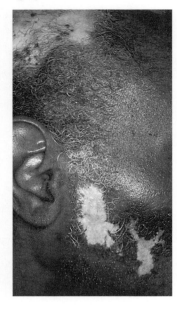

Figure 2–9. Discoid lupus erythematosus. Well-demarcated lesions with central atrophy surrounded by red edges.

▶ Pathology

Arteriole vasospasm. May exist with infection, vasculitis, or hematologic conditions. May be drug-induced.

▶ Treatment Steps
1. Avoid cold exposure.
2. Treat coexisting medical conditions.

F. Lupus Erythematosus

▶ Description

Autoimmune disease involving vasculature and connective tissue. May be cutaneous (discoid) and/or systemic. (See also Chapter 7.)

▶ Symptoms

Skin changes include malar erythema (butterfly rash), vasculitis, Raynaud's phenomenon, alopecia, and others (Fig. 2–9).

▶ Diagnosis

History, physical exam; skin biopsy, serum autoantibody testing (antinuclear antibody [ANA], double-stranded DNA).

▶ Pathology

Epidermal basal cell destruction. Autoantibodies against DNA. Immune complexes damage glomeruli and lead to vasculitis.

▶ Treatment Steps
1. Avoid sun exposure.
2. Topical corticosteroids.
3. Antimalarials.
4. Systemic corticosteroids.

G. Amyloidosis

▶ Description

Extracellular amyloid deposition. Can be systemic and associated with myeloma or localized cutaneous amyloidosis.

▶ Symptoms

Macroglossia, waxy papules/nodules on face. Carpal tunnel syndrome.

▶ Diagnosis/Pathology

Amyloid deposition in dermis and around vascular walls. **Congo red stain is used on biopsy specimen.**

▶ Treatment Steps
1. Prednisone(?).
2. Colchicine(?).
3. Rule out multiple myeloma.

H. Scleroderma

▶ Description

May be localized to the skin (morphea) or systemic disease, also called **progressive systemic sclerosis.** Etiology unknown.

▶ Symptoms

Raynaud's, dysphagia, masklike face, thin lips, tight skin.

▶ Diagnosis

History, physical exam; skin biopsy.

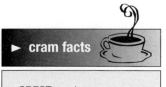

▶ **cram facts**

CREST syndrome: calcinosis, Raynaud's, esophageal dysfunction, sclerodactyly, telangiectasia.

► Treatment Steps
Symptomatic. D-Penicillamine.

I. Tuberous Sclerosis

► Description/Symptoms
A multisystem autosomal dominant disorder characterized by **retinal phacomas, seizures, mental retardation, sebaceous adenomas. Ash-leaf hypopigmented macules.**

► Diagnosis
History, physical exam; biopsy. Facial angiofibromas, periungual fibromas, hypomelanotic "ash leaf" macules.

► Treatment Steps
None. Control seizures. Supportive measures.

J. Necrobiosis Lipoidica Diabeticorum

► Description
Chronic skin disorder, some cases associated with diabetes.

► Symptoms/Diagnosis
Yellow plaques, usually legs and ankles. Clinical diagnosis. Consider skin biopsy.

► Pathology
Granulomatous reaction and necrobiosis of collagen and loss and fragmentation of elastic fibers.

► Treatment Steps
1. Topical and intralesional corticosteroids.
2. Aspirin.
3. Dipyridamole.
4. Clofazimine.

K. Porphyria Cutanea Tarda (PCT)

► Description
Heme pathway defect disorder. Deficiency of urogen decarboxylase. Autosomal dominant.

► Symptoms
Vesicles on the back of hands, fragile skin.

► Diagnosis
Urine will fluoresce orange/red under Wood's light; hyperpigmentation. Blood/urine/stool studies for porphyrins, biopsy.

► Pathology
May be induced by chemicals, drugs, alcohol, ethyl alcohol, estrogen hormones, hexachlorobenzene, iron, polychlorinated biphenyls. **Also seen with hepatitis C.**

► Treatment Steps
1. Stop alcohol use, chloroquine.
2. **Phlebotomy.**

L. Acanthosis Nigricans

► Description
Gray-brown thickening of the skin, often on back of neck or axilla.

► Symptoms/Diagnosis
Asymptomatic black, velvetlike axillary/neck patch. Clinical diagnosis.

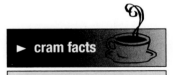

► **cram facts**

PCT is most common porphyria; association with heavy drinking, diabetes. No abdominal crises in PCT. Abdominal/neurologic symptoms are found in variegate porphyria, acute intermittent and hereditary coproporphyria.

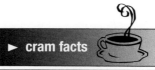

1. Polycystic ovaries, hirsutism, and acanthosis nigricans are a triad associated with hyperinsulinemia.
2. Malignant acanthosis nigricans is usually of sudden onset; rapidly progressive and usually secondary to an intra-abdominal adeno-carcinoma.

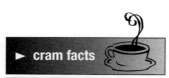

SIGNS OF TTP

The classic pentad is described, but very rare for all five to be present:

- Fever
- Thrombocytopenia
- Microangiopathic hemolytic anemia
- Renal dysfuncion and/or hematuria
- Neurologic dysfunction

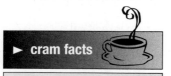

CAUSES OF DIC

There are many, but commonly cited causes include:

- Trauma/crush injury
- Sepsis/septic shock
- Malignancy
- Abruptio placenta
- Eclampsia
- Retained products of conception
- Hyperthermia

► **Pathology**

May associate with malignancy, endocrine disease, obesity, or be familial.

► **Treatment Steps**

Rule out coexisting pathology.

M. Peutz–Jeghers Syndrome

► **Description**

Autosomal dominant familial polyposis markedly increases a patient's risk of cancer, primarily of gastrointestinal (GI) tract, pancreas, lung, and reproductive system.

► **Symptoms**

Pigmented macules on **lips** and **oral mucosa. Lentigines, pigmentation. GI polyps, GI bleeding, melena.**

► **Diagnosis**

History, physical exam; biopsy.

► **Treatment Steps**

1. Monitor for malignancy.
2. Surgery (GI tract lesions).

N. Thrombotic Thrombocytopenic Purpura (TTP)

► **Description**

TTP is a thrombotic microangiopathy and is likely closely related to hemolytic–uremic syndrome (HUS).

► **Symptoms**

Sudden onset of **petechiae** and **ecchymosis.** Legs and mucous membranes typically.

► **Diagnosis**

TTP is a clinical diagnosis with no pathognomonic laboratory test findings. Common lab findings include: thrombocytopenia, anemia, and schistocytes; elevated lactic dehydrogenase (LDH); elevated indirect bilirubin; and normal fibrinogen, D-dimer, prothrombin time (PT), and partial thromboplastin time (PTT). Urinalysis: Proteinuria and microscopic hematuria.

► **Treatment Steps**

Standard of care is plasmapheresis. Prior to instituting plasmapheresis, steroids (prednisone) and fresh frozen plasma can be given.

O. Disseminated Intravascular Coagulation (DIC)

► **Description**

Bleeding disorder with many possible etiologies.

► **Symptoms**

Cutaneous hemorrhage and ecchymosis.

► **Diagnosis**

Low plasma fibrinogen and **elevated fibrin split products.** Elevated PT, PTT. Skin biopsy.

► **Pathology**

Endothelial surface injury and tissue injury resulting in coagulation activation.

▶ Treatment Steps
1. Treat primary cause.
2. Heparin.
3. Control coagulation abnormality.

XVII. NAIL SIGNS AND DISEASE

A. Onycholysis
Nail lifting off nail bed, **hyperthyroidism, psoriasis, injury.**

B. Terry's Nails
Proximal two-thirds of nail is white, **congestive heart failure (CHF), low albumin, cirrhosis.**

C. Splinter Hemorrhages
Trauma, subacute bacterial endocarditis (SBE).

D. Beau's Lines
Horizontal nail depression, **nail growth cessation from stress.**

E. Clubbed Fingers
Cardiopulmonary disease, cancer, or abnormal trait.

F. Muehrcke's Nails
Two horizontal white stripes, **low albumin/nephrotic syndrome.**

G. Yellow Nails
Lung disease, cancer.

H. Half-and-Half Nails
Normal proximal half, distal brown, **chronic renal failure.**

XVIII. NEWBORN AND INHERITED DISORDERS

A. Erythema Toxicum Neonatorum
Newborn macule and pustule dermatitis; self-limited.

B. Port-Wine Stain
Termed *nevus flammeus;* often facial and **unilateral red lesion;** treatment is usually **inadequate,** and **the 585-nm flash lamp pulse dye laser is used.**

C. Café au Lait Spots
Pigmented macule; typical of neurofibromatosis.

D. Mongolian Spot
Blue discoloration near sacral area; no clinical significance or treatment.

E. Miliaria
Dermatitis secondary to sweat gland/duct blockage; avoid heat and ensure **cool room/patient to treat.**

F. Ataxia–Telangiectasia
Telangiectases and **ataxia, bronchiectasis;** autosomal recessive.

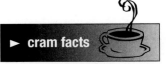

▶ **cram facts**

- General treatment tools include antihistamines for itch, moisturizers for itch and lubrication, corticosteroids, antibiotics, antifungals, and antivirals.
- If the lesion is wet, use soaks. If the lesion is dry, use an ointment. Anti-itch compounds include menthol and phenol, Aveeno baths.
- Wet dressing might use Burow's solution or boric acid solution.

BIBLIOGRAPHY

Freedberg I, et al. *Fitzpatrick's Dermatology in General Medicine,* 5th ed. Vols. 1 and 2. New York: McGraw-Hill, 1999.

Rassner G. *Atlas of Dermatology,* 3rd ed. Philadelphia: Lea & Febiger, 1994.

Sams WM Jr., Lynch P. *Principles and Practice of Dermatology,* 2nd ed. New York: Churchill Livingstone, 1996.

Thiers BH. *Yearbook of Dermatology and Dermatologic Surgery.* St. Louis: Mosby, 2005.

Endocrine and Metabolic Disorders | 3

I. HEALTH AND HEALTH MAINTENANCE

A. Hyperlipidemia

Impact includes an elevated **risk of atherosclerotic disease** and other disorders (**pancreatitis,** tendinous xanthoma). **Screening** should be performed on all adult patients, and in younger individuals where there is increased family risk. **Prevention** of morbidity and mortality includes adequate treatment and follow-up, along with education (including the benefits of diet and exercise).

B. Diabetes Mellitus

Impact includes U.S. incidence of about 5%, and resulting complications (**nephropathy, neuropathy, retinopathy,** cataracts, etc.). Incidence increases with age, African-American, Hispanic population. **Screening** is useful, especially in **high-risk** cases, by fasting blood glucose, or random glucose. Fasting glucose $\geq$ 126 ng/dL twice, random glucose > 200 ng/dL with symptoms of polyuria, polydipsia, polyphagia. **Prevention** of morbidity and mortality includes adequate education (value of diet and exercise), and treatment (prevent ketosis and abnormal blood glucose values/fluctuations). Early detection and treatment of complications may reduce potential severity (microvascular complications). In addition, comorbidities need to be addressed (hypertension, hyperlipidemia).

C. Addisonian Crisis

Prevention of **morbidity** and **mortality** includes **early recognition** and management of high-risk patients (Addison patients with stress: infection, surgery, trauma, glucocorticoids). Recognition includes both physician alertness and patient education. **Preventive therapy** includes additional glucocorticoid doses during patient stress and emergency bracelet use.

D. Neonatal Hypothyroidism

Prevention of **morbidity** and **mortality** secondary to neonatal hypothyroidism (**cretinism**) includes **screening** for **family history** (and medications ingested by the mother), and **routine newborn thyroxine (T_4), and thyroid-stimulating hormone (TSH) studies.**

II. MECHANISMS OF DISEASE AND DIAGNOSIS

A. Thyroid Disorders

1. Thyroid Tests

- *TSH*—ultrasensitive assay; most important test.
- *Free T_4*—(FT$_4$), active circulating T_4.
- *T_4RIA*—changes with thyroxine-binding disorders.
- *T_3RU*—excess thyroxine binding (estrogen use) results in T_3RU decrease, T_4 elevated. Reduced binding states (malnutrition) results in T_3RU increased, T_4 decreased.
- *FTI* equals $T_4 \times T_3$RU.
- Thyroid antibodies.

2. Thyroid Nodule

▶ Description
Solitary thyroid lesion.

► **differential diagnosis**

RISK FACTORS USEFUL IN DISTINGUISHING BENIGN FROM MALIGNANT THYROID LESIONS

	More Likely Benign	More Likely Malignant
History	Family history of benign goiter Residence in endemic goiter area	Family history of medullary cancer of thyroid Previous therapeutic irradiation of head or neck Recent growth of nodule Hoarseness, dysphagia, or obstruction
Physical characteristics	Older woman Soft nodule Multinodular goiter	Child, young adult, male Solitary, firm nodule clearly different from rest of gland ("dominant nodule") Adenopathy Vocal cord paralysis, firm lymph nodes, distant metastases
Serum factors	High titer of thyroid autoantibodies	Elevated serum calcitonin Elevated serum thyroglobulin (?)
Scanning techniques 123I	"Hot nodule"	"Cold nodule"
Ultrasound	Cyst (pure)	Solid or semicystic
Biopsy (needle)	Benign appearance on cytologic examination	Malignant or suggestion of malignancy
Levothyroxine therapy (0.2 md/day or more for 3 months or longer)	Regression	No regression

► Symptoms

May be asymptomatic, or exhibit thyroid dysfunction, known as a "hot" nodule.

► Diagnosis

History and physical exam, needle aspiration or thyroid scan (most malignant nodules are nonfunctioning, cold), ultrasound and surgical removal.

► Pathology

Most common benign lesion: follicular adenoma. Most common malignant nodule: papillary cancer. History of irradiation: very important to ask. Increased chance of malignancy if young. Poor outcome—male gender, over 40 years old, distant metastases, large primary tumor over 1.5 cm in diameter, extrathyroidal invasion.

► Treatment Steps

1. Cyst: aspirate/follow.
2. Carcinoma: surgical/radioiodine (^{131}I) (see Chapter 6).

3. Goiter

► Description/Symptoms

Enlarged thyroid gland. May be asymptomatic or cause compressive symptoms secondary to large gland size.

► Diagnosis

History and physical exam, T_4 normal, TSH may be normal or slightly elevated, ultrasound examination. No autoimmune antibodies present.

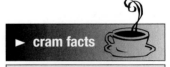

► **cram facts**

THYROID NODULE
AND MALIGNANCY

History of prior irradiation to the head and neck increases the risk of malignancy by 25%.

▶ Pathology
Inadequate iodine or excessive iodine. Lithium use, familial goiter, adolescent goiter.

▶ Treatment Steps
1. **Levothyroxine.**
2. If inadequate iodine in iodine deficiency countries, give iodine.
3. Surgery (rare).

4. Thyroiditis

▶ Description
Thyroid gland inflammation.

▶ Symptoms
- **Acute suppurative**—thyroid pain/erythema/dysphagia, and fever.
- **de Quervain's**—lethargy, migratory neck pain, fever, malaise, may be asymptomatic.
- **Hashimoto's**—goiter.
- **Riedel's**—tracheal compression/sclerosing fibrosis (rare).
- Painless thyroiditis (postpartum).
- May have type I diabetes.

▶ Diagnosis
History and physical exam, thyroid scan, lab (thyroid peroxidase autoantibodies-autoimmune), **elevated** T_4 and T_3RU, in de Quervain's. **de Quervain's: Elevated sed rate,** biopsy.

▶ Treatment Steps
Suppurative: antibiotics. de Quervain's: aspirin/NSAIDs, prednisone. Autoimmune: thyroxine. Riedel's: thyroxine.

5. Congenital Hypothyroidism (Cretinism)

▶ Symptoms
Dry skin, lethargy, umbilical hernia, slow teething/sexual development (see Fig. 3–1).

▶ Diagnosis
History and physical exam, **elevated TSH, low T_4, bone stippling,** and **delayed maturation.**

▶ Pathology
Thyroid absent, or ineffective hormone secreted due to enzyme deficiency (familial goiter).

▶ Treatment Steps
Levothyroxine (synthetic L-thyroxine).

6. Adult Hypothyroidism

▶ Description
Failure of the thyroid gland. Usually idiopathic (see Fig. 3–2). Two to three percent of general population. Subclinical hypothyroidism can occur.

▶ Symptoms
Fatigue, myxedema of tissue, cold intolerance, dry skin, lateral **eyebrow thinning,** constipation, lethargy, bradycardia, carpal tunnel syndrome, depression, menorrhagia.

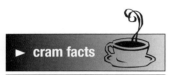

▶ **cram facts**

HASHIMOTO'S THYROIDITIS

- Most common type of thyroiditis.
- Autoimmune etiology.
- Serum antithyroid antibodies may be present.
- Although can cause transient hyperthyroidism, more often causes hypothyroidism requiring treatment with thyroxine.

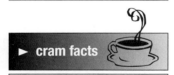

▶ **cram facts**

Myxedema may result in an enlarged heart/heart failure, ascites.

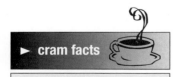

▶ **cram facts**

Pendred syndrome: congenital goiter and deafness.

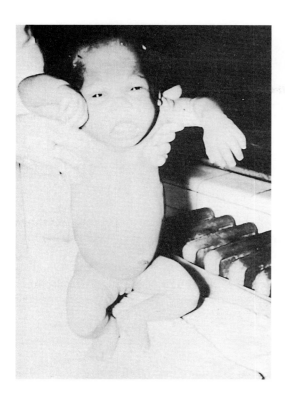

Figure 3–1. A 9-month-old infant with hypothyroidism (cretinism). Note the puffy face, protuberant abdomen, umbilical hernia, and muscle weakness (infant cannot sit up unassisted).

▶ Diagnosis

Elevated TSH, low T_4, low free T_4.

▶ Pathology

The two most common causes are autoimmune thyroid disease (Hashimoto's thyroiditis) and prior treatment of hyperthyroidism (including thyroidectomy and prior radioactive iodine for Graves' disease). Other less common causes include postpartum necrosis of the pituitary gland (Sheehan's syndrome), use of antithyroid medications (propothiouracil and methimazole), iodine deficiency or excess, and other medications (amiodarone, lithium).

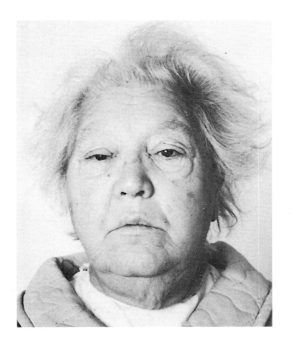

Figure 3–2. Hypothyroidism in adult (myxedema). Note puffy face, puffy eyes, frowsy hair, and dull and apathetic appearance.

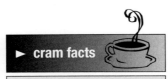

► **cram facts**

HYPO- VERSUS HYPER-THYROIDISM

- One major difference between the two conditions is that in hypothyroidism, treatment should be started immediately, but in hyperthyroidism, the etiology of the hyperthyroidism needs to be established to determine the course of treatment.
- For example, in Graves' disease, radioactive iodine (RAI) may be needed. However, if a patient had surreptitious ingestion of thyroxine, RAI would not be curative (but stopping ingestion of the hormone would!).

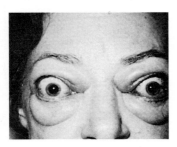

Figure 3–3. Severe ophthalmopathy of Graves' disease. Note marked periorbital edema, injection of corneal blood vessels, and proptosis. There was also striking limitation of upward and lateral eye movements and reduced visual acuity.

► **Treatment Steps**
Levothyroxine. Low dose if history of heart disease. Follow TSH levels approximately every 6–8 weeks and adjust dose of levothyroxine accordingly.

7. Hyperthyroidism/Thyrotoxicosis/Graves' Disease

► **Symptoms**
Anxiety, tremors, diarrhea, weight loss, heat intolerance, diaphoresis, palpitations, insomnia, menstrual irregularities.

► **Diagnosis**
Physical findings may include tremor, tachycardia, goiter, onycholysis. Thinning of hair may occur. High-output congestive heart failure (CHF) is rare but can occur.

Labs show a depressed TSH (classically "undetectable," which is < 0.01) and an elevated free T_4. (Although classically thyroid panels will include testing for total thyroxine, T_3 and T_3 resin uptake (T_3RU), the findings of an elevated free T_4 with low TSH are diagnostic.)

► **Pathology**
Causes of an overactive thyroid gland are many, but most people think first of Graves' disease (see below). Other causes: See Table 3–1.

Graves' Disease—Graves' disease is a type of autoimmune hyperthyroidism caused by circulating antibodies, known as thyroid-stimulating immunoglobulins (TSIs). The TSIs bind to the TSH receptor, causing excess production of thyroxine and growth of the thyroid gland. This causes symptoms of hyperthyroidism as well as goiter. Goiter is present in virtually all patients with Graves'.

One classic finding of Graves' disease is ophthalmopathy, which can manifest as eye changes ranging from proptosis and lid retraction to diplopia and, rarely, visual loss (see Figs. 3–3 and 3–4).

► **Treatment of Hyperthyroidism**
Treatment varies with etiology; can include:
- β-Blockers may be used to help with symptoms (tremor, tachycardia).
- Antithyroid medications used in certain cases (propylthiouracil, methimazole).
- Radioactive iodine or subtotal thyroidectomy.

8. Thyroid Storm

► **Description**
Severe thyrotoxicosis. Usually in individuals inadequately treated or new-onset hyperthyroidism. **This is a medical emergency.**

3-1

CAUSES OF HYPERTHYROIDISM

- Graves' disease
- Thyrotoxicosis factitia (surreptitious ingestion of thyroxine, commonly in persons attempting to lose weight). On boards, this is often a young woman, and is described as a nurse or a patient with a family member with hypothyroidism, which would mean she would have some access to thyroxine.
- Subacute thyroiditis (which is often self-limited)
- Hydatidiform mole
- Toxic multinodular goiter

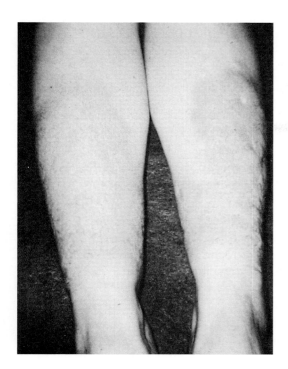

Figure 3–4. Dermopathy of Graves' disease.
Marked thickening of the skin is noted, usually over the pretibial area. Thickening will occasionally extend downward over the ankle and the dorsal aspect of the foot but almost never above the knee.

► **Symptoms**
Hyperthermia (very high fever), delirium, nausea, vomiting, abdominal pain.

► **Diagnosis**
Physical exam findings can include diaphoresis, tachycardia, hypertension in early stage, hypotension and shock in later stages, signs of high-output heart failure. Labs: Elevated T_4, elevated free T_4, and T_3-RIA. TSH suppressed.

► **Pathology**
Thyroid storm can be precipitated by multiple causes in individuals who already have hyperthyroidism, including infection/sepsis, trauma, surgery, radioactive iodine therapy, medications (pseudoephedrine, anticholinergics). Rarely, thyroid storm can be the presentation of a patient with new-onset hyperthyroidism.

► **Treatment Steps**
1. Supportive care (control of hyperthermia, arrhythmias, hyper- or hypotension).
2. β-Blockers will help minimize symptoms.
3. Glucocorticoids to minimize peripheral conversion of T_4 to T_3.

9. **Euthyroid Sick Syndrome**
This refers to abnormal finding on thyroid testing that occurs in the setting of a sick, usually hospitalized patient. The thyroid function abnormalities can vary, but the most common are low T_3 and elevated reverse T_3. These abnormalities should reverse as the patient improves.

10. **Thyroid Cancer**
See Chapter 6.

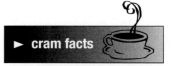

► **cram facts**

THYROTOXICOSIS

Other symptoms include onycholysis, bruit, high-output failure, thin hair, and confusion.

B. Diabetes Mellitus

1. Type 1

► **Description**
Absolute insulin deficiency, due to autoimmune islet cell antibodies.

► **Symptoms**
Polyuria, polyphagia, polydipsia, hyperglycemia, urine/blood ketones.

► **Diagnosis**
Two or more fasting plasma glucose levels over 126 mg/dL. May have **islet cell antibodies** and **human leukocyte antigen (HLA) present,** low C-peptide.

► **Pathology**
No insulin production by pancreatic β cells under stimuli. A result of **genetic predisposition to pancreatic immune and/or environmental injury.** Human leukocyte antigen markers common.

► **Treatment Steps**
1. Insulin (see Table 3–2).
2. Diet (monitor carbohydrates and be consistent with snacks/timing of meals), **exogenous insulin.**
3. Exercise—aerobic, approximately 30 minutes three times per week.

2. Type 2

► **Description**
Most commonly due to insulin resistance. Occasionally due to insulin secretory defect.

► **Symptoms**
Polyuria, polydipsia, blurred vision. **May be asymptomatic,** skin/vaginal infections noted.

► **Diagnosis**
Two or more **fasting plasma glucose levels over 126 mg/dL, or random glucose over 200 mg/dL** × 2 with polyuria, polydipsia, polyphagia. Finally, although not commonly performed, a level ≥ 200 mg/dL 2 hours after a 75-g glucose load is diagnostic of diabetes.

► **Pathology**
Increased hepatic glucose production, decreased peripheral glucose utilization. Insulin resistance.

3-2

TYPES OF INSULIN

Types of insulin will differ with respect to their time of onset, peak, and duration. Besides those listed below, others include lente, ultralente, and aspart. Also, mixtures of insulin exist, usually long-acting and short-acting insulin combination. (Example: 70/30 is 70% NPH and 30% regular.)

Of note: Insulin Glargine (Lantus) must never be mixed in the same syringe with other types of insulin.

- Insulin Glargine (Lantus) onset about 1 hour, no peak, and duration approximately 24 hours.
- NPH insulin onset 1–2 hours, peak 6–12 hours, duration 18–24 hours.
- Regular (R) insulin onset 30 minutes, peak 2–4 hours, duration 6–8 hours.
- Insulin Lispro (Humalog) onset 5–15 minutes, peak 1 hour, duration 3–4 hours. Given about 5 minutes before a meal.

► Treatment Steps
1. Diet (restrict calories and carbohydrates to reach ideal body weight) and patient education.
2. **Oral agents** (secretagogue, biguanides, α-glucosidase inhibitors, glitazone) (see Table 3–3).
3. Exercise.
4. Insulin alone or in combination with oral agents.

3. Diabetic Ketoacidosis

► Symptoms
Lethargy, nausea/vomiting, polyuria, abdominal pain, confusion, **Kussmaul's** respiration, dehydration, fruity breath.

► Diagnosis
History and physical exam, **elevated glucose** (400–600 mg/dL), ketonuria/ketonemia, low pH on arterial blood gas (ABG), **metabolic acidosis** with **increased anion gap.**

► Pathology
May be the presentation of a new-onset diabetic. May result from infection/illness/not taking insulin, stress, hyperthyroidism; is associated with lack of insulin.

► Treatment Steps
1. **Insulin** (continuous infusion 5–10 U/hr or 0.1 U/kg/hr).
2. **Correction of fluid/electrolyte abnormality. Use isotonic saline to start;** check glucose, electrolytes frequently.
3. **Replace potassium as necessary** and monitor blood pressure (BP), electrocardiogram (ECG), and electrolytes.

4. Hyperosmolar Coma

► Description
Extracellular hyperosmolality associated with hyperglycemia.

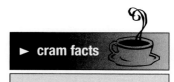

cram facts

Glycosylated hemoglobin (HbA$_{1C}$) elevation indicates **hyperglycemia over prior 2 to 3 months.** Recommend every 3 months.

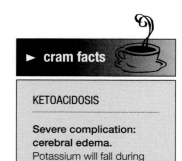

cram facts

KETOACIDOSIS

Severe complication: cerebral edema. Potassium will fall during treatment if not replaced.

3-3

COMMONLY USED ORAL MEDICATIONS FOR DIABETES

Glipizide (Glucotrol), Glyburide (Micronase)
- Sulfonylurea class of medications.
- Stimulates insulin secretion from β cells of the pancreas.
- Can cause hypoglycemia.

Metformin (Glucophage)
- Biguanide class of medications.
- Decreases gluconeogenesis in the liver and decreases insulin resistance in hepatic and peripheral tissues.
- Does not cause hypoglycemia.
- Excellent to use in overweight/obese patients as metformin can cause weight loss.
- Contraindicated in patients with prior congestive heart failure or renal insufficiency, as these conditions can increase the risk of lactic acidosis, a rare but potentially fatal side effect.
- Stop medication prior to and for at least 48 hours after surgery and intravenous dye.
- Despite side effects, very commonly used medication.

Acarbose (Precose)
- α-Glucosidase inhibitor, delays digestion of complex carbohydrates.
- May cause flatulence, diarrhea.
- Must take with first bite of each meal.

Pioglitazone (Actos), Rosiglitazone (Avandia)
- Thiazolidinedione class of medications.
- Act by enhancing insulin sensitivity in muscle and adipose tissue and, to a lesser extent, inhibiting gluconeogenesis in the liver.
- Use with caution in patients with congestive heart failure as the drugs can increase plasma volume.
- Follow serial liver function tests.

► Symptoms
Severe dehydration, lethargy, confusion, coma.

► Pathology
Elevated glucose without ketosis resulting in cellular fluid loss.

► Treatment Steps
1. **Fluids—water** (hypotonic saline).
2. **Insulin** (lower doses required than in ketoacidosis).
3. Treat infection, malignancy, and other underlying illness.

5. Lactic Acidosis

► Description
Excess lactic acid in the blood, may be combined with diabetic ketoacidosis.

► Symptoms
Coma, confusion, hyperventilation.

► Diagnosis
History and physical exam [critically ill diabetic with complication(s)], **elevated plasma lactate, negative ketonuria, positive anion gap.**

► Pathology
Overproduction or inadequate removal of lactic acid, noted rarely with biguanides.

► Treatment Steps
1. **Treat etiology.**
2. Sodium bicarbonate.
3. Supportive.

6. Chronic Complications

► Description

Renal—Nephropathy (see Chapter 17).

Neurologic—Neuropathy (sensory: Charcot joint, motor-nerve palsy).

Ophthalmic—Retinopathy (nonproliferative, proliferative), cataracts (subcapsular, **senile most common**).

Other—Peripheral vascular disease, dermopathy, infection, cardiovascular.

C. Hypoglycemia, Pancreatic β-cell Tumors

► Description
Fasting hypoglycemia; **insulinoma,** Addison's disease, hypopituitarism. Reactive hypoglycemia (postprandial): treat with frequent meals, reduced simple carbohydrates.

► Symptoms
Lethargy, diplopia, headache, in A.M. or when fasting.

► Diagnosis
History and physical exam, **typical** hypoglycemic **symptoms, blood glucose under** 40 mg/dL, **response to glucose.** Elevated serum insulin level during hypoglycemic episode. **Elevated proinsulin level,** and **lack of C-peptide suppression.**

► Pathology

Islets of Langerhans adenoma most often; usually benign.

► Treatment Steps
1. **Surgical excision of insulinoma;** preop give diazoxide (Proglycem).
2. **Emergency therapy: give 50 mL 50% dextrose IV.**

D. Parathyroid Disorders

1. Primary Hyperparathyroidism

► Symptoms

Often asymptomatic and found on routine blood work (elevated calcium). Occasionally **kidney stones,** bone pain/lesions **(osteitis fibrosa cystica).** Symptoms of elevated calcium (memory loss, depression, **proximal muscle weakness,** nausea, weight loss, polyuria).

► Diagnosis

Elevated serum calcium, and **elevated intact parathyroid hormome (iPTH).** May see **subperiosteal bone resorption on x-ray.** Parathyroid scan may localize an adenoma.

► Pathology

Etiology unknown; **single chief cell adenoma most common. Hyperplasia in multiple endocrine neoplasia (MEN) syndromes.**

► Treatment Steps
1. **Surgical resection;** for parathyroid adenoma: parathyroid neck exploration.
2. If severe hypercalcemia is present, medical therapy—saline, furosemide, calcitonin, pamidronate.

2. Hypoparathyroidism

► Description

Decreased parathyroid hormone amount or effect. Can include thyroid surgery or genetic.

► Symptoms

Symptoms of **hypocalcemia (positive Chvostek's** and **Trousseau's** signs), **circumoral paresthesia, tetany,** cataracts, intracranial calcifications, laryngeal stridor, seizures.

► Diagnosis

History and physical exam, **hyperphosphatemia, hypocalcemia, normal renal function,** parathyroid hormone (PTH), and urinary cyclic adenosine monophosphate (cAMP) level.

► Treatment Steps

Vitamin D and **calcium.**

E. Pituitary and Hypothalamic Disorders

1. Diabetes Insipidus

► Description

Water-loss syndrome. Nephrogenic vasopressin resistant: kidney does not respond to vasopressin. Neurogenic vasopressin responsive/central: inadequate vasopressin.

► Symptoms

Polyuria, nocturia, thirst. May crave ice.

► Diagnosis

History and physical exam, routine urinalysis and labs, **urine specific gravity under 1.005, urine osmolality under 250, water loss more than 3 L/day.**

Water-Deprivation Test—Vasopressin injection followed by plasma/urine osmolality studies.

Nephrogenic Diabetes Insipidus—Cannot concentrate urine (not responsive to vasopressin).

Primary Polydipsia—No urine osmolality change (or minimum increase) after injection.

Central Diabetes Insipidus—Urine osmolality greater than plasma osmolality (responsive to vasopressin).

► Pathology

Insufficient antidiuretic hormone (ADH), or lack of response to ADH, resulting from pituitary injury, tumor, or other disorder (tuberculosis, sarcoid, etc.). Drugs—demeclocycline, lithium (nephrogenic).

► Treatment Steps

Antidiuretic hormone replacement (pitressin tannate, 1-deamino-8-D-arginine vasopressin [DDAVP]), subcutaneous or oral.

2. Syndrome of Inappropriate Secretion of Antidiuretic Hormone (SIADH)

► Symptoms

Confusion, lethargy, seizures, coma.

► Diagnosis

Hyponatremia, serum hypo-osmolality, urine hyperosmolarity.

► Pathology

Associated with **malignant/nonmalignant lung disease, other tumors, endocrinopathy, central nervous system (CNS) disease, drugs.**

► Treatment Steps

1. **Fluid restriction.**
2. Demeclocycline and/or hypertonic saline in certain cases.

3. Panhypopituitarism

► Description

Reduced or lacking pituitary hormone secretion. Affecting single or several hormones.

► Symptoms

Lack of TSH: hypothyroid symptoms. Lack of adrenocorticotropic hormone (ACTH): adrenocortical insufficiency symptoms (hypotension, nausea/vomiting, confusion). Lack of **gonadotropins:** impotence/amenorrhea. Evidence of lack of **prolactin and/or growth hormone.**

► Diagnosis

History and physical exam, thyroid functions, serum testosterone, growth hormone, insulin-like growth factor (IGF)-1, endocrine stimulation testing.

► Pathology

Infarction (Sheehan's syndrome), tumor, infection, trauma, and other causes; use of clofibrate, vincristine, vinblastine, chlorpropamide.

► Treatment Steps

Replacement of appropriate hormone deficiency (glucocorticoids, thyroxine, estrogen, testosterone, growth hormone).

4. Acromegaly

► Description

Excessive **growth hormone** secretion postpuberty, from a pituitary adenoma.

► Symptoms

As Adult—Enlarging hands/feet, coarse features, deep voice, wide teeth, large tongue, joint pain, hypertension, headache, hyperhydrosis (see Fig. 3–5).

► Diagnosis

Clinical features, labs, and magnetic resonance imaging (MRI) of the brain.

- IGF-1 levels are elevated in acromegaly and it is a sensitive screening test for acromegaly
- Glucose suppression test: An oral glucose load is given (1.75G/kg, maximum dose 75G). Failure to suppress serum growth hormone (GH) levels to < 5 ng/dL is diagnostic of acromegaly.
- Random measurements of GH are **not** useful because GH is secreted in a pulsatile fashion.
- MRI can confirm the presence of a pituitary adenoma.

► Treatment Steps

1. Surgical (transsphenoidal) to resect a pituitary adenoma. May be curative.
2. Radiation and medications are used if surgery not curative.

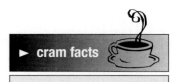

► cram facts

Sheehan's syndrome: postpartum pituitary necrosis.

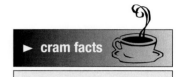

► cram facts

GIGANTISM

- Gigantism is caused by excess growth hormone in childhood
- Features include excessively tall stature (7–8 feet tall)
- Extremely rare, with about 100 reported cases to date

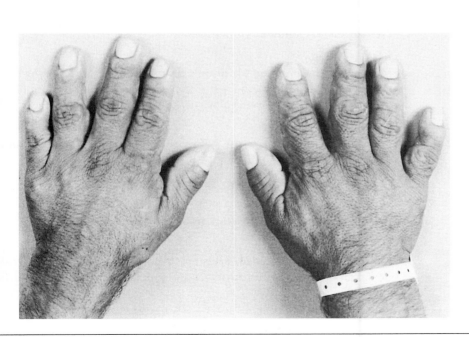

Figure 3–5. Markedly increased soft tissue bulk and blunt fingers in a middle-aged man with acromegaly.

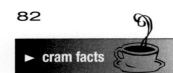

► **cram facts**

COSYNTROPIN STIMULATION TEST

- Can be done at any time of day.
- First, check baseline plasma cortisol level.
- Inject (IV or IM) 250 mg of cosyntropin (synthetic ACTH).
- Check repeat plasma cortisol level 30 minutes later.
- Normal response is a plasma cortisol level > 20 μg/dL.
- Note: There is also a low-dose cosyntropin (1 μg) test that can be used, but the traditional test utilizes 250 μg.

► **cram facts**

Corticosteroid use complications: hypokalemia, peptic ulcer, hyperglycemia, hypertension (sodium retention), psychosis, infection. Give potassium as necessary. **Sudden discontinuance of corticosteroids may result in adrenal insufficiency,** as noted previously.

► **cram facts**

Primary adrenocortical insufficiency: elevated plasma ACTH. Secondary adrenocortical insufficiency: plasma ACTH normal or low.

Increase hydrocortisone during periods of stress/illness.

---

3. Medications (bromocriptine, octreotide, cabergoline). Goal is normalization of GH.

F. Adrenal Disorders

1. Adrenocortical Insufficiency—Acute

► **Description**
Abrupt lack of adrenocortical hormones.

► **Symptoms**
Patients can present with severe hypotension (shock), which can be mistaken for septic shock. Other symptoms include fever, nausea, vomiting, abdominal pain, fatigue, weakness, and hypoglycemia.

► **Diagnosis**
One needs to have a high clinical suspicion as it is often mistaken for other illnesses. **Cosyntropin testing** (see Cram Facts). Often, steroids are given empirically (particularly if patient is not responding to other treatments) and clinical response to steroids is virtually diagnostic.

► **Pathology**
Trauma, infection, gland necrosis, glucocorticoid withdrawal (in steroid-dependent patient).

► **Treatment Steps**
1. **Hydrocortisone sodium succinate** 100 mg IV, infusion, then taper.
2. Fludrocortisone as mineralocorticoid supplement may be indicated.

2. Adrenocortical Insufficiency—Chronic

► **Symptoms**
Lethargy, skin pigmentation, hypotension, nausea/vomiting, dehydration, salt craving.

► **Diagnosis**
History and physical exam, **hyponatremia, hyperkalemia,** low plasma cortisol, ACTH stimulation test.

► **Pathology**
Most often autoimmune (Addison's disease) and history of long-term glucocorticoid use as etiology. Other causes: human immunodeficiency virus (HIV), cytomegalovirus, hemorrhage, tuberculosis (TB).

► **Treatment Steps**
Usually both hydrocortisone (glucocorticoid), and **fludrocortisone** (mineralocorticoid) needed.

3. Cushing's Syndrome

► **Description**
Clinical state caused by glucocorticoid overabundance.

► **Symptoms**
Centripetal **obesity, striae/bruising, hypertension, hirsutism,** weakness, osteoporosis, supraclavicular fat pad, buffalo hump, moon facies, facial plethora.

► **Diagnosis**
Clinical, **overnight dexamethasone suppression test, 24-hour urine for free cortisol,** elevated urine 17-hydroxysteroids.

► Pathology

Most commonly iatrogenic. Other causes: **Cushing's disease most common** (pituitary adenoma), also adrenal tumor, or ectopic ACTH hypersecretion.

► Treatment Steps
1. Iatrogenic—use smallest effective steroid dose possible.
2. Cushing's disease—surgery/radiation.
3. Medications include ketoconazole, metyrapone, mitotane.

4. **Adrenogenital Syndrome**

► Description
Virilizing female disorder.

► Symptoms
Hirsutism, amenorrhea, deep voice, acne, enlarged clitoris (ambiguous genitalia as newborn).

► Diagnosis
History and physical exam, **high urinary 17-ketosteroids,** ultrasound, laparoscopy, high 17-hydroxyprogesterone.

► Pathology
In child: usually due to congenital adrenal hyperplasia (21-hydroxylase deficiency) (see Cram Facts).
In adult: ovarian disease (polycystic ovary), or adrenal disease (attenuated forms).

► Treatment Steps
1. Surgical excision (if tumor).
2. Estrogen spironolactone, metformin (for polycystic ovary syndrome).
3. For congenital adrenal hyperplasia, give glucocorticoid replacement/possible mineralocorticoid replacements.

5. **Hyperaldosteronism**

► Symptoms
May be **asymptomatic** or show evidence of **hypokalemic symptoms,** weakness, hypertension.

► Diagnosis
History and physical exam, **sodium retention, hypokalemia, hypertension, low plasma renin, elevated plasma/urine aldosterone.**

► Pathology
Aldosterone overproduction by zona glomerulosa, from **adenoma (Conn's syndrome),** or **hyperplasia.**

► Treatment Steps
Adrenalectomy, give spironolactone preop.

6. **Pheochromocytoma**

► Description
Catecholamine-producing chromaffin cell tumor.

► Symptoms
Episodes of headache, flushing, diaphoresis, diplopia, weight loss, paroxysmal hypertension.

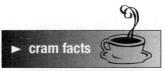

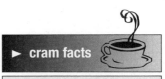

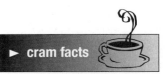

► cram facts

Cushing's syndrome refers to all conditions that caue excess glucocorticoid. *Cushing's disease* refers to glucocorticoid excess due to a pituitary adenoma.

► cram facts

Congenital adrenal hyperplasia: due to 11- or 21-β-hydroxylase deficiency (most common). Diagnosis by high levels of 11-deoxycortisol or 17-hydroxyprogesterone.

► cram facts

Differential diagnosis between adenoma and hyperplasia: after salty diet, A.M. plasma aldosterone over 20 ng/dL in adenoma; under 20 ng/dL in hyperplasia.

Pseudohyperaldosteronism: Liddle syndrome, (?)renal tubule defect results in hyperaldosteronism symptoms without excess aldosterone production.

Overindulgence in licorice may cause hyperaldosteronism-like picture, but aldosterone excess is absent. Treatment: switch to another junk food!

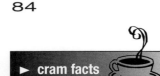

COMMON SYMPTOMS IN PATIENTS WITH HYPERTENSION DUE TO PHEOCHROMOCYTOMA

Symptoms during or following paroxysms
- Headache
- Sweating
- Forceful heartbeat with or without tachycardia
- Anxiety or fear of impending death
- Tremor
- Fatigue or exhaustion
- Nausea and vomiting
- Abdominal or chest pain
- Visual disturbances

Symptoms between paroxysms
- Increased sweating
- Cold hands and feet
- Weight loss
- Constipation

Things to remember:
- The hypertension can be lethal.
- The tumor can be a carcinoma.
- It may be a part of MEN-1 or -2.

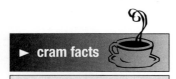

► cram facts

Pituitary dwarf has low FSH.

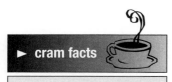

► cram facts

The first test that should be done in a woman with amenorrhea is a pregnancy test.

► Diagnosis

History and physical exam, tachycardia, **24-hour urinary vanillylmandelic acid (VMA), or metanephrines,** serum catecholamines. **Urinary catecholamines may be elevated by Aldomet and other meds.** MRI.

► Pathology

Tumor, may be intra-adrenal or extra-adrenal. May be familial or sporadic.

► Treatment Steps
1. **Surgical excision** (difficult procedure).
2. **Give phenoxybenzamine preop,** hydration.

G. Ovarian Disorders

1. Turner's Syndrome
See Chapter 14.

2. True Hermaphroditism

► Symptoms
Ambiguous genitalia.

► Diagnosis
History and physical exam, chromosome studies, histologic evaluation of ovatestes tissue.

► Pathology
Ovarian and testicular tissue present (ovatestes).

► Treatment Steps
Varies with age and genitalia development.

3. Polycystic Ovarian Syndrome (PCOS)
See Chapter 13, section II.G.2.

4. Premature Ovarian Failure

► Description
Cessation of menses in a woman younger than age 35.

► Diagnosis
Amenorrhea, negative pregnancy test, elevated follicle-stimulating hormone (FSH) and leutinizing hormone (LH).

► Pathology
Autoimmune (antiovarian antibodies).

► Treatment Steps
Supportive treatment. Hormone therapy controversial.

5. Amenorrhea/Galactorrhea
See also Chapter 13 for amenorrhea.

► Symptoms
No menses, abnormal flow of milk from breasts. If pituitary tumor present, may have visual field cut or headache.

► Diagnosis
Clinical, **elevated prolactin level, MRI of head** with gadolinium (reveals pituitary adenoma).

► Pathology
Most common cause is a pituitary adenoma that produces excess prolactin. Galactorrhea can be an uncommon side effect of some medications (haloperidol, thorazine).

► differential diagnosis

DIFFERENTIAL DIAGNOSIS OF DELAYED PUBERTY

	Serum Gonadotropins	Serum Gonadal Steroids	Miscellaneous
Constitutional delay in growth and adolescence	Prepubertal (low)	Low	Patient usually has short stature for chronologic age but appropriate height and growth rate for bone age. Adrenarche and gonadarche are delayed.
Hypogonadotropic hypogonadism	Prepubertal (low)	Low	Patient may have anosmia (Kallmann syndrome) or other associated pituitary hormone deficiencies. If gonodotropin deficiency is isolated, patient usually has normal height and growth rate. Adrenarche may be normal in spite of absent gonadarche (serum dehydroepiandrosterone [DHEA] sulfate may be pubertal).
Hypergonadotropic hypogonadism	Elevated	Low	Patient may have abnormal karyotype and stigmas of Turner's or Klinefelter's syndrome.

► Treatment Steps

1. Surgery/radiation to resect adenoma.
2. Medications include bromocriptine, cabergoline.

H. Lipid Metabolism Disorders

See Chapter 1, section X.

I. Mineral Metabolism Disorders

1. Hereditary Hemochromatosis

► Description

Hereditary disorder of iron excess. Autosomal recessive inheritance. Also known as bronze diabetes. (See also Chapter 5.)

► Symptoms

Hepatomegaly, skin pigmentation, cardiomegaly, pancreatic disease (diabetes mellitus).

► Diagnosis

May be diagnosed due to screening of family members with the disease. Genetic testing is available. Labs include abnormal aspartate transaminase (AST) and alanine transaminase (ALT), elevated iron, ferritin, and percentage of saturation. Liver biopsy may be indicated.

► Treatment Steps

1. Phlebotomy.
2. Deferoxamine.

2. Wilson's Disease

See Chapter 11.

▶ **cram facts**

EXAMPLES OF MANIFESTATIONS OF ENDOCRINE DISEASE
(THE MANIFESTATIONS DO NOT OCCUR IN ALL CASES, AND THE SEVERITY CAN VARY MARKEDLY)

Abdominal pain	Addisonian crisis; diabetic ketoacidosis; hyperparathyroidism
Amenorrhea or oligomenorrhea	Adrenal insufficiency, adrenogenital syndrome, anorexia nervosa, Cushing's syndrome, hyperprolactinemic states, hypopituitarism, hypothyroidism, menopause, ovarian failure, polycystic ovaries, pseudohermaphroditic syndromes
Anemia	Adrenal insufficiency, gonadal insufficiency, hypothyroidism, hyperparathyroidism, panhypopituitarism
Anorexia	Addison's disease, diabetic ketoacidosis, hypercalcemia (e.g., hyperparathyroidism), hypothyroidism, anorexia nervosa
Constipation	Diabetic neuropathy, hypercalcemia, hypothyroidism, pheochromocytoma
Depression	Adrenal insufficiency, Cushing's syndrome, hypercalcemic states, hypoglycemia, hypothyroidism
Diarrhea	Hyperthyroidism, metastatic carcinoid tumors, metastatic medullary thyroid carcinoma
Fever	Adrenal insufficiency, hyperthyroidism (severe thyroid storm), hypothalamic disease
Hair changes	Decreased body hair (hypothyroidism, hypopituitarism, Cushing's syndrome, thyrotoxicosis); hirsutism (androgen excess states, Cushing's syndrome, acromegaly)
Headache	Hypertensive episodes with pheochromocytoma, hypoglycemia, pituitary tumors
Hypothermia	Hypoglycemia, hypothyroidism
Libido changes	Adrenal insufficiency, Cushing's syndrome, hypercalcemia, hyperprolactinemia, hyperthyroidism, hypokalemia, hypopituitarism, hypothyroidism, poorly controlled diabetes mellitus
Nervousness	Cushing's syndrome, hyperthyroidism
Polyuria	Diabetes insipidus, diabetes mellitus, hypercalcemia, hypokalemia
Skin changes	Acanthosis nigricans (obesity, polycystic ovaries, severe insulin resistance, Cushing's syndrome, acromegaly); acne (androgen excess); hyperpigmentation (adrenal insufficiency, Nelson's syndrome); dry (hypothyroidism); hypopigmentation (panhypopituitarism); striae, plethora, brusing, ecchymoses (Cushing's syndrome); vitiligo (autoimmune thyroid disease, Addison's disease)
Weakness and fatigue	Addison's disease, Cushing's syndrome, diabetes mellitus, hypokalemia (e.g., primary aldosteronism, Bartter's syndrome), hypothyroidism, hypercalcemia (e.g., hyperparathyroidism, panhypopituitarism, pheochromocytoma)
Weight gain	Central nervous system disease, Cushing's syndrome, hypothyroidism, insulinoma, pituitary tumors
Weight loss	Adrenal insufficiency, anorexia nervosa, endocrine cancer, hyperthyroidism, insulin-dependent diabetes mellitus, panhypopituitarism, pheochromocytoma

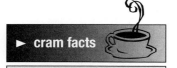

▶ **cram facts**

No true endocrine etiology for obesity. Syndromes including obesity include **Prader–Willi** (mental retardation, hypogonadism), hypotonia and Laurence–Moon–Biedl (nerve deafness, retinal pathology).

J. Other Disorders

1. **Klinefelter's Syndrome**
   See Chapter 14.

2. **Fabry's Disease**
   See Chapter 11.

3. **Gaucher's Disease**
   See Chapter 11.

4. **Obesity**

   ▶ **Description**
   Excess adipose tissue storage of triglyceride. (See Clinical Pearls.)

   ▶ **Treatment Steps**
   1. Reduce calories/nutrition consultant/weight loss programs..
   2. Exercise.
   3. Drugs include sibutramine (Meridia) and orlistat (Xenical).

4. Gastric bypass increasing in popularity, but significant mortality associated with the procedure.

5. Gestational Diabetes

▶ Description
Gestational diabetes mellitus (GDM) refers to abnormal levels of hyperglycemia occurring in pregnant women. (It does not address pregnant women who have preexisting diagnoses of type I or type II diabetes mellitus.) Women are often asymptomatic and diagnosis is made during prenatal screening.

▶ Diagnosis
Screening test: In pregnant women who are not high risk for GDM, a glucose tolerance test is given at 26–28 weeks. Serum glucose is checked after a 50-g glucose load. If this initial screening test is abnormal, a 3-hour (100-g) glucose tolerance test is given. (Fasting glucose should be < 95, 1 hour < 180 mg/dL, 2 hours < 155 mg/dL, 3 hours < 140 mg/dL.)

In women who are at higher risk for GDM, screening should be done in the first trimester. This includes women with GDM in a prior pregnancy, maternal age > 35 years, prior unexplained fetal demise, prior infant weighing less than 4,000 g, obesity, or strong family history of type 2 diabetes.

▶ Treatment Steps
1. Diabetic diet, counseling with a nutritionist.
2. Insulin in certain cases.

6. Carcinoid Syndrome

▶ Description
Serotonin-secreting, argentaffin cell tumor.

▶ Symptoms
Diarrhea, flushing, bronchospasm, and heart valve lesions.

▶ Diagnosis
History and physical exam, **urinary 5-hydroxyindoleacetic acid (5-HIAA).**

▶ Pathology
Tumors from enterochromaffin cells. Pulmonary and gastrointestinal (GI) tract sites common.

▶ Treatment Steps
1. Surgery.
2. Cyproheptadine.

7. Mastocytosis

▶ Description/Symptoms
Mast cell disorder causing **flushing,** vomiting, diarrhea, tachycardia, hypotension, syncope, in episodic attacks.

▶ Diagnosis
History and physical exam, may have **urticaria pigmentosa,** histamine and histamine metabolite studies, skin/bone marrow biopsy. May show **Darier's sign** (stroking skin lesion results in elevated/erythematous reaction: dermographism).

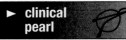

▶ clinical pearl

OBESITY

- Currently a serious public health concern.
- World Health Organization definitions:
  - Overweight: Body mass index (BMI) 25–29.0 kg/m^2
  - Obese: BMI 30–39.9 kg/m^2
  - Morbidly obese: BMI ≥ 40 kg/m^2
- Multiple comorbidities including diabetes, hypertension, hyperlipidemia, depression, obstuctive sleep apnea, osteoarthritis with joint replacement.

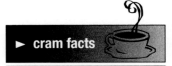

▶ cram facts

COMPLICATIONS OF GDM

- Fetal macrosomia
- Shoulder dystocia
- Miscarriage/stillbirth
- Birth defects
- Neonatal polycythemia
- Neonatal hypoglycemia

► Pathology

Release of mast cell mediators (heparin, histamine, enzymes). Cutaneous and systemic types.

► Treatment Steps

Epinephrine, antihistamines (block both H_1 and H_2 receptors), and antiprostaglandins.

BIBLIOGRAPHY

Expert Panel on Detection, Evaluation, and Treatment of High Blood Cholesterol in Adults. Executive Summary of the Third Report of the National Cholesterol Education Program (NCEP) Expert Panel on Detection, Evaluation, and Treatment of High Blood Cholesterol in Adults (Adult Treatment Panel III). JAMA 2001;285:2486–2497.

Felig P. *Endocrinology and Metabolism*, 3rd ed. New York: McGraw-Hill, 1995.

Ingbar SH. *The Thyroid: A Fundamental and Clinical Text*, 6th ed. Philadelphia: J.B. Lippincott, 1992.

McDermott MD. *Endocrine Secrets*. Philadelphia: Mosby, 1995.

Scriver CR. *The Metabolic Basis of Inherited Disease*, 7th ed. New York: McGraw-Hill, 1994.

Wilson JD. *Textbook of Endocrinology*, 8th ed. Philadelphia: W.B. Saunders, 1992.

Gastroenterology

4

I. GASTROINTESTINAL (GI) BLEEDING

A. Acute Upper GI Bleeding

▶ Description

Site of bleeding is esophagogastric (EG) junction (esophageal varices, esophagitis, Mallory–Weiss tears), **one-third; stomach** (ulcers, gastritis), **one-third;** and **pyloroduodenal region** (ulcers, duodenitis), **one-third.**

▶ Symptoms

Vomiting blood (hematemesis) or melena.

▶ Diagnosis

Esophagogastroduodenoscopy (EGD) identifies source in 95%. In ulcers, visible vessel in ulcer base indicates rebleed of 50%, and clean ulcer base, rebleed of 1%.

▶ Treatment Steps

Mortality unchanged at 10% in past 40 years.

Bleeding ulcer:
1. Intravenous proton pump inhibitor (IV Protonix 80 mg IV (stat), then 8 mg/hr IV),
2. Correct coagulopathy if present.
3. Transfuse as needed.
4. Urgent endoscopy when indicated.
5. Epinephrine injected into visible vessel spurting in an ulcer may stop acute bleeding.
6. Surgery if bleeding is uncontrolled after medical interventions.

Esophageal varices:
1. Octreotide 50 μg IV bolus, then 50 μg/hr IV constant infusion, or
2. Banding and/or sclerotherapy.
3. Endotracheal intubation may be needed in rapidly bleeding patient.
4. Transjugular intrahepatic portosystemic shunt (TIPS) (can fix varices but very often cause/worsen encephalopathy).

B. Acute Lower GI Bleeding

▶ Description

Common causes include diverticulosis, angiodysplasia, neoplasm, colitis.

▶ Symptoms

Bright red blood per rectum.

▶ Diagnosis

Colonoscopy when bleeding stops. Angiography if bleeding persists.

▶ Treatment Steps
1. Replace blood.
2. Correct coagulation factors if needed.
3. Vasopressin infusion at angiographic bleeding site.

▶ **differential diagnosis**

GASTROINTESTINAL BLEEDING

Upper
- Nasogastric (NG) positive.
- Upper endoscopy.

Lower
- NG tube negative, bile no blood.
- Colonoscopy if bleeding stops.
- Bleeding scan if bleeding continues.
- If positive, surgical evaluation—possible angiography with vasopressin at bleeding site.

▶ **cram facts**

SIGN OR SYMPTOM: HEMATEMESIS AND LOWER GI BLEED

Think of: Defined as bleeding above or below the ligament of Trietz, respectively: **UGIB** (gastritis, peptic ulcer disease, Mallory–Weiss tear, cancer, esophageal varices, to mention only a few of the most common ones); **LGIB** (atriovenous malformations, malignancies, hemorrhoids, trauma, diverticulitis, colitis [Crohn's disease, ulcerative, pseudo-membranous], and a few others).

II. INFLAMMATORY BOWEL DISEASE

▶ General Description

Inflammatory bowel disease (IBD) refers to ulcerative colitis (UC) and Crohn's disease (CD), two chronic inflammatory gastrointestinal disorders of unknown etiology.

In UC, inflammation always begins in the rectum, extends proximally, and then abruptly stops. (A demarcation can be seen via endoscopy between involved and uninvolved mucosa.) The rectum is always involved in UC and no "skip areas" (normal areas in between disease areas) are present. In UC, only the mucosa and the submucosa are involved, except in very rare cases. Crypt abscesses and mucosal ulceration can occur. The small intestine is never involved, except when "backwash ileitis" occurs: when the distal terminal ileum is inflamed as a result of proximal colonic involvement. As the disease becomes chronic, the colon loses its usual haustral markings, leading to the lead pipe appearance seen on barium enema.

CD, on the other hand, consists of segmental involvement by a nonspecific granulomatous inflammatory process. In contrast to UC, one of the most important pathologic features is involvement of all layers of the bowel, not just the mucosa and the submucosa. "Skip areas" are present. Late in the disease, the mucosa develops a cobblestone appearance. The small intestine can be involved. Rectal sparing is a typical but not constant feature of CD. However, anorectal complications (e.g., fistulas, abscesses) are common. CD causes three patterns of involvement: (1) inflammatory disease, (2) strictures, and (3) fistulas.

Diagnosis of UC and CD use a combination of clinical findings, along with colonoscopy and biopsies. However, no single finding is absolutely diagnostic for one disease or the other, and about one-fifth of patients have a clinical picture that falls between CD and UC; they are said to have indeterminate colitis (see Table 4–1).

4-1

DIFFERENTIATING ULCERATIVE AND CROHN'S COLITIS

	Ulcerative Colitis	Crohn's Colitis
Clinical findings		
Perianal disease	Rare	Common (1/3 of patients)
Fistulas	Rare	Common (up to 40% of patients)
Abscess	Rare	20% of patients
Stricture	Rare	Common
Colonoscopic findings		
Rectal involvement	Always	Usually spared
Pattern	Continuous, proximal extension from rectum	Usually skip lesions
Radiologic findings		
Ileal involvement	Rare, nonspecific "backwash ileitis"	75% of patients with Crohn's disease
Histologic findings		
Depth of inflammation	Usually limited to mucosa or submucosa, except in fulminant cases	Typically transmural
Granulomas	Only associated with crypts in severe colitis	20% of endoscopic biopsies

A. Ulcerative Colitis

▶ Symptoms
Small, frequent, bloody diarrheal stools often associated with **tenesmus.** Abdominal pain, fever, and leukocytosis. Fulminant colitis is associated with worsening systemic toxicity and may show colonic dilatation (transverse diameter > 5 cm).

▶ Diagnosis
Rule out antibiotics and other drugs, stool for ova and parasites, culture and sensitivity (O&P, C&S), and *Clostridium difficile* toxin (*Escherichia coli* O157:H7-culture negative hemorrhagic colitis, after raw beef or milk causes hemolytic anemia syndrome, 35% mortality in elderly). Histologic exam of mucosa. Colonoscopy and ileoscopy, barium enema if not megacolon, and small bowel series (see Table 4–1).

▶ Pathology
Crypt abscesses and superficial ulceration compatible with diagnosis.

▶ Treatment Steps
Azulfidine 4 q/day; folic acid 1 mg daily for 2–3 weeks. Amebiasis should be excluded before beginning steroid therapy. Oral prednisone (30–60 mg daily) responds usually in 2 weeks, taper by 5 mg weekly. **Maintenance** prophylactic therapy: **sulfasalazine** 500 mg PO qid and **folate** 1 mg daily. 6-Mercaptopurine for steroid sparing in steroid-dependent disease, 1–1.5 mg/kg/day.

B. Crohn's Disease

▶ Description
Chronic idiopathic inflammation.

▶ Symptoms
Small intestinal sites cause pain, bloating, diarrhea, weight loss, fever. Obstruction causes crampy abdominal pain followed by vomiting. Perianal disease (fistula, perianal abscess, fissures), fistulae (to the bladder, vagina, colon, skin, among loops of bowel), or abdominal masses due to abscesses.

▶ Diagnosis
Stomach or small bowel involvement, rectal sparing, fistulization. Deep fissures, ulcer, granulomas, or patchy distribution of colonic inflammation. Upper GI/small bowel, barium enema with flexible sigmoidoscopy versus colonoscopy (see Fig. 4–1).

▶ Pathology
Transmural, "fat wrapping" on serosal surface, noncaseating granulomas.

▶ Treatment Steps
1. **Sulfasalazine:** 4 g/day, and if confined to the colon, 1 mg folic acid for 2–4 weeks, if sulfa allergic. Asacol 800 mg tid.
2. **Metronidazole:** 10 mg/kg/day. If no response in 4 weeks, then
3. **Prednisone:** 30–60 mg/day should be used instead (start with prednisone if symptoms are severe). If patient responds to treatment 1 or 2, continue for 4–6 months; then stop if symptoms gone. Maintenance prophylactic therapy: Asacol (mesalamine) (5ASA) 800 mg PO tid. Twenty percent of cases of IBD are neither

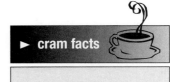

▶ **cram facts**

There is an increased incidence of gallstones and calcium oxalate kidney stones in Crohn's disease.

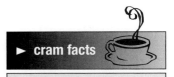

▶ **cram facts**

Extraintestinal manifestations of IBD include arthritis, iritis, episcleritis, dermatologic manifestations, and sclerosing cholangitis.

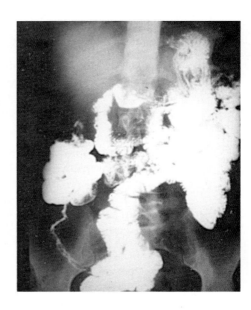

Figure 4–1. Crohn's disease. Small-bowel barium contrast x-ray shows marked narrowing of the terminal ileum as a result of transmural inflammation.

specifically ulcerative colitis nor Crohn's disease. Sulfasalazine and prednisone appear safe in pregnancy and during lactation.
4. 6-Mercaptopurine in steroid-dependent case (1–1.5 mg/kg/day).
5. Infliximab (Remicade) 5 mg/kg IV over 2 hrs. One infusion for active disease. Three infusions (0, 2, 6 wks) for fistulous disease.

III. PEPTIC ULCER (DUODENAL AND GASTRIC ULCER)

► Description
Peptic ulcers are defects in GI mucosa extending to the submucosa, into the muscle layers, and require acid and pepsin. The major complications of duodenal ulcers are bleeding, perforation, gastric outlet obstruction, and penetration into the pancreas.

► Symptoms

► cram facts

PEPTIC ULCER DISEASE

Risk factors for NSAID ulcers

• > 70 years old
• History of prior ulcer disease or complications
• Co-therapy with corticosteroids or with anticoagulants
• Misoprostol (200 mg qid) is the only drug approved by the Food and Drug Administration (FDA) to prevent NSAID-induced ulcer, proton pump inhibitors (PPIs) may be helpful.

H. pylori

• Urease of CLO-test, H. pylori on gastric biopsy, (+) C_{14} urea breath test clarithromycin 500 mg bid, omeprazole 20 mg or lansoprazole 30 mg bid, and amoxicillin 1 g bid (with penicillin allergy—metronidazole 500 mg bid) for 2 weeks (other regimens exist).
• C_{14} urea breath test no earlier than 1 month after treatment to check for cure.
• Occurs in 90% of patients with duodenal ulcers and 70–80% of patients with gastric ulcer.

Burning epigastric pain, dull ache, often associated with heartburn/gastroesophageal reflux disease (GERD).

Bleeding ulcers may be painless, but cause hematemesis, melena, anemia, or hematochezia.

Gastric outlet obstruction may present with repeated vomiting and dehydration.

▶ **Diagnosis**

Upper endoscopy, biopsy and brush of gastric ulcers to rule out cancer). Radiographic exam (upper GI series) somewhat less accurate. Assess for *Helicobacter pylori* via biopsy, CLO test, or breath test.

▶ **Treatment Steps**

If *H. pylori* infection positive, multiple regimens exist. One example: clarithromycin 500 mg bid, omeprazole 20 mg, or lansoprazole 30 mg bid, and amoxicillin 1 g bid (or with penicillin allergy—metronidazole 500 mg bid) for 2 weeks.

1. Stop caustics: alcohol, nonsteroidal anti-inflammatory drugs (NSAIDs), caffeine, nicotine.
2. Proton pump inhibitors initially given bid (omeprazole, lansoprazole, others).

IV. MOTOR DISORDERS OF THE GI TRACT

A. Oropharyngeal Dysphagia

▶ **Description**

Neuromuscular control of oral and oropharyngeal stage of **swallowing is impaired.** Skeletal muscle is primarily involved; 50% of nursing home patients in the United States have difficulty with eating and drinking.

▶ **Diagnosis**

Barium video swallow with liquid to solid foods, neurological evaluation. Occasionally, esophageal manometry (ear, nose, and throat [ENT]) evaluation.

▶ **Pathology**

Cerebrovascular accident **(CVA) (most common),** Alzheimer's, bulbar and pseudobulbar palsy. Cranial nerve paralysis, myasthenia gravis, skeletal myopathies.

▶ **Treatment Steps**

Treat underlying condition where possible. If patient aspirates more than 10% of barium test bolus and develops barium residue in oropharynx with sequential swallows, needs endoscopic (percutaneous endoscopic gastrostomy [PEG]) or surgical gastrostomy for feeds.

B. Achalasia

▶ **Description**

Achalasia is characterized by **increased basal pressure of the lower esophageal sphincter (LES),** incomplete LES relaxation after a swallow, and aperistalsis of the distal two-thirds of the esophageal body.

▶ **Symptoms**

Dysphagia for liquids, then solids; chest pain, vomiting frequently without sour taste, nocturnal cough, pneumonia, lung abscess.

▶ **differential diagnosis**

OROPHARYNGEAL DYSPHAGIA

• Usually caused by CVA, Parkinson's, or Alzheimer's.
• Evaluate with video swallow.
• If aspirates, depending on clinical course and/or family wishes, PEG or G tube

ESOPHAGEAL DYSPHAGIA

Structural

• Schatzki's ring—shown on video swallow with tablet; when symptomatic, usually has superficial inflammation or erosion; brush cytology, balloon dilatation, and treatment with PPIs
• Stricture, benign—brush cytology, balloon dilatation, and treatment with PPI
• Carcinoma—biopsy diagnosis; resection if lower, radiation if upper; chemotherapy showing recent promise

Nonstructural

• Achalasia—aperistalsis, incomplete relaxation of LES with a high resting LES pressure. Botox injection in LES if ≥ 50 years old; pneumatic dilatation; if failed, then surgical myotomy with fundoplication
• Scleroderma—aperistalsis, incompetent LES treatment for GERD

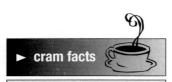

GERD AND BARRETT'S ESOPHAGUS

- Long-term sequelae of GERD include dysphagia, stricture, and Barrett's esophagus.
- Barrett's esophagus is a metaplastic lesion—normal epithelium is replaced by columnar epithelium.
- Patients with long-standing GERD need endoscopic surveillance for Barrett's.
- Barrett's increases the risk of adenocarcinoma of the esophagus.

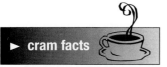

TREATMENT OF GERD

1. Lifestyle changes include not lying down after eating (and not eating close to bedtime) and reduction in foods that trigger GERD (often fatty foods, alcohol, spicy foods).
2. Empiric treatment with PPI (although H_2 blockers are less expensive, the PPIs are more effective, therefore cost effective, in the end.
3. If symptoms refractory despite compliance with above, may use esophageal pH monitoring to look at physiologic response.
4. Refractory cases of GERD may respond to surgery (Nissen fundoplication).

► **Diagnosis**

Air–fluid level near aortic arch with widened mediastinum on **chest x-ray. Barium swallow** may show dilated distal two-thirds of the esophagus and smooth tapering at EG junction.

All patients with achalasia should have **upper endoscopy** to exclude tumors and to enter the stomach to differentiate the tonically contracted LES from a malignant stricture.

Esophageal manometry should be done and is the "gold standard" (see Description).

Computed tomography may be used to exclude extrinsic circumferential lesions simulating achalasia.

► **Pathology**

Abnormalities are found in the dorsomotor nucleus of the vagus nerve and in the postganglionic neurons, which innervate the circular smooth muscle of the esophagus (myenteric plexus).

► **Treatment Steps**

1. Botoxin injection (80 U) into the lower esophageal sphincter if > 50 years old; if no help, then can be repeated in one month; if no help then #2.
2. **Pneumatic dilation**—transmural rupture of esophagus is an uncommon complication—if no help, then
3. **Surgical myotomy** (modified Heller's) with fundoplication, attempting to avoid esophageal stricture (20%) or Barrett's esophagus.

C. Gastroesophageal Reflux Disease (GERD)

► **Description**

Reflux of gastric acid into lower esophagus causing irritative symptoms.

► **Symptoms**

Heartburn (can manifest as chest/epigastric pain), occasionally chronic cough, nocturnal cough, choking, wheezing, laryngospasm, hoarseness, earache.

► **Diagnosis**

Upper GI endoscopy to rule out ulcers, Barrett's esophagus. However, can diagnose GERD clinically and start empiric therapy.

► **Treatment Steps**

See Cram Facts.

D. Scleroderma Esophagus

► **Description**

A patulous esophagus leads to reflux disease and dysphagia associated with Raynaud's phenomenon in 90% of cases.

► **Symptoms**

Heartburn, dysphagia for liquids, then solids.

► **Diagnosis**

Air-filled esophagus on chest film. Prone view of esophagogram fails to empty. Esophageal manometry in advanced state includes decreased LES pressure, low amplitude or absent contractions in the smooth muscle esophagus, normal peristalsis in the striated muscle esophagus, and a normal upper esophageal sphincter (UES).

► Treatment Steps
See treatment for GERD. Surgery is unnecessary and probably contraindicated here because of the limited ability to empty the esophagus.

E. Gastroparesis

► Description
Delayed gastric emptying without mechanical cause.

► Symptoms
Nausea, vomiting, bloating, upper abdominal discomfort.

► Diagnosis
Retained barium in stomach on upper GI series (UGI). Delayed nuclear medicine gastric emptying scan. Upper endoscopic exam within normal limits.

► Pathology and Associated Conditions
Acute with intact vagi (blood sugar > 300 mg/dL, acute pancreatitis, trauma, abdominal surgery, porphyria, severe hypokalemia, or drugs [opiates, digitalis, ganglionic blockers, anticholinergic]). **Chronic** (most frequently caused by neuropathy [postvagotomy or diabetic] **or myopathy** [scleroderma]).

► Treatment Steps
Metoclopramide (a dopaminergic antagonist, 30% neurologic, and psychiatric side effects). Erythromycin (oral).

F. Constipation

► Description
Symptomatic decrease in frequency of bowel movements and may also mean (to some patients) passage of dry stools, excessive straining, lower abdominal fullness, and a sense of incomplete evacuation.

► Diagnosis
Rule out organic disease (endocrine pharmacologic, neurologic, and structural).

► Treatment Steps
Insoluble dietary bulk 15 g of crude fiber (e.g., wheat bran [methylcellulose] or commercial psyllium products with 32 oz of water per day). Lactulose can be tolerated well for long periods. Occasionally, mineral oil enemas can help relieve distal fecal impaction.

G. Diarrhea

► Description
Twenty-four-hour excretion weight or volume greater than 200 g/24 hours and greater than 10 g/kg in infants, and change in consistency—more liquid.

Not incontinence (the involuntary release of rectal contents).

► Diagnosis
Osmotic diarrhea stool: 290 − 2 (Na + K) = > 50 (Osm gap). Diarrhea should disappear when patient fasts.

H. Infectious Diarrhea

There are a multitude of organisms that can cause infectious diarrhea. It is helpful to divide the organisms into two groups—inflam-

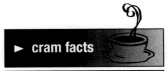
► cram facts

SIGN OR SYMPTOM: DIARRHEA

Always think of the common ones first: gastroenteritis, food intoxication/poisoning, infections (bacterial—*Salmonella, Shigella, Vibrio, Clostridium*), parasitic (*Giardia, Entamoeba*), as well as human immunodeficiency virus (HIV)-related; absorption syndromes (sprue, tropical sprue, lactose intolerance).

matory vs. noninflammatory diarrhea. Inflammatory diarrhea has white blood cells in the stool. Blood may also be present.

Noninflammatory	**Inflammatory**
Enterotoxigenic *E. coli* (ETEC)	*Campylobacter jejuni*
Clostridium perfringens	*Shigella* species
Staphylococcus aureus	Enterohemorrhagic *E. coli*
Bacillus cereus	(EHEC)
Vibrio cholera	*Clostridium difficile*
Rotavirus	*Vibrio parahaemolyticus*
Norwalk virus	*Entamoeba histolytica*
Giardia lamblia	*Salmonella* species
Cryptosporidium	

Please see Chapter 9 for more on presentation and management of specific conditions.

I. Pseudomembranous Colitis (*Clostridium difficile* Diarrhea)

► Description
Prior antibiotic use alters the normal GI flora and *C. difficile* causes diarrhea. Can occur with any antibiotic (even one dose as long as 2 months before).

► Diagnosis
Identifying ***C. difficile*** toxin in the stool. On colonoscopy: **yellow adherent plaques on the colonic mucosa.**

► Treatment Steps
1. **Remove the offending antibiotic whenever possible.**
2. Oral metronidazole is the treatment of choice, although patients can have recurrence.
3. If multiple recurrences, use oral vancomycin.
4. Alternatives include cholestyramine and *Saccharomyces boulardii* 500 mg PO bid.

V. COLORECTAL CANCER

► Description
Cancer of colon is the most frequent neoplasm of the GI tract and is the second most common cause of cancer mortality in the United States. Early detection may lead to a substantial improvement in outcome (see Fig. 4–2).

► Symptoms
Rectal bleeding, change in bowel habits. Sometimes asymptomatic, but found on routine screening colonoscopy.

► Diagnosis
American Cancer Society recommends fecal occult blood testing (FOBT) of passed stool yearly after age 50 and flexible sigmoidoscopy every 4 years. Start earlier age with colonoscopy if genetic predisposition or prior disease. More recent studies have suggested screening all normal-risk individuals with colonoscopy starting at age 50, regardless of results of FOBT.

The presence of heme in an asymptomatic person at risk is an indication for colonoscopy.

► **cram facts**

COLORECTAL CARCINOMA (CRC)

- Second leading cause of cancer deaths in the United States.
- 140,000 cases and 55,000 deaths/year.
- 80% sporadic, 20% hereditary.
- 6% of all cases HNPCC (hereditary nonpolyposis colorectol cancer, also known as the Lynch syndromes).
- 1% of all cases FAP (familial adenomatous polyposis).
- < 1% of all cases mutation of APC gene (at 1307 codon) noted in 6% Ashkenazi Jews (95% of American Jews are Ashkenazi). If the gene is present, 30% chance of colon cancer in patient's lifetime. This chance goes up to 50% if family history of a first-degree relative with colon cancer.
- Dot blot gene testing with genetic counseling leads to colonoscopic surveillance if positive.
- Asymptomatic individuals with colon cancer in first-degree relatives have a 2 to 4 times higher risk for colorectal cancer.
- Recommend: colonoscopic screening.
- **Asymptomatic individuals without family history of cancer should have annual fecal occult blood testing and flexible sigmoidoscopy every 5 years (after a negative initial study). If heme positive or if adenomatous polyp found, colonoscopy is recommended.**
- Over 50 years old average risk, colonoscopy every 10 years.

Colonoscopy is more sensitive, a biopsy can be made (and polyps can be removed); especially in high-risk patients whose first-degree relatives have colorectal cancer or who themselves have IBD, previous breast or genital cancer, prior colonic adenomas, or familial polyposis.

Finding even one adenoma on flex sig should lead to total colonoscopy and polypectomy. Repeat colonoscopy in 3 years; if normal, can be followed by exams every 5 years depending on the completeness of the exam and type of polyp.

► Pathology

Ninety-five percent of malignancies of the colon and rectum are adenocarcinoma.

► Treatment Steps

The **only curative therapy is surgical resection of the primary tumor** and of the isolated hepatic metastases. Rule out synchronous lesions by doing full colonoscopy preop. Colonoscopy in 1 year to exclude

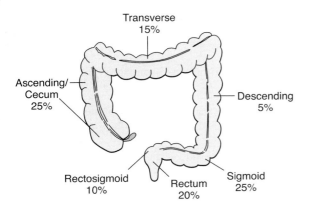

Transverse
15%

Ascending/
Cecum
25%

Descending
5%

Rectosigmoid
10%

Rectum
20%

Sigmoid
25%

Figure 4–2. Distribution of colorectal cancers within the large intestine. Only half of the cancers are found within reach of the flexible sigmoidoscope.

recurrence and at 3–5 years to prevent the 8–10% incidence of second cancers, which occur within 10 years of the initial surgery. Chemotherapy for metastatic disease. (See also Chapter 6, section VII.E.9 and 10.)

VI. HEPATOBILIARY SYSTEM

A. Chronic Liver Disease

▶ **Description**

A variety of conditions can cause chronic liver disease (see Cram Facts). With recent increases in hepatitis C and obesity (and therefore fatty liver disease) the incidence of liver disease is increasing. If chronic liver disease progresses to end-stage liver disease, the patient can have a multitude of problems, including hepatic encephalopathy, coagulopathy (elevated prothrombin time [PT] and international normalized ratio [INR] due to impaired synthesis of coagulation factors), thrombocytopenia (due to portal hypertension causing hepatosplenomegaly and consumption of platelets), esophageal varices (due to portal hypertension), and hepatorenal syndrome (renal failure due to liver disease).

▶ **Symptoms**

See Cram Facts.

▶ **Treatment Steps**

Varies according to the underlying condition. With any etiology, if cirrhosis/end-stage liver disease is present, patients may be considered for liver transplantation if they are abstaining from alcohol.

1. Autoimmune Hepatitis

▶ **Description**

Chronic active autoimmune hepatitis (CAAH) can present with striking increases in enzymes resembling viral hepatitis, but stigmata of chronic liver disease or marked elevations in gamma globulins may help identify it as chronic without evidence of other causes. A positive antinuclear antibody (ANA) strongly suggests the diagnosis.

▶ **Symptoms**

CAAH is suspected when physical examination reveals signs of chronic liver disease (e.g., spider angiomata, ascites, and elevated serum glutamic oxaloacetic transaminase [SGOT] or serum glutamate pyruvate transaminase [SGPT]). Often, the patient may have only increased fatigue and persistent elevated enzymes for 6 months or more.

▶ **Pathology**

Piecemeal necrosis and bridging necrosis (fibrosis can lead to cirrhosis).

This disease is associated with three important patterns of autoantibodies in serum:

1. The first pattern characteristically has positive ANA, anti-smooth muscle antibody (ASMA) liver membrane autoantibodies.
2. The second pattern is associated with antibodies to a soluble liver antigen (antisoluble liver antigen [anti-SLA]).
3. The third is associated with anti-liver-kidney microsomal-1 antibody (mainly in Europe).

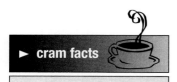

▶ **cram facts**

CAUSES OF CHRONIC LIVER DISEASE

- Autoimmune hepatitis
- Hereditary hemochromatosis
- Chronic alcohol use
- Fatty liver disease (non-alcoholic steatohepatitis)
- Wilson's disease
- Viral (hepatitis B, C)

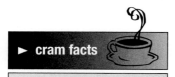

▶ **cram facts**

CHRONIC LIVER DISEASE

Symptoms

- Fatigue
- Increasing abdominal girth (due to ascites)
- Jaundice
- Spider angiomas
- Bleeding (GI bleeding due to hemorrhoids or esophageal varices)

Signs

- Palmar erythema
- Hepatosplenomegaly
- Gynecomastia
- Testicular atrophy

Labs

- Elevated AST and ALT
- Elevated PT and INR
- Thrombocytopenia, anemia (often macrocytic), or pancytopenia
- Hyponatremia
- Hypoalbuminemia

Drugs producing a hepatitis that mimics CAAH are α-methyldopa and nitrofurantoin (especially women).

▶ **Treatment Steps**

Steroid therapy achieves symptomatic, clinical, and histologic remission, but relapse occurs in 90% over 2 years, requiring long-term maintenance therapy leading to increases in life expectancy, but does not appear to stop progression to cirrhosis. 6-Mercaptopurine may be used with steroids.

2. Hereditary Hemochromatosis

▶ **Description**

A genetic condition (usually autosomal recessive with variable penetrance) that causes iron overload. Iron can be deposited in many organs. The classic tetrad includes cirrhosis, diabetes, skin hyperpigmentation, and cardiac failure. Sometimes called **"bronze diabetes."**

▶ **Treatment Steps**

Removal of excess iron through phlebotomy. Chelation therapy (with deferoxamine) is usually indicated only when phlebotomy is inappropriate.

3. Chronic Alcohol Use

▶ **Description**

Liver disease due to alcohol consumption. Can range from asymptomatic liver function test (LFT) abnormalities to alcoholic hepatitis to cirrhosis/end-stage liver disease. Women are at higher risk from liver damage due to alcohol than are men because ethanol is metabolized differently. Any chronic liver condition will be worsened by alcohol use.

▶ **Treatment Steps**

Cessation of drinking alcohol, which can be very difficult. Support groups (Alcoholics Anonymous) have been effective. A patient must demonstrate cessation of alcohol before he/she can be considered for a liver transplant.

4. Fatty Liver Disease (Nonalcoholic Steatohepatitis [NASH])

▶ **Description**

A condition in which lipids accumulate in the hepatocytes. Fatty change in the liver is known as steatosis, and steatosis with inflammation is called steatohepatitis. Because steatohepatitis is common in patients who drink alcohol, this particular subset (NASH) occurs in people who do not ingest alcohol. There is often a common clinical picture: Patients have obesity, diabetes, hyperlipidemia, and/or high-fat diet.

Unfortunately, this condition is becoming exceedingly common in the United States, as the number of people with diabetes and obesity is higher now than ever before. It is now felt that many people who have presented with cryptogenic cirrhosis may have actually had NASH that was undiagnosed.

▶ **Diagnosis**

Technically, NASH is a pathologic diagnosis seen on liver biopsy. However, patients are suspected of having NASH, or "fatty liver disease" in the correct clinical setting (overweight/obese, diabetes, hyperlipidemia), and elevated LFTs. Ultrasound of the liver can show

▶ **differential diagnosis**

HYPERBILIRUBINEMIA

Conjugated

1. Bilary obstruction: choledocholithiasis, biliary atresia, malignancy, pancreatitis, sclerosing cholangitis, others.
2. Hereditary: Gilbert syndrome, Crigler–Najjar syndrome, Dubin–Johnson syndrome.
3. Hepatocellular dysfunction: hepatitis, hepatic cirrhosis, biliary cirrhosis, sepsis, postop, drugs, infections, mononucleosis, cholangitis, sarcoidosis, toxins, lymphomas.

Unconjugated

1. Hemolytic anemias.
2. Posthepatitis.
3. Gilbert syndrome.

changes consistent with fatty liver. All other causes of chronic liver disease should be ruled out.

► Treatment Steps

1. Varying opinions exist as to whether all patients should have a liver biopsy. The argument is that pathology (inflammation, fibrosis/cirrhosis) can be followed serially.
2. Evidence exists that a low-fat diet, weight loss, and control of diabetes and hyperlipidemia will help fatty liver. However, if cirrhosis develops, supportive care and consideration of liver transplant are needed.

5. Wilson's Disease

► Description

Wilson's disease (hepatolenticular degeneration) is an inherited (autosomal recessive) genetic disorder. While it is rare, it is important to recognize as it can be fatal if unrecognized/untreated. (See also Chapter 11, section IX.C.)

► Diagnosis

Patients may present with acute hepatitis. Psychiatric manifestations may include confusion, aggression. Labs that are basically diagnostic for Wilson's include serum ceruloplasmin (< 20 mg/dL), low total serum copper, and increased urinary copper excretion. One clue to the diagnosis is the presence of hemolytic anemia. Computed tomographic (CT) scan of the brain can reveal hypodense regions in the basal ganglia. Liver biopsy can confirm the diagnosis: a hepatic copper content > 250 μg dry weight of the liver in the correct clinical setting.

► Treatment Steps

Copper chelating medications include penicillamine. The disease is uniformly fatal if untreated.

6. Viral Hepatitis

► Description

Almost any virus can cause an acute and often self-limited hepatitis. Classically, hepatitis viruses B and C are capable of causing chronic liver disease. Hepatitis A virus is never a cause of chronic liver disease. However, acute hepatitis A infection can worsen a patient's condition in the setting of chronic liver disease.

► Treatment Steps

See later in this chapter, section V.G.

B. Complications of Cirrhosis

- Portal hypertension causes hepatosplenomegaly, hemorrhoids, abdominal and esophageal varices.
- In a patient with chronic liver disease, endoscopy should be performed, and if esophageal varices are present, β-blockers should be started to decrease portal pressures and decrease risk of bleeding. Bleeding esophageal varices can be a significant cause of morbidity and mortality.
- Pancytopenia can occur, due to hypersplenism—the spleen consumes cells from all three cell lines. (Alcohol can also suppress bone marrow.)
- Coagulopathy—elevated PT and INR due to the lack of production of the vitamin K–dependent clotting factors in the liver (factors II, VII, IX, X).

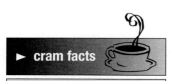

► **cram facts**

WILSON'S DISEASE

Two clues to the diagnosis:
- Hemolytic anemia.
- Kayser–Fleischer rings—asymptomatic color changes that occur in the Descemet membrane of the eye. They are always found if there is neurologic involvement. The rings can disappear with appropriate treatment.

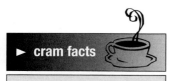

► **cram facts**

Immunization against hepatitis A and B is indicated in patients with chronic liver disease if they are not already immune.

► cram facts

CIRRHOSIS—COMPLICATIONS

Fourth most common (25–45%) cause of death in U.S. urban areas.

- Ascites: Na, fluid restriction and diuretics; Aldactone 50–400 mg/24 hr; if no help, furosemide; if no help, large-volume paracentesis can be done one to three times a month for life, if no help TIPS may help.
- Spontaneous bacterial peritonitis: > 250 polys; 10–100 mL blood culture bottles at bedside; treat with cefotaxime 2 g IV q8 to 12h for 5–10 days. If polys not decreased 50% by 48 hr, change med and reevaluate problem.
- Encephalopathy: protein restriction, lactulose 30 cc qh until diarrhea, then q6h; if PO not available, then 300 mL lactulose plus 700 mL tap water enema one to three times daily if deemed safe to give enemas. Treat underlying condition.

- Ascites, spontaneous bacterial peritonitis, hepatic encephalopathy (see next three sections).
- See also Cram Facts.

C. Ascites

► Description
Fluid in peritoneal cavity.

► Diagnosis
Ultrasound (US) or CT more sensitive than physical exam.

Paracentesis 10 mL into blood culture bottles, acid-fast bacteria (AFB), fungal cultures, cytology, amylase, total protein, white blood count (WBC) and differential.

► Pathology
All the factors in ascites mechanism and formation are not known.

► Treatment Steps
1. Sodium and fluid restriction and diuretics.
2. Initially with spironolactone 50–400 mg/24 hr.
3. If no help in 3–4 days, start furosemide 40 mg daily.
4. If no response, double daily up to 240–320 mg daily.
5. Failure: other drugs, bumetanide, ethacrynic acid, or metolazone, watch for large diuresis.
6. If no help, large-volume paracentesis if > 5 L needed to give albumin 6–8 g/L of fluid removed. Can be done one to three times per month for life.
7. Patient with intractable ascites who has bled from varices may benefit from intrahepatic shunting by a stent radiologically placed through hepatic vein to the portal vein (TIPS).

D. Spontaneous Bacterial Peritonitis

► Description
Bacteria most likely reaches ascites through hematogenous spread; *E. coli* is most common pathogen. Mortality and recurrence is high even with antibiotics.

► Symptoms
Fever, abdominal pain, encephalopathy in cirrhotic patient with ascites, but many patients may be asymptomatic.

► Diagnosis

Greater than 250/mL polys is reliable even if fluid is sterile, if symptoms are suggestive.

Best ascites culture yields (> 80%) obtained by inoculation of 10 mL of ascites into each of three 100-mL blood culture bottles (aerobic, anaerobic, and microaerophilic) at the bedside, protein usually less than 1 g/mL. WBC greater than 10,000/mL, protein greater than 2.5 with free air suggests ruptured viscus.

► Treatment Steps

1. Cefotaxime 2 g IV every 8–12 hours for 5–10 days.
2. Repeat paracentesis in 48 hours after initiation of antibiotics; if ascitic fluid poly count not decreased by at least 50%, antibiotics should be changed and the problem reevaluated.

E. Hepatic Encephalopathy

► Description

Abnormal mental state and neuromuscular dysfunction **due to hepatic failure.** Often associated with elevated ammonia level.

► Symptoms

Starting with **lethargy** and progressing to **stupor** or **coma,** with dropping things and making mistakes as early signs.

► Diagnosis

Can be spontaneous. Seek precipitating cause (e.g., diuretics, hypokalemic alkalosis, hypovolemia, hyponatremia, azotemia, tranquilizer, sedative, analgesic drugs, infection, severe constipation, hypoxia, excessive dietary protein, and progressive liver damage).

► Treatment Steps

Lactulose 30 cc PO hourly until diarrhea, then every 6 hours. If PO not available, then 300 cc lactulose plus 700 cc tap water enema one to three times daily if deemed safe to give enemas. Treat underlying condition. If refractory to lactulose, consider oral neomycin.

F. Liver Transplantation

► Description

For end-stage liver disease, usually in postnecrotic cirrhosis, primary biliary cirrhosis (PBC), primary sclerosing cholangitis (PSC). Five-year survival from 55 to 85%. **Absolute contraindication:** active **sepsis** outside biliary tree, **metastatic hepatobiliary malignancy, advanced cardiopulmonary disease,** and **acquired immune deficiency syndrome (AIDS).**

Relative contraindications: active alcohol (EtOH)-induced liver disease (only 13–16% resume EtOH after), portal vein thrombosis, or previous portacaval shunt surgery. Clinically apparent hepatocellular carcinoma or cholangiocarcinoma, Hepatitis B surface antigen (HBsAg)-positive liver disease, and advanced chronic renal disease. In fulminant hepatic failure, decide before stage IV coma (e.g., drug-induced, hepatitis C viral hepatic failure, and fulminant Wilson's disease).

G. Viral Hepatitis

► Description

Five viruses are clearly identified, and a sixth is suggestive epidemiologically (like non-B, non-C) (see Table 4–2).

► **clinical pearl**

ACETAMINOPHEN TOXICITY

- Acute liver injury occurs after a toxic ingestion of acetaminophen.
- In the acute setting, it is often taken by a patient as a suicide attempt in a large dose, with or without alcohol.
- It is the drug most commonly ingested in overdoses.
- Acetaminophen-induced liver failure is the second most common cause of liver transplantation.
- Immediate treatment with N-acetylcysteine needed.

4-2

SEROLOGIC DIAGNOSIS OF VIRAL HEPATITIS

Significance	Anti-HAV IgM	HBsAg	HBeAg	Anti-HBc IgG	Anti-HBc IgM	Anti-HBs IgG	Anti-HCV IgM/IgG	Anti-HDV IgM	Anti-HEV IgM
Acute HAV	+	–	–	–	–	–	–	–	–
Acute HBV	–	+	+	–	+	–	–	–	–
Chronic HBV, active replication	–	+	+	+	–	–	–	–	–
Chronic HBV, quiescent	–	+	–	+	–	–	–	–	–
Resolved HBV	–	–	–	–	+	+	–	–	–
Post-vaccine immune	–	–	–	–	–	+	–	–	–
Chronic or recent HCV	–	–	–	–	–	–	+	–	–
Acute or chronic HDV	–	+	–	–	–	–	–	+	–
Acute HEV	–	–	–	–	–	–	–	–	+

1. Hepatitis A (HAV)

▶ Description

The RNA virus: almost exclusive **fecal–oral routes, usually early childhood. Rarely fulminant and fatal. Chronic A not described.**

▶ Symptoms

Easy fatigability, jaundice, anorexia, fever, but often not diagnosed because of mild anicteric disease.

▶ Diagnosis

Immunoglobulin M (IgM) anti-HAV (+) indicates acute infection; immunoglobulin G (IgG) indicates previous infection with A. SGPT greater than SGOT, usually > 1,000.

▶ Treatment Steps
1. Prevent with vaccination. Vaccines of killed and attenuated types produced.
2. Immune serum globulin within 2 weeks of close contact.
3. Supportive care for acute infection.

2. Hepatitis B (HBV)

▶ Description

DNA virus: Transmitted perinatally, parenterally, and sexually, but not fecal–oral.

HBsAg is earliest marker, can be negative in fulminant hepatitis B. IgM anti-hepatitis B core (HBc) will become rapidly positive and diagnostic.

HBsAg > 6 months = chronic B. Hepatitis Be antigen (HBeAg): whole virus replication (likely HBV DNA is detectable in serum and is highly infective).

IgM anti-HBc AB titer can become low and persist in chronic hepatitis.

IgG anti-HBc with normal enzymes and no anti-HBs may have had viral B in the past, but failed to develop anti-HBs or lost it.

IgG anti-HBc found alone in a case may be associated with HBV detectable by polymerase chain reaction (PCR) technique.

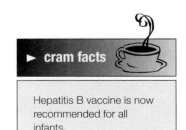

▶ cram facts

Hepatitis B vaccine is now recommended for all infants.

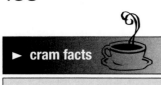

► **cram facts**

- A patient with immunity from hepatitis B due to vaccination has a + hepatitis B surface antibody, but a – hepatitis B core antibody.
- If the core antibody is positive, it means the patient has been exposed to the virus.

► Symptoms

Flulike illness, jaundice in one-third. Incubation a few weeks to 6 months. Ten percent to 20% (high) incidence of serum sickness—fever, arthralgia or arthritis, or skin rash, most frequently maculopapular or urticarial.

► Diagnosis

Clinical picture and serologies.

► Pathology

Cytotoxic T cells recognize hepatitis B core antigen receptors on liver cells. T cells attach to receptors, leading to cellular necrosis.

► Treatment Steps

Prevent with active (vaccine) and passive hepatitis B immunoglobulin (HBIG) immunization. Interferon-α stops replications in chronic hepatitis. HBV DNA and HBeAg disappear from serum. Patient is less infective in 35% of cases. In 10%, cure, HBsAg gone, and anti-HBs appeared; or lamivudine 100 mg PO qd for 12 months (and possible adefovir 10 mg/day); limitation resistance and mutation.

3. **Hepatitis C (HCV)**

► Description

Ribonucleic acid (RNA) viral infection.

► Symptoms

Similar to B, but the acute attack is usually unrecognized. No features predicting chronicity, except for concomitant alcohol use.

► Diagnosis

Anti-HCV antibody and positive HCV RNA by PCR.

► Pathology

Direct viral cytopathic injury postulated. Fatty change in 75% of cases. Mild chronic hepatitis is characteristic.

► Treatment Steps

1. Goals of treatment: Sustained virologic response (absence of HCV RNA in serum) and prevention of cirrhosis.
2. PEG interferon-α-2b (1.5 μg/kg/wk) plus ribavirin (800 mg/day).
3. If normal serum alanine aminotransferase (ALT) and negative HCV RNA by PCR does not occur by 3 months, treatment is stopped.
4. Continue regimen for 12 months in responders.

4. **Hepatitis D**

► Description

Unique RNA, requiring outer envelope of HBsAg for replication, coinfection, or superinfection (which is more likely to produce fulminant hepatic failure). **Prevalent among parenteral drug addicts, hemophiliacs, and homosexual men.**

► Treatment Steps

Interferon-α treats D but relapses after therapy. **Immunity to B prevents D.**

5. **Hepatitis E**

► Description

Transmitted by fecal–oral route—waterborne epidemics, especially in India, Nepal, Pakistan, and Southeast Asia.

► Symptoms

The disease is self-limited and does not evolve into chronic hepatitis, but has often been observed to be cholestatic; unique fulminant disease in pregnant women.

► Treatment Steps

Standard gamma globulin is ineffective and there are no active vaccines available.

H. Drug-Induced Liver Disease

► Description

Acute hepatitis (isoniazid [INH]), chronic active hepatitis (nitrofurantoin, α-methyldopa), cirrhosis (methotrexate), cholestasis (sulfonamides), fatty liver (corticosteroids), granuloma (allopurinol), benign and malignant neoplasms (estrogens), vascular lesions (vitamin A) and sclerosing cholangitis (5-fluorodeoxyuridine [5-FUDR]).

Acetaminophen is suicide—> 15 g causes massive necrosis; generates toxic metabolites through P_{450} cytochrome. Cimetidine competes for oxidation by cytochrome P_{450}.

Alcohol increases P_{450} activity and toxic metabolites. Doses averaging 6 to 7 g/day (acetaminophen) taken by alcoholic have been associated with severe hepatotoxicity characterized by increased aspartate aminotransferase (AST) > 3,000 to 10,000. The mortality in one series was 20%.

Antiarrhythmic amiodarone like alcoholic hepatitis (e.g., steatosis, hepatocellular necrosis, and Mallory bodies).

Verapamil and captopril mixed hepatocellular cholestatic patterns; ketoconazole variable hepatocellular and in 40% cholestatic.

Methotrexate cirrhosis > 1.5 g total dose; low dose 7.5 mg/week for 2 years; not associated with bridging fibrosis or cirrhosis.

Most NSAIDs are found to be associated with some form of hepatotoxicity.

Total parenteral nutrition (TPN) associated with fragment cholestatic jaundice, much mixed origin but not characterized.

I. Primary Biliary Cirrhosis

► Description

Autoimmune disease characterized by **antimitochondrial antibodies in the serum.**

Anti-M2 are the major marker-specific mitochondrial antibodies against the inner mitochrondrial membrane (see Fig. 4–3).

► Symptoms

Most common symptoms are insidious onset of **pruritus** and **fatigue,**

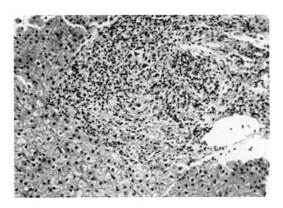

Figure 4–3. Primary biliary cirrhosis. Percutaneous liver biopsy specimen shows bile duct surrounded by dense lymphoid infiltrate typical of stage 1 disease.

early **hepatomegaly,** and elevation of serum alkaline phosphatase before symptoms.

▶ Pathology

Destruction of intrahepatic bile ducts in the first stage with progression to macronodular cirrhosis in the final stage, with mononuclear infiltrate in the portal tracts and paucity of bile ducts.

▶ Treatment Steps

No specific effective treatment; ursodeoxycholic acid; transplantation in advanced stages. Benadryl for pruritus.

VII. GALLSTONES

▶ Description

Twenty percent with asymptomatic gallstones develop biliary colic, cholecystitis, or pancreatitis.

No indication for prophylactic cholecystectomy or nonsurgical treatment in asymptomatic patient.

Cholecystectomy standard or laparoscopic cholecystectomy best therapy for symptomatic disease.

For symptomatic gallstones, if no major contraindications to surgery, operative mortality overall 1%. Lower for elective in 50-year-old, and as high as 10% in emergency situation in elderly.

▶ Symptoms

Epigastric pain, which can be colicky, advances to prolonged constant pain, lasting more than 30 minutes, and usually moderately severe. May radiate to the midscapular area or to the top of the right scapula, the right shoulder, or neck. May be mistaken for angina.

▶ Diagnosis
- US is often diagnostic.
- Hepatobiliary scan (Disida) is used when ultrasound is nondiagnostic.

▶ Treatment Steps

Laparoscopic cholecystectomy in qualified hands and appropriate cases is treatment of choice; second, open cholecystectomy (less frequently used).

1. Magnetic resonance cholangiopancreatography (MRCP) if suspected common bile duct stone and/or pancreatitis.
2. Endoscopic retrograde cholangiopancreatography (ERCP), sphincterotomy (where safe and feasible), and stone removal to remove common bile duct stones; subsequent cholecystectomy in selected cases.
3. Transhepatic techniques with radiologic guidance may be used as well.

VIII. MESENTERIC ISCHEMIA

▶ Description/Symptoms

Strangulation obstruction of the small bowel—most common form of mesenteric ischemia. Splanchnic vasospasm: nonocclusive mesenteric ischemia. Classic presentation is severe abdominal pain with a paucity of clinical findings.

► Diagnosis

Angiography is the standard. Leukocytosis, acidosis, abdominal pain and tenderness.

► Treatment Steps

Prompt laparotomy: reestablish arterial flow; assess bowel viability; resect frankly ischemic segments. Embolectomy or revascularization with second-look laparotomy 24–48 hours later to reveal intestine left in situ; 50–90% mortality from acute intestinal arterial occlusion.

IX. ACUTE PANCREATITIS

See also Chapter 18.

► Description

Inflammation from escape of active pancreatic enzymes, causing necrosis of pancreatic tissue, and peripancreatic fat.

Mortality is about 5–10%, **major causes are alcohol and gallstones.**

► Symptoms

Epigastric pain radiating to midback, better sitting up. Jaundice and fever are possible.

► Diagnosis

Elevated serum amylase; swollen, inflamed pancreas on CT scan (Fig. 4–4). Elevated amylase also seen in perforated ulcer, mesenteric infarction, intestinal obstruction, pancreas, pseudocyst, and chronic pancreatitis; also in mumps parotitis, renal failure (if creatinine > 3, serum amylase can be three times normal on that basis), ovarian and oat cell tumor of lung, ruptured ectopic pregnancy, and macroamylasemia.

Lipase is slower to rise and fall and may also become elevated due to renal failure.

► Treatment Steps

1. Supportive care with NPO.
2. Analgesia.
3. Nasogastric tube if nausea and vomiting or ileus with abdominal distention.
4. Watch for poor prognostic signs: hypotension, serum calcium < 8, Cr > 2 , WBC > 20,000, Po_2 < 60, decreased Hgb.
5. If hyperalimentation used, use H_2 blocker and avoid IV lipids.
6. With severe gallstone pancreatitis, a gallstone impacted at duodenal ampulla may benefit from early ERCP with sphincterotomy and stone extraction, or if unsuccessful. (MCRP may be helpful preliminarily.)
7. Surgical intervention, especially in the nonalcoholic with pancreatitis.

X. COMPLICATIONS OF ACUTE PANCREATITIS— PSEUDOCYST VERSUS ABSCESS

► Description and Symptoms

Worsening of pain, nausea, and vomiting after initial improvement, with fever, increased WBC, and positive blood culture.

► Diagnosis

CT of pancreas with Chiba aspiration, culture, and Gram stain. If cyst without significant pancreatitis, rule out cystic neoplasm.

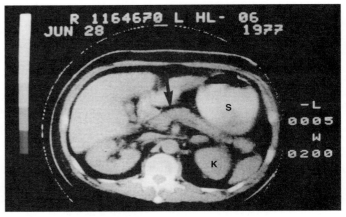

A

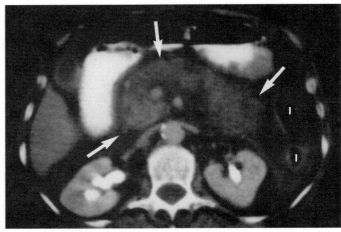

B

Figure 4–4. A: The normal pancreas on computed tomography. The gland (arrows) is homogeneous in appearance and, like the adjacent stomach (S) and left kidney (K), sharply demarcated. **B:** The pancreas on computed tomography in acute pancreatitis (arrows) is enlarged and inhomogeneous because of edema and inflammation. In addition, inflammatory changes have increased the density of the tissue surrounding loops of intestine (I) near the tail of the pancreas.

► Treatment Steps
1. Antibiotics for proven abscess and possibly for phlegmon.
2. Surgical drainage of abscess reduces mortality from > 50% to 10–20%, if aspiration used for early diagnosis.
3. Present thinking is that pseudocysts that are asymptomatic should be managed medically. Report pain, chills, or fever immediately.
4. *Late* surgery for sterile necrosis if asymptomatic—4–6 weeks of TPN.
5. If extrapancreatic pseudocyst is associated with significant pancreatic necrosis, it may need surgical evacuation.

XI. PANCREATIC CANCER

► Description
Fifth leading cause of cancer deaths in United States. **Five-year survival of 1–5%.**

► Symptoms

Vague midabdominal pain, anorexia, and weight loss. Jaundice can occur in the absence of pain. Nausea and vomiting.

► Diagnosis

US or CT biopsy of mass. If negative, ERCP, because 90–95% of pancreatic cancers arise from the pancreatic duct system. Rare to do laparotomy for tissue diagnosis. CA 19-9 in nonjaundiced patient has some validity and can be used as tumor marker after apparently curative surgery.

► Pathology

Adenocarcinoma arising from ductular epithelium account for **three-fourths** of pancreatic cancer; 60–80% arise in the head; 10–20%, body; 5–7%, tail. At surgery, 85% have disseminated disease.

► Treatment Steps

Ten to 20% are candidates for attempted curative resection with small tumor in head of pancreas and no evident spread. Modified Whipple (pancreaticoduodenectomy) 5–10% mortality in the best centers. Endoscopic and percutaneous stent for biliary obstruction. Palliative gastric bypass and pain control.

XII. MALABSORPTION

► Description

Any condition in which nutrients are not properly absorbed by the GI tract. Abnormal labs; anemia; low serum iron, folate, vitamin C, vitamin B_{12}, calcium, phosphorus, magnesium, zinc, and other trace metals; elevated alkaline phosphatase (bone disease or cholestasis), or folate (blind-loop syndrome), and a prolonged protime.

► Diagnosis

Steatorrhea (excess fat in stool): 100 g fat/diet/day × 3, after which stool is collected for another 3 days; greater than 7 g/24 hr is abnormal. D-xylose, if abnormal, suggests small bowel disease. Normal value suggests focus on pancreatic disease: CT scan of the abdomen, serum amylase, γ-glutamyl transferase. If overgrowth considered, note response of malabsorption to antibiotic therapy. Celiac sprue panel: antiendomysial antibody, tissue transglutaminase, total serum IgA; antigliadin antibody IgA and IgG; at least three biopsy specimens from distal duodenum—gold standard.

► Treatment Steps

Treat underlying condition.

XIII. ESOPHAGEAL CANCER AND BARRETT'S ESOPHAGUS

See Chapter 6, section VII.E.3.

BIBLIOGRAPHY

AGA Position Statement. *Gastroenterology* 2001;120:1522–1525.

Sherlock S, Dooley J. *Diseases of the Liver and Biliary System*, 10th ed. London: Blackwell Science, 1997.

Silen W. *Cope's Early Diagnosis of the Acute Abdomen*. Oxford University Press, 2005.

Sleisenger MH, Feldman M, Scharschmidt BF. *Sleisenger and Fordtran's Gastrointestinal and Liver Disease*. Philadelphia: W.B. Saunders, 1998.

I. ANEMIA

A. General

1. Definition

Reduction in red cell mass. In women, hemoglobin (Hb) < 12 g, hematocrit (Hct) < 36%; in men < 14 g and < 42%.

2. Basic Measurements

Mean corpuscular volume (MCV): normal 80 to 100 cubic microns; separates anemias into microcytic, normocytic, macrocytic, but combined deficiencies may be normocytic. Use RDW (red cell distribution width) to assess anisocytosis (see Fig. 5–1).

a. *Pancytopenia* (a reduction in all three cell lines—white blood cells [WBCs], red blood cells [RBCs], and platelets). Primary marrow disease, megaloblastic anemia, hypersplenism, alcohol, or human immunodeficiency virus (HIV).

b. *Reticulocytes.* A typical RBC survives 120 days. Therefore, approximately 1% of RBCs are new each day, giving a normal reticulocyte count of 1%. The corrected reticulocyte count (CRC) adjusts for severity of anemia and assesses marrow response.

$$CRC = reticulocyte \% \times \frac{patient\ Hct}{45}$$

> 4% indicates adequate response

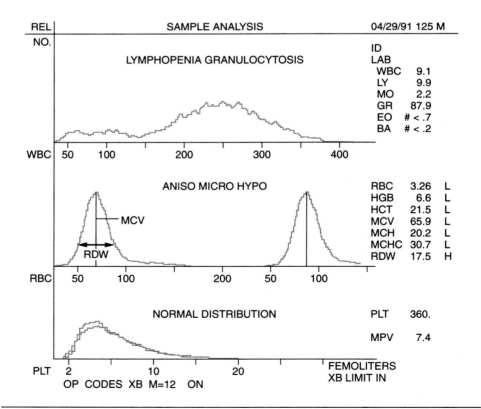

Figure 5–1. Example of cell distribution curves generated by a typical Coulter counter. Demonstrates calculation of MCV, RDW, and MPV. (Personal collection, C.M. Clay, M.D.)

3. **Red Cell Morphology**

Rouleaux (myeloma); Burr cells (renal failure); tear drops and nucleated red cells (myelophthisic anemias); hypochromia and microcytosis (iron deficiency); targets (thalassemias, other hemoglobinopathies; obstructive jaundice); oval macrocytes (vitamin B_{12} or folate deficiency). Basophilic stippling (lead poisoning, see Fig. 5–2); spherocytes (hereditary spherocytosis); schistocytes (microangiopathic hemolysis, see Fig. 5–9).

4. **Value of Bone Marrow Sampling**

- *Assess iron stores and presence of megaloblastic processes in combined deficiencies, chronic diseases, and alcoholism.*
- *Look for primary blood dyscrasias (e.g., leukemias) or invasion by metastatic tumor or infection.* A *core biopsy* to evaluate cellularity or invasive processes.
- Culture for opportunistic infections in HIV and fevers of unknown origin.

B. The Major Types of Anemia

1. **Hypoproliferative**

Marrow aplasias; anemia of chronic disease; drug causes (include alkylating agents, chloramphenicol, phenytoin, benzene, gold, and azidothymidine [AZT]). Insufficient erythropoietin and testosterone.

2. **Maturation Defects**

Hypochromic anemias, megaloblastic; drug causes include alcohol, trimethoprim, triamterene, isoniazid (INH), lead.

3. **Hyperproliferative**

Hemorrhagic, hemolytic.

4. **Dilutional Anemias**

Pregnancy.

C. Blood Loss (Acute and Chronic)

▶ Description

Chronic is usually gastrointestinal (GI) or uterine.

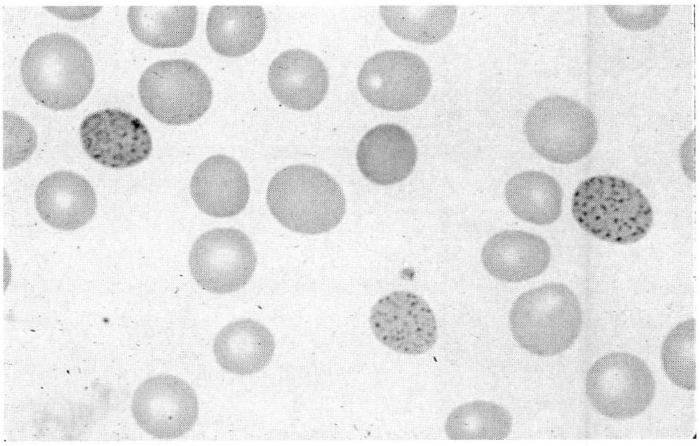

▶ **differential diagnosis**

ANEMIA

Microcytic (MCV < 80)

- Iron deficiency
- Thalassemia
- Anemia of chronic disease
- Sideroblastic anemia

Normocytic (MCV 80–100)

- Anemia of chronic desease
- Uremia
- Endocrinopathy (i.e., hypothyroid)
- Bone marrow failure (i.e., aplastic anemia)

Macrocytic (MCV > 100)

- Vitamin B_{12} deficiency
- Folate deficiency
- Myelodysplastic syndrome
- Drug induced
- Hepatic dysfunction
- Reticulocytosis

Figure 5–2. Lead poisoning demonstrates basophilic stippling.

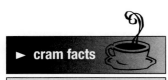

▶ **cram facts**

Testing for anemia should include:

- Iron studies (iron, TIBC, % saturation, and ferritin)
- Folate
- B_{12}
- Thyroid-stimulating hormone
- LDH, billirubin, and haptoglobin (helps diagnose hemolysis)
- Reticulocyte count
- PT/INR/PTT

▶ Symptoms

Acute presents with signs of **hypoxia** and **hypovolemia:** weakness, hypotension, tachycardia. Significant hypovolemia (blood loss > 1,000 cc) is manifest by postural signs. *Chronic* presents with fatigue, dyspnea, pallor, but often can be asymptomatic.

▶ Diagnosis

If acute, no significant drop in hematocrit initially. Increased blood urea nitrogen (BUN) if GI bleeding. Hemoccult can detect 5 mL bleeding in 24 hours. Do three to six specimens. Remember false positives (e.g., broccoli, turnips, rare meat).

▶ Treatment Steps

1. **Correct hypovolemia.** Packed red blood cells and intravenous fluids (normal saline, lactated Ringer's).

2. **Look for source** of bleeding.

3. **Remember to check** coagulation tests and order tests **before** transfusing (see Cram Facts).

D. Iron Deficiency Anemia (IDA)

▶ Description

The most common anemia; almost always due to **blood loss. Men** and **postmenopausal women** must be evaluated for **GI bleeding.** Premenopausal females: Etiology can include normal menses, menorrhagia, and uterine fibroids. Other causes include pregnancy; diagnostic venipunctures; soft tissue bleeding after hip fracture/surgery (see Fig. 5–3).

▶ Symptoms

Fatigue, palpitations, dizziness, dyspnea, headache. Angular stomatitis; glossitis. Thinning and flattening of nails, spoon-shaped nails (koilonychia) in advanced disease. Pica.

▶ Diagnosis

Anisocytosis (increased RDW), decreased MCV, mean corpuscular hemoglobin (MCH), MCH concentration (MCHC). Central red cell pallor. Thrombocytosis. Low serum ferritin (< 12 µg/dL). Decreased serum iron (< 60); increased total iron-binding capacity (TIBC)

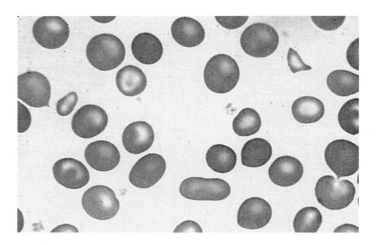

Figure 5–3. Iron deficiency anemia demonstrates microcytosis and anisocytosis.

(> 360). Marrow not usually needed, but iron stores absent or severely reduced.

► Treatment Steps

1. Find the source of iron loss and correct.
2. Supplement with oral iron daily for 6–12 months.
3. Parenteral iron for special circumstances (e.g., patient unable to tolerate oral iron).
4. Check reticulocyte count in 5–10 days (to assess response).

E. Nutritional Deficiencies: Pernicious, Other Megaloblastic Anemias

1. General

► Description

A **macrocytic** nutritional anemia (with **pancytopenia**) due to impaired deoxyribonucleic acid (DNA) synthesis. Etiology usually **cobalamin (vitamin B$_{12}$) or folate deficiency,** drugs.

► Symptoms

Of anemia; neurologic changes in cobalamin and folate deficiency.

► Diagnosis

Macro-ovalocytic anemia, leukopenia, thrombocytopenia; increased bilirubin, iron, and iron saturation; decreased haptoglobin and uric acid. Increased RDW and MCV. **Hypersegmented** polys. **Increased** lactate dehydrogenase (LDH).

    Marrow biopsy needed to rule out myelodysplastic syndrome, hematologic malignancy. **Nuclear–cytoplasmic asynchrony** (mature cytoplasm, immature nucleus). Marrow very cellular; increased mitotic figures; decreased M:E ratio (1:1); megaloblastic changes in erythrocytic and granulocytic series (see Fig. 5–4).

► Pathology

Impaired DNA, but normal ribonucleic acid (RNA) synthesis leads to **ineffective erythropoiesis** and nonimmune **hemolysis.**

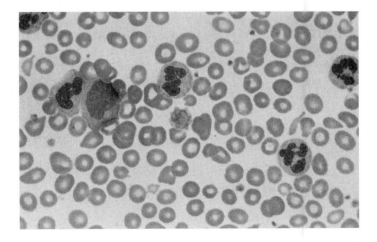

Figure 5–4. Megaloblastic anemia—the characteristic findings in a peripheral blood smear in megaloblastic anemia are hypersegmentation of neutrophils, macro-ovalocytes, schistocytes, teardrop cells, and giant platelets. The hypersegmented neutrophils have six or more nuclear lobes.

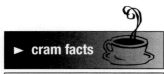

NEUROLOGIC SYMPTOMS IN B_{12} DEFICIENCY

Neurologic symptoms can precede anemia:

- Symmetric paresthesias in feet and fingers
- Disturbed proprioception and vibratory sense
- Irritability
- Somnolence
- Abnormal taste or smell
- Central scotomas (vision)

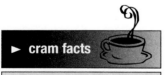

► **cram facts**

Folate supplementation is important in pregnant women. It is thought that folate deficiency may increase the incidence of neural tube defects.

2. Cobalamin (B_{12}) Deficiency

► Description

Usually pernicious anemia, rarely dietary deficiency, gastrectomy, pancreatic disease, blind loop syndrome. Takes several years to develop.

► Symptoms

Of **anemia. Neurologic symptoms:** See Cram Facts.

► Diagnosis

Decreased serum cobalamin. Responds within hours to cobalamin therapy. Folate usually increased. (Increased serum and urine methylmalonic acid and homocysteine, but not routinely measured.)

3. Pernicious Anemia

► Description

A **gastric atrophy** condition, autoimmune, leading to **decreased intrinsic factor** (IF) and cobalamin deficiency. Typically in older, fair-skinned, northern Europeans. Blocking and binding anti-IF antibodies.

► Diagnosis

Presence of antiparietal cell antibodies in serum. **Achlorhydria after histamine stimulation.** Decreased cobalamin absorption (**Schilling test** = decreased urinary excretion of [^{657}Co]cyanocobalamin in 24 hours, corrected by oral IF).

► Treatment Steps

1. **Cobalamin** to replete the normal stores and to provide daily need for life. 1,000 micrograms IM daily for 1 week; two times per week for 4 more weeks; then **monthly for life.**
2. Must also give iron if deficient. Folate given alone may worsen neurologic picture.

4. Folate Deficiency

► Description

Usually a dietary deficiency of folic acid. Folic acid is found in green vegetables, liver, kidney, yeast, mushrooms. Takes 4 months to become deficient. Causes include

- *Inadequate diet*—as in chronic alcohol use
- *Malabsorption (sprue)*
- *Phenytoin*
- *Oral contraceptives*
- *Pregnancy*
- *Chronic hemolytic anemias*
- *Altered folate metabolism—alcohol, methotrexate, 5-FU*

► Diagnosis

Decreased serum folate; response to therapy; history of precipitating factors.

► Treatment Steps

Folic acid, 1 mg PO daily (4–5 weeks to replace stores). Patients with chronic hemolysis may require more.

F. Hemolytic Anemias: General

► **Description**

Premature destruction of red cells due to **defective red cells,** or **toxic factors.** Can be intravascular or extravascular (more common)—cells sequestered by liver or spleen and destroyed.

► **Symptoms**

Of anemia, jaundice, pallor, splenomegaly.

► **Diagnosis**

Reticulocytosis, polychromatophilia, marrow hyperplasia; increased indirect bilirubin, LDH, free hemoglobin, urine hemosiderin and hemoglobin.

G. Hemolytic Anemias: Immune Hemolysis

1. General

Binding of antibodies and/or complement to RBC membrane. *Two types:* Immunoglobulin M (IgM)—agglutinating and work at colder temperatures; and immunoglobulin G (IgG)—nonagglutinating and work at 37°C. The **direct Coombs'** (direct antiglobulin) test detects immunoproteins on the **membrane** and is positive in nearly all immunohemolytic disorders. The **indirect Coombs'** (indirect antiglobulin) test detects serum antibodies (see Fig. 5–5).

2. Autoimmune Hemolytic Anemia (AIHA) Due to IgG Warm Antibodies

► **Description**

Anemia that may be secondary to underlying neoplastic or collagen vascular disease. Symptoms of anemia and underlying disorder.

► **Diagnosis**

Variable anemia, increased MCV, occasionally decreased WBCs and platelets. Spherocytosis, rouleaux formation, anisocytosis, reticulocytosis. **Positive direct Coombs'.**

► **Treatment Steps**

1. **Treat the underlying disorder.**

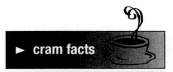

► cram facts

AUTOIMMUNE HEMOLYSIS

- Women > men
- Midlife
- 50% idiopathic
- 50% associated with:
  - Drugs
  - Other autoimmune disorders (i.e., systemic lupus erythematosus [SLE])
  - Evans syndrome (hemolytic anemia and immune thrombocytopenic purpura)
  - B-cell lymphoma
  - Chronic lymphocytic leukemia

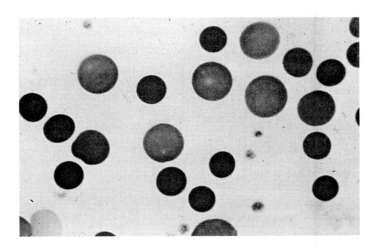

Figure 5–5. Autoimmune hemolytic anemia demonstrates spherocytosis and reticulocytosis.

2. If hemolysis mild, no treatment. If severe, **glucocorticoids.** 75% obtain control with steroids.
3. IV **gamma globulin.**
4. **Immunosuppressive drugs.**
5. **Splenectomy.**
6. **Transfusion** anytime if necessary to stabilize hemodynamics.

3. Autoimmune Hemolytic Anemia Due to Cold-Reacting Antibodies

3–1. Cold-Agglutinin Disease

▶ Description

IgM cold agglutinins are increased by **infection** (mycoplasma, Epstein–Barr, trypanasomiasis, malaria), but only rarely cause hemolysis. **Lymphomas** (especially B-cell lymphoma). **Idiopathic** in some elderly.

▶ Symptoms

Mild if from infection, worse if idiopathic or from lymphoma. Hemoglobinuria with severe chilling.

▶ Diagnosis

Jaundice. Anticoagulated blood clumps. Warming to 37°C corrects. **Positive cold agglutinin titer and direct Coombs'.**

▶ Treatment Steps
1. **Treat underlying disorder.**
2. **Avoid cold.**
3. Transfuse if necessary with blood warmer.
4. Plasma exchange in critical situations.
5. Steroids/splenectomy no value.

3–2. Paroxysmal Cold Hemoglobinuria (Donath–Landsteiner Hemolytic Anemia)

Rare. Transient. Caused by **IgG** cold-reacting antibodies. In syphilis, infectious mononucleosis, measles, and mumps.

3–3. Drug Mechanisms

- Hapten-type **drug binds to red cell (penicillin).**
- Immune complex type complement-fixing antibodies against drug-protein complex on cell surface (sulfonamides, phenothiazines, quinine, quinidine).
- α-**Methyldopa–type** antibodies against altered cell membrane. Positive direct Coombs' (α-methyldopa, levodopa, mefenamic acid). Treat by stopping drug.

3–4. Paroxysmal Nocturnal Hemoglobinuria (PNH)

▶ Description

Rare acquired disorder of an intrinsic membrane protein which acts as an anchor for other membrane proteins, thereby predisposing to complement-mediated membrane damage. May develop **aplastic anemia** or **acute leukemia.** Most die within 10 years, usually from thrombotic events, some with aplastic anemia or acute myelogenous leukemia.

► Symptoms

Pallor, jaundice. **Veno-occlusive events.** Abdominal/back pain.

► Diagnosis

Chronic hemolysis, **hemoglobinuria after periods of sleep,** variable pancytopenia. Increased LDH and decreased to absent haptoglobin. Hemosiderinuria. **Ham's test (more specific), sucrose hemolysis test.** Decreased to absent iron stores.

► Treatment Steps

1. Correct anemia with glucocorticoids, folate, iron, and transfusion.
2. Treat and prevent thrombosis.
3. Bone marrow transplantation.

H. Hemolytic Anemias: Nonimmune

1. Glucose-6-Phosphate Dehydrogenase (G6PD) Deficiency

► Description

Enzyme deficiency leading to hemolysis. The G6PD deficiency decreases production of glutathione. Precipitating causes of acute hemolysis; infection of fava beans or certain medications can precipitate hemolysis (see Cram Facts).

► Symptoms

Acute intravascular hemolysis with jaundice 1–3 days after exposure. Abdominal and back pain. Symptoms of anemia. Occasional renal failure.

► Diagnosis

Hemoglobinemia, hemoglobinuria, jaundice, **Heinz bodies,** increased RBC methemoglobin. Can **assay enzyme levels.**

► Pathology

Oxidation of hemoglobin produces **methemoglobin,** with characteristic Heinz bodies (denatured hemoglobin), which lead to red cell fragility and splenic "bites."

► Treatment Steps

1. **Avoid offending agents.**
2. Support with pRBC transfusion.

2. Hemoglobinopathies

2–1. General Structure

Hemoglobin is **tetramer of globin polypeptide chains** (a pair of "α-like" and pair of "non-α" chains). Adult Hb is hemoglobin A ($\alpha_2 \beta_2$), and hemoglobin A$_2$ ($\alpha_2 \delta_2$). Fetal Hb is Hb F ($\alpha_2 \gamma_2$).

► Symptoms

Symptoms vary depending on particular hemoglobinopathy, ranging from mild anemia to chronic cyanosis, constant fatigue, and intrauterine death.

► Diagnosis

• With high oxygen affinity hemoglobins—cyanosis with normal Po$_2$.

• With methemoglobin level > 30%—chocolate brown serum.

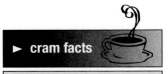

► **cram facts**

DRUGS THAT CAUSE HEMOLYSIS IN G6PD DEFICIENCY

Antimalarials:
• Primaquine
• Pamaquine
• Dapsone

Sulfonamides:
• Sulfamethoxazole

Nitrofurantion

Analgesics:
• Acetanilid

Miscellaneous:
• Vitamin K
• Doxorubicin
• Methylene blue
• Furazolidone
• Niridazole
• Phenazopyridine

▶ Pathology

Usually inherited; rarely acquired (toxin, neoplasms). Classification[1]:

a. **Structural hemoglobinopathies**—mutated amino acid sequences, as in
   (1) **Abnormal polymerization**—(hemoglobin S) see section H.3.
   (2) **Reduced solubility**—(unstable hemoglobin).
   (3) **Altered oxygen affinity**—two types:
      (a) Increased oxygen affinity (e.g., Hb Zurich).
      (b) Decreased oxygen affinity (e.g., Hb Kansee).
   (4) **M hemoglobins—(methemoglobinemia).**
b. **Thalassemias**—see sections H.2–2 and 2–3.
c. **Hereditary persistence of hemoglobin F.**
d. **Acquired hemoglobinopathies**—methemoglobinemia.

▶ Description

Oxidation of hemoglobin from ferrous (Fe^{++}) to ferric (Fe^{+++}) state, which doesn't transport oxygen. May be due to:

a. **Globin mutation** leading to methemoglobin formation (M hemoglobin).
b. **Methemoglobin reductase deficiency** (very rare).
c. **"Toxic" oxidation to methemoglobinemia** by foreign substances (acetanilid, phenacetin, nitrites, aniline, and many others).

▶ Treatment Steps

1. M hemoglobin: No treatment.
2. Reductase deficiencies: Oral methylene blue (1 mg/kg IV in emergency situations or orally if milder), or ascorbic acid.

2–2. Thalassemia

Hypochromic, microcytic hemolytic anemia due to defective globin synthesis, leading to **unbalanced production** of α or β chains. Thalassemia trait believed to be protective against malaria (see Fig. 5–6).

▶ Description

Defective β-globin synthesis can be severe—thalassemia major, moderate—thalassemia intermedia, or very mild—thalassemia trait. **Defective α-globin synthesis** also has variations depending on the number of genes deleted (mild—1 or 2, moderate—3, not compatible with life ex utero—4)

▶ Symptoms

In those patients with severe defects or multiple gene deletions they may appear normal at birth but by 6 to 9 months have severe anemia, failure to thrive, hepatosplenomegaly, and bone changes secondary to expanding marrow. Mild to moderate defects are generally asymptomatic, manifesting only as a mild to moderate microcytic anemia.

▶ Diagnosis

In severe disease, **thalassemia major,** the hemoglobin is 3–6 g. There is severe microcytosis, hypochromia, and cell fragmentation (see Fig. 5–7). Thalassemia trait is usually found in both parents. In the patient, if β-thalassemia, there is low or absent Hb A, large amount of Hb F, and increased Hb A_2 of 4–10%. Fetal DNA analysis from chori-

---

[1] Benz EJ Jr. Classification and basic pathophysiology of the hemoglobinopathies. In: Wyngaarden JB, Smith LH, Bennett JC, eds. *Cecil Textbook of Medicine.* 19th ed. Philadelphia, PA: WB Saunders, 1992: Classification of Hemoglobinopathies: Table 136-2, p 878.

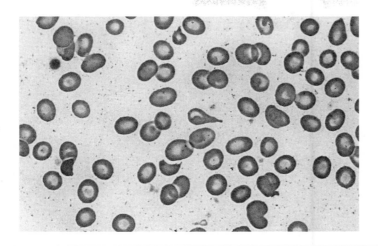

Figure 5–6. Thalassemia is caused by an excessive production of one of the globin chains. In peripheral blood smears, there is an increase in the number of microcytic red blood cells; target cells, which exhibit a dense zone of hemoglobin in the red blood cell center surrounded by a zone of pallor; teardrop cells; and schistocytes, fragmented red blood cells.

onic villus biopsy (early pregnancy), or amniotic fluid (later pregnancy) allows option of therapeutic abortion.

► Pathology

Ineffective erythropoiesis leads to severe anemia, hypercellular marrow, osteoporosis, compression fractures.

► Treatment Steps

1. **Transfusion** to keep Hb > 9 g/dL.
2. **Iron chelation** to prevent iron overload—start early.
3. Administer Pneumovax, penicillin prophylaxis, and folate supplementation.
4. **Splenectomy**—delay until 5–6 years old if necessary because of high transfusion needs.
5. In thalassemia intermedia or with mild α-thalassemia, treatment is not always needed unless other issues arise, such as iron deficiency, pregnancy, or other sources of blood loss. Some patients with thalassemia intermedia do require transfusion if their ane-

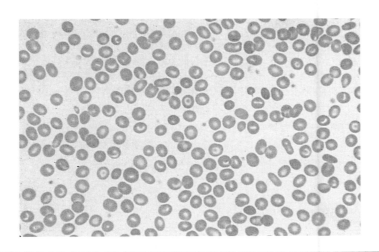

Figure 5–7. β-Thalassemia intermedia demonstrates microcytosis without anisocytosis.

mia is more significant, and can develop hemochromatosis, Organ damage from iron overload generally occurs later but should be monitored as this is a preventable complication.

3. Sickle Cell Anemia

▶ **Description**

Hemolytic anemia with red cells assuming characteristic **sickle cell shapes (drepanocytes)** due to abnormal β globin subunit of adult hemoglobin β chain of Hb S ($\alpha_2\beta^s_2$) (see Fig. 5–8). Associated with other abnormal hemoglobins. People of African descent, but also in those around the Mediterranean, Saudi Arabians, Indians. May be malaria protective. In the United States, trait in 8–10% of blacks.

▶ **Pathology**

Aggregation or polymerization of hemoglobin S molecules, leading to **gel state** when in the deoxy conformation (reversible, to a point), chronic hemolysis, tissue damage, and **acute painful vaso-occlusive crises.**

▶ **Symptoms**

Sickle cell trait. **Asymptomatic. Not anemic.** If anemia present, search for *other* causes.

Sickle cell anemia. **Chronic compensated hemolytic anemia.** Hb 6.5–10 g. Retics 10–25%. Mild jaundice. Increased indirect bilirubin. **Vaso-occlusive crisis** (pain in back, chest, extremities) precipitated by infection, dehydration, acidosis, hypoxia. Can see cerebrovascular accident (CVA), seizures, pulmonary infarction, priapism. Occasional **hypoplastic** or **aplastic crisis,** especially with infection (parvovirus B$_{19}$). **Megaloblastic crisis** due to folate deficiency. Aseptic necrosis of hip.

Sickle/β-thalassemia and **sickle cell** anemia less severe, less sickling. Fewer vaso-occlusive events. (More eye complications, aseptic necrosis of femoral head in sickle cell anemia.)

Splenic sequestration crisis. Seen in children who still have an enlarged spleen. Uncontrolled hemorrhage into the spleen.

▶ **Diagnosis**

Screening: **sickle cell prep** (sodium metabisulfate) or **solubility test. Hemoglobin electrophoresis** for precise diagnosis (may need special

---

▶ **differential diagnosis**

Patient with sickle cell anemia and pain. Consider:

1. Vaso-occlusive crisis
2. Acute chest syndrome
3. Sequestration crisis
4. Aplastic crisis

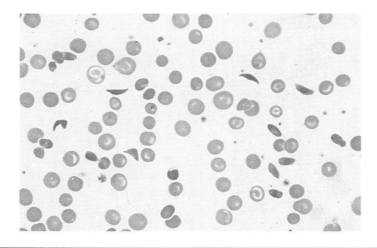

Figure 5–8. Homozygous hemoglobin S disease (sickle cell anemia), demonstrates sickled cells and microcytosis.

electrophoresis). May be diagnosed at birth with screening hemoglobin electrophoresis.

► Treatment Steps
Prevention. Genetic counseling. Prenatal diagnosis with fetal DNA analysis.

In childhood:
1. Prophylactic Pen VK.
2. Immunizations critical—usual ones plus *Haemophilus influenza* and pneumoccal.
3. Consider chronic transfusions.

Vaso-occlusive crisis:
1. Analgesics—oral if possible, morphine IV if necessary. Avoid Demerol.
2. Identify and treat infections.
3. Oral and IV fluids.
4. Oxygen if hypoxic.
5. Consider hydroxyurea or hypertransfusion if frequent.

Aplastic crisis:
1. Early recognition by checking reticulocyte count (should be elevated in sickle cell disease).
2. Transfuse.

Splenic sequestration:
1. Treat as any significant bleed.
2. Last resort—resect.

4. Hereditary Spherocytosis

► Description
Inherited hemolytic anemia with **increased osmotic fragility. Autosomal dominant** in 75%. Instability of the red cell membrane.

► Symptoms
Anemia, jaundice, splenomegaly. Hemolysis at all ages; worsened with some infections (mono) and intense physical activity. **Crises: hemolytic** (mild). **Aplastic** (severe)—frequently caused by human parvovirus. **Megaloblastic** (with pregnancy)—maintenance folic acid. Gallstones (bilirubin), gout, ankle ulcers.

► Diagnosis
Reticulocytosis. Microspherocytosis. Incubated osmotic fragility test.

► Treatment Steps
1. **Splenectomy** for anemia or significant hemolysis; defer until age 6 to 7 because of sepsis potential.
2. Pneumococcal vaccine.

5. Hereditary Elliptocytosis
A spherocytosis variant with autosomal dominant inheritance and membrane skeleton defect. Several types exist.

6. Other Nonimmune Hemolytic Disorders
1. **Hypersplenism**—excessive trapping and destroying of even normal (nonsenescent) RBCs by an **enlarged spleen of any cause.** Cytopenias correlate poorly with spleen size.

2. **Chemicals**—inorganic cations (arsenic, copper), organic substances (e.g., chloroamine from water purification with alum and chlorine), amphotericin B. Toxins from *Clostridium welchii,* spiders, snake venom.

3. **Metabolic abnormalities**—spur cell hemolytic anemia: in severe liver disease with poor prognosis.

4. **Red cell parasites**
   a. **Malaria**—especially *Plasmodium* species. A major cause of hemolysis worldwide. Splenomegaly, fevers (see Chapter 9).
   b. **Babesiosis.** Protozoans in red cells. Thrombocytopenia, disseminated intravascular coagulation (DIC). Deer tick vector. More common in northeastern United States. Coinfection with Lyme disease is possible.
   c. **Bartonellosis.** *Bartonella bacilliformis.* South America. Sand fly vector. Fever, chills, headache, musculoskeletal pain. Hemolysis. Responds to antibiotics.

5. **Trauma to red cells** (e.g., dialysis, pheresis, cardiac bypass).

6. **March hemoglobinuria**—seen with marching, running, other repetitive contact (karate). See hemoglobinemia and hemoglobinuria.

7. **Fragmentational hemolysis**—due to cardiac or large vessel abnormality. Usually **left side of heart** etiology; *mild* hemolysis from severe aortic stenosis (AS) or aortic insufficiency (AI), ruptured sinus of Valsalva, traumatic arteriovenous fistula, aortofemoral bypass surgery. More *severe* hemolysis from **prosthetic valves** (especially with aortic, artificial, metallic, defective, or poorly functioning valves).

► Diagnosis

Increasing anemia. Slight reticulocytosis, schistocytes. Chronic urinary iron loss (hemosiderin) may lead to iron deficiency. Elevated LDH, depressed haptoglobin.

► Treatment Steps

Based on specific etiology.

7. **Microangiopathic Hemolytic Disorders**
See also Chapter 2, section XVI.N.

► Description

Red cells are injured flowing through partially blocked channels. *Three main types:*

1. **Disseminated intravascular coagulation (DIC)**—Thrombocytopenia. Prolonged prothrombin time (PT), partial thromboplastin time (PTT), and thrombin time. Increased fibrin degradation products (FDP) and D-dimers. May be caused by gram-negative endotoxin-containing bacteria, amniotic fluid embolus, metastatic cancer, and HIV.

2. **Vascular lesions**—cavernous hemangioma, organ transplant undergoing rejection, malignant hypertension, eclampsia.

3. **Thrombotic thrombocytopenic purpura (TTP) and hemolytic–uremic syndrome** are characterized by hemolysis, thrombocytopenia, renal failure, fever, and neurologic changes.

► Diagnosis

Schistocytes, helmet cells. Hemolysis revealed as: increased indirect bilirubin and LDH, decreased haptoglobin, hemosiderinuria. Also, elevated reticulocyte count (see Fig. 5–9).

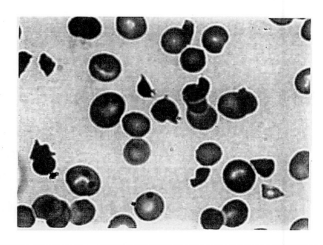

Figure 5–9. Peripheral smear of microangiopathic hemolytic anemia (MAHA) seen in TTP and hemolytic uremic syndrome (HUS). Demonstrates fragmented RBCs and reticulocytes. (Personal collection C.M. Clay, MD.)

► Treatment Steps
1. Treat the cause.
2. Steroids, fresh frozen plasma (FFP), and plasmapheresis for TTP.
3. Transfusion of blood products.
4. Rarely, anticoagulation with heparin may help.

I. Anemia Associated with Chronic Disease (ACD)

► Description
A very common condition in patients with chronic medical conditions. A usually **normocytic,** normochromic anemia, but often hypochromic and occasionally microcytic, seen with **chronic infection, inflammatory disease,** or **cancer.**

► Symptoms
Of anemia and the underlying disease.

► Diagnosis
Decreased iron, transferrin, and transferrin saturation (but usually > 10%). Normal or increased ferritin and marrow iron stores.

► Pathology
Impaired iron utilization, shortened RBC life span, mild hemolysis.

► Treatment Steps
1. Correct underlying problem.
2. Erythropoietin injections.
3. Additional iron supplementation should not be used.

J. Anemia Associated with Chronic Renal Insufficiency

► Description
Due to decreased erythropoietin production, but worsened by poor nutrition, blood loss, hemolysis.

► Diagnosis
Hemoglobin 5–8 g. MCV normal. Burr cells.

► Treatment Steps

Erythropoietin injections. Iron stores need to be adequate prior to starting erythropoietin. Intravenous iron is given in certain instances.

K. Aplastic Anemias, Pancytopenias

► Description

Marrow failure, which may be due to

Aplastic Process—Failure of stem cells to undergo differentiation.

Myelophthisic Process—Destruction of the marrow environment by invaders or inflammatory tissue. May see isolated deficiency (e.g., pure red cell aplasia [PRCA], agranulocytosis, thrombocytopenia).

► Symptoms

Bleeding (petechial, retinal), fatigue, pallor, infections.

► Diagnosis

Pancytopenia. Bone marrow biopsy. Ham test or sucrose hemolysis test (paroxysmal nocturnal hemoglobinuria); serum immunoglobulins (hypoglobulinemia); CT chest (thymoma). Must distinguish from leukemia, myelofibrosis, or myelodysplasia.

► Pathology

Peripheral pancytopenia and marrow replaced with fat. Pathogenesis:

1. **Idiopathic** (50%).
2. **Dose-dependent, drug-related** (cytotoxic drugs, phenytoin, phenothiazines, chloramphenicol, thiouracil).
3. **Idiosyncratic, drug related** (chloramphenicol).
4. **Environmental toxins** (solvents such as benzene; insecticides).
5. **Infections** (hepatitis, parvovirus).
6. Myelodysplastic syndromes.

► Treatment Steps

1. **Bone marrow transplantation.**
2. **Antilymphocyte globulin.**
3. **High-dose steroids.**
4. **Immunosuppressive therapy.**
5. **Androgens.**
6. **Red cell and platelet transfusions**—try to minimize if patient is transplant candidate.

L. Anemia Associated with Intestinal Parasites, Especially in Children

1. Hookworm

► Description

Hookworm disease is an infection by *Necator americanus* ("New World hookworm"), *Ancylostoma duodenale* ("Old World hookworm"), or *A. ceylonicum* (Far East). Adults live in upper part of small intestine. Each adult extracts 0.2 mL blood daily (equal to 0.1 mg iron).

► Symptoms

Erythematous maculopapular rash, edema, severe pruritus (especially around toes). Cough, pneumonia, fever if severe pulmonary involvement.

► Diagnosis

Iron deficiency anemia, hypoalbuminemia. In young children, may see severe anemia; cardiac insufficiency; anasarca; retarded physical, mental, and sexual development. **Hookworm eggs** in fecal smear. **Eosinophilia** (as high as 70–80%).

► Treatment Steps

1. Antihelmintic agents (mebendazole).
2. Iron replacement.
3. Transfusion.
4. Maintain good nutrition.

II. BLEEDING DISORDERS, COAGULOPATHIES, THROMBOCYTOPENIA

A. Mechanisms of Hemostasis

Normal hemostasis has three phases: vasoconstriction, platelet adhesion and aggregation, fibrin formation and stabilization; followed by clot destruction (fibrinolysis). Trauma → reflex constriction → platelet adhesion → release of tissue factor (TF) → activation of clotting cascade (TF VIIa activates factor X ["extrinsic pathway"] and IX ["intrinsic pathway"]). Various platelet factors are released to further aggregation (adenosine diphosphate [ADP], prostaglandin G_2, thromboxane A_2).

Pathologic hemostasis is activated in response to an abnormality in the:

Vessel Wall—e.g., atherosclerosis.

Platelets—e.g., myeloproliferative disorder.

Coagulation System—e.g., antithrombin III deficiency.

Infection—e.g., endotoxin.

Malignancy—e.g., pancreatic.

Diagnostic Tests—Platelet count, PT, PTT (with mixing studies), D-dimers, fibrin-split products, fibrinogen, antithrombin III, protein C, protein S, anticardiolipin antibodies, lupus-type inhibitor, factor V_{Leiden} mutation, and prothrombin gene mutation.

B. Platelet Disorders

1. General

► Description

Normal count 130,000–400,000 per mL. Megakaryocyte growth is stimulated by interleukin-6 (IL-6), granulocyte and macrophage colony-stimulating factor (GM-CSF), and thrombopoietin. Platelet circulation is 9 to 10 days. Spleen is usual site of destruction.

► Diagnosis/Testing

Platelet function tests: **bleeding time** reflects platelet and vascular components of coagulation; is normal in coagulation factor deficiencies (except von Willebrand's disease). Should not be routinely ordered because of poor reproducibility and poor correlation with clinically significant bleeding. **Platelet aggregometry** for congenital qualitative platelet disorders much more sensitive.

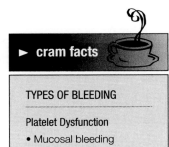

► cram facts

TYPES OF BLEEDING

Platelet Dysfunction

• Mucosal bleeding
• Petechial rash

Disseminated Intravascular Coagulation

• Mucosal bleeding
• All puncture wounds bleed
• Soft tissue

Factor VIII and IX Deficiency

• Soft tissue and joints

2. Abnormal Platelets—Mechanisms

Two major mechanisms for abnormal platelets: qualitative and quantitative (thrombocytopenia).

1. **Qualitative defect:** Platelets may be normal in number but do not function normally. Acquired qualitative defects include:
   - Medications (aspirin, clopidogrel [Plavix], nonsteroidal anti-inflammatory drugs [NSAIDs], heparin, penicillins, dipyridamole)
   - Uremia
   - Cirrhosis
   - Paraproteinemias (multiple myeloma, macroglobinemia)

   Hereditary qualitative defects include von Willebrand's disease.
2. **Quantitative defect:** Low platelet count (thrombocytopenia)
   - < 10,000—high risk for spontaneous bleeding
   - < 20,000—may have spontaneous bleeding
   - > 50,000—rare bleeding, even with major surgery (if platelet functioning normally)

3. Thrombocytopenia

Two major mechanisms for thrombocytopenia: decreased production and increased destruction.

Decreased production:
- Aplastic anemia.
- Bone marrow damage/suppression by alcohol, chemicals, drugs, radiation, viral infection.
- Marrow replacement by leukemia, metastatic disease, myelofibrosis.
- Ineffective thrombopoiesis.

Increased destruction:
- Immune (idiopathic thrombocytopenic purpura [ITP], platelet antibodies in systemic disorders).
- Nonimmune (DIC, TTP, hemolytic–uremic syndrome [HUS]).

3–1. Increased Destruction: Immune

a. Idiopathic Thrombocytopenic Purpura (ITP)

► Description

Autoimmune bleeding disorder with antibodies to one's platelets. In children there is usually an acute onset; seen after viral illness; 70% recover in 4–6 weeks. In adults it can be drug related (e.g., sulfas) but usually is more chronic; onset more gradual.

► Symptoms

Petechiae, ecchymoses, epistaxis, menorrhagia.

► Diagnosis

By exclusion of other disorders. Platelet antibody tests rarely helpful. Bone marrow exam usually shows increased megakaryocytes, but can be normal or have decreased megakaryocytes.

► Treatment Steps

1. **Observation.** If count > 50,000 and asymptomatic.
2. **Prednisone.**
3. **Intravenous gamma globulin.**
4. **WinRhoD.**
5. **Splenectomy.**
6. **Danazol.**
7. **Alkylating agents.**

b. Platelet Antibodies in Systemic Disorders

Cancer—lymphoproliferative disorders (chronic lymphocytic leukemia [CLL], lymphoma).

Systemic Autoimmune Disorders—SLE, rheumatoid arthritis.

Viral Illnesses—infectious mononucleosis, HIV, cytomegalovirus (CMV). HIV thrombocytopenia may be multifactorial—treat the HIV, avoid steroids, consider WinRhoD.

Drug-Induced Antibodies—many drugs implicated, but common ones are quinine, quinidine, sulfa drugs, hydrochlorothiazide (HCTZ), phenytoin, methyldopa, heparin (3–5% of heparin users), digitalis derivatives.

3–2. Increased Destruction: Nonimmune Disorders

a. Disseminated Intravascular Coagulation (DIC)
See section H.7–8.

b. Thrombotic Thrombocytopenic Purpura (TTP)
See Chapter 2.

c. Hemolytic Uremic Syndrome (HUS)

▶ Description
Thrombocytopenic and **hemolytic** syndrome with **renal failure,** usually in infants and young children. Often follows an infection (diarrhea in about 90% of cases, upper respiratory infection in 10%). Mitomycin is the drug most commonly associated with HUS.

▶ Diagnosis
Microangiopathic hemolytic anemia; mild to moderate thrombocytopenia; **prominent renal failure, severe hypertension,** no neurologic signs, fever less common.

▶ Pathology
Thrombosis and necrosis of intrarenal vessels.

▶ Treatment Steps
1. **Correct hypovolemia.**
2. Establish **diuresis.**
3. **Dialysis.**
4. Plasmapheresis.
5. FFP if pheresis not available.
6. Transfuse if needed.

4. Thrombocytosis
Two types:
- *Essential.* A myeloproliferative disorder (1–2 million platelets). Complications include thrombosis and/or bleeding. Also seen in early agnogenic myeloid metaplasia, polycythemia vera, chronic myelocytic leukemia.
- *Reactive.* In iron deficiency, hemorrhage, postsplenectomy, inflammatory bowel disease, leukemoid reactions. Platelets increase as an acute-phase reactant. No treatment needed.

5. Platelet Transfusions
For surgery, bring platelets to > 50,000 (> 90,000 if in central nervous system). Prefer single donor for each transfusion but inadequate supply, therefore often reserved for patients expected to need

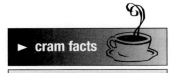

▶ cram facts

The most common pathogen in HUS is *E. coli* 0157:H7. Other pathogens include *Salmonella, Shigella, Yersinia,* and *Campylobacter.*

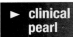

▶ clinical pearl

If antibiotics are used in the tretment of *E. coli* 0157:H7, they can increase the risk of acquiring HUS.

frequent platelet transfusions. One single donor pheresis equals 5 to 7 random donor units. On average, 1 unit random donor raises count 10,000.

C. Vascular Disorders

1. Congenital

1–1. Hereditary Hemorrhagic Telangiectasia (Rendu–Osler–Weber Disease)

► Description

The most common genetic cause of vascular bleeding; autosomal dominant.

► Symptoms

Epistaxis; telangiectases on face, mucous membranes, GI tract; serious GI bleeding, cerebrovascular accident.

► Treatment Steps

Can treat some lesions surgically or with laser.

1–2. Congenital: Cavernous Hemangioma (Kasabach–Merritt Syndrome)

► Diagnosis

Hemangioma with thrombocytopenia, mild DIC.

► Treatment Steps

Surgery, laser, radiation, induced thrombosis; may involute spontaneously. Choice depends on size and location of lesion.

2. Acquired

2–1. Scurvy

Vitamin C deficiency. Lower extremity, perifollicular bleeding.

2–2. Purpura with Immunoglobulin Disorders

Cryoglobulinemia; benign hyperglobulinemia (Waldenström's purpura may evolve into Sjögren syndrome or SLE); **amyloidosis** (periorbital hemorrhages); **Waldenström's macroglobulinemia** and **multiple myeloma; Henoch–Schönlein purpura** (a childhood vasculitis with purpura, arthralgias, abdominal pain).

D. Coagulation Disorders

1. General

Normal hemostasis requires interaction between blood vessels, platelets and monocytes, and coagulation factors. This activates the **coagulation cascade,** as shown in Figure 5–10.

2. Evaluation of Coagulation Disorders

History—family history; response to trauma; menstrual history; response to meds (especially aspirin); joint problems.

Lab—**complete blood count; bleeding time;** PT measures only **extrinsic** and common pathway; international normalized ratio (INR) standardizes values from various laboratories and reagent lots; **activated partial thromboplastin time** (aPTT) measures the **intrinsic and common pathway.** When doing PT and aPTT, mixing of normal and abnormal plasma is used to distinguish **defi-**

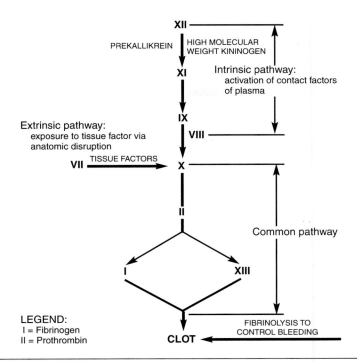

Figure 5–10. Evaluation of coagulation disorders. (Adapted from Mosher D. Disorders of blood coagulation. In: Wyngaarden JB, Smith LH, Bennett JC, eds. *Cecil Textbook of Medicine,* 19th ed. Philadelphia, PA: WB Saunders, 1992: Diagrams of interactions among coagulation factors: Figure 155-1, p 1001.)

ciencies of clotting factors from presence of **inhibitors.** Measuring specific coagulation factors.

3. Inherited Disorders of Blood Coagulation

3–1. Hemophilia A (Factor VIII Deficiency)

▶ Description

X-linked recessive inheritance. Of affected male: daughters will be carriers; sons will be normal. Of carrier female: 50% chance of producing a hemophiliac male or carrier daughter. Extreme lyonization can result in symptomatic heterozygous females.

▶ Symptoms

Level of factor VIII correlates with bleeding frequency. **Hematomas** in muscle or soft tissue (retroperitoneum). **Hemarthroses** (elbow, knee, ankle) may lead to crippling. Bleeding after surgery (must prep with factor VIII).

▶ Diagnosis

Factor VIII level < 5% and usually < 1% of normal. History of joint and soft tissue bleeding. Must distinguish from factor IX deficiency (hemophilia B), von Willebrand's disease. Have normal PT, abnormal aPTT. Factor VIII level.

▶ Treatment Steps

1. **Factor VIII**—Prophylactic infusion beginning in childhood significantly decreases bleeding and increases long-term function.

2. Physical activity counseling.

3. Acquired immune deficiency syndrome (AIDS) risk: Use of recombinant factor VIII has virtually eliminated new cases of HIV, but most older factor VIII–deficient patients have the infection.

3–2. von Willebrand's Disease

▶ **Description**

The **most common hereditary bleeding disorder,** due to deficient or abnormal von Willebrand's factor (vWf). Autosomal dominant. Types:

- I—decreased synthesis of vWf.
- IIa—synthesize only small multimers.
- IIb—synthesize only large, abnormal multimers.
- III—virtually absent vWf.
- Pseudo-vWd—abnormal affinity of platelets for plasma vWf.

▶ **Symptoms**

Variable. Usually superficial bleeding, epistaxis, easy bruising. Postop bleeding a major hazard; postdental extraction common. Menorrhagia.

▶ **Diagnosis**

Low levels of activated factor VIII (rarely < 5%, so bleeding generally mild); low level of immunoreactive vWf; long bleeding time. Abnormal platelet aggregation in response to ristocetin. Levels can be variable within the same person.

▶ **Treatment Steps**

1. Desmopressin (1-deamino-8-D-arginine vasopressin, DDAVP) is effective in type 1. Useless or harmful in IIa, IIb, and pseudo-vWD.
2. Replacement with single-donor cryoprecipitate (contains factors VIII and vWf).
3. Platelets in pseudo-vWD.
4. EACA (epsilon aminocaproic acid) useful addition to dental or minor surgery.

3–3. Hemophilia B (Factor IX Deficiency; Christmas Disease)

▶ **Description**

Similar to factor VIII deficiency with inheritance, with fewer symptoms, but with potential for severe bleeding.

▶ **Symptoms**

Similar symptoms as in hemophilia A.

▶ **Diagnosis**

Normal PT, prolonged aPTT. Factor IX level.

▶ **Treatment Steps**

1. Recombinant factor IX.
2. FFP.

4. Acquired Abnormalities of Blood Coagulation

4–1. Heparin

Heparin is a universally used anticoagulant for thromboembolic conditions. Regulate heparin anticoagulation with aPTT, aiming for 1.5–2 times control. Minimize bleeding complications by giving drug by continuous infusion, regular checking of aPTT, avoidance of use in patients with bleeding diathesis or occult bleeding site, avoidance of aspirin or IM injection. Low-molecular-weight heparin inhibits factor Xa with reduced thrombin inhibitory effect. Does not affect aPTT.

► **Treatment Steps**

If uncontrolled bleeding occurs, stop heparin, reverse with protamine.

4–2. Therapeutic Fibrinolysis (Thrombolysis)

Streptokinase, urokinase, alteplase (recombinant tissue plasminogen activator, rt-PA) are used in treating deep vein thrombosis, pulmonary embolus, acute myocardial infarction, peripheral arterial thromboembolism. May cause hemorrhage. Minimize bleeding complications by selecting appropriate patients, avoidance if bleeding disorder, recent GI or genitourinary (GU) bleed, severe hypertension, history of CVA, recent head trauma, major surgery or invasive procedure in last 2 weeks, or pregnant.

► **Treatment Steps**

1. **Pressure.**
2. **Discontinue drug.**
3. **FFP.**

4–3. Vitamin K Deficiency and Coumarin Anticoagulants

Normally adequate vitamin K in diet (green leafy vegetables). May be deficient in malabsorption states, bile-salt deficient states, poor dietary intake, and with use of antibiotics.

► **Diagnosis**
Increased PT.

> *Vitamin K Deficiency of Newborn*—Routinely give vitamin K (1 mg IM at delivery) to avoid hemorrhagic disease of the newborn.

> *Malabsorption Syndromes*—Vitamin K deficiency seen with impaired fat absorption (adult celiac disease, regional enteritis, cholestyramine or neomycin use, biliary tract obstruction).

► **Treatment Steps**
Daily PO vitamin K.

> *Antibiotics in Debilitated Patients*—Prevent with vitamin K.

> *Coumarin Anticoagulants*—Therapeutic level of PT INR varies from 1.8 to 3 depending on the indication. More bleeding seen at INR > 2.0. Requirement can change with diet (vitamin K intake) and drugs that affect warfarin. Avoid aspirin. (Avoid coumarin in pregnancy between 6th and 12th week and after the 38th week.)

► **Treatment Steps**

1. Vitamin K PO or SQ.
2. FFP.

> *Liver Disease*—Since the liver makes fibrinogen, plasminogen, vitamin K–dependent proteins, and antithrombin, bleeding is common with liver disease.

► **Diagnosis**
Hypofibrinogenemia; acquired dysfibrinogenemia; increased fibrinolysis; DIC.

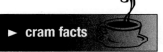

► **cram facts**

HYPERCOAGULABLE STATES

- Most common hypercoagulable state is pregnancy. Other commonly related processes are obesity, immobility, and malignancy (usually adenocarcinoma).
- Increasing numbers of defects in thrombosis regulation: protein C deficiency, protein S deficiency, antithrombin III deficiency, antiphospholipid antibodies (lupus inhibitors and anticardiolipin antibodies), factor V_{Leiden} mutation.
- Majority of thrombi now associated with some stimulus or defect.

► Treatment Steps

Normalize the PT, fibrinogen concentration, platelet count prior to high-risk procedures (give vitamin K, platelets, FFP). No treatment of DIC unless clinically significant bleeding treat the underlying disorder.

4–4. Renal Disease

Prolonged bleeding time. Platelet function abnormal; platelet count occasionally low.

► Treatment Steps

1. Correct the anemia.
2. DDAVP.
3. Platelets.

4–5. Factor VIII Inhibitors

Commonly seen in factor VIII deficiency (hemophilia A) or spontaneously in elderly patients.

► Treatment Steps

If patient is actively bleeding:

1. Increase doses of factor VIII if titer is < 5 Bethesda units (BU).
2. Plasmapheresis followed by factor VIII if titer is 5–30 BU.
3. If titer > 30, very hard to control; try porcine factor VIII or factor XI concentrate.

4–6. Lupus-Type Inhibitors (Antiphospholipid Antibodies)

Predispose to venous and arterial clotting.

4–7. DIC, Hypofibrinogenemia

Clinical types:

Compensated DIC—ongoing **thrombosis** and **fibrinolysis** in traumatized or inflamed tissues in chronic serious diseases. Normal PT, platelets, **increased fibrinogen.** No bleeding seen.

► Treatment Steps

May require long-term heparin or low-molecular-weight heparin (Trousseau syndrome of "migratory" arterial and/or venous thrombosis; underlying neoplasm). Coumadin often ineffective.

Defibrination Syndrome—massive release of tissue factor causing depletion of fibrinogen, other factors, leading to thrombosis and/or bleeding, low platelets and fibrinogen, increased FDP, increased PT. Seen with shock, sepsis (Waterhouse–Friderichsen syndrome in meningococcemia), cancer, burns, obstetric complications, rhabdomyolysis.

► Treatment Steps

1. Support with blood products as needed.
2. Treat underlying cause (i.e., evacuate the uterus).
3. Possibly heparin if poor response and thrombosis predominates.

Primary Fibrinolysis—primary release of plasminogen activator. Seen in cancer of prostate, acute promyelocytic leukemia (APML), hemangiomas, snake venoms.

► Symptoms

Diffuse bleeding.

► Diagnosis

Decreased fibrinogen, increased FDP, increased PT.

► Treatment Steps

1. In APML, treat with all-trans retinoic acid (ATRA) followed by standard chemotherapy.
2. Other causes: FFP, cryoprecipitate, and epsilon aminocaproic acid (EACA).

Microangiopathic Thrombocytopenia

► Description

Syndrome seen in sepsis, malignancy, immune complex disease, vasculitis, malignant hypertension, eclampsia (HELLP syndrome).

► Diagnosis

Low platelet count, fragmented RBCs, increased FDP, but PT and fibrinogen normal.

► Treatment Steps

In eclampsia: deliver. In other causes:

1. Treat underlying disorder.
2. Support with blood products.

Snake Bite—Venom contains toxic proteins and enzymes that cause tissue injuries.

► Treatment Steps

Antivenom, platelets, plasma.

Hemolytic–Uremic Syndrome—See Microangiopathic Hemolytic Disorders.

III. LEUKOPENIC DISORDERS, AGRANULOCYTOSIS

A. Neutropenia

► Description

Usual WBC 4–10 10^9/L (varies with ethnicity, sex, hormonal status). Neutropenia = neutrophils < 2.0 10^9 (in blacks < 1.5 10^9), but usually no clinical problems until < 1.0 10^9, and especially if < 0.5 10^9. Causes:

1. **Marrow failure**—many are drug induced.
2. **Marrow invasion**—by cancer, infection.
3. **Maturation arrest**—in folate or B_{12} deficiency.

► Symptoms

Range from asymptomatic to signs of severe infection. Signs of infection may be absent because WBCs mediate the inflammatory response.

► Diagnosis

Must distinguish primary versus secondary neutropenia. Vacuolization suggests infection. Bandemia > 20% suggests good marrow. Need bone marrow exam (aspiration and biopsy).

► Treatment Steps

1. **Determine the cause.**
2. **Antibiotics.**

3. **Glucocorticoids.**

4. **GM-CSF: colony-stimulating factor, granulocyte,** bone marrow transplant.

B. Lymphocytopenia

▶ Description

Causes:

1. **Decreased production**—protein-calorie malnutrition, radiation, immunosuppressive agents, congenital lymphocytopenic immunodeficiency states, viruses (measles, polio, varicella-zoster, HIV).

2. **Increased lymphocyte destruction**—from antilymphocyte antibodies, or in thoracic duct fistula, protein-losing enteropathy, severe congestive heart failure (CHF).

▶ Symptoms

Of the underlying condition.

▶ Treatment Steps

Treat underlying cause.

IV. NEOPLASTIC DISORDERS

A. Plasma Cell Disorders

1. General

▶ Description

Neoplastic or potentially neoplastic disorders with proliferation of **monoclonal plasma cells of B-cell series** producing **monoclonal gammopathies, paraproteinemias, dysproteinemias,** or **immunoglobulinopathies** due to secretion of **monoclonal proteins.** Each monoclonal protein is composed of two heavy and two light chains. Heavy chains include G, A, M, D, E. The light chains include kappa (κ) and lambda (λ).

▶ Diagnosis

Serum protein electrophoresis (SPEP) is good for screening, but **immunoelectrophoresis** is needed for confirmation. Do SPEP if multiple myeloma, macroglobulinemia, amyloidosis is suspected, and for unexplained weakness or fatigue, anemia, back pain, renal insufficiency, osteoporosis, osteolytic lesions, or spontaneous fracture. **Must distinguish monoclonal (usually neoplastic) from polyclonal (usually reactive or inflammatory) gammopathy.** Do serum **viscosity** for high globulins or if patient has blurred vision, mucosal bleeding, or other symptoms suggesting hyperviscosity. Urine: Do urine immunoelectrophoresis or immunofixation rather than Bence Jones. **Be aware that one can have negative urine protein test and electrophoresis, but have positive immunoelectrophoresis or immunofixation.** Rarely totally nonsecreting.

2. Monoclonal Gammopathy of Undetermined Significance (MGUS; Benign Monoclonal Gammopathy)

▶ Description

M-protein in serum **without evidence** of systemic disease. Significance: 25% go on to develop myeloma, macroglobulinemia, amyloidosis, or lymphoma.

139

HEMATOLOGY Neoplastic Disorders

► Diagnosis

M-protein < 3 g; < 5% plasma cells in marrow; insignificant M-proteinuria; **no lytic lesions or anemia, no hypercalcemia or renal insufficiency;** stable M-protein and no other abnormalities. Must distinguish from myeloma. **Follow-up of evolution** may be the only way to distinguish.

► Treatment Steps

Follow.

3. Multiple Myeloma

► Description

A neoplastic proliferation of **plasma cells producing a monoclonal immunoglobulin.**

► Symptoms

Bone pain in back, chest; vertebral collapse. Weakness, fatigue; symptoms and signs of anemia, renal failure, hypercalcemia, amyloidosis.

► Diagnosis

The diagnosis of myeloma is made with these three criteria:

1. At least 10–15% of a bone marrow aspirate demonstrates plasma cells.
2. Radiographic survey demonstrating lytic lesions.
3. Monoclonal immunoglobulins in the urine or blood.

The monoclonal gammopathy most commonly seen is IgG, followed by IgA, which is usually diagnosed using SPEP. Less commonly, the monoclonal band (M-protein) is not seen on SPEP and urine protein electrophoresis is indicated. Overall, 99% of patients have M-protein in serum or urine at time of diagnosis. Other labs include elevated erythrocyte sedimentation rate (ESR), hypercalcemia, elevated alkaline phosphatase, proteinuria, and renal failure. β_2-Microglobulin level is associated with activity and progression of disease.

► Pathology

Renal involvement caused by "myeloma kidney," hypercalcemia, amyloidosis, hyperuricemia, acquired Fanconi syndrome, or light-chain deposition. Radiculopathy in thoracic and lumbosacral areas. **Myeloma variants** include **smoldering myeloma** and **plasma cell leukemia.**

► Treatment Steps

1. Can defer treating minimal disease.
2. Chemotherapy includes melphalan + prednisone, M2 protocol (melphalan, cyclophosphamide, carmustine [BCNU], vincristine, prednisone), or VAD (vincristine, adriamycin, decadron).
3. Transfusions and erythropoietin.

Treat until M-protein is stable in urine and serum, and no other evidence of disease. α-Interferon is of value in maintaining remission. *Refractory disease:* other chemotherapy combinations, bone marrow transplant, thalidomide.

Begin all stage 2 and 3 patients on prophylactic pamidronate to decrease risk of fracture; improves quality of life and survival.

Special complications include:

1. **Hypercalcemia**—hydration, bisphosphonates, prednisone, calcitonin, increased physical activity.

► **clinical pearl**

If a patient has a normal albumin but an elevated total protein level, SPEP will help diagnose what type of protein is causing the elevation. Asymptomatic multiple myeloma may be found in its earliest stages if SPEP is done.

2. **Renal failure**—allopurinol, hemodialysis if symptomatic, plasmapheresis.

3. **Lytic lesions in weight-bearing bones**—consider prophylactic orthopedic procedure.

4. **Pain**—liberal use of analgesics. Combine narcotics with NSAIDs. Radiation to painful spots. May be helped by bisphosphonates.

4. Waldenström's Macroglobulinemia

▶ Description

Production of large **monoclonal** IgM protein by abnormal proliferation of plasmacytoid lymphocytcs.

▶ Symptoms

Weakness, fatigue, bleeding, pallor; impaired vision, weight loss; **hepatosplenomegaly; lymphadenopathy;** neurologic symptoms (sensorimotor peripheral neuropathy); infection; CHF.

▶ Diagnosis

Normocytic, normochromic anemia; γ-globulin spike (IgM type on immunoelectrophoresis). About 75% have κ light chains. Bone marrow biopsy shows hypercellular marrow, **infiltrated with plasmacytoid lymphocytes.**

▶ Treatment Steps

1. Treat if anemic, if constitutional symptoms, hyperviscosity problems, or significant hepatosplenomegaly or lymphadenopathy.

2. **Chemotherapy** (chlorambucil [Leukeran]; M2 protocol; α_2-interferon).

3. **Transfusions** and erythropoietin.

4. **Plasmapheresis** for hyperviscosity.

5. Bone marrow transplant.

5. Hyperviscosity Syndrome

▶ Description

Syndrome of increased serum viscosity seen in Waldenström's macroglobulinemia, and occasionally in multiple myeloma.

▶ Symptoms

Occur if relative viscosity is > 4 centipoises (cp). Manifest by mucosal bleeding, retinal hemorrhages, papilledema, decreased vision, dizziness, headaches, coma, aggravation of CHF.

▶ Treatment Steps

1. **Plasmapheresis** until patient asymptomatic.

2. Treat underlying disorder.

6. Heavy-Chain Disease

▶ Description

Due to a monoclonal protein composed of only the heavy chain. There are γ, α, and μ types.

1. γ—**lymphoma-like illness. Results fair with cyclophosphamide, vincristine, and prednisone (CVP) chemotherapy.**

2. α—**the most common type. Common involvement of the GI tract. Poor prognosis. Some response to chemotherapy.**

3. μ—**seen in chronic lymphocytic leukemia or lymphoma. Bence Jones proteinuria in two thirds. Treat with steroids and alkylating agents.**

B. Polycythemia Rubra Vera; Other Cythemias, Including Eosinophilias

1. General
Must differentiate **relative polycythemia** (decreased plasma volume) from **absolute polycythemia** (increased red cell mass). Distinguish absolute from relative by measuring red cell mass (with ^{51}Cr-labeled RBCs) or plasma volume (with ^{125}I-albumin). Normal red cell mass is 30 ± 3 mL/kg in men, 27 ± 2 mL/kg in women. Normal hematocrit up to 54% in men, 48% in women.

2. Relative Polycythemia (also called Stress Polycythemia, Gaisbock Syndrome)

► Description
Consider relative polycythemia after ruling out dehydration, the most common cause of polycythemia.

► Diagnosis
Hypertensive, smoking, middle-aged male.

► Symptoms
May have no symptoms; risk of increased incidence of thromboembolic events.

► Pathology
Common factors are smoking and diuretics (in hypertensives).

► Treatment Steps
1. Discontinue smoking.
2. May need phlebotomy.
3. Use nondiuretic antihypertensives.

3. Absolute Polycythemia
May be secondary or primary.

3–1. Secondary Polycythemia
Two types: **Physiologically appropriate** response to tissue hypoxia. Increased erythropoietin. Seen in:
1. High altitude. Diagnosis: increase anterioposterior diameter of chest, ruddy cyanosis, engorged capillaries of skin, mucous membranes.
2. Cardiopulmonary disease. Right-to-left shunts, chronic obstructive pulmonary disease (COPD).
3. Alveolar hypoventilation (e.g., pickwickian syndrome).
4. Abnormalities of oxygen-hemoglobin dissociation curve. High oxygen–affinity hemoglobinopathies; hereditary methemoglobinemias; carbon monoxide exposure (smoking, industrial exposure).

Physiologically inappropriate.
1. Neoplasms and non-neoplastic renal disease. Neoplastic includes renal and adrenal cancer, cerebellar hemangioblastoma, hepatocellular carcinoma; non-neoplastic includes renal cysts and hydronephrosis. Increased erythropoietin production.
2. Drug-induced. Testosterone, adrenal corticosteroids.

► Symptoms
Ruddy cyanosis, headache, tinnitus, fullness in head and neck, lightheadedness; increased thrombotic events; epistaxis; upper GI (UGI) bleeding.

▶ Diagnosis

Serum erythropoietin. O_2 level to evaluate hypoxia. Computed tomography (CT) of abdomen and chest x-ray. Bone marrow biopsy with chromosomal analysis.

▶ Treatment Steps

1. In "inappropriate" group, phlebotomize to hematocrit < 50%.
2. In "appropriate" group, phlebotomy may do more harm, so aim for hematocrit < 60%.

3–2. Polycythemia Rubra Vera

▶ Description

Malignant proliferative disorder of **erythroid, myeloid, and megakaryocytic** elements of marrow leading to **increased red cell mass** and often to increased granulocytes and platelets in blood. Related to myeloproliferative disorders. If treated, median survival increased from 1 to 10 years. **Thrombosis** the major cause of death closely followed by infection.

▶ Symptoms

Headache, tinnitus, lightheadedness, vertigo, blurred vision. Thrombotic and hemorrhagic episodes (epistaxis, **easy bruising,** UGI bleeding). Increased incidence of peptic ulcer disease and pruritus. Severe pain in the feet and hands (erythromyalgia).

▶ Diagnosis

Splenomegaly in 75%. Hepatomegaly in 40%. Increased hemoglobin, hematocrit, red cell count. Low mean corpuscular volume (MCV). Low serum iron. Hematocrit is best guide to red cell mass (> 60% is very suggestive). Increased red cell mass (> 36 in men; > 32 in women). Increased WBCs, platelets, trending to higher levels and more immature forms later in disease. Increased numbers of basophils and eosinophils. **Increased leukocyte alkaline phosphatase, B_{12},** and lysozyme levels. **Normal O_2 saturation** (> 92%). Low or absent erythropoietin.

▶ Pathology

Hypochromic, microcytic cells. Leukocytosis to leukemoid picture. Often marked thrombocytosis (> 400,000). Marrow hyperplastic, panmyelosis, megakaryocytic hyperplasia. Absent iron stores.

▶ Treatment Steps

1. Phlebotomy to Hct < 45%.
2. Myelosuppression with hydroxyurea if < 70 years old, p^{32} if > 70 or with significant medical problems.

Comment: Phlebotomy alone associated with increased risk of thrombosis. Increased long-term risk of second malignancies.

3–3. Eosinophilic Syndromes

1. **Parasitic diseases**—especially multicellular helminthic parasites. Diagnosis: often three or more stool specimens needed to diagnose.
2. **Other infections**—allergic bronchopulmonary aspergillosis, coccidioidomycosis. Eosinophils depressed by bacterial and viral infections.
3. **Allergic diseases**—allergic rhinitis, asthma, hypersensitivity drug reaction, drug-induced interstitial nephritis.
4. **Myeloproliferative disease**—idiopathic hypereosinophilia syndrome. Treatment: steroids; chemotherapy.
5. **Neoplastic diseases**—eosinophilic leukemia; chronic myelocytic leukemia; occasionally in Hodgkin's disease; some carcinomas.

6. **Cutaneous diseases**—scabies, bullous pemphigoid, episodic angioedema with eosinophilia.
7. **Pulmonary eosinophilias**—see Pulmonary section.
8. **Gastrointestinal disease**—eosinophilic gastroenteritis; inflammatory bowel disease.
9. **Immunologic disease**—hypersensitivity vasculitis; allergic granulomatous angiitis (Churg–Strauss syndrome); some immunodeficiency syndromes (Wiskott–Aldrich syndrome, graft-versus-host disease).
10. **Other**—Dressler syndrome; chronic peritoneal dialysis; eosinophilia–myalgia syndrome secondary to contaminated L-tryptophan; Addison's disease; hypopituitarism.

C. Reactions to Transfusion of Blood Components

1. Acute Hemolytic Transfusion Reaction

▶ Description

Reaction occurs within minutes or hours of exposure. Intravascular destruction caused by complement activation. Extravascular destruction caused by antibodies without complement activation. Rare.

▶ Symptoms

Fever, chest pain, wheezing, back pain, hypotension, DIC, bleeding diathesis, renal impairment.

▶ Treatment Steps

1. **Discontinue transfusion.**
2. **Correct hypotension.**
3. **Control bleeding.**
4. **Prevent acute renal failure** (use IV fluids, mannitol, diuretics to maintain output at 100 cc/hr).
5. Follow blood bank protocol for returning unit and checking urine and serum.

2. Febrile Nonhemolytic Transfusion Reaction

▶ Description

Reaction occurs within minutes or hours of exposure. In 0.5% of transfusions, relatively common. Less common since most units of pRBCs are now filtered.

▶ Symptoms

Transient flushing, palpitations, tachycardia, cough, chest discomfort, neutropenia. Latent period of 15–60 minutes; then increased blood pressure, headache, chills, rigors.

▶ Pathology

Cytotoxic or agglutinating antibodies from prior transfusion, reacting to transfused WBCs.

▶ Treatment Steps

1. **Discontinue transfusion** and test for hemolysis.
2. Antipyretics.
3. WBC filter if not already done.

3. Acute Lung Injury

▶ Symptoms

Fever, chest pain, dyspnea, cyanosis, cough, blood-tinged sputum, hypoxemia. Resembles CHF, but noncardiogenic.

► Pathology

Anti–human lymphocyte antigen (HLA) antibody.

► Treatment Steps

1. **Respiratory support, mechanical ventilation.**
2. **Fluid replacement.**

4. Allergic Reactions

Urticaria and pruritus in approximately 1%. Is reaction of donor protein and patient immunoglobulin E (IgE). Is usually mild. Anaphylaxis very rare.

5. Hypervolemia

6. Bacterial Sepsis—Very rare.

7. Delayed Reactions

7–1. Delayed Hemolytic Transfusion Reaction

► Description

Reaction occurs days after exposure. Antibodies occur as anamnestic response. History of prior transfusion or pregnancy. Positive direct Coombs'.

7–2. Graft-versus-Host Disease

► Description

Reaction seen in immunocompromised patient or in patients getting treatment for lymphoma or leukemia, 4–30 days after transfusion.

► Symptoms

Fever, erythema, diarrhea, liver function test (LFT) abnormalities, pancytopenia. **Mortality 84%.**

► Pathology

T-lymphocyte mediated.

► Prevention

Pretransfusion irradiation of blood or components in high-risk patients.

7–3. Iron Overload

See Hemochromatosis.

7–4. Post-transfusion Purpura

► Description/Pathology

Thrombocytopenia 5–9 days after transfusion, caused by alloantibodies to platelet antigens.

► Treatment Steps

1. **Steroids.**
2. **IV gamma globulin.**
3. **Plasma/blood exchange.**

7–5. Transfusion-Transmitted Infection

a. Hepatitis

Hepatitis C most common, although excellent screening exists. Illness 7–8 weeks after transfusion; 50% of hepatitis C patients develop chronic hepatitis; 10–20% of these get **cirrhosis** or **hepatocellular carcinoma.** Aim for **prevention** with donor screening.

b. Retroviral Infection

Three percent of AIDS is from transfusion. Seven-year latency. Aim for **prevention** with donor screening. New cases extremely rare. Risk is about one case per million units of transfused packed red blood cells.

c. Cytomegalovirus (CMV)

Infection not serious if immunocompetent. Bone marrow recipients may be more severely affected and die; therefore, these patients should be tested and receive CMV-negative blood.

V. HEMOCHROMATOSIS (IRON-STORAGE DISEASE)

► Description

Primary ("idiopathic") hemochromatosis is a common autosomal recessive genetic disease in Europeans. Secondary hemochromatosis is seen in anemias with ineffective erythropoiesis, increased iron absorption, and multiple transfusions.

► Symptoms

Hepatomegaly, splenomegaly, **skin pigmentation,** weakness, lethargy, **chronic abdominal pain,** arthralgia, loss of libido, impotence. Atrial tachyarrhythmias, dilated cardiomyopathy, and congestive heart failure. Insulin-dependent diabetes mellitus. Cancer of liver occurs late.

► Diagnosis

Requires presence of these symptoms and signs, family history, index of suspicion, and **demonstration of iron overload** (saturated iron-binding capacity [60–100%], and high plasma ferritin level [> 300 μg/L in male, and > 200 in female]). **Liver biopsy is diagnostic.** The gene has been identified.

► Pathology

The excess iron stored as **hemosiderin** is damaging to the parenchymal tissue, and leads to **fibrosis and cirrhosis** (in liver) of the organ. Slate-gray skin. Testicular atrophy.

► Treatment Steps

1. Early detection so phlebotomies started before organ damage occurs.

2. Treat with weekly phlebotomy as needed to restore iron to normal in full-blown disease; then at 2- to 3-month intervals. Treatment increases 5-year survival from 18–92%.

3. In secondary hemochromatosis, treat with deferoxamine.

See also Chapter 4, section VI.A.2.

BIBLIOGRAPHY

Beutler E, et al. *Hematology.* New York: McGraw-Hill, 2000.

Hoffman R, et al. *Hematology: Basic Principles and Practice,* 4th ed. New York: Churchill Livingstone, 2000.

Mosher D. Disorders of blood coagulation. In: Wyngaarden JB, Smith LH, Bennett JC, eds. *Cecil Textbook of Medicine,* 22nd ed. Philadelphia: W.B. Saunders, 2004: Drugs and conditions that influence response to warfarin: Table 155-2, p 1014.

Oncology | 6

I. GENERAL

A. General Statistics

In 2002, more than 1,285,000 new cancer cases were diagnosed in the United States, with over 550,000 deaths—25% of all deaths. These numbers do not include the more than 1 million cases of basal and squamous cell cancers of the skin, 54,300 cases of breast carcinoma in situ, and 34,300 cases of melanoma in situ. Though the absolute numbers continue to increase yearly, the overall incidence and mortality rates have been declining steadily since 1992. For example, the incidence of male lung and bronchus cancer between 1992 and 1998 decreased by 2.4% per year. The incidence of female lung and bronchus cancer have been stable, but for women under 65 the rate decreased from 28.3/100,000 in 1991 to 22.7/100,000 in 1998. African-American males have shown the most dramatic deline in both incidence and mortality. Though the mortality rate for female lung cancer continues to rise, the rate of rise is slowing. For men, the three most common cancers remain prostate, lung and bronchus, and colon and rectum. For women they are breast, lung and bronchus, and colon and rectum. (*Source: CA Cancer J Clin* 2002;52:23–47)

B. Etiologic Factors

Multiple steps and factors are now known to exist. Carcinogens and cocarcinogens are acting with genetic assistance. Implicated agents include:

- **Chemicals** (e.g., chemotherapy for other malignancies or after immunosuppressive treatment in transplants).
- **Viruses** (e.g., human papillomavirus [HPV] and cervical cancer [CA]; human herpesvirus-8 and Kaposi's sarcoma).
- **Physical agents** (ionizing radiation, ultraviolet light).
- **Diet** (**high-fat, low-fiber,** and **low-calcium diet** [colon]).
- **High alcohol** (oral, breast).
- **Cocarcinogens (tobacco products are a major public health hazard.** One-third of cancer in United States and Europe is related to tobacco products).
- **Genetic** (via **oncogenes** [pieces of cellular deoxyribonucleic acid, or DNA, found in oncogenic retroviruses], **proto-oncogenes** [DNA sequences in normal cells related to oncogenes]). **Oncogenes:** Human genome has a set of genes (20–100 loci) called proto-oncogenes. The first studies were from viruses causing animal tumors. Retroviruses (ribonucleic acid [RNA] genes are copied into RNA by reverse transcriptase into the host). Retroviral oncogenes are misplaced copies of cellular genes acquired by a process known as transduction. May be tumorogenic because their usual controls were lost, or there may have been mutations. At least 78 proto-oncogenes have been identified in humans.

C. Histology

Cancer cells: **large, irregular, more numerous nuclei** with **increased mitotic figures.** Necrosis and hemorrhage (outgrow vascular supply). "Tumor blush" in angiograms. Carcinomas: epithelial origin. Sarcomas: mesenchymal origin.

D. Cytogenetics

Most common is **band deletion** or **reciprocal translocation** between two chromosomes. **Aneuploidy, addition, deletion, translocation.** Example: Philadelphia chromosome (Ph^1) in chronic myelocytic leukemia is classically a translocation.

E. Growth Kinetics

A particular "doubling time" is characteristic of particular tumors. Clinically detectable (1-cm) tumors have undergone 30 doublings to reach 10^9 cells. Ten further doublings will produce a lethal 1 kg of tumor.

F. Predicting Outcome

1. Staging

The TNM system (tumor, node, metastases) is generally used but is not always clinically useful (good in head and neck, breast, lungs, colon, not so good in lymphomas).

2. Other Determinants of Prognosis

Biologic characteristics of the tumor (e.g., DNA index, Ki67 index, S-phase); **host resistance; host-tumor interaction; toxic:therapeutic ratio; hormone receptors** (breast), **genetic mutations** (her-2).

G. Tumor Markers

See Cram Facts and section VI.

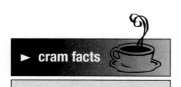

► cram facts

TUMOR MARKERS

- β-hCG: Testicular cancer
- AFP: Hepatocellular cancer
- CEA: Cancers of the GI tract
- PSA: Prostate cancer
- CA-125: Ovarian cancer
- CA 19-9: Colorectal/GI and pancreatic cancer

II. DETECTION AND SCREENING

See Table 6–1.

III. MANAGEMENT

A. General

Define therapeutic strategies, do periodic reassessment after diagnosis and staging, and share with patients and family. Consider physical, psychological, and social situation.

B. Therapeutic Modalities

1. Biological Response Modifiers: Modulation of Host Immune System

Interleukin-2 (IL-2) effective in renal cell CA. α-Interferon (α-IFN) prolongs remission in myeloma, used with IL-2 ± 5-fluorouracil (5-FU) in renal cell CA and in melanoma. Effective in **renal cell CA, malignant melanoma.**

2. Chemotherapy

a. Can be given orally, or injected into veins, arteries, and pleural, pericardial, peritoneal, or thecal spaces.

b. **Measuring responses:** complete (no measurable tumor) versus partial (50% reduction).

3. Surgery

The **primary therapeutic modality** for most early cancers.

6-1

SUMMARY OF AMERICAN CANCER SOCIETY RECOMMENDATIONS FOR THE EARLY DETECTION OF CANCER IN ASYMPTOMATIC PEOPLE[1]

Test or Procedure	Sex	Age	Frequency
Sigmoidoscopy, flexible	M & F	50 and over	Every 3–5 years
Fecal occult blood test	M & F	50 and over	Every year
Digital rectal examination	M & F	40 and over	Every year
Prostate-specific antigen	M	Normal risk: 50 and over	Every year
		High risk: 40 and over	Every year
Pap test	F	All women who are or who have been sexually active, or have reached 18, should have annual Pap and pelvic. After three or more consecutive satisfactory exams, the Pap may be done less often, at discretion of physician.	
Pelvic exam	F	18–40	Every 1–3 years
		Over 40	Every year
Endometrial tissue sample	F	At menopause, women at high risk*	
Breast self-exam	F	20 and over	Every month
Clinical breast exam	F	20–40	Every 3 years
		Over 40	Every year
Mammography	F	40–49	Every 1–2 years
		50 and over	Every year
Health counseling	M & F	Over 20	Every 3 years
Cancer checkup	M & F	Over 40	Every year

* History of infertility, obesity, failure to ovulate, abnormal uterine bleeding, or estrogen therapy. Screening mammography should begin by age 40. To include exam for cancers of thyroid, testicles, prostate, ovaries, lymph nodes, oral region, and skin.

[1] Levin B, Murphy GP. Revision in American Cancer Society recommendations for the early detection of colorectal cancer. *CA—A Cancer Journal for Clinicians.* 1992;42(5):296–299.

Updated recommendations:

- At age 50 screening colonoscopy, repeat every 10 years if normal.
- High risk for colorectal cancer (therefore, earlier and more frequent screening needed for ulcerative colitis, prior adenomas, prior history of colorectal cancer, familial syndromes (adenomatous polyposis, family history of colorectal cancer), history of female genital cancer, breast cancer, or prior radiation for cervical cancer.
- CEA is unsuitable for screening.

4. Radiation

Usually an adjuvant therapy but sometimes primary treatment for brain metastases, low-stage Hodgkin's, unresectable lung CA.

C. Supportive Care

Antibiotics, transfusions, antiemetics, anxiolytics.

D. Nutritional Problems

Reasons for anorexia and hypercatabolism include anatomical, dysphagia secondary to mucosal breakdown, paraneoplastic syndromes, chemotherapy, depression, secretion of peptides. **Improved nutrition** may permit use of chemotherapy (may require parenteral or tube feedings).

E. Hyperuricemia and Hyperuricosuria

In lymphocytic leukemia and lymphomas. Treat with **allopurinol** and **hydration.**

F. Deconditioning, Hypercalcemia, Fractures

1. Prevention: **Keep mobile.**
2. Use **bisphosphonates** prophylactically in myeloma and metastatic bone involvement.

G. Psychosocial Issues

Supportive family, physician, and staff. Support groups and individual therapy.

H. Pain Control

Liberal use of narcotics for severe generalized pain. **Radiotherapy.** Physical therapy. Acupuncture. Anti-inflammatories for bone pain. Strontium for blastic lesions. Epidural anesthetics.

I. Hospice and Home Care

Much preferred over continued hospitalization or nursing home for palliative and end-of-life care.

IV. EPIDEMIOLOGY AND PREVENTION

Great variation in incidence among countries, regions, and cultures within countries suggests environmental and genetic factors. Most cancers result from multiple exposures and susceptibility states.

A. Major Factors

1. Tobacco

The main hazard in Western countries. In lung, larynx, mouth, pharynx, esophagus, bladder, pancreas, kidney, and possibly **cervix.** Two packs per day leads to 20-fold increase in lung CA rate. Passive smoking is also carcinogenic.

2. Alcohol

Multiplies the effect of tobacco in CA of mouth, pharynx, esophagus, larynx. **Liver CA** in cirrhotics. Not carcinogenic alone. Increases risk of breast CA.

3. Solar Radiation

Skin CA (squamous and basal cell; melanoma).

4. Ionizing Radiation

Accounts for 3% of all CA. Mainly **breast, thyroid,** and **bone marrow.**

5. Occupational and Environmental Pollution Hazards
See Cram Facts.

6. Medication

Synthetic Estrogen—adenocarcinoma of **vagina** and **cervix** occurring several years later in daughters **exposed in utero to diethylstilbestrol.**

Oral Contraceptives—possible role in benign liver tumors. However, note **decreased risk** reported in endometrial and ovarian CA with **combined oral contraceptive.**

Alkylating Agents—acute myelogenous leukemia. **Immunosuppressives** such as azathioprine and corticosteroids in transplant patients: lymphoma.

7. Infectious Agents

Papillomavirus (HPV) and Herpesvirus—Cervical cancer.

Epstein–Barr (EBV)—Nasopharyngeal and Burkitt's lymphoma.

Hepatitis C—Hepatocellular cancer.

► cram facts

OCCUPATIONAL HAZARDS
AND CANCER

- Aromatic amines: Bladder cancer
- Arsenic: Lung, skin, liver cancer
- Asbestos: Malignant mesothelioma
- Benzene: Leukemia
- Mustard gas: Lung, larynx, and sinus cancer
- Vinyl chloride: Liver cancer

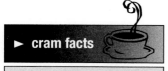

► cram facts

Unopposed estrogen (i.e., estrogen without progesterone) should never be given to a woman with an intact uterus because it increases the risk of endometrial cancer.

Human T-cell Leukemia Virus (HTLV-I)—Adult T-cell leukemia.

Human Immunodeficiency Virus (HIV)—Non-Hodgkin's lymphoma.

8. Nutrition

Fat—Colon and breast CA.

Fat and Caloric Excess—Endometrial CA.

Decreased Fiber—Colon CA.

Decreased Vitamin A, β-Carotene, and Selenium—Lung CA.

Decreased Fruits and Vegetables and Vitamin C—Stomach CA.

Increased Alcohol—Esophageal and breast CA.

Aflatoxin (from Fungus *Aspergillus flavus*)—Liver CA.

9. Genetic
Chinese: nasopharyngeal CA. Native Americans and **Hispanic** groups: gallbladder CA. **Caucasians:** skin CA. Autosomal dominant heredity: **retinoblastoma, polyposis coli.** Hereditary preneoplastic syndromes (neurofibromatosis leading to sarcomatous change, gliomas of brain and optic nerve, acoustic neuroma, meningioma, and acute leukemia).

B. Chemoprevention Trials Currently in Progress
Nonsteroidal anti-inflammatory drugs (NSAIDs) (colon and rectum); retinoids (oral cavity, lung, skin, breast, bladder).

V. PARANEOPLASTIC SYNDROMES

A. General
Syndromes due to **remote or biologic effects of proteins or hormones secreted by tumor.** Often improve after treatment of tumor.

B. Syndromes

1. Wasting of Host (Tumor Cachexia)
Most common paraneoplastic syndrome. Possibly multifactorial. Tumor necrosis factor (cachexin).

▶ **Treatment Steps**
Treat the malignancy; hyperalimentation if surgery planned or if hope of significant remission or cure with therapy.

2. Endocrine

2–1. Ectopic Adrenocorticotropic Hormone (ACTH)

▶ **Description**
Cushing's syndrome: about 50% from the lung. Adrenal tumors produce cortisol, but not ACTH. Increased production by cancer cells of pro-opiocortin (prohormone molecule of ACTH).

▶ **Symptoms**
Often subtle. Mild weakness, hypokalemia, psychosis, abnormal glucose tolerance curve.

ONCOLOGIC EMERGENCIES

Spinal Cord Compression
- Symptoms: Back pain in at-risk patient, bowel or bladder incontinence, loss of sphincter tone.
- Treatment: Steroids, radiation, surgical decompression.

Hypercalcemia
- Symptoms: Mental status changes, polyuria, constipation.
- Treatment: IV hydration (normal saline), loop diuretics (furosemide), IV bisphosphonates.

Tumor Lysis Syndrome
- Symptoms: Elevated uric acid, potassium, and phosphate cause hypocalcemia and renal failure in rapidly growing tumors.
- Treatment: Allopurinol, hydration with alkalinizatin of the urine, close monitoring of electrolytes, dialysis.

Cerebral Herniation
- Symptoms: Change in mental status, papillary edema.
- Treatment: Steroids, radiation, decompression.

► **Diagnosis**
Extremely high plasma ACTH that **does not suppress with dexamethasone.**

► **Treatment Steps**
1. Treat the malignancy.
2. If unable to treat CA, then try aminoglutethimide or metyrapone.

2–2. Hypercalcemia

► **Description**
Seen in solid tumors **(lung, breast, kidney, ovary),** and hematological disease **(multiple myeloma and adult T-cell lymphoma).** Mechanisms include release of osteoclast-activating factor, increased renal calcium absorption.

► **Symptoms**
Polyuria, constipation, lethargy, personality change.

► **Treatment Steps**
Acutely: Saline, loop diuretics (furosemide), IV bisphonates, glucocorticoids, calcitonin.

Chronically: Treat malignancy, mobilize patient, bisphosphonates, avoid dehydration.

2–3. Chorionic Gonadotropin
Cleared rapidly from serum; little clinical effect; rarely see gynecomastia.

2–4. Hypoglycemia
Most commonly in mesotheliomas, hepatic carcinomas, adrenal cortical carcinomas. Due to factors with insulin-like activity.

2–5. Growth Hormone and Growth Hormone-Releasing Hormone (GHRH)

Acromegaly in bronchial carcinoid or pancreatic islet cell tumor.

2–6. Calcitonin

Little or no biologic effect in normal adults, so no symptoms. **Good hormonal marker for medullary carcinoma of thyroid.**

2–7. Vasopressin

Causes syndrome of inappropriate antidiuretic hormone (SIADH). Seen in carcinoma of the lung.

2–8. Erythropoietin

Benign and malignant **renal conditions** (hypernephroma, renal cysts, hydronephrosis). Nonrenal conditions include hemangioblastomas, uterine fibromas, adrenal cortical neoplasms, ovarian neoplasms, hepatomas, pheochromocytomas.

3. Neurologic

Subacute cerebellar degeneration, subacute motor neuropathy, sensory neuropathy, Eaton–Lambert syndrome, dermatomyositis.

4. Hematologic

4–1. Erythrocytosis

From erythropoietin secretion, renal or liver tumors (see Endocrine section).

4–2. Leukemoid Reactions

From colony-stimulating factor (CSF) secretion. Also see granulocytosis (lung, gastric, pancreatic, brain, melanomas, lymphomas) or eosinophilia (lymphomas, Hodgkin's, gastrointestinal [GI] carcinomas).

4–3. Anemia

See differential diagnosis in margin.

4–4. Microangiopathic Hemolytic Anemia

In stomach, breast, lung cancers.

4–5. Granulocytopenia

Usually from chemotherapy, radiation therapy, infection, marrow involvement.

4–6. Idiopathic Thrombocytopenic Purpura (ITP)

In lymphomas.

5. Thromboembolic Paraneoplastic Syndromes

▶ **Description**

Hypercoagulable state. Three types:

  a. Migratory thrombophlebitis (Trousseau's syndrome). Usually GI neoplasm, but also lung, breast, ovarian, prostate.

▶ **Treatment Steps**

Difficult; may require long-term heparin or enoxaparin if warfarin doesn't work.

  b. Disseminated intravascular coagulation (DIC). **May be common and subclinical.**

▶ **differential diagnosis**

CHANGE IN MENTAL STATUS IN AN ONCOLOGY PATIENT

1. Metabolic— hypercalcemia, hypoglycemia, hyperkalemia
2. Neurologic—cerebral metastases with edema, cerebral thrombosis, cerebral hemorrhage
3. Pulmonary—hypoxia
4. Drug-related—opioids
5. Infection
6. Dehydration

▶ **differential diagnosis**

ANEMIA IN THE ONCOLOGY PATIENT

Anemia of Chronic Disease

• Normo- or microcytic
• Elevated ferritin, low total iron-binding capacity (TIBC)

Chemotherapy Related

• Cisplatin
• Hydroxyurea
• Cytarabine (Ara-C)

Hemolytic Anemia

• Immune mediated in chronic leukemias and low-grade lymphomas
• Microangiopathic secondary to mitomycin

Renal Insufficiency

• Obstruction by tumor
• Chemotherapy toxicity (i.e., cisplatinum)
• Tumor lysis (hyperproliferative state)

Iron Deficiency

• Chronic GI or genitourinary (GU) bleed

► Treatment Steps

Treat the tumor. May use heparin.

c. **Nonbacterial thrombotic endocarditis (marantic endocarditis).** Usually mucin-secreting adenocarcinomas. May embolize.

► Treatment Steps

Treat the tumor.

6. Renal
   a. SIADH.
   b. Nephrotic syndrome. Hodgkin's (lipoid nephrosis, minimal change glomerulopathy). Non-Hodgkin's lymphoma (immune complex).
   c. Myeloma and amyloid kidney.
   d. Hypokalemia. Myelogenous leukemia (lysozyme related).

7. Dermatologic
   Acanthosis nigricans (hyperkeratosis and pigmentation of axillae, neck, and groin), **dermatomyositis, flushing in carcinoid.** Leser–Trelat (sudden onset of seborrheic keratoses), porphyria cutanea tarda (photosensitive skin lesions), pruritus.

8. Gastrointestinal
   Protein-losing enteropathy, malignant hepatopathy.

9. Miscellaneous
   Fever (lymphomas, hypernephromas). **Lactic acidosis** (acute leukemias, lymphomas). **Hypokalemia and hypertension** (lung, hypernephroma, Wilms'). **Hypertrophic pulmonary osteoarthropathy** (lung, mesothelioma, other metastases to lung). **Amyloidosis** (myeloma, lymphoma, carcinomas). **Systemic lupus** (lymphomas, leukemias, thymomas, testicular, lung, ovarian).

VI. TUMOR MARKERS

Usefulness: screening, early detection, assessing **tumor burden** and **prognosis,** assessing **response to therapy,** evaluating **early recurrence. Examples:**

Hormones—β subunit of human chorionic gonadotropin (β-hCG): testicular cancer, choriocarcinomas, hydatidiform mole. The level assesses response to therapy. *Others:* Human placental lactogen, ACTH, vasopressin, calcitonin, gastrin-releasing peptide.

Oncofetal Proteins—α-Fetoprotein (AFP): hepatoma and testicular CA. The level has predictive value in follow-up.

Carcinoembryonic Antigen (CEA)—GI tract, breast, lung, ovarian tumors. Increased by smoking and inflammatory processes, so should not be used for screening. Used to assess response and recurrence (colon).

Immunoglobulins—myeloma and some other lymphoproliferative disorders; good for following response to treatment. Heavy chains and light chains in myeloma and Waldenström's macroglobulinemia.

Enzymes—**Prostatic acid phosphatase:** one-third of occult prostate and 75% of more advanced prostate cancer.

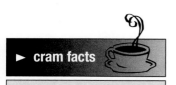

► cram facts

Marker for medullary cancer is calcitonin level. Thyroid lymphoma: use x-ray therapy. Largest percentage of thyroid cancer death is due to anaplastic CA. Risk of leukemia with increasing ^{131}I use.

Thyroglobulin level marker for recurrence of papillary cancer.

Tumor Antigens—**CA-125:** ovarian. **CA 19-9:** biliary. β_2 **Microglobulin** (a human leukocyte antigen [HLA] class I antigen): assessing response in myeloma therapy. **Prostate-specific antigen (PSA):** prostate. **CA 27-29:** breast.

VII. SPECIFIC TYPES OF NEOPLASTIC DISORDERS

A. Blood and Blood-Forming Organs

1. Hodgkin's Disease

▶ Description
Lymph node malignancy of centroblast (proliferating germinal center cell); average age 32; male more than female.

▶ Symptoms
Painless cervical or other **adenopathy.** Chest x-ray may show mediastinal mass, infiltrates, effusions. **Fever,** sometimes cyclic (Pel–Ebstein fever). **Night sweats. Pruritis.** Superior vena cava obstruction. Spinal cord compression. Hepatic and splenic enlargement. Infections (herpes zoster, cryptococcosis, *Pneumocystis carinii* pneumonia, toxoplasmosis). Immunologic abnormalities common.

▶ Diagnosis
Use computed tomography **(CT) of chest and abdomen, lymphangiography. Bilateral bone marrow biopsy** in all patients suspected of diffuse or bone disease. Gallium scans can be useful. (See Fig. 6–1.)

    Biospsy of an involved node, needle aspiration generally not adequate. CT of chest, abdomen, and pelvis. Lymphangiography less commonly used now. **Bilateral bone marrow biopsy** in patients suspected of diffuse or bone disease. Positron-emission tomography (PET) and gallium also helpful. (See Fig. 6–1.)

    Staging:
    I. Single lymph node or group.
    II. More than one node or group; same side of diaphragm.
    III. Spleen and nodes; both sides of diaphragm.
    IV. Liver or marrow.

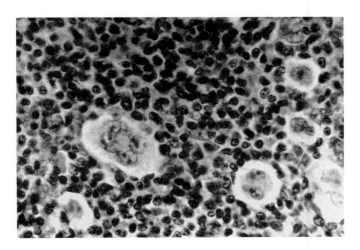

Figure 6–1. Hodgkin's disease—demonstrates lymphocytic background, Reed–Sternberg cells.

► B Symptoms

Fever > 38.5; night sweats; 10% weight loss over 6 months. A—absence of "B" symptoms. B—presence of 1 or more.

► Pathology

Anemia of chronic disease, but occasionally due to hypersplenism, marrow invasion, Coombs'-positive hemolytic anemia. Leukocytosis, eosinophilia. Pathognomonic **Reed–Sternberg cell** (large, bilobed cell with prominent eosinophilic nucleoli), is pathognomonic but not necessary as variants exists.

► Treatment Steps

Biopsy first. Staging before treatment. **Staging laparotomy (with splenectomy)** is not used as frequently but still has a place in staging. Treat with **radiotherapy:** 3,600 to 4,000 rads. Radiation alone initially in stage I. Stages IIA and IIIA either radiation or chemotherapy. **Chemotherapy:** in advanced (IIB, IIIB, and IV) disease. Standard is changing and could be ABVD (adriamycin, bleomycin, vinblastine, dacarbazine) or less commonly now MOPP (mechlorethamine, vincristine [oncovin], procarbazine, prednisone), four to six cycles. Radiation can be added to involved fields. Produces complete remission in 70–80%; disease free 10–20 years later in 50% of these. Greatly improved prognosis due to staging, radiotherapy, and chemotherapy advances.

2. Non-Hodgkin's Lymphoma

► Description

The largest group of immune system neoplasms, characterized by monoclonal proliferation of B or T lymphocytes. An immune dysfunction may contribute (e.g., acquired immune deficiency syndrome [AIDS]). Possible viral etiology in Burkitt's, adult T-cell leukemia.

► Symptoms

Similar to Hodgkin's.

► Diagnosis

Node pathology; B- and T-cell typing studies. Use CT of abdomen, pelvis, and chest. Immunoglobulins, bone scan, upper GI studies (UGI), bone marrow biopsies, PET scan, gallium scan.

► Pathology

Classifying systems: Rappaport Classification, Lukes and Collins, The NCI Working Formulation (1982), REAL classification.

► Treatment Steps

Depends on grade and stage. Modalities include multiagent **chemotherapy** (CHOP—cytoxan, adriamycin, vincristine, prednisone) or **combined chemo/irradiation,** and **immunotherapy** (rituxamab).

► Special Problems

Superior vena cava obstruction: chemotherapy or irradiate. Gastric lymphoma: resect. Central nervous system (CNS) disease: irradiate. Urate nephropathy: allopurinol to prevent, if severe may require dialysis support.

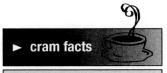

3. Acute Leukemia in Children

3–1. Acute Lymphoblastic Leukemia (ALL)

▶ **Description**

Malignant proliferation of lymphoid precursors, with replacement of normal cells; 75% of the 2,500 new acute leukemias.

▶ **Symptoms**

Pallor, fatigue, bleeding, fever, bone pain, adenopathy, arthralgias, hepatosplenomegaly.

▶ **Diagnosis**

Marrow **morphology, cytochemical staining, immunologic cell surface markers, cytogenetics.**

▶ **Pathology**

Marrow infiltrated or replaced with lymphoblasts.

▶ **Treatment Steps**

Cure rate 65–70%. **Multiple-drug chemotherapy** (prednisone, vincristine, doxorubicin, methotrexate, asparaginase) + **intrathecal chemotherapy** (methotrexate or cytarabine) or **cranial irradiation.** Because of high cure rate, no marrow transplant usually with first remission unless patient has poor prognostic factors, but is recommended after second remission.

3–2. Acute Myeloblastic Leukemia (AML)

▶ **Description**

Malignant proliferation of myelocytic precursors, with replacement of normal cells; 15–20% of acute leukemias.

▶ **Symptoms**

Similar. Usually sicker than patients with ALL.

▶ **Diagnosis**

Bone marrow biopsy.

▶ **Pathology**

Marrow infiltrated or replaced with myeloblasts (see Fig. 6–2).

▶ **cram facts**

LYMPHOMAS

Hodgkin's

- Bimodal age distribution
- Contiguous spread
- Very high cure rate
- Linked to EBV

Four basic types— nodular sclerosing (60–75%), mixed cellularity (20–35%), lymphocyte predominant (5–10%), lymphocyte depleted (2–5%)

Non-Hodgkin's

- Increasing frequency with age
- Variable spread
- Variable cure rates—most common types not curable
- Over 30 different types
- NCI working formulation: low grade, intermediate grade, high grade

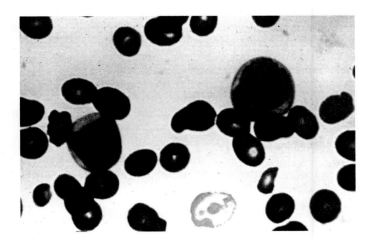

Figure 6–2. Acute myeloblastic leukemia—demonstrates myeloblasts: large nuclei, multiple nucleoli, scant cytoplasm.

▶ Treatment Steps

Intensive **chemotherapy** with daunorubicin and cytarabine, sometimes combined with other agents. **Intrathecal chemo** or **irradiation** in some cases. Produces 80% complete remission (CR) rate, 65% remain in continuous CR.

4. Acute Leukemia in Adults

▶ Description

Malignant unregulated proliferation of immature myeloid or lymphoid precursors, with replacement of normal cells. Inciting agents include ionizing radiation, oncogenic viruses, genetic and congenital factors, chemical agents.

▶ Symptoms

Anemia, hemorrhage, infection, leukemic infiltrates (bone pain, meningitis, mediastinal mass, chloromas), lymphadenopathy, splenomegaly.

▶ Diagnosis

Anemia, thrombocytopenia, and abnormal bone marrow. Immunohistochemical stains and flow cytometry. Must distinguish from infections, other cancers, drug effects.

▶ Pathology

Bone marrow: **morphologic, histochemical techniques, surface markers** (immunologic techniques), **cytoplasmic markers** (enzymes), chromosomal changes. Eighty percent are acute myelogenous leukemia (AML).

▶ Treatment Steps

1. Correct complications.
2. Allopurinol.
3. **Chemotherapy.**

   Acute Myelogenous (AML)—remission achieved in majority of patients older than 60 with one course of cytosine arabinoside (ara-C) and daunomycin or doxorubicin. Bone marrow transplant for relapse after first remission or in first remission if prognostic factors are unfavorable. Age limits vary from center to center and with physiologic age. Cure rate 20% in AML.

   Acute Promyelocytic Leukemia (APML)—induce remission with all-trans retinoic acid (ATRA), then consolidate with standard chemotherapy. Cure rates of 35–45% are clearly better than typical AML.

   Acute Lymphoblastic (Acute Lymphocytic, ALL)—vincristine, prednisone, and a third drug, such as L-asparaginase, doxorubicin, or daunorubicin, gives 80% remission in adults. Need CNS prophylaxis (cranial irradiation or intrathecal methotrexate), then maintenance or continuation therapy. For relapse, give systemic chemo and local irradiation. Bone marrow transplant (30% survival rate in allogeneic transplant).

5. Myelodysplastic Syndromes

Characterized by normal to increased marrow cellularity and ineffective erythropoiesis: refractory anemia (RA), refractory anemia with ringed sideroblasts (RARS), refractory anemia with excess blasts (RAEB), and RAEB-in transition (RAEB-IT).

6. Chronic Leukemic States

6–1. Chronic Myelogenous Leukemia (CML)

► **Description**

Originates in primitive myeloid stem cell. Characteristic **Philadelphia (Ph¹) chromosome** (see Fig. 6–3).

► **Symptoms**

Fatigue, anorexia, weight loss, sense of abdominal fullness. Headaches, fever, sweats, bone pain. Hemorrhages, thromboses, fever.

► **Diagnosis**

Splenomegaly. Leukocytosis with immature cells. **Thrombocytosis. Anemia** with marked leukocytosis. Markedly decreased leukocyte alkaline phosphatase. Elevated uric acid, lactic dehydrogenase (LDH), vitamin B_{12}. **Myelofibrosis.** Enters a **blastic** or **accelerated phase** (myeloblastic or lymphoblastic) after 3 years in 80%.

► **Pathology**

Bone marrow aspiration reveals hypercellular marrow, increase in eosinophils, basophils, megakaryocytes. Diagnosis confirmed by Philadelphia chromosome.

► **Treatment Steps**

1. **Treat** with imatinib mesylate (Gleevec), a tyrosine kinase inhibitor.
2. For relapsing disease, **hydroxyurea,** and α-interferon are the main drugs, though cyclophosphamide and busulfan are also effective.
3. Acute leukostatic or thrombotic complications require leukapheresis, or plateletpheresis. Good hydration and allopurinol.
4. Splenic radiation to reduce spleen size and white count.
5. Treatment of blastic phase very difficult.
6. In younger patients, consider bone marrow transplant in chronic phase if donor available.

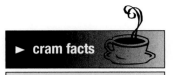

► **cram facts**

Philadelphia chromosome is a translocation between chromosomes 9 and 22, designated t(9;22). The translocation results in an abnormal gene (bcr-abl).

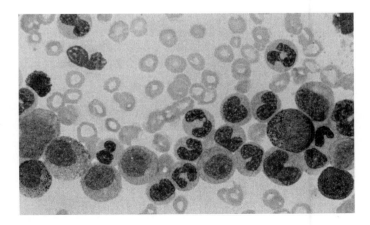

Figure 6–3. Chronic myelogenous leukemia—An important prognostic indicator seen in approximately 90% of patients with chronic myelogenous leukemia is the Philadelphia (Ph¹) chromosome. The peripheral smear is characterized by a "left shift" toward immature granulocytic cells, with myelocytes predominating. Basophils are increased in number.

6–2. Chronic Lymphocytic Leukemia (CLL)

▶ Description
Twenty-five percent of all leukemias. Monoclonal proliferation of long-lived, usually B **lymphocytes.** Unknown etiology. May be asymptomatic. High incidence of **second malignancies.**

▶ Symptoms
Symptoms vary by extent of disease. **Asymptomatic** lymphocytosis. **Adenopathy, splenomegaly.** Malaise, fatigue, weight loss, anorexia, fever, night sweats, bacterial infections; herpes zoster is common.

▶ Diagnosis
Lymphocytosis, with > 50% of small lymphs with round nuclei in the marrow. Peripheral blood flow cytometry for monoclonality of lymphocytes (CD5+) (see Fig. 6–4).

Stage 0—lymphocytosis only
Stage 1—lymphocytosis with lymphadenopathy
Stage 2—lymphocytosis with splenomegaly
Stage 3—lymphocytosis with anemia
Stage 4—lymphocytosis with throbocytopenia

▶ Pathology
Lymphocytosis can be massive. Anemia, thrombocytopenia, neutropenia. Coombs'-positive **autoimmune hemolytic anemia** is common.

▶ Treatment Steps
1. Should **avoid vaccination** with live vaccines.
2. **Treat only if progressive** and symptomatic. Chlorambucil or fludarabine.
3. Corticosteroids for acute symptoms, hemolytic anemia, thrombocytopenia.
4. Local radiotherapy to splenomegaly or massive adenopathy.

6–3. Hairy Cell Leukemia (Leukemic Reticuloendotheliosis)

▶ Description
A chronic **B-cell leukemia;** 2% of all leukemias.

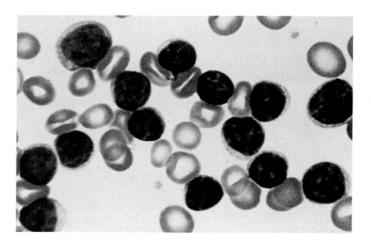

Figure 6–4. Chronic lymphocytic leukemia—demonstrates proliferation of mature lymphocytes.

► Symptoms

Of marrow suppression and hypersplenism.

► Diagnosis

Progressive splenic enlargement. Pancytopenia. **Hairy cells** in blood and marrow are CD10+ and TRAP+ (tartrate-resistant acid phosphatase). May need marrow biopsy (see Fig. 6–5).

► Pathology

Medium to large lymphocyte with hairy projections. Surface monoclonal immunoglobulin.

► Treatment Steps

1. **May observe,** as it is slowly progressive.
2. **Cladribine** drug of choice; 75% effective.
3. Also used after relapse are α-interferon, pentostatin, and splenectomy.

6–4. Mycosis Fungoides

► Description

A **cutaneous T-cell lymphoma.** The Sézary syndrome is the leukemic form of mycosis fungoides.

► Symptoms

Skin eruption with **appearance of eczema or psoriasis.**

► Diagnosis

Multiple biopsies necessary.

► Pathology

Prolonged course, beginning with **nonspecific lesions** (premycotic stage) that slowly evolve into **cutaneous plaques and patches** (mycotic stage), and then into **ulcerative nodules and tumors** (tumor stage). May involve lymph nodes and internal organs later.

► Treatment Steps

Local therapy:

1. Topical chemotherapy.

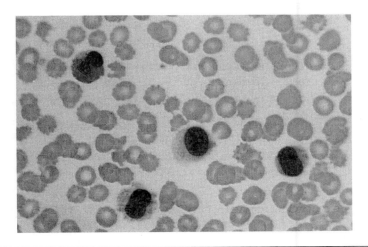

Figure 6–5. Hairy cell leukemia—In the peripheral smear in hairy cell leukemia, the neoplastic lymphocytes have hairlike cytoplasmic projections, the nucleus may be cleaved, and nucleoli are present.

2. PUVA (psoralen plus irradiation).

3. Radiotherapy.

Systemic therapy:

1. Interferon.

2. Retinoids.

3. Cytotoxics—methotrexate, adriamycin, cladribine.

6–5. Polycythemia Rubra Vera
See Chapter 5, section IV B.3-2.

B. Nervous System

1. Primary Neoplasms of the Brain

► **Description**
Most common CA in children. "Benign" brain tumors can be lethal. **Cerebral edema** is a major cause of morbidity.

► **Symptoms**
Headache (morning), mental changes, generalized convulsions, papilledema (25%), vomiting, vasomotor/autonomic, hormonal changes.

► **Diagnosis**
Magnetic resonance imaging (MRI) of head. Must distinguish from benign intracranial hypertension (nonfocal), stroke (acute event), subdural hematoma, Alzheimer's.

► **Pathology**
Types:

1. **Neuroectodermal** are the most common. These include **astrocytoma** (more benign), **glioblastoma multiforme** (more malignant).
2. **Mesodermal meningioma** ("benign," though grow very large and can cause death).
3. **Pituitary adenoma** and **craniopharyngioma.**
4. **Pineal** (produce endocrinopathies).
5. **Metastatic.**
6. **Vascular** arteriovenous malformations (AVMs), hemangioblastomas.

► **Treatment Steps**

1. **Surgery** for **cure** in meningioma, benign cerebellar tumors, or acoustic schwannomas.
2. **Radiation** for malignant tumors or symptomatic unresectable "benign" tumors.
3. *Medical therapy:* **steroids** relieve edema; **anticonvulsants; chemotherapy,** local and systemic.

2. Metastases to the Brain

► **Description**
Most CNS tumors are metastatic. Brain metastases are from **lung** and **breast;** melanoma has high propensity to spread to brain.

► **Symptoms**
Neurologic symptoms, seizures, headaches, motor weakness.

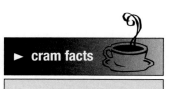

► **cram facts**

- Suspect brain tumor in an adult presenting with new-onset headache.
- Also, if a patient with chronic headaches has a sudden change in the quality or severity of headaches, consider brain tumor.

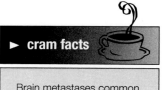

► **cram facts**

Brain metastases common in:
- Lung cancer
- Breast cancer
- Melanoma

► Diagnosis

Use **MRI** with gadolinium or **CT with contrast.** Distinguish from seizure, meningeal carcinomatosis, paraneoplastic syndrome.

► Treatment Steps

Depends on the primary tumor and the extent of disease. Options include

1. **For solitary lesions, surgery and steroids.**
2. **For multiple metastases, irradiation chemotherapy** (for small-cell lung and testicular CA).

3. Leptomeningeal Metastases

► Description

About 8% of CA patients develop meningeal spread.

► Symptoms

Headaches, altered mentation, cranial nerve defects, lumbosacral radiculopathies, seizures.

► Diagnosis

Lumbar puncture (LP) (5–100 cells, increased protein, decreased glucose). **Positive cytology** (repeat LPs may be needed) to confirm diagnosis. MRI and CT are usually normal, but gadolinium contrast can be suggestive.

► Treatment Steps
1. **Cranial irradiation.**
2. **Intrathecal chemotherapy.** Usually combined.

4. Acoustic Neuroma

► Description

Schwannoma of eighth nerve.

► Symptoms

Hearing loss, tinnitus, less often vertigo.

► Diagnosis

Brain stem auditory-evoked responses (BAERs); MRI or CT with contrast.

► Treatment Steps

Microsurgery or **radiosurgery** yields 85–95% control rate.

5. Retinoblastoma

An **autosomal dominant hereditary** tumor of the retina. The most common intraocular tumor of children.

C. Circulatory System (Kaposi's Sarcoma)

► Description

Seen after **immunosuppressive therapy** and **HIV infection** (50% of homosexual men with AIDS). Originally described in elderly male of Mediterranean origin. Cause now felt felt to be human herpesvirus-8.

► Symptoms

Hemorrhagic **nodules** with violaceous, dark brown lesions. Before AIDS epidemic, primarily on lower extremities. With AIDS, see **mucocutaneous and lymph node involvement.**

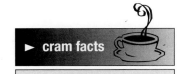

► **cram facts**

Leptomeningeal spread common in:
- Hodgkin's disease
- Leukemia
- Melanoma
- Breast cancer
- Lung cancer
- GI tract adenocarcinoma

▶ Diagnosis
Clinical picture; biopsy (see Fig. 6–6).

▶ Treatment Steps
Local: Topical chemotherapy, intralesional injections, local radiation.

Widespread: α-Interferon, cytotoxics (e.g., vinblastine, vincristine, Adriamycin).

D. Respiratory System

1. Carcinoma of the Nasopharynx

▶ Symptoms
Pharyngitis, lymphoid hypertrophy, voice change, conductive hearing loss, dysphagia, odynophagia, halitosis, weight loss.

▶ Diagnosis
Endoscopy, biopsy.

▶ Pathology
Most common is **squamous cell.** Also lymphoma, lymphoepitheliomas (Schmincke's tumor), anaplastic carcinoma.

▶ Treatment Steps
1. **Surgery.**
2. **Radiation.**
3. Chemotherapy as radiation sensitizer or for recurrent disease.

2. Tumors of the Larynx (Malignant)

▶ Symptoms
Hoarseness, pain, dysphagia, odynophagia, cough, hemoptysis, halitosis.

▶ Diagnosis
Direct laryngoscopy, pharyngoscopy, biopsy.

▶ Pathology
Squamous cell carcinoma, neuroendocrine, salivary gland.

▶ Treatment Steps
1. **Radiation.**
2. **Laryngectomy.**

3. Tumors of the Larynx (Benign)

▶ Symptoms/Diagnosis
Hoarseness, later dyspnea, dysphagia, pain. Diagnosed via endoscopy.

▶ Pathology
Papilloma (caused by papillomavirus), hemangioma, angiofibroma.

▶ Treatment Steps
Carbon dioxide laser (for papillomas).

4. Carcinoma of the Lung

▶ Description
Produces 180,000 new cases per year in United States; 150,000 deaths. Eighty to ninety percent associated with **smoking and passive**

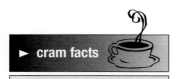

▶ cram facts

Laryngeal and nasopharyngeal carcinoma are strongly associated with tobacco and alcohol use.

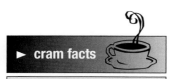

▶ cram facts

SYNDROMES ASSOCIATED WITH LUNG CANCER

• Pancoast syndrome: Tumor of thte superior sulcus, brachial plexus symptoms
• Horner's syndrome: Unilateral ptosis, meiosis, and anhidrosis (due to compression of the ipsilateral superior cervical ganglion by lung tumor, particularly squamous cell cancer)
• SVC syndrome: Obstruction of the superior vena cava causes facial swelling/plethora, dyspnea, and cough. Dilated veins of neck and chest are often seen.

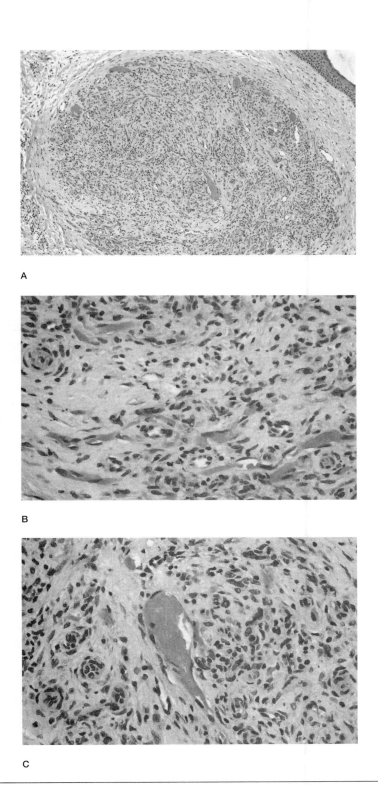

A

B

C

Figure 6–6. Kaposi's sarcoma—the most common neoplasm in AIDS. A: In this example involving the skin, there is a dermal nodule. The nodule is composed of a proliferation of atypical spindle cells lining slitlike vascular channels. **B:** There is red blood cell extravasation, and eosinophilic globules are present extracellularly in macrophages and in tumor cells. **C:** In older lesions of Kaposi's sarcoma, hemosiderin is also present.

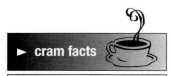

smoke inhalation. Occupational risks include **uranium, halo-ethers, arsenical fumes, asbestos. Asbestos and radon** (heavily insulated homes) may be cocarcinogens with cigarette smoke.

► Symptoms

Cough, hemoptysis, weight loss, weakness, wheezing, fever, chest pain.

► Diagnosis

Chest x-ray (mass in lung). Need **tissue** via sputum cytology, bronchoscopic biopsy or brushings, transbronchial biopsy or needle aspiration, CT-guided transthoracic biopsy, thoracotomy.

► Pathology

Four types make up 95% (see Cram Facts).

► Treatment Steps

Depends on stage and histology.

   Non–small cell: TNM stages I and II: **surgery.**

   Stage III: **Surgery** and **irradiation.** Surgery results: 10–35% 5-year survival (squamous 37%, adeno 27%). Since very radiosensitive, give radiation therapy (XRT) in I, II, and III who do not have surgery. Unresectable (disseminated) non–small cell can be treated with concomitant XRT and **chemotherapy;** XRT also to palliate SVC syndrome, hemoptysis, cough, pain.

   Chemotherapy: 30–40% response rate.

   Small cell: Low survival, despite high initial response rate. Treat with **chemotherapy** (very sensitive) and **irradiation.** Not a surgical disease. Useful programs include a platinum plus a second agent (paclitaxel, etoposide).

5. **Metastases to the Lung**

► Symptoms

Can be asymptomatic, dyspnea, chest pain, cough, cor pulmonale. Can occur via lymphatic or hematogenous spread.

► Diagnosis

Sputum cytology, bronchoscopy, thoracotomy.

► Treatment Steps

1. **Treat the primary.**
2. **Consider resection** if solitary metastasis from colon, melanoma or sarcoma.

6. **Mesothelioma**

► Description

Main primary pleural tumor. Benign or malignant. Malignant related to **asbestos** in 80–90%.

► Symptoms

Cough, chest pain, dyspnea occur late.

► Diagnosis

Malignant cells in pleural fluid or pleural biopsy.

► Pathology

Benign associated with hypertrophic pulmonary osteoarthropathy and clubbing (responds to surgical removal).

► Treatment Steps

No standard treatment. Prognosis very poor.

E. Digestive System

1. Salivary Gland Neoplasms

Most common is pleomorphic **adenoma** (benign). Malignancies include mucoepidermoid **carcinoma,** adenoid cystic carcinoma, adenocarcinoma.

► Symptoms/Diagnosis

Slow-growing mass leading to ulceration, invasion of nerves, numbness or facial paralysis. Diagnose via biopsy.

► Treatment Steps

Surgery and/or radiation.

2. Carcinoma of the Mouth

► Description

Smoking and **alcohol** are risk factors. Tongue most common.

► Symptoms

Painful indurated ulceration.

► Diagnosis

Biopsy.

► Pathology

Mostly **squamous,** with 20% chance of a **second head and neck cancer.**

► Treatment Steps

1. **Radiation and surgery in combination** can be curative.
2. **Chemotherapy** in more advanced cases (methotrexate, bleomycin, cisplatin).
3. Rehabilitation and prostheses important; 50% survival rate.

3. Carcinoma of the Esophagus

► Description

Barrett's esophagus, smoking, and alcohol are risk factors. Survival has been increased to 40% by combined modality therapy.

► Symptoms

Progressive **dysphagia;** steady, boring pain; halitosis; weight loss; cough after drinking fluid.

► Diagnosis

Esophagogram, endoscopy with biopsy and brushings, CT of chest, chest x-ray. (See Figure 6–7.)

► Pathology

Squamous (more common; associated with head and neck cancer, lye strictures, inadequately treated achalasia). **Adenocarcinoma** arises in columnar epithelium (Barrett's esophagus—see Cram Facts).

► Treatment Steps

1. Surgery: much morbidity.
2. Combined radiation and a platinum and 5-FU regimen.

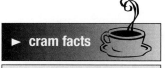

► cram facts

BARRETT'S ESOPHAGUS

- Arises in the distal esophagus.
- Healthy squamous epithelium is replaced by columnar epithelium.
- Occurs in patients with long-standing gastroesophageal reflux disease (GERD).
- Serial endoscopies recommended for patients with long-standing GERD or who are high risk.
- It is a metaplastic disorder that confers an increased risk of adenocarcinoma of the esophagus.

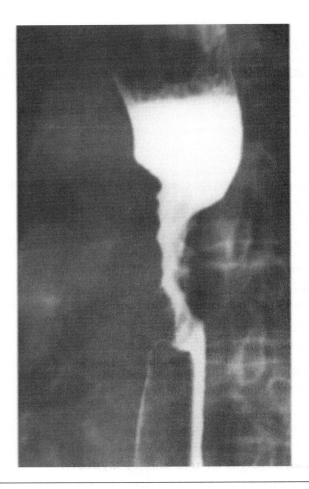

Figure 6–7. Barium swallow, showing mid-esophageal stricture. The abrupt change in caliber, irregular mucosa, and near circumferential narrowing are highly suggestive of an esophageal cancer.

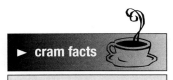

► cram facts

**RISK FACTORS FOR
GASTRIC CANCER**

- Blood type A
- Atrophic gastritis
- Pernicious anemia
- Nitrosamines (in food)
- Familial adenomatous
  polyposis
- *H. pylori* associated with
  mucosa-associated
  lymphoid tissue (MALT)

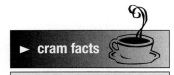

► cram facts

Gastric cancer associated
with:
- **Virchow's node:**
  Enlarged supraclavicular
  node
- **Blumer's shelf:**
  Metastatic tumor felt via
  rectal exam
- **Sister Mary Joseph's
  node:** Enlarged
  periumbilical node
- Acanthosis nigricans

4. Carcinoma of the Stomach

► Description
Majority are malignant; 5% are lymphomas.

Incidence decreasing in the United States. Common in Japan. Low incidence where colorectal cancer is high. See Cram Facts.

► Symptoms
Early are asymptomatic. **Anorexia, weight loss, early satiety,** bloating, dysphagia, epigastric pain, vomiting.

► Diagnosis
Epigastric mass. Recurrent thrombophlebitis (Trousseau's syndrome). Air-contrast UGI x-rays. Endoscopy with biopsy and brush cytology. Culture for *H. pylori*.

► Pathology
Usually **adenocarcinoma.** Spread to esophagus, liver, pancreas, transverse colon, lung, brain, bone.

► Treatment Steps
1. **Surgery** for cure or palliation.
2. **Chemotherapy** for unresectable disease.
3. **Radiotherapy.**
4. Antibiotics for *H. pylori* if culture positive in MALT.

5. Carcinoma of the Pancreas

► **Description**

Slowly progressive, **highly malignant. Second most common GI tumor after colon.** Risk factors include smoking; high-fat, high-meat diet; exposure to manufacturing of paper, oil refining, gasoline. Usually not curable but can control symptoms.

► **Symptoms**

Epigastric pain, weight loss, vomiting, hematemesis, melena, jaundice, palpable mass, palpable gallbladder (Courvoisier's sign), thrombophlebitis, psychiatric disturbances, diabetes, anemia, blood in stool.

► **Diagnosis**

Ultrasound and/or CT, followed by **needle aspiration.** If negative, endoscopic retrograde cholangiopancreatography (ERCP) (very sensitive and tissue for cytology helpful). The UGI is poor in early detection. Occasional amylase elevation. Elevated CA 19-9.

► **Pathology**

Usually adenocarcinoma. Occasionally endocrine tumors (apudomas and carcinoids).

► **Treatment Steps**

1. **Whipple's resection** (pancreaticoduodenectomy) for small focal mass lesions. High operative mortality; 5% 5-year survival.
2. Chemotherapy with gemcitabine improves quality of life.
3. Radiation with 5-FU may improve survival by weeks.

6. Carcinoma of the Biliary System

► **Description**

Associated with tobacco use and cholelithiasis.

► **Symptoms**

Obstructive jaundice, acute cholecystitis, palpable mass, right upper quadrant pain, or disseminated carcinoma.

► **Diagnosis**

Ultrasound. Must distinguish from cholesterol polyp or stone. Elevated CA 19-9.

► **Pathology**

Adenocarcinoma.

► **Treatment Steps**

Surgery; 5% 5-year survival, even with optimal surgery.

7. Carcinoma of the Liver/Hepatocellular Cancer

► **Description**

Uncommon, but **increasing in United States.** Median survival 6 months.

► **Symptoms**

Abdominal pain, mass, weight loss, deterioration of patient with cirrhosis.

► **Diagnosis**

Ultrasound, CT, or MRI. Elevated alkaline phosphatase, transaminase, CEA, and AFP. **Needle biopsy, wedge biopsy** at laparotomy.

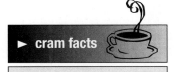

► **cram facts**

RISK FACTORS FOR HEPATOCELLULAR CANCER

- Cirrhosis
- Hepatitis B and/or C
- Aflatoxins (toxic metabolites from *Aspergillus flavus* [peanuts and grains])
- Very common in Asia

▶ Treatment Steps

1. **Hepatic resection** effective if early.
2. **Chemotherapy** with doxorubicin (Adriamycin), 5-FU, cisplatin regimens yield 50% response rate, but minimal survival advantage.
3. Chemoembolization.
4. Cryosurgery or radioablation (RITA).

8. **Metastases to the Liver**

The majority of hepatic tumors are **metastatic** in adults. Mostly stomach, colon, pancreas. Isolated metastases can be resected for improved survival.

9. **Carcinoma of the Colon**

See also Chapter 4, section V.

▶ Symptoms

Silent; **bleeding,** obstruction, **change in bowel habits,** pain, symptoms of localized perforation. Right-side lesions rarely obstruct. Left-side polypoid lesions cause diarrhea and signs of obstruction.

▶ Diagnosis

In suspected case, **digital rectal exam** followed by **colonoscopy.** Brushings and/or biopsy. Must distinguish from angiodysplasia, diverticulosis, benign tumors.

▶ Pathology

About **60% occur from splenic flexure down,** and almost all are adenocarcinomas.

▶ Treatment Steps

1. **Surgery** with curative intent.
2. **Chemotherapy** for metastatic disease (especially liver) with irinotecan (Camptosar) and 5-FU. Evidence for effectiveness of adjuvant chemo in Duke's C colon carcinoma with 5-FU plus levamisole or leucovorin. Follow with colonoscopy, CEA if elevated preoperatively. Two new medications approved for metastatic colorectal cancer are cetuximab (Erbitux) and bevacizumab (Avastin). Both are monoclonal antibodies.
3. **Radiation** for recurrent disease.

▶ Screening

See *American Cancer Society Recommendations for the Early Detection of Cancer in Asymptomatic People.* High-risk patients require annual sigmoidoscopy beginning at puberty.

10. **Carcinoma of the Rectum**

If below the peritoneal reflection, it commonly recurs, and postop radiation + 5-FU is recommended. Anal: chemotherapy + radiation is better than surgery as primary treatment.

11. **Carcinoid Tumors**

▶ Description

Tumors that arise from **enterochromaffin cells** (Kulchitsky) and **produce biologically active amines and peptides** (serotonin, bradykinin, histamine, prostaglandins). Survival variable but if metastatic, < 5 years.

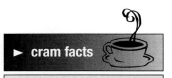

▶ **cram facts**

RISK FACTORS FOR
COLORECTAL CANCER

- Increased fat
- Animal protein
- Decreased fiber
- Increasing age
- Inflammatory bowel disease
- Family history of female genital or breast cancer
- History of colonic cancer or adenoma (especially villous adenomas)
- History of familial colon cancer syndromes (familial polyposis, Gardner syndrome, Peutz–Jeghers syndrome, generalized juvenile polyposis)

► Symptoms

Cutaneous **flushing** (precipitated by alcohol, food, stress), facial telangiectasias, tachycardia and decreased blood pressure, headache after the flush, **diarrhea,** symptoms of peritoneal fibrosis, right-sided endocardial fibrosis (with congestive heart failure). Bronchoconstriction and wheezing less common.

► Diagnosis

Clinical suspicion; markedly **increased urinary 5-hydroxyindoleacetic acid (5-HIAA)** hepatomegaly. Of less help are CT, ultrasound, scans.

► Pathology

Often arise in ileum and metastasize to the liver. Excrete **serotonin** and 5-HIAA. Carcinoids can arise in almost all organs, including appendix, rectum, stomach, and lung.

► Treatment Steps

1. Surgery if resectable or symptomatic.
2. If not resectable, no treatment for mild symptoms. Symptomatic treatment (antidiarrheal agents, bronchodilators, nutritional support).
3. Chemotherapy not very effective.

12. Colon Polyps

► Description

Importance: **bleeding** or **malignant potential.**

► Symptoms/Diagnosis

Asymptomatic, bleeding, pain, diarrhea. Seen on colonnoscopy; biopsy needed to assess benign vs. malignant.

► Pathology

Four main types:

1. **Hyperplastic**—(majority of rectal polyps; not considered neoplastic).
2. **Tubular adenomas.**
3. **Villous adenomas**—(neoplastic; villous have high malignant transformation rate than tubular).
4. **Mixed type**—cancer rate much higher in larger polyps.

► Treatment Steps

1. **Removal.**
2. **Follow with colonoscopy.**

13. Polyposis Syndromes

a. *Familial polyposis:* Autosomal dominant; will nearly all develop carcinoma.
b. *Gardner syndrome:* Dominantly transmitted; associated with bone tumors (osteomas), and soft tissue tumors (lipomas, sebaceous cysts, fibromas, fibrosarcomas); high malignant potential.
c. *Munro syndrome:* Colon adenomas plus central nervous system tumors; high malignant potential.
d. *Peutz–Jeghers syndrome:* Autosomal dominant; polyps plus mucocutaneous hyperpigmentation; low malignant potential.
e. *Generalized juvenile polyposis:* Autosomal dominant; hamartomas; possible increased carcinoma incidence.

► Treatment Steps

Subtotal colectomy. Also genetic counseling and intensive screening of family members.

F. Endocrine and Reproductive Systems

1. Pituitary Adenoma

► Description

Adenomas form 90% of all pituitary tumors; **most are functioning; benign,** but may have aggressive local growth pattern.

► Symptoms

Variable **headaches, visual disturbances** (blindness, optic atrophy), temperature instability, hyperphagia, emotional disturbance, disturbed sleep patterns, hypopituitarism, hypogonadism.

► Diagnosis

Enlarged sella by x-ray, **mass** on CT or MRI, visual fields, visual evoked response.

► Treatment Steps

1. Transsphenoidal pituitary **surgery.**
2. Optionally, can **irradiate.**
3. Will require endocrine replacement (see Chapter 3).

2. Thyroid Nodules and Cancer

2–1. Benign Nodules

► Symptoms/Diagnosis

Asymptomatic. Large functioning adenomas produce hyperthyroidism. Diagnose via needle aspiration.

► Treatment Steps

Follow *warm* (nonclinically thyrotoxic) nodules with **annual thyroid function tests.** *Hot* (clinically toxic) nodules are treated with **surgery** or **radioactive iodine.**

2–2. Thyroid Cancer

► Description

Risk factors include **childhood exposure to radiation** and **heredity;** 11,000 cases per year; 1,000 deaths; 3–4% of solitary thyroid nodules are cancer.

► Symptoms

Thyroid nodule; symptoms of local invasion.

► Diagnosis

Needle aspiration may reduce the need for surgery by 60%. Optionally, thyroid scanning and ultrasound. Thyroxine to suppress thyroid-stimulating hormone (TSH).

► Pathology

May occur as part of familial thyroid carcinoma (multiple endocrine neoplasia [MEN] types 2 and 3). *Four histologic types:*

1. **Papillary**—(the most benign and the most common; pathognomonic is the **psammoma body).**
2. **Follicular.**

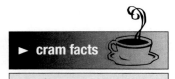

► **cram facts**

- About 96% of thyroid nodules are benign.
- A "functioning" or "hot" nodule is also almost always benign.

► **cram facts**

FACTORS THAT WORSEN PROGNOSIS IN THYROID CANCER

- Male gender
- Age > 40 years old
- Anaplastic histological type
- Large primary tumor > 1.5 cm in diameter
- Distant metastases
- Extrathyroidal invasion

3. **Medullary**—(produces calcitonin). Can be associated with MEN-2.

4. **Poorly differentiated (anaplastic)**—(the most highly malignant).

▶ Treatment Steps

1. **Needle aspiration.**
2. **Surgical resection** (if hypo- or euthyroid)
3. **Radiation therapy** with ^{131}I (if hyperfunctional).
4. **Thyroxine suppression.**
5. Irradiation and chemotherapy for thyroid lymphoma.

3. Adrenal Neoplasms

3–1. Cushing's Disease

▶ Description
A primary adrenal tumor secreting cortisol, causing signs and symptoms of glucocorticoid excess.

▶ Symptoms
Abdominal mass. **Obesity, plethora, hirsutism,** menstrual disorders, **hypertension, weakness** (hypokalemia), back pain (from osteopenia), **striae, acne,** depression, bruising.

▶ Diagnosis
Use **24-hour urine free cortisol;** overnight 1 mg **dexamethasone-suppression test;** basal plasma ACTH levels. Tumor localization with CT and ultrasonography.

▶ Pathology
Adenoma and carcinoma equally. Spread to liver and lung.

▶ Treatment Steps

1. **Adrenalectomy.**
2. **Mitotane** for residual or nonresectable carcinoma.
3. Other cytotoxics—doxorubicin.
4. Control hypersecretion—aminoglutethimide, metyrapone.
5. **Steroid replacement** therapy.

3–2. Pheochromocytoma
See Chapter 3, section II.F.6.

4. Endometrial Carcinoma
See Chapter 13, section V.E.3.

5. Carcinoma of the Cervix and Cervical Dysplasia
See Chapter 13, section V.E.1.

6. Carcinoma of the Ovary
See Chapter 13, section V.E.4.

7. Carcinoma of the Vulva
Must biopsy early to help. Surgery. Also see Chapter 13, section V.E.6.

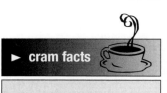

▶ **cram facts**

In anaplastic thyroid cancer, the patient may have hoarseness due to a rapidly growing mass.

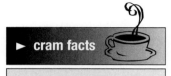

▶ **cram facts**

Cushing's syndrome refers to any and all conditions that cause an excess of glucocorticoids.

Cushing's disease refers specifically to a pituitary tumor causing excess glucocorticoids.

8. Neoplasms of the Vagina

Female offspring of women given **diethylstilbestrol** during pregnancy may get adenosis of vagina and have increased risk of vaginal cancer (adenocarcinoma, clear cell type).

9. Carcinoma of the Breast

▶ Description

203,500 new cases in 2002; 12% of women will get it; 85% are older than 40 years old. *Risk factors:* prior breast cancer, family history, early menarche, late menopause, late or no pregnancy; moderate alcohol intake; radiation exposure; western society diet. Oral contraceptives do not increase the risk, nor does estrogen given for osteoporosis.

▶ Symptoms

Painless lump. Hard, irregular mass, skin dimpling, or nipple retraction.

▶ Diagnosis

• **Screening.** See *American Cancer Society Recommendations for the Early Detection of Cancer in Asymptomatic People.*
• **Mammograms** (90% accuracy), **fine-needle biopsy, excisional biopsy.**

▶ Pathology

Assume distant metastases. Size of tumor, and presence of axillary nodes correlates with risk of recurrence. The presence of estrogen receptors (ER) and progesterone receptors (PR) indicates better prognosis. High Ki67 and the presence of the her-2 mutation a poorer prognosis. About 80% are infiltrating ductal; others are infiltrating lobular, medullary, comedocarcinoma, colloid carcinoma (see Fig. 6–8).

▶ Treatment Steps

Two steps: outpatient fine-needle biopsy or excisional biopsy under local; discuss options, then do definitive treatment.

Stage I and II Disease—local resection (lumpectomy and axillary node dissection or modified radical) followed by irradiation. Ad-

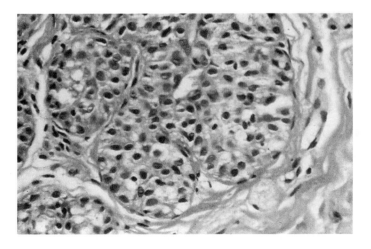

Figure 6–8. Lobular carcinoma in situ—demonstrates proliferation of cells forming glands within but not invading through a lobule.

juvant systemic therapy for poor prognosis stage I and all stage II. Tamoxifen if postmenopausal and ER positive. Chemotherapy if ER negative.

Lobular—higher risk of bilateral disease.

Resectable Stage III—do mastectomy followed by radiation and chemotherapy. If patient strongly wishes breast conservation, consider preoperative chemotherapy.

Unresectable Stage III or Inflammatory Breast Carcinoma—give chemotherapy followed by irradiation (and possible resection).

Stage IV (Metastatic)—**hormonal** (bone, soft tissue, and mild pulmonary spread respond) or **chemotherapy** (liver, brain, and extensive lung).

9–1. Premenopausal

Chemotherapy if adjuvant therapy indicated using such drugs as cyclophosphamide, 5-FU, methotrexate, and Adriamycin. Consider adding a taxane if positive lymph nodes. Hormonal therapy of benefit if ER positive.

9–2. Postmenopausal

Tamoxifen if ER/PR positive (anastrazole also an option); chemotherapy if resistant to hormone.

Adjuvant chemotherapy. National Institutes of Health (NIH) Consensus says adjuvant chemotherapy and hormonal therapy (tamoxifen) are effective in axillary node-positive patients (especially if ER positive).

If CEA or CA 27-29 elevated preoperatively, can be used to monitor. No follow-up apart from mammogram proven to improve survival.

10. Gestational Trophoblastic Disease
See Chapter 13, section II.A.13.

11. Neoplasms of Testes

11–1. Nonseminomatous

▶ Description
Germ cell tumors that include embryonal cell carcinomas, choriocarcinomas, and teratomas. Stages I and II, 99% cure rate. Stage III, 70%.

▶ Symptoms
Painless testicular **mass.** May have dyspnea, abdominal or back pain, gynecomastia, supraclavicular adenopathy, or ureteral obstruction.

▶ Diagnosis
Stage with chest x-ray, CT chest and abdomen, AFP, β-hCG. Do *not* perform percutaneous biopsy.

▶ Treatment Steps
1. **Inguinal orchiectomy and retroperitoneal lymph node dissection** for staging and initial treatment.
2. **Cisplatin-based aggressive chemotherapy.**

11–2. Seminoma

▶ Description

Rare; most are malignant, derived from germ cells, 20–35 years old. *Risk factor* is cryptorchidism.

▶ Diagnosis

Evaluate with AFP, β-hCG, CT of abdomen and pelvis.

▶ Treatment Steps

1. Inguinal orchiectomy and radiation produce 80–95% cure rates.
2. If increased AFP, treat like nonseminomatous germ cell tumor (GCT).

G. Kidney and Urinary System

1. Hypernephroma (Renal Cell Carcinoma, Renal Adenocarcinoma)

▶ Description

Risk factors include male gender and tobacco use.

▶ Symptoms

Gross or microscopic **hematuria, flank pain, abdominal mass.** Symptoms of paraneoplastic syndrome (fever, hypertension, anemia, hepatic dysfunction [Stauffer syndrome]). Many unusual symptoms. Erythrocytosis.

▶ Diagnosis

Intravenous pyelogram (IVP), ultrasound, CT, MRI. Rule out renal vein thrombus. (See Figs. 6–9 and 6–10.)

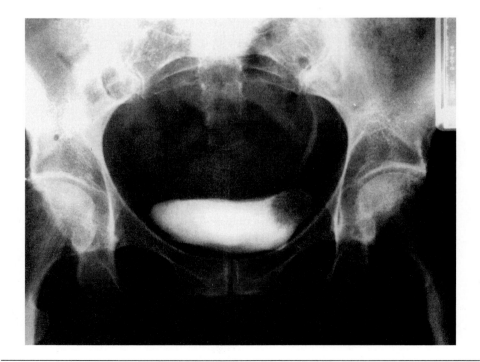

Figure 6–9. Superficial bladder tumor demonstrated on intravenous urogram.

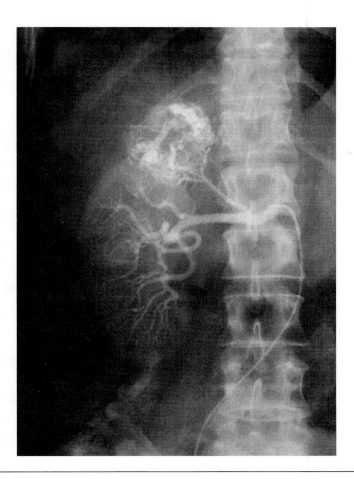

Figure 6–10. Renal angiogram displays tumor neovascularization.

► Pathology
Three histologic types: clear cell, granular cell, and sarcomatoid.

► Treatment Steps
1. Stages I, II, and IIIA require **radical nephrectomy** and yield 50–70% 5-year survival. No significant benefit to adjuvant therapy.
2. Stage IV—combination therapies of α-interferon, IL-2, and 5-FU are used.

2. Wilms' Tumor (Nephroblastoma)

► Description
Most patients are under 4 years old.

► Symptoms
Asymptomatic palpable abdominal mass, hematuria, hypertension, abdominal pain.

► Diagnosis
IVP, ultrasound, or CT. Must distinguish from neuroblastoma (with urinary vanillylmandelic acid [VMA]).

► Pathology
About 80% are localized and resectable.

▶ Treatment Steps

1. Limited disease: **surgery + chemotherapy** (doxorubicin, actinomycin D, vincristine) yields 85% disease-free survival.
2. Advanced disease: **irradiation + chemotherapy.**

3. Carcinoma of the Bladder

▶ Description

About 50,000 new cases per year; men predominate. Chemical carcinogens are implicated (including those in cigarette smoke).

▶ Symptoms

Hematuria, bladder irritability (frequency, dysuria).

▶ Diagnosis

Cystoscopy and transurethral bladder **biopsy.**

▶ Pathology

Transitional cell. Rarely squamous if *Schistosoma haematobium* infestation.

▶ Treatment Steps

Stage A:

1. Transurethral resection of bladder tumor (TURBT).
2. **Cystoscopic surveillance** for multiple recurrences.
3. **Intravesical chemotherapy:** bacillus Calmette–Guérin.

Stages B and C:

1. **Pelvic lymphadenectomy and radical cystectomy.** *Metastatic disease.*
2. **Chemotherapy** (e.g., methotrexate, vinblastine, platinums, doxorubicin, paclitaxel).

4. Carcinoma of the Prostate

▶ Description

Second leading cancer cause in males. No relationship to benign prostatic hypertrophy (BPH); little relationship to smoking or alcohol. Of 30,000 deaths per year, 30–50% of men older than 50 have at least a focus of adenocarcinoma of prostate. African Americans' risk two times that of Caucasians.

▶ Symptoms

Asymptomatic early, urinary retention symptoms, bone pain.

▶ Diagnosis

Digital rectal exam, transrectal prostatitic ultrasound (TRUS), confirmation with TRUS-guided **needle biopsy. Do PSA** before biopsy. IVP, bone scan, if biopsy positive.

▶ Pathology

About 50% of prostate nodules are malignant; **95% are adenocarcinomas.** Bone metastases common (pelvis, lumbar spine, femurs, thoracic spine, ribs); lung and liver metastases the most common visceral spread.

▶ Treatment Steps

Will vary with physiologic age of patient, being more aggressive in younger patients. Also considering importance of sexual function. Suppression with leuprolide preoperatively.

- *A1.* **Observation and rebiopsy.**
- *A2 and B1.* **Radical prostatectomy.**
- *B2 and C.* **Transurethral resection of prostate (TURP) followed by radiation** (40% post-XRT impotence; 2% incontinence).
- *D (metastatic).* **Hormonal therapy** (orchiectomy or luteinizing hormone–releasing hormone [LHRH] analog), which should be delayed until symptoms appear. **Chemotherapy** if hormone independent not very effective.

Treating complications. **Radiation** for pain; erythropoietin or transfusion for anemia, *strontium* for painful blastic lesions.

After treatment. Follow with periodic digital rectal exam (DRE) and PSA.

H. Skin and Musculoskeletal Systems
See Chapter 2.

1. Actinic Keratosis
See Chapter 2, section XV.A.

2. Basal Cell Carcinoma
See Chapter 2, section XV.C.

3. Squamous Cell Carcinoma
See Chapter 2, section XV.B.

4. Melanoma
See Chapter 2, section XV.D.

5. Nevi
See Chapter 2, sections XIV.C and D.

6. Hemangioma
See Chapter 2, section XII.A.

7. Osteosarcoma
See Chapter 10, section II.G.1.

8. Metastases to Bone
High rate from **breast, lung, prostate, kidney, thyroid.** Metastatic more common than primary bone. **Bone scans** very sensitive in detection. Prostate 90% blastic; breast 50% blastic; lung 25% blastic. Exception is purely lytic lesions of multiple myeloma where skeletal survey is preferred. *Treatment:* **radiation;** open reduction and internal fixation of threatened or fractured bone.

I. Head and Neck Tumors

▶ Description
Risk factors: tobacco and alcohol. Premalignant lesions include leukoplakia, erythroplakia.

▶ Pathology
Usually squamous (epidermoid). Oral 44%; laryngeal 32%.

▶ Treatment Steps
1. **Surgery.**
2. **Irradiation.**
3. Chemotherapy for palliation (e.g., cisplatin and 5-FU). High response rates seen but not sustained.

BIBLIOGRAPHY

Casciato DA, Lowitz BB. *Manual of Clinical Oncology.* Boston: Little, Brown & Co., 1995.

DeVita VT Jr., Hellman S, Rosenberg S. *Cancer: Principles and Practices of Oncology.* Philadelphia: J.B. Lippincott, 2001.

Pazdur R, et al. *Cancer Management: A Multidisciplinary Approach,* 2nd ed. Huntington, NY: PRR, 1997.

Immunology and Allergy 7

I. HEALTH AND HEALTH MAINTENANCE

A. Epidemiology and Prevention of Food and Drug Reactions

General information:

- **Type I immediate hypersensitivity reaction:** anaphylaxis.
- **Type II cytotoxic reaction:** drug and transfusion reactions.
- **Type III immune complex–mediated reaction:** serum sickness, glomerulonephritis.
- **Type IV cell-mediated delayed hypersensitivity reaction:** tuberculin skin test reactions, contact dermatitis.

1. Epidemiology

Includes a wide range of reactions (minimal to anaphylactic) to any food, medication, or foreign substance. No increased incidence by gender or geographic location. Shellfish, nuts, and milk products are common offenders (drugs include antibiotics, vaccines, hormones, dyes, and allergic extracts; foreign substances include venom from *Hymenoptera* insects).

Allergic (Eosinophilic) Gastroenteropathy—Rare disorder of immunoglobulin E (IgE) production and rapid-onset food allergy (nausea/vomiting, etc.).

Anaphylactic Reactions—IgE antibody mediated (type 1), widespread organ disorder.

Contact Dermatitis—Mediated via T-cell hypersensitivity.

Drug Reaction—Mediated via IgE (penicillin anaphylaxis), T cell (contact dermatitis), immune complex (serum sickness), or cytotoxic-antibody systems (nephritis and Coombs'-positive hemolytic anemia).

2. Prevention

Includes allergy testing, allergen avoidance, and desensitization to inhalant allergens, drugs, and hymenoptera venom. Accurate history taking and skin testing prior to medication use are important. Testing includes wheal-and-flare prick (epicutaneous), intradermal skin testing and radioallergosorbent test (RAST) serum testing. Patients with known allergies are advised to wear Medic Alert bracelets. Medical facility protocols to avoid drug allergy reactions, transfusion reactions, and so on. Use of preventive medication when risk of allergic reaction is significant (prednisone, benadryl, and an H_2 blocker prior to contrast dye injection).

B. Human Immunodeficiency Virus (HIV) Infections and Acquired Immune Deficiency Syndrome (AIDS)

1. Diagnosis

A presumptive diagnosis of AIDS can be made if certain opportunistic infections are present such as candidiasis of the esophagus, trachea, bronchi, or lungs or toxoplasmosis of the brain is present, for example. Definitive diagnosis incorporates finding antibody to HIV. Viral load is then usually checked.

2. Epidemiology

Ribonucleic acid (RNA) retrovirus HIV-induced pandemic (possible 15–20% population infected in Africa, and cases throughout the

---

► **differential diagnosis**

ANAPHYLAXIS

1. Type I Immediate hypersensitivity reaction:
   a. Food or food-additive allergy.
   b. Hymenoptera (bee sting) allergy.
   c. Drug allergy.
2. Disorders associated with sudden collapse but without urticaria and angioedema:
   a. Arrhythmia.
   b. Myocardial infarction.
   c. Food aspiration.
   d. Pulmonary embolism.
   e. Seizure disorders.
   f. Vasovagal collapse.
3. Miscellaneous:
   a. Hereditary angioedema.
   b. Serum sickness.
   c. Cold urticaria.
   d. Idiopathic urticaria.

world), with increased frequency in Blacks/Hispanics (compared to population figures), and pockets of increased frequency among drug users noted (New York). Adult risk of infection by needle sharing, broken skin/mucosal exposure, unprotected vaginal/anal intercourse, and by transfusion of blood products. Newborns and children by birth most often (infected mother), child abuse, and blood products.

There is an estimated one in a million chance of transmission of HIV via receipt of a blood transfusion due to donation from people who are HIV-infected but have not yet developed antibodies to HIV. These donors are therefore not picked up by enzyme-linked immunosorbent assay (ELISA) screens, by may be identified by lifestyle screens. However, newer blood testing involves checking for HIV antigens (like p24).

HIV infects lymphocytes and other cells bearing the CD4 surface marker. HIV infection leads to impaired cell-mediated and humoral immunity. AIDS is due to HIV infection and is characterized by immune dysfunction, opportunistic infections, and unusual malignancies. The incubation period between HIV infection and the onset of AIDS is about 10 years in adults. (See Fig. 7–1.)

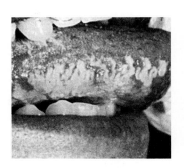

Figure 7–1. Hairy leukoplakia in an HIV-positive man. (Reprinted, with permission, from *Medical Immunology*, 9th ed., by Daniel P. Stites. Copyright 1997 by Appleton & Lange.)

3. Impact

A significant public health concern with increasing frequency of reported AIDS cases (AIDS is the leading cause of death in men between the ages of 25 and 44 years in the United States), with resulting impact (medical, financial, social/psychological, legal) on the patients, the patients' families, the health care system (including social service, home health, and foster care systems), and the insurance industry.

AIDS remains 100% fatal. There is no cure, although vaccines are being tested. However, with newer drugs, patients are living much longer than in the 1980s, when the virus was first discovered in humans.

4. Screening

Screening includes detection of HIV infection by an ELISA, and confirmation by Western blot.

Screening of high-risk patients and blood products/blood donors is critical. Screening via voluntary screening sites, and by most insurance companies for life insurance policies, is in effect. Universal premarital or populace screening may prove costly, with low yield and increased false-positive reports, but research is ongoing to see if more widespread screening could save lives.

U.S. blood donation centers began screening in March 1985. Minimal transfusion-related HIV/AIDS risk remains. Initial lab testing for patients who test positive for HIV should include absolute CD4 lymphocyte count and CD4 lymphocyte percentage. Counts less than 500 cells/mm^3 may indicate HIV-associated immunodeficiency. CD4 < 200 is associated with a high risk for opportunistic infections or malignancy.

5. Prevention

Cornerstone is **education** (including safe sex and effective use of condoms, types of high-risk behavior). Special effort to address high-risk groups (homosexuals, intravenous (IV) drug users/parenteral exposure, prostitutes, promiscuous individuals, hemophiliacs, partners of high-risk individuals) are needed. Education and regulation to protect health care workers and their patients (decontamination, gloves, reduction of needlesticks). Screening will provide both patient education/treatment and partner tracing/treatment. Distribution of condoms and bleach has been attempted. Distribution of sterile needles has been proposed.

► Treatment Steps
Antiretroviral therapy inhibits viral replication by inhibiting transcriptase. Nucleoside analogue (stavudine, abacavir) and non-nucleoside (delaviridine, efavirenz) reverse transcriptase inhibitors can be used in conjunction with protease inhibitors (amprenavir, indinavir). (See also Chapter 9.)

C. Prevention of Newborn Hemolytic Disease

► Description
Also termed *erythroblastosis fetalis.* **Fetal red blood cell antigens attacked by maternal immunoglobulin G (IgG)** (isoimmune disease) or **anti-A** or **anti-B** (ABO disease) **antibodies,** after transplacental passage.

Prevention includes maternal testing for **type, Rh, and antibody screen;** Rh$_o$(D) immune globulin (RhoGAM) injection; more accurate screening for maternal sensitization/fetal disease (amniocentesis), with intervention (labor induction) as necessary.

Give Rh immune globulin injection for Rh-negative mothers (see Table 7–1).

Kleihauer test: determines amount of fetal cells in maternal serum. Perform after traumatic delivery to determine amount of Rh immune globulin to give.

D. Prevention of Transfusion Reactions

► Description
Usually ABO incompatibility. Prevention includes proper blood-bank specimen handling and technique, along with accurate patient and specimen identification. Other factors include close patient observation during transfusion (major hemolytic reactions occur early during transfusion), and observation of the blood itself (abnormal color may indicate bacterial contamination).

Patient history of atopy or asthma may predispose to allergic transfusion reactions, so additional caution/observation is indicated. Pretransfusion treatment with antihistamines may be of value, along with the use of washed erythrocytes.

Patient history of multiple transfusions or pregnancies may predispose to febrile transfusion reactions. May try infusing leukocyte-depleted infusions (donor leukocyte antigens may result in the reaction).

Patient history and examination will assist in dictating rate and amount of volume to be infused (thus avoiding congestive heart failure).

7-1

RhoGAM INJECTIONS

If mother is Rh negative: Give injection at 28 weeks, within 3 days of delivery, after any bleeding, after amniocentesis.
If baby is Rh positive: Give another dose postpartum.
Standard dose: 1 mL (300 µg); counteracts 10 mL antigenic fetal cells.

E. Immunization

Passive (antibodies given for short-acting protection) or **active** (antigen given).

1. Infants and Children

a. **Hepatitis B**
#1 from birth to 2 months
#2 from 1 month to 4 months (at least 1 month after the first dose)
#3 from 6 months to 18 months (at least 4 months after the first dose and at least 2 months after the second dose, but not before 6 months of age for infants)

Infants born to hepatitis B surface antigen (HbsAg)-positive mothers should receive the hepatitis B vaccine and hepatitis B immune globulin (HBIG) within 12 hours of birth.

Infants born to mothers whose HBsAg status is unkown should receive the hepatits B vaccine within 12 hours of birth.

b. **Diptheria and Tetanus Toxoids and Acellular Pertussis (DTaP)**
#1 at 2 months
#2 at 4 months
#3 at 6 months
#4 at 15–18 months
#5 at 4–6 years

c. **Tetanus and Diptheria Toxoids (TD) at 11–12 Years of Age and Every 10 Years**

d. *H. influenzae* **Type b (Hib)**
#1 at 2 months
#2 at 4 months
#3 at 6 months
#4 at 12–15 months

e. **Inactivated Polio (PV)**
#1 at 2 months
#2 at 4 months
#3 at 6–18 months
#4 at 4–6 years

Oral polio vaccine (OPV) should only be used in selected situations.

f. **Pneumococcal Conjugate (PCV)**
#1 at 2 months
#2 at 4 months
#3 at 6 months
#4 at 12–15 months

g. **Measles–Mumps–Rubella (MMR)**
#1 at 12 to 15 months
#2 at 4 to 6 years

h. **Varicella**
12–18 months
Susceptible patients 13 years of age or older should receive two doses at least 4 weeks apart.

i. **Hepatitis A Vaccination**—Recommended in selected states and for high-risk groups after 2 years of age.

2. **Adults**
   - Tetanus, diphtheria (Td) every 10 years.
   - Influenza (yearly in elderly or chronic cardiopulmonary disease patients).
   - Pneumococcus vaccine (high-risk chronic cardiopulmonary disease, asplenia, diabetes, and elderly).
   - Hepatitis vaccine if in higher-risk group.

   Other specific vaccines for travel and/or work: rabies, cholera, typhoid.

3. **Postexposure Therapy**
   Hepatitis: HBIG.
   Rabies: rabies immune globulin (RIG).
   Tetanus: tetanus immune globulin (TIG).
   Varicella: Zovirax tablets 800 mg qid for 5 days.

4. **Compromised Immune System Patients**
   Give zoster immune globulin (ZIG) to prevent chickenpox, if exposed.

   Avoid live, attenuated vaccines (increased risk of paralysis with trivalent oral polio vaccine [TOPV]). **Avoid bacillus Calmette–Guérin (BCG) vaccine.**

   Okay to give influenza, inactivated polio, and pneumococcal vaccines.

5. **Severe Egg Allergy**
   Controversy exists about avoiding vaccines grown on chick or duck embryos, which include vaccines for yellow fever and influenza. Influenza vaccines may be tolerated by egg-allergic individuals. Measles and mumps vaccines are grown on chick or duck fibroblast tissue cultures and are generally free of egg albumin. Measles and mumps vaccines can therefore be used in the severe egg allergic individual but caution should be taken.

F. Prevention of Allergic-Related Morbidity

▶ Description

Key is **education,** along with early detection (both of the disease and of hypoxia/respiratory distress), and treatment of asthma/allergic rhinitis.

Education includes avoiding specific triggers (sulfites, aspirin, home/environmental/occupational triggers, allergens and irritants, gastroesphageal reflux).

Preventive treatment includes desensitization and medication.

Inhaled bronchodilators and/or cromolyn sodium prior to exertion in exercise-induced asthma may prevent attacks. Cromolyn sodium, nedocromil sodium, long-acting β-agonists, leukotriene modifiers, and inhaled corticosteroids are effective as preventive therapy for asthmatics. Other considerations include evaluation and treatment of emotional components.

Early intervention may prevent ventilatory failure.

Allergic rhinitis prevention: avoidance, desensitization, oral antihistamines, nasal cromolyn sodium/corticosteroids/antihistamines/anticholinergics.

▶ **clinical pearl**

Patients with anaphylaxis or severe allergic reactions should always carry an EpiPen. Parents and caregivers of children with severe allergies should carry and know how to use the EpiPen.

▶ **cram facts**

Difference between DT and Td—Children with pertussis vaccine reaction are given DT. Children older than 7 and adults are given Td vaccine (less diphtheria toxoid dose).

► **cram facts**

IMMUNOLOGIC PULMONARY DISEASE

- Hypersensitivity pneumonitis—IgE or IgG-mediated reaction to organic dust; cough, fever, chills, dyspnea; peripheral neutrophilia (no eosinophilia); nodular or fibrotic radiograph.
- Allergic bronchopulmonary aspergillosis—IgE-mediated and immune complex–mediated reaction to *Aspergillus;* history of asthma; fever, wheezing, productive cough; leukocytosis, sputum and blood eosinophilia, elevated total serum IgE, serum precipitins for *Aspergillus;* radiographic infiltrates from proximal bronchiectasis.
- Goodpasture's syndrome—Type II or antigen–antibody reaction; pulmonary hemorrhage and nephritis; hemoptysis, dyspnea, lethargy, hematuria, proteinuria; positive serum anti-GBM antibody; acinar consolidation or reticular radiographic pattern; restrictive lung defect.
- Pulmonary eosinophilia (Löffler syndrome)—IgE-mediated reaction or idiopathic; eosinophilia with migratory infiltrates; mild cough, wheeze, low-grade fever, myalgias; good prognosis.

II. MECHANISMS OF DISEASE, DIAGNOSIS, AND TREATMENT

A. Allergic Dermatopathies

1. Hereditary Angioedema

► **Symptoms**
Slow-onset, swelling attacks without hives (lasting 1–4 days).

► **Diagnosis**
History and physical examination, lab studies, **no hives present,** no pruritus.

C4 levels are diminished during asymptomatic periods and are undetectable during an attack. C2 levels are normal during asymptomatic periods and are diminished during an attack. C1-esterase inhibitor levels (functional or qualitative rather than quantitative levels) are most specific. C1 may be low in acquired angioneurotic edema states but not in hereditary angioneurotic edema.

► **Pathology**
Autosomal dominant; C1 esterase inhibitor deficiency. Rare.

► **Treatment Steps**
1. Supportive.
2. Danazol or stanozolol.

2. Angioedema

► **Symptoms/Diagnosis**
Swelling; may be associated with hives and pruritus. Clinical diagnosis.

► **Pathology**
Cutaneous anaphylaxis resulting from **IgE-mediated reaction** (though may also result from unknown causes).

► **Treatment Steps**
1. Antihistamines (Benadryl, Claritin).
2. H_2 blockers (Zantac).

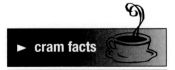

► **cram facts**

Attacks may affect laryngeal area resulting in airway obstruction. Epinephrine/ corticosteroids of little value.

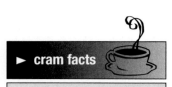

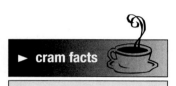

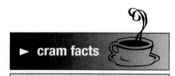

3. Leukotriene modifiers.
4. Tricyclic antidepressants in low doses (Sinequan).
5. Oral adrenergics (Proventil Repetab).
6. Corticosteroids.
7. Epinephrine.

3. Urticaria (Hives)

► **Symptoms/Diagnosis**
Hives (wheal and flare), **pruritus.** Clinical diagnosis.

► **Treatment Steps**
See treatment steps for angiodema above.

B. Allergic Rhinitis, Hay Fever, and Asthma

1. Allergic Rhinitis

► **Description**
Seasonal or continuous eye, nose, and throat symptoms. Caused by histamine release (and other immune mediators) in response to allergens.

► **Symptoms**
Itchy nose/eyes, rhinitis, dry cough, and sneezing.

► **Diagnosis**
History and physical examination, allergy testing (skin and/or RAST, including IgE level), nasal smear for eosinophils.

► **Treatment Steps**
1. Avoidance techniques.
2. Medicines:
   a. Oral antihistamines (Benadryl or Zyrtec) may be added to oral decongestants (Sudafed).
   b. Oral antihistamine/decongestant combination preparations (Allegra D or Claritin D) may be used instead of individual antihistamines and decongestants.
   c. Nasal corticosteroids (Nasonex).
   d. Nasal antihistamines (Astelin).
   e. Nasal ipratropium bromide (Atrovent 0.03%).
   f. Nasal cromolyn sodium (Nasalcrom).
   g. Nasal decongestants (Afrin) should be avoided for extended periods as they may cause rhinitis medicamentosa.
   h. Oral corticosteroids (prednisone).
3. Desensitization, also known as immunotherapy, to inhaled allergens.

2. Asthma

► **Description**
Usually, reversible airway obstructive disorder, characterized by inflammation and bronchospasm. Asthma can be classified into the following categories depending on the degree of symptomatology such as frequency of awakenings, absenteeism, need for inhalers and emergent intervention:
1. **Mild intermittent**—symptoms $\leq$ 2/week, nighttime symptoms $\leq$ 2/month, forced expiratory volume in 1 second (FEV_1) $\geq$ 80% of predicted.
2. **Mild persistent**—symptoms > 2/week but < 1/day, nighttime symptoms > 2/month, $FEV_1 \geq$ 80% of predicted.

3. **Moderate persistent**—daily symptoms, symptoms affect activity, daily use of short-acting β_2-agonist, nighttime symptoms > 1/week, FEV_1 > 60% but ≤ 80% of predicted.

4. **Severe persistent**—continual symptoms, limited physical activity, frequent nighttime symptoms, FEV_1 ≤ 60% of predicted.

► Symptoms

Wheezing, cough, and **dyspnea.**

► Diagnosis

History and physical examination, chest x-ray, pulmonary function testing (pre- and postbronchodilator), provocation testing (with methacholine), allergy testing.

► Pathology

Airway inflammation and hyperreactivity (triggered by allergen exposure or emotional/environmental factors).

► Treatment Steps

Education, avoid inciting agents, home peak flow monitoring. Pharmaceutical treatment consists of **quick-relief** and **long-term-control** medicines. Start with a quick-relief medicine (e.g., Proventil HFA prn), and then consider adding a long-term-control medicine (e.g., Pulmicort Turbuhaler) if the quick-relief medicine is necessary more than twice weekly.

Quick-Relief Medicines

1. Inhaled short-acting β_2-adrenergic (Proventil HFA or albuterol solution via nebulizer or inhaler).
2. Inhaled ipratropium bromide (Atrovent).
3. Subcutaneous epinephrine.
4. Oral corticosteroids.
5. Intravenous corticosteroids (prednisone, methylprednisolone).
6. Intravenous aminophylline.
7. Oxygen.

Long-Term-Control Medicines

1. Inhaled corticosteroid (fluticasone, beclomethasone).
2. Inhaled long-acting β_2-adrenergic (salmeterol).
3. Inhaled cromolyn sodium (Intal).
4. Inhaled nedocromil sodium (Tilade).
5. Oral sustained-release theophylline (UniDur).
6. Oral leukotriene modifiers (Singulair, Accolate, Zyflo).
7. Combination inhaled corticosteroid and long-acting β-adrenergic (Advair).

All patients should always have a metered-dose inhaler (MDI) with a short-acting β_2-agonist (albuterol) to be used as a rescue medication.

Treatment of Mild Intermittent Asthma

1. Daily medication not needed. Inhaled short-acting β_2-adrenergic (albuterol) 2 puffs qid, prn.
2. For exercise-induced asthma, treat with an inhaled short- or long-acting β_2-adrenergic (as above) 15–20 minutes prior to exercise.

Treatment of Mild Persistent Asthma

Daily medication for long-term control: low-dose inhaled corticosteroids. Alternatives include cromolyn, leukotriene-modifying drugs, nedocromil, or theophylline.

► **differential diagnosis**

ASTHMA

1. Emphysema
2. Chronic bronchitis
3. Congestive heart failure
4. Pulmonary embolism
5. Intraluminal lesions (e.g., foreign body, carcinoma, adenoma)
6. Carcinoid
7. Mastocytosis
8. Parasitic infestations
9. Extraluminal lesions (e.g., lymphoma, aortic aneurysm)
10. Gastroesophageal reflux
11. Allergic rhinitis/sinusitis
12. Vocal cord dysfunction
13. Cystic fibrosis
14. Cough secondary to drugs (e.g., angiotensin-converting enzyme [ACE] inhibitors)

► **cram facts**

- Child with large foul stools and wheezing: rule out cystic fibrosis.
- Wheezing with diarrhea and flushing: rule out carcinoid.
- Child with unilateral sudden wheezing: rule out foreign body.

Treatment of Moderate Persistent Asthma

Daily medications for long-term control should include low- to medium-dose inhaled corticosteroid *and* long-acting inhaled β_2-agonist (can be accomplished using one inhaler, Advair). Alternatives include increasing inhaled corticosteroid dose or adding either a leukotriene modifier or theophylline.

Treatment of Severe Persistent Asthma

1. Daily mediations for long-term control should include high-dose inhaled corticosteroids *and* long-acting inhaled β_2-agonist.
2. If needed, oral corticosteroids can be used with repeated attempts to reduce the systemic dose and maintain control with inhaled corticosteroid.

Management of Asthma Exacerbations

- Often occurs in the hospital. Oxygen will be utilized, as well as nebulized solutions of albuterol, usually with ipratropium bromide (Atrovent).
- Systemic corticosteroids (prednisone or solumedrol) used as well as empiric antibiotics.
- Peak flows should be followed, as well as oxygenation and CO_2 retention. Due to rapid respiratory rate, CO_2 levels on arterial blood gases (ABGs) should be low. If patient is acutely ill and CO_2 is returning to normal or is elevated, mechanical ventilation may be needed, as the patient may be heading toward acute respiratory failure.
- Subcutaneous epinephrine and magnesium are sometimes given in the emergency department.
- Alternative methods used include heliox, a mixture of oxygen and helium, to improve oxygenation.

Adjunctive Therapy in Asthma

- Seasonal allergies/allergic rhinitis can worsen asthma. Nasal corticosteroids are very effective, as well as newer antihistamines, which are less sedating: loratidine (Claritin), cetirizine (Zyrtec), or fexofenadine (Allegra) (see prior section, Allergic Rhinitis).
- Gastroesophageal reflux disease (GERD) can worsen asthma, particularly causing nighttime cough. Treatment with proton pump inhibitors can be very effective.
- Educating patients on proper use of inhalers, careful monitoring of peak flows and symptoms, what to do in an acute attack, avoidance of triggers, and importance of maintenance medications is very important to minimize morbidity and mortality.

C. Immunologic Pulmonary Disease

1. Hypersensitivity Pneumonitis

▶ Description

Allergic pulmonary disorder, from organic dust inhalation (see Table 7–2).

▶ Symptoms

Cough, fever, chills (4–6 hours after exposure to offending allergen).

▶ Diagnosis

History and physical examination, chest x-ray, pulmonary function testing, inhalation challenge testing, lung biopsy.

7-2

ALLERGENS CAUSING HYPERSENSITIVITY PNEUMONITIS

Allergen	Source	Disease
BACTERIA		
Thermophilic actinomycetes	Contaminated hay or grains	Farmer's lung
	Contaminated bagasse	Bagassosis
	Mushroom compost	Mushroom worker's lung
Bacillus subtilis	Contaminated walls	Domestic hypersensitivity pneumonitis
Streptomyces albus	Contaminated fertilizer	*Streptomyces* hypersensitivity pneumonitis
FUNGI		
Aspergillus spp.	Moldy barley	Malt worker's lung
	Moldy tobacco	Tobacco worker's lung
	Compost	Compost lung
Aureobasidium, Graphium spp.	Redwood bark, sawdust	Sequoiosis
	Contaminated sauna water	Sauna worker's lung
	Contaminated humidifier	Humidifier lung
Cryptostroma corticale	Maple bark	Maple bark disease
Penicillium casei	Moldy cheese	Cheese worker's lung
Sacchoromonospora viridis	Dried grass	Thatched roof disease
Various undetermined puffball spores	Moldy dwellings	Domestic hypersensitivity pneumonitis
	Mold in cork dust	Suberosis
	Lycoperdon puffballs	Lycoperdonosis
Alternaria, Penicillium spp.	Wood pulp, dust	Woodworker's lung
INSECTS		
Sitophilus granarius (wheat weevil)	Infested flour	Wheat miller's lung
ORGANIC CHEMICALS		
Isocyanates	Various industries	Chemical worker's lung
MISCELLANEOUS		
Pituitary snuff	Medication	Pituitary snuff taker's lung
Coffee bean protein	Coffee bean dust	Coffee worker's lung
Rat urine protein	Laboratory rats	Laboratory worker's lung
Animal fur protein	Animal pelts	Furrier's lung
Unknown	Contaminated tap water	Tap water hypersensitivity pneumonitis

Reprinted, with permission, from *Medical Immunology*, 9th ed., by Daniel P. Stites. Copyright 1997 by Appleton & Lange.

► **Pathology**

IgE- or IgG-mediated reaction to dust inhalation. Includes wide variety of antigens (wood, hair, mold, trees).

► **Treatment Steps**

1 Avoid inciting agent.
2. See the treatment of asthma.

2. **Allergic Bronchopulmonary Aspergillosis**

See Chapter 16.

3. **Goodpasture's Syndrome**

► **Description/Symptoms**

Autoimmune disease causing both pulmonary and renal disease. Symptoms include **hemoptysis, hematuria, cough,** anemia, lethargy, proteinuria.

► **Diagnosis**

History and physical examination, **renal biopsy,** chest x-ray, **positive serum anti–glomerular basement membrane (anti-GBM) antibody,** and antialveolar basement membrane antibody (see Fig. 7–2).

► **Pathology**

Linear immunoglobin deposits noted on glomerular basement membrane.

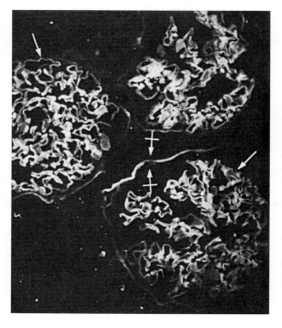

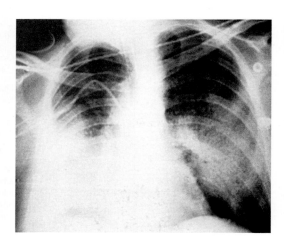

A

B

Figure 7–2. A: Smooth linear deposits of IgG (arrows) representing anti-GBM antibodies are seen outlining the GBM of three glomeruli from a young man with Goodpasture syndrome. The antibody also had reactivity with Bowman's capsule (opposed hatched arrows). (Original magnification ×160.) **B:** Chest x-ray of a patient with Goodpasture syndrome, showing extensive bilateral pulmonary infiltrates typical of intra-alveolar hemorrhage. (Reprinted, with permission, from *Medical Immunology,* 9th ed., by Daniel P. Stites. Copyright 1997 by Appleton & Lange.)

► Treatment Steps
1. Plasmapheresis.
2. Prednisone (1 mg/kg/day).
3. Cyclophosphamide (1–2 mg/kg/day).

4. Pulmonary Eosinophilia (Löffler Syndrome)

► Symptoms
Eosinophilia, cough, pulmonary infiltrates, or asymptomatic.

► Pathology
IgE-mediated reaction to various agents, or idiopathic.

► Treatment Steps
1. Eliminate exposure to the offending agent.
2. Corticosteroids—a brief tapering course of prednisone.

D. Transfusion Reactions

See Chapter 5.

E. Immunologically Mediated Drug Reactions

1. Anaphylactic Shock

► Description
Acute, life-threatening allergic reaction.

► Symptoms/Diagnosis
Shock, hypotension, airway obstruction/bronchoconstriction, urticaria, angioedema. Clinical diagnosis.

► **Treatment Steps**
1. Control airway.
2. Cardiopulmonary resuscitation (CPR).
3. Epinephrine 1:1,000 (0.3–0.5 cc SQ).
4. Repeat epinephrine twice every 15–20 minutes.
5. Volume replacement.
6. Corticosteroids.
7. Antihistamines.
8. β-Agonists.

2. Hemolytic Drug Reactions

► **Description**
Hemolysis secondary to medication ingestion.

► **Symptoms**
Dyspnea, hypotension, lethargy (symptoms of anemia).

► **Diagnosis**
Clinical, serologic studies (direct Coombs').

► **Pathology**
Etiology includes immune complex formation, medication antibodies, and autoimmune hemolytic anemia, methyldopa (Aldomet).

► **Treatment Steps**
1. Stop offending medication.
2. Corticosteroids have limited benefit in autoimmune-type hemolysis.

F. Autoimmune Disorders

1. Chronic Thyroiditis—Hashimoto's
See Chapter 3.

2. Graves' Disease
See Chapter 3.

3. Addison's Disease

► **Description**
Adrenocortical insufficiency due to autoimmune destruction of adrenal gland. See Chapter 3.

4. Pernicious Anemia
See Chapter 5.

5. Idiopathic Thrombocytopenic Purpura (ITP)
See Chapter 5.

6. Immune Hemolysis

6–1. Warm Autoimmune—Hemolytic Anemia
See Chapter 5.

6–2. Paroxysmal—Cold Hemoglobinuria
See Chapter 5.

6–3. Cold-Agglutinin Disease
See Chapter 5.

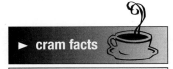

► cram facts

Anaphylactoid reactions: Etiology is direct mediator release (contrast dye, for example), presentation/ treatment similar to anaphylaxis.

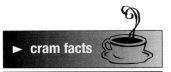

► cram facts

THYROIDITIS TYPES

- *Acute:* bacterial (fever/pain).
- *Subacute* (de Quervain's): **viral?** (fever/pain/large gland/high sed rate).
- *Chronic* (Hashimoto's): **autoimmune.** Chronic type also includes Reidel's thyroiditis (unknown cause). **Increased incidence of systemic lupus erythematosus (SLE), scleroderma and pernicious anemia with Hashimoto's disease.**
- *Schmidt syndrome:* **Hashimoto's disease plus Addison's disease.**

► **cram facts**

AUTOIMMUNE DISORDERS

1. Chronic thyroiditis—Hashimoto's, thyroid inflammation; female preponderance; hyper- or euthyroid at first; positive antimicrosomal antibody; treat with thyroid hormone replacement.
2. Graves' disease—hyperthyroidism; thyrotoxicosis; antithyroid antibodies, homogeneous thyroid scan; treat with β-adrenergic blockers followed by antithyroid medications.
3. Addison's disease—adrenocortical insufficiency; weight loss, lethargy, metabolic acidosis; diagnose with adrenocorticotropic hormone (ACTH) stimulation test; treat with corticosteroids.
4. Pernicious anemia—autoimmune B_{12} deficiency; anemia, antiparietal cell and anti-intrinsic factor antibodies; treat with parenteral vitamin B_{12}.
5. Idiopathic thrombocytopenic purpura—thrombocytopenia due to antiplatelet antibodies; purpura; petechia; treat with corticosteroids, possibly splenectomy.
6. Immune hemolysis—includes warm autoimmune hemolytic anemia (most common), paroxysmal cold hemoglobinuria (cold induced), cold-agglutinin disease (cold induced), and newborn hemolytic disease (due to D antigen Rh).
7. Chronic active hepatitis—jaundice, ascites, extrahepatic symptoms; due to virus, medication, or other etiology; treat with corticosteroids.
8. Glomerulonephritis—hematuria, edema, hypertension due to poststreptococcal infection, SLE, and vasculitis.
9. Multiple sclerosis—demyelinating central nervous system (CNS) disease; vertigo, nystagmus, incoordination; diagnose with magnetic resonance imaging (MRI), lumbar puncture; treat with immunosuppressives.
10. Myasthenia gravis—neuromuscular disorder; ptosis, diplopia; diagnose with electromyogram (EMG), tensilon test; positive acetylcholine receptor antibodies; treat with thymectomy, corticosteroids.

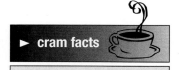

Acute ITP: usually children, often postviral, self-limited disease usually. *Chronic ITP:* usually adults.

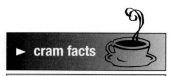

- Direct Coombs': detects red blood cell surface antibody.
- Indirect Coombs': serum antibody.

6–4. Newborn—Hemolytic Disease

► **Description**
Newborn immune hemolytic disorder **(erythroblastosis fetalis)**. See Table 7–1.

► **Symptoms**
Early-onset **jaundice,** anemia, kernicterus.

► **Diagnosis**
History and physical examination, prenatal lab studies, amniocentesis, **positive direct Coombs'.**

► **Pathology**
Mother's antibodies (most often **D antigen Rh**), attack fetal blood cells.

► **Treatment Steps**
1. Prevention.
2. *Predelivery:* **fetoscopic transfusion.**
3. *After delivery:* **exchange transfusion,** phototherapy.

7. Chronic Active Hepatitis (Fig. 7–3)
See Chapter 4.

8. Glomerulonephritis
See Chapter 17.

9. Multiple Sclerosis
See Chapter 11.

10. Myasthenia Gravis
See Chapter 11.

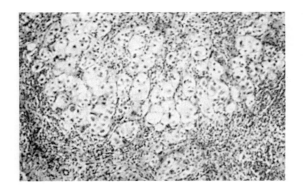

Figure 7–3. Chronic HBV infection. Liver biopsy specimen shows ballooning of hepatocytes and piecemeal necrosis typical of chronic active hepatitis. (Reprinted, with permission, from *Medical Immunology,* 9th ed., by Daniel P. Stites. Copyright 1997 by Appleton & Lange.)

G. Immunization Against Infectious Agents

See section I.E.

H. Connective Tissue Disorders

1. Systemic Lupus Erythematosus (SLE)

▶ **Description**

Multisymptom inflammatory immune disorder.

▶ **Symptoms**

Since SLE is a multisystem disorder, symptomatology is variable. For exam purposes, the patient is often a young female with joint pain. Also may have malar rash (see Fig. 7–4), symptoms of fatigue.

▶ **Diagnosis**

See Cram Facts.

▶ **Pathology**

Immune mediated with increased incidence in females, and those with positive family histories of SLE.

▶ **Treatment Steps**

1. Corticosteroids.
2. Immunosuppressives.
3. Antimalarials.

▶ **cram facts**

DIAGNOSIS OF LUPUS

- Malar rash
- Discoid rash
- Photosensitivitiy
- Oral ulcers
- Arthritis (nonerosive, in two or more joints)
- Serositis (pleuritis or pericarditis)
- Renal disorder (proteinuria or casts)
- Neurologic disorder (seizures or psychosis)
- Hematologic disorder (hemolytic anemia, leukopenia, lymphopenia, thrombocytopenia)
- Positive ANA
- Immunologic disorder (positive anti-double-stranded DNA, positive anti-SM, positive antiphospholipid antibody, or false-positive syphilis test (Venereal Disease Research Laboratory [VDRL]).

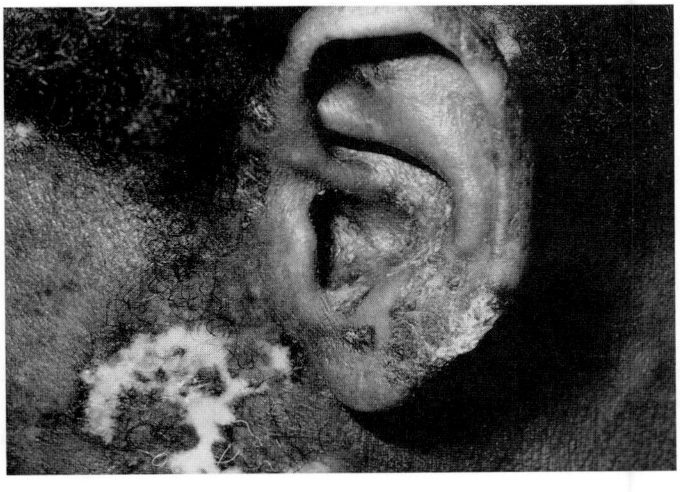

Figure 7–4. Active scaly areas and old depigmented, scarred areas on the face and pinna in a patient with discoid lupus erythematosus. (Reprinted, with permission, from *Medical Immunology,* 8th ed., by Daniel P. Stites. Copyright 1994 by Appleton & Lange.)

► **cram facts**

CONNECTIVE TISSUE DISORDERS

1. Systemic lupus erythematosus—multisystem disorder; malar rash, arthritis, proteinuria, vasculitis, alopecia; positive ANA, antiphospholipid antibodies; treat with corticosteroids.
2. Juvenile rheumatoid arthritis—asymmetric joint pain, fever, morning stiffness; abnormal erythrocyte sedimentation rate (ESR), RF, ANA, joint x-rays; systemic, polyarticular or pauciarticular; treat with salicylates, NSAIDs, gold, corticosteroids.
3. Adult rheumatoid arthritis—chronic synovitis, symmetric joint swelling, subcutaneous nodules, extraarticular symptoms; abnormal ESR, RF, x-rays; immune-complex formation; treat with salicylates, NSAIDs, gold, corticosteroids.
4. Rheumatic fever—poststreptococcal multisystem inflammatory disease; polyarthritis, chorea, carditis, erythema marginatum, subcutaneous nodules; abnormal ASO, CRP, ESR, leukocytosis; treat with penicillin, NSAIDs, corticosteroids.
5. Scleroderma—progressive systemic sclerosis; multisystem, anemia, dyspnea, arthritis; abnormal ANA, single-stranded RNA, biopsy; treat with corticosteroids.
6. Polymyalgia rheumatica—severe shoulder and pelvis pain/stiffness in elderly, fever, lethargy; no decreased joint motion; abnormal cortisol secretion rate, human lymphocyte antigen (HLA)-associated; treat with corticosteroids.

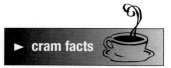

► **cram facts**

Disorders that may coexist with SLE: psoriasis, porphyria cutanea tarda, Sjögren's syndrome.

► **cram facts**

Systemic JRA: Still's disease; adenopathy, fever.
• Polyarticular: ≥ 5 joints affected.
• Pauciarticular: ≤ 4 joints, most frequent type, iridocyclitis is most significant complication.

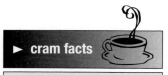

► **cram facts**

Felty syndrome: RA, granulocytopenia, and splenomegaly.

2. Juvenile Rheumatoid Arthritis (JRA)

► **Description**
Most frequent childhood rheumatic disorder (peak age 1–2 years). Also called **juvenile chronic arthritis or Still's disease.**

► **Symptoms**
Asymmetric joint pain, tenderness and swelling, for > 6 weeks' duration, fever, morning stiffness.

► **Diagnosis**
History and physical examination, lab studies (sed rate, rheumatoid factor [RF], antinuclear antibody [ANA], etc.), x-ray.

► **Pathology**
Autoimmune-induced synovitis—three types: systemic, polyarticular, and pauciarticular.

► **Treatment Steps**
1. Salicylates.
2. Nonsteroidal anti-inflammatory drugs (NSAIDs).
3. Gold.
4. Antimalarials.
5. Corticosteroids.

3. Adult Rheumatoid Arthritis

► **Description**
Chronic adult immune-mediated synovitis.

► **Symptoms**
Symmetric joint swelling, morning stiffness, subcutaneous nodules, extra-articular symptoms (episcleritis, neuropathy, pulmonary fibrosis/pleuritis, vasculitis, lethargy) (see Fig. 7–5).

► **Diagnosis**
History and physical examination (with attention to American Rheumatism Association criteria), lab (RF, sed rate), x-ray (marginal erosions/osteoporosis), synovial fluid analysis.

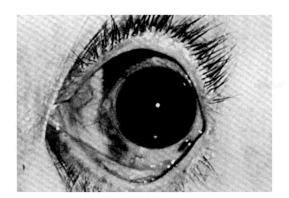

Figure 7–5. Scleral thinning in a patient with rheumatoid arthritis. Note the dark color of the underlying uvea. (Reprinted, with permission, from *Medical Immunology*, 9th ed., by Daniel P. Stites. Copyright 1997 by Appleton & Lange.)

▶ Pathology

Chronic synovitis resulting from **immune complex formation** with **joint/tissue** injury.

▶ Treatment Steps

1. NSAIDs.
2. Corticosteroids.
3. Disease-modifying antirheumatic drugs (DMARDs) including penicillamine, gold salts, immunosuppressants (methotrexate, immuran), and hydroxychloroquine.
4. Physical therapy/occupational therapy (PT/OT).
5. Surgery.
6. New "biologic" medications (see Cram Facts).

4. Rheumatic Fever

▶ Description

Poststreptococcal multisystem inflammatory disorder.

▶ Symptoms

Major: polyarthritis, chorea, carditis, erythema marginatum, and **subcutaneous nodules.**
Minor: fever, abnormal lab studies (antistreptolysin-O [ASO] titer, C-reactive protein [CRP], sed rate, leukocytosis).

▶ Diagnosis

History and physical examination, streptococcal infection plus Jones criteria (two major symptoms or one major plus two minor).

▶ Pathology

Multisystem tissue inflammation; a possible result of host versus streptococcal antigen reaction.

▶ Treatment Steps

1. Penicillin (eliminates strep, but will not alter RF disease course).
2. NSAIDs.
3. Prednisone (for carditis).

5. Scleroderma

▶ Description

Multisystem connective tissue disorder (progressive systemic sclerosis).

▶ Symptoms

Affects **skin/vascular** system (Raynaud's phenomenon), GI **tract, renal, pulmonary,** and **cardiac systems.** Also anemia, dyspnea, and arthritis.

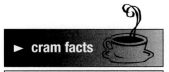

▶ cram facts

RHEUMATOID ARTHRITIS TREATMENT

Three new biologic medications are used in the treatment of rheumatoid arhritis. All three work to block TNF-α:
- Etanercept (Enbrel)
- Adalimumab (Humira)
- Infliximab (Remicade)

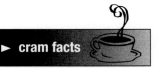

▶ cram facts

RA therapy side effects:
- *Gold*—rash, liver/renal abnormalities, hematologic disorders.
- *Methotrexate*—marrow toxicity, teratogenic.
- *Penicillamine*—rash, hematologic toxicity, teratogenic.
- *Hydroxychloroquine*—rash, retinal damage.

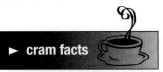

▶ cram facts

- **Most frequent cause for scleroderma death: renal disease.**
- **Most frequent internal organ affected: esophagus.**

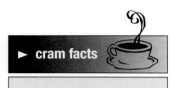

► Diagnosis

History and physical examination, lab studies (single-strand RNA, ANA), biopsy.

► Pathology

Increased skin and organ collagen deposition, along with vascular narrowing. May be localized (morphea), or generalized.

► Treatment Steps
1. Supportive.
2. Corticosteroids.

6. Polymyalgia Rheumatica

See Chapter 10, section II.F.1.

I. HIV Infections and AIDS

See Chapter 9, section I.C.3.

J. DiGeorge Anomaly

► Description

Genetic disorder characterized by abnormal facies, congenital heart disease, hypocalcemia, and increased susceptibility to infections.

► Pathology

Hypoplasia or aplasia of the thymus occurs, causing defective T cells.

► Treatment Steps

Early thymus transplantation may promote immune reconstitution.

K. Humoral Immunity Deficiency

1. Severe Combined Immunodeficiency Disease (SCID)

SCID refers to several genetic diseases that result in B- and T-cell disorders. The most common type is X-linked. The other forms are autosomal recessive or due to spontaneous mutations. One of these forms is linked to a deficiency of the enzyme adenosine deaminase (ADA).

Patients are at increased risk of infection and if SCID is not diagnosed and treated early, it can result in severe infection and death by age 2. Treatment includes prophylaxis against PCP (*Pneumocystis carinii* pneumonia). In certain genetic causes, bone marrow transplantation is offered. If caused by ADA deficiency, ADA replacement may be warranted. Gene therapy is being investigated.

L. Transplantation Rejection

► Description

Immunological transplant rejection.

► Symptoms

Fever, pain, lethargy. Dysfunction of transplanted organ.

► Diagnosis

History and physical examination, additional studies (kidney: blood urea nitrogen [BUN], creatinine, renal biopsy).

▶ Pathology

Lymphocyte- and antibody-induced reaction, with T-cell graft tissue injury (acute reaction). Renal transplant may also present as hyperacute or chronic reaction.

▶ Treatment Steps

Immunosuppressive medication (corticosteroids, cytotoxic medications, antimetabolites).

BIBLIOGRAPHY

American Academy of Pediatrics, Commitee on Infectious Diseases, Recommended Childhood Immunization Schedule—United States January–December 2001. *Pediatrics* 2001;107:202.

Beers MH. *Merk Manual of Diagnosis and Therapy,* 17th ed. Whitehouse Station, NJ: Merk Research Laboritories, 1999.

Behrman RE. *Nelson Textbook of Pediatrics,* 16th ed. Philadelphia: W.B. Saunders, 2000.

Braunwald, E. *Harrison's Principles of Internal Medicine,* 15th ed. New York: McGraw-Hill, 2001.

Busse, WW. Advances in Allergic Disease Supplement to the *Journal of Allergy and Clinical Immunology* June 2000;105(6, Part 2):5593–5644.

DaVita VT. *AIDS Etiology, Diagnosis, Treatment and Prevention.* Philadelphia: Lippincott-Raven, 1997

Fleisher TA. Primary Immune Deficiencies. *Pediatric Clinics of North America* 2000:47(6): 1197–1407.

Grevnik A. *Textbook of Critical Care,* 4th ed. Philadelphia: W.B. Saunders, 2000.

Hall JC. *Sauer's Manual of Skin Diseases,* 8th ed. Philadelphia: Lippincott Williams & Wilkins, 2000.

National Asthma Education and Prevention Program. Clinical Practice Guidelines. Expert Panel Report 2: *Guidelines for the Diagnosis and Management of Asthma.* NIH Publication No. 97-4051, July 1997. www.nhlbi.nih.gov.

Tierney LM. *Current Medical Diagnosis and Treatment,* 41st ed. New York: Lange Medical Books/McGraw Hill, 2002.

Injury and Toxicology 8

I. MECHANISMS OF DISEASE, DIAGNOSIS, AND TREATMENT

A. Fractures

Note: The diagnosis of all fractures starts with a history and physical, then usually an evaluation with plain film (x-ray). Computed tomographic (CT) scan may also be used.

1. Facial

▶ Description

Fractures of the zygomatic arch, mandible, maxilla, orbits, or nose.

▶ Symptoms

Pain, swelling, deformity, and ecchymosis.

> *Orbital Fracture*—Diplopia and facial paresthesias.
>
> *Ethmoid*—May have cerebrospinal fluid (CSF) rhinorrhea.
>
> *Nasal Bones*—Deformity, epistaxis, septal hematoma.
>
> *Mandible/Maxilla*—Airway compromise, malocclusion.

▶ Treatment Steps
1. Antibiotics, fracture reduction.
2. *Nasal*—drain septal hematoma, reduction in fracture cases with cosmetic deformity.
3. *Maxillary*—reduction, interdental or other wiring.
4. *Mandibular*—interdental or other wiring.
5. *Orbital*—surgical to resupport orbit.

2. Skull

▶ Description

Closed (simple) or **open** (compound) fractures of linear or depressed type involving calvarium or basilar skull.

▶ Symptoms

Asymptomatic or **pain/swelling,** CSF leak (nose or ears).

▶ Treatment Steps
1. Rule out brain/cervical spine injury.
2. *Simple linear*—observation. Temporal location across middle meningeal artery at risk for epidural hematoma.
3. *Compound linear*—antibiotics.
4. *Depressed*—surgical treatment (fragment elevation).

3. Vertebral Column

▶ Description

Vertebral body fracture, pedicle fracture, transverse process fracture, spinous process fracture. If posterior elements are involved, it may be unstable with risk of cord injury. Caused by trauma or osteoporosis.

▶ Symptoms

Pain, neurologic abnormalities, including motor and sensory deficits, bowel and bladder disturbances.

▶ Diagnosis

CT scan to evaluate stability, hematoma, or bone fragment intrusion into spinal cord.

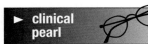

▶ **clinical pearl**

Signs of basilar skull fracture:
- Hemotympanum (blood behind tympanic membranes)
- CSF leak from nose or ear
- Ecchymosis behind ear (Battle's sign)
- Periorbital ecchymoses (raccoon eyes)

► **Treatment Steps**

Depends on location and extent of fracture.

The cervical spine with an unstable fracture or neurologic deficit requires immediate cranial traction with application of a halo device **followed by surgical internal fixation.**

4. Thorax

► **Description**

Rib or sternum fracture.

► **Symptoms**

Pain, increased with inspiration/palpation.

► **Treatment Steps**

Simple rib fracture same as contusion—analgesics, ice initially, injection of local anesthetic (into intercostal nerve) as an option.

5. Pelvis

► **Description**

Fracture of innominate bone (ilium, ischium, or pubis), sacrum.

► **Symptoms**

Pain; major trauma can cause hypotension from bleeding fracture site(s) (see Cram Facts).

► **Diagnosis**

History and physical examination, **x-ray studies,** CT scan.

► **Pathology**

Trauma; via falls, motor vehicle accidents, sports injuries.

► **Treatment Steps**

Depends on multiple factors, with open reduction and internal fixation, traction, and external fixation as choices. Need to evaluate for coexisting injuries/trauma and treat accordingly.

6. Extremities

6–1. Tibia/Fibula

► **Description**

Tibia fracture can involve tibial plateau (knee), shaft or distal (medial malleolus of ankle). Fibula fracture can involve shaft or distal (lateral malleolus of ankle).

► **Symptoms**

Pain, swelling, ecchymosis.

► **Treatment Steps**

Depends on nature and location of fracture.
1. **Closed reduction immobilization, cast.**
2. Certain cases of tibia fracture need open reduction and internal fixation (ORIF).

6–2. Femur

► **Description**

Femur fracture can involve shaft, distal (epicondyles at knee), or proximal (hip joint).

► **Symptoms**

Pain, swelling, deformity.

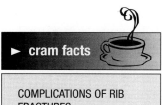

► **cram facts**

COMPLICATIONS OF RIB FRACTURES

- Pneumothorax
- Pulmonary contusion
- Mediastinal injury
- Cardiac contusion

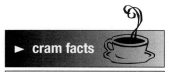

► **cram facts**

PELVIC FRACTURE

Most important complication of pelvis fracture: hemorrhage. Angiography/embolization may be required for severe persisting hemorrhage.

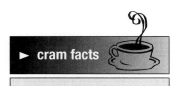

► **cram facts**

FEMUR FRACTURE

In child, rule out child abuse.

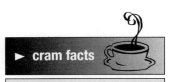

► **cram facts**

- Colles' fracture—fall on extended wrist, **fracture of distal radius and often ulnar styloid** (volar angulation/dorsal displacement).
- Smith's fracture fall on flexed wrist—dorsal angulation/volar displacement.

► Treatment Steps

Majority of femur fractures require ORIF for definitive care. Traction is used to stabilize prior to surgery.

6–3. Radius

► Description

Radius fracture most commonly involves proximal (radial head) and distal (wrist). Diagnose with history and physical, x-ray.

► Symptoms

Pain, swelling, reduced joint motion.

► Treatment Steps

Radial Head—**Hemarthrosis aspiration and mobilization** if simple, **surgical** (ORIF) **if complete/displaced fracture.**

Distal Radius—**Cast 4–6 weeks, therapy.**

6–4. Ulna

► Description

Ulna fracture most often involves proximal (elbow) and distal ulnar styloid at wrist.

► Symptoms

Pain, swelling, decreased joint motion.

► Treatment Steps

Proximal ulna fractures of the olecranon at the elbow are treated with immobilization or ORIF if displaced.

6–5. Humerus

► Description

Humerus fracture includes proximal (shoulder), shaft, and supracondylar (elbow).

► Symptoms

Pain, swelling, decreased joint motion.

► Treatment Steps

1. Proximal humeral fractures have numerous classifications and are treated by immobilization or ORIF.
2. Humeral shaft fractures are frequently associated with radial nerve injuries.
3. Supracondylar fractures in children often result in distal vascular compromise and may require closed reduction in addition to immobilization.

6–6. Scaphoid Fracture

- The scaphoid is the most frequently fractured carpal bone.
- Cause most often is a fall on an outstretched hand.
- If clinical concern persists despite normal radiographic results, the clinician has two main options:
  - The patient's hand and wrist can be immobilized, and radiographs can be repeated after 2 weeks to detect an initially occult fracture.
  - Additional imaging modalities may be used (bone scan, CT, and magnetic resonance imaging [MRI]).

- A complication of scaphoid fracture is avascular necrosis (AVN). AVN is more common in scaphoid fractures than most other bones because of its blood supply.

B. Sprains and Dislocations

Note: These conditions are also usually diagnosed clinically, and x-ray may be used to rule out fracture.

1. Hands

1–1. Distal Interphalangeal (DIP) Sprain

► **Description**
Disruption or avulsion of the extensor tendon attached to base of distal phalanx produces a mallet finger.

► **Symptoms**
Patient unable to extend at DIP joint.

► **Diagnosis**
X-ray may show chip avulsion at base of distal phalanx.

► **Pathology**
Traumatic extensor tendon disruption.

► **Treatment Steps**
Dorsal splint of DIP in extension for 6 weeks.

1–2. Interphalangeal (IP) Dislocations

► **Description**
Dislocation of DIP or proximal interphalangeal (PIP) joints are usually dorsal due to blows to tip of the flexed digit.

► **Symptoms**
Pain, deformity, joint immobility. On exam, displaced digit, motion loss.

► **Treatment Steps**
1. Closed reduction.
2. Exam for collateral ligament injury.
3. Immobilization in flexion.

1–3. Metacarpophalangeal (MCP) Injuries

► **Description**
MCP joint dislocations fail closed reduction more often than IP joints because of entrapment of volar plate. Recognition of injury to ulnar collateral ligament of thumb MCP (gamekeeper's thumb) is critical to preserve ability to pinch (requires urgent hand surgeon consultation).

► **Symptoms**
Pain, deformity, motion loss.

► **Treatment Steps**
1. Closed reduction.
2. Surgery if unsuccessful and if required for ulnar collateral ligament tear.
3. Immobilization.

2. Ankle Sprain

► **Description**
Ankle ligament injury classified into first-, second-, and third-degree sprains.

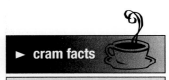

► cram facts

OTTAWA ANKLE RULES

Ankle x-rays are not
indicated if:
- The patient is < 55 years
  old.
- The patient is able to
  walk four steps at time of
  injury and time of
  evaluation.
- There is no tenderness
  over the posterior edge
  (distal 6 cm) or tip of
  either malleolus.
- There is no tenderness
  over the base of the fifth
  metatarsal.
- There is no tenderness
  over the navicular bone.

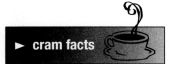

► cram facts

- Elbow dislocation—
  check vascular/
  neurologic status;
  **urgent reduction
  indicated,** usually
  closed, then immobilize.
- If elbow effusion,
  immobilize and repeat
  examination on followup
  to detect occult radial
  head fracture.

► Symptoms

Pain, swelling, ecchymosis.

► Pathology

Lateral Pain—Injury to anterior/posterior talofibular ligament.
May also include injury to calcaneofibular and posterior talofibular
ligaments.

Medial Pain—Deltoid ligament injury.

► Treatment Steps

1. Rest, ice, compression, elevation (RICE).
2. Early mobilization for minor injury, or casting for more severe ankle splint.

3. Elbow

► Description

Elbow dislocation is usually posterior with a hyperextension injury.
Elbow joint effusion/hemarthrosis may be associated with an occult
radial head fracture.

► Symptoms

Pain, decreased joint mobility. X-ray may show posterior/anterior fat
pad sign indicating an effusion.

► Treatment Steps

See Cram Facts.

4. Shoulder

► Description

Sprain or dislocation injury. **Anterior-inferior dislocation most common.**

► Symptoms

Shoulder pain, protruding acromion/shoulder deformity with anterior dislocation.

► Treatment Steps

Dislocation—reduction, usually closed, immobilization for 4–6
weeks.

5. Spine

► Symptoms

Pain. Increased pain with muscle stretch (strain). Head in extension
or tilted, muscle spasm and more pain (sprain). Stiff neck/back.

► Diagnosis

MRI if disk/cord involvement is suspected.

► Pathology

Trauma, flexion/extension injury (cervical spine); overuse common
in thoracic/lumbar spine injury.

► Treatment Steps

1. Rest.
2. Ice for first 24 hours, moist heat after 48 hours.
3. Nonsteroidal anti-inflammatory drugs (NSAIDs).
4. Muscle relaxants.
5. Rehabilitation.

C. Burns, Electrical Injuries, and Environmental Thermal Injuries

1. Burns

► **Description**

Heat injury to skin and underlying tissues. May be first, second, or third degree.

► **Symptoms/Diagnosis**

Erythema (first degree), **blisters** (second degree), painless eschar (third degree). Diagnose clinically.

► **Pathology**

Epidermal destruction, with partial dermal destruction in second degree. Epidermal and dermal destruction in third-degree burn.

► **Treatment Steps**

1. Remove patient from source of burn. Cool the burned area.
2. Clean/debride burn.
3. Fluids (crystalloids initially).
4. Tetanus prophylaxis.
5. Grafting.

2. Electrical Injuries/Burns

► **Description**

Burns and trauma secondary to electrical injury.

► **Symptoms**

Entry/exit wound (high voltage, lightning). Massive tissue and bone destruction. Initial presentation may not reflect extent of injury to deep structures.

► **Diagnosis**

History and physical examination. Observation or surgical exploration for deep injury.

► **Pathology**

Tissue necrosis with myoglobinuria, hyperkalemia. Cardiac arrhythmias.

► **Treatment Steps**

1. Remove patient from source safely.
2. Supportive care and monitoring.
3. Fluids.
4. Clean/debride burns.
5. Surgical evaluation (fasciotomy, amputation).

3. Environmental Thermal Injuries

3–1. Frostbite

► **Description**

Most severe cold injury.

► **Symptoms**

Blistering, tissue cold/hard without feeling. Necrosis.

► **Diagnosis**

History and physical; affected area may be white, blistered (superficial injury), or firm and frozen (deep injury).

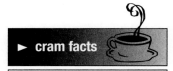

► **cram facts**

RISK FACTORS ASSOCIATED WITH ENVIRONMENTAL HEAT INJURIES

1. Age: infants and elderly.
2. Environmental factors: high temperature and humidity.
3. Drugs: phenothiazine, other anticholinergics such as benztropine (Cogentin), cyclic antidepressants, monoamine oxidase inhibitors (MAOIs), amphetamines.

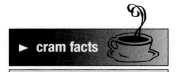

► **cram facts**

Rule of nines to estimate burn extent: each leg is 18%, each arm is 9%, body front is 18%, back is 18%, head is 9%, groin is 1%.

► **Pathology**

Skin/tissue damage from ice crystal formation. May be superficial or deep. Line of demarcation may develop.

► **Treatment Steps**

1. **Rapid but gentle rewarming.**
2. Surgical evaluation/amputation.

3–2. Hypothermia

► **Description/Diagnosis**

Reduced **core temperature** (under 35°C).

► **Symptoms**

Confusion, coma, hypotension, bradycardia. Electrocardiogram (ECG) findings (Osborn [J] wave, bradycardia) (see Fig. 8–1).

► **Pathology**

Reduced core temperature from cold exposure resulting in decreased cardiac output, hypotension. Respiratory depression, central nervous system (CNS) depression.

► **Treatment Steps**

1. Supportive care and monitoring.
2. Apply passive or active rewarming techniques.
   - Passive: insulation.
   - Active external: warming blankets, radiant heat.
   - Active core: heated lavage of bladder, stomach, pleura, pericardium, cardiopulmonary bypass.

3–3. Heatstroke

► **Description**

Most severe type of heat injury, with elevated core temperature and neurologic symptoms.

► **Symptoms/Diagnosis**

Confusion, elevated core temperature, tachycardia, syncope, coma. Clinical diagnosis.

► **Pathology**

Tissue injury from elevated temperature; children and elderly at most risk.

► **Treatment Steps**

Rapid cooling (water-soaked sheets/fans/ice packs).

D. Lacerations

► **Description**

Skin/soft tissue mechanical disruption.

► **Diagnosis**

History and physical examination to include distal neurovascular evaluation, foreign bodies, and deep structure involvement.

► **Treatment Steps**

1. Irrigation and debridement, antibiotics, tetanus prophylaxis, and primary closure.
2. Use 1–2% lidocaine for anesthesia. Remove sutures in 7–14 days. Utilize deep and subcutaneous sutures to reduce tension on skin edges. Try to remove facial sutures in 5 days.

► **clinical pearl**

HYPOTHERMIA

- Profound hypotension can mimic clinical death.
- However, some patients have a good neurologic outcome if resuscitated and rewarmed.
- The old adage that is repeated: "Patients are not dead until they are warm and dead."

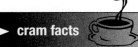

► **cram facts**

- Heat cramps—cramps in multiple muscle groups from **salt depletion; rest and electrolyte replacement.**
- Heat exhaustion—volume depletion; nausea/weakness/headache/thirst; rest and volume replacement.
- Complications of heat stroke—disseminated intravascular coagulation, rhabdomyolysis, cardiovascular collapse.

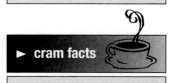

► **cram facts**

Human bites—increased infection with primary closure.

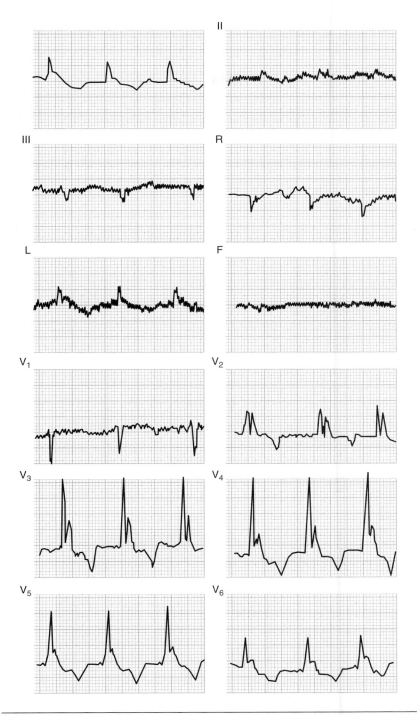

Figure 8–1. Typical ECG seen in hypothermia. This patient was a 69-year-old man with a core temperature of 24°C (75.2°F). Note the typical J wave abnormalities (Osborn waves) in the terminal phase of the QRS complex. This patient's ECG returned to the premorbid state on rewarming. (Reprinted, with permission, from Goldfrank's *Toxicologic Emergencies,* 6th ed., by Lewis R. Goldfrank. Copyright 1998 by Appleton & Lange.)

E. Chest, Abdominal, and Pelvic Injuries

1. Pneumothorax

▶ **Description**
Air in pleural cavity.

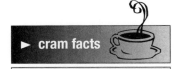

PUNCTURE WOUND

- Excellent opportunity to update someone's tetanus status.
- Give tetanus booster if patient has not had one in the last 10 years.

► Symptoms

Dyspnea, chest pain. Tachycardia and hypotension may occur in tension pneumothorax.

► Diagnosis

History and physical examination (absent breath sounds, hyperresonance), **chest x-ray** (see Fig. 8–2).

► Pathology

A result of blunt or penetrating trauma (including iatrogenic trauma). May also be spontaneous, especially in patients with pulmonary disease.

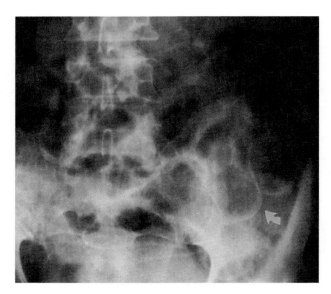

A

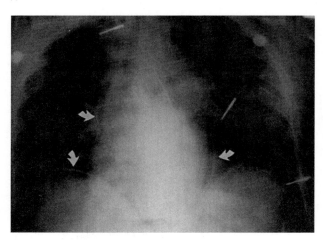

B

Figure 8–2. GI perforation following gastric lavage with a large-bore orogastric tube.
A: Free intraperitoneal air, which outlines the outer side of the small bowel wall, is seen on the supine abdominal radiograph (arrow). **B:** The upright chest radiograph shows air under the right hemidiaphragm and pneumomediastinum (arrows). An esophagram with water-soluble contrast did not reveal the site of perforation. Laparotomy revealed a perforation of the anterior wall of the stomach. Gastric lavage is not always without complication. This patient had had endotracheal intubation prior to lavage to prevent aspiration. (Reprinted, with permission, from Goldfrank's *Toxicologic Emergencies,* 6th ed., by Lewis R. Goldfrank. Copyright 1998 by Appleton & Lange.)

► Treatment Steps

1. **Small pneumothorax**—with good pulmonary reserve may require only close observation. Most require catheter or tube thoracotomy.

2. **Tension pneumothorax requires urgent intervention—insert large-bore needle into second intercostal space, midclavicular line (MCL) followed by tube thoracotomy.**

2. Hemothorax

► Description/Symptoms

Blood in pleural cavity. Causes dyspnea, chest pain.

► Diagnosis

History and physical examination (absent breath sounds), **chest x-ray.**

► Treatment Steps

1. **Large-bore tube thoracotomy.**

2. **Open thoracotomy for persisting hemorrhage, or massive initial blood loss.**

3. Flail Chest

► Description

Multiple rib fractures resulting in a flail chest wall segment with ineffective, paradoxical inspiratory motion.

► Symptoms

Paradoxical chest wall segment motion, respiratory distress.

► Diagnosis

History and physical, **x-ray examination.**

► Pathology

Traumatic segmental rib fractures (two or more on same rib) of three or more consecutive ribs create a flail segment that moves inward on inspiration.

► cram facts

COMMONLY USED INOTROPIC DRUGS IN CRITICAL CARE

- **Dopamine:** For treatment of hypotension. Acts at β receptor. Low dose to help increase renal perfusion. Pressor dosages increase cardiac output (CO) and also act on α receptors peripherally.
- **Dobutamine:** For treatment of certain scenarios of hypotension (decreased CO). Acts in mostly β receptors but also in some α receptors. Increases CO. Careful, low dose initially can cause hypotension depending on patient's volume status.
- **Norepinephrine:** For treatment of severe hypotension. Acts at cardiac β receptors and very strongly at α peripheral receptors. Increases systemic vascular resistance (SVR), helping to improve CO. Watch for renal hypoperfusion.
- **Epinephrine:** For treatment of hypotension. Very strong cardiac and peripheral β agonist and also activates peripheral α. Increases SVP and CO.
- **Phenylephrine:** For refractory hypotension or for instances of severe tachycardia. Very strong exclusive α agonist. Increases SVP. Watch for renal hypoperfusion.

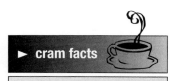

cram facts

- Blunt abdominal trauma—spleen most often injured.
- Penetrating abdominal trauma—small bowel most often injured.
- Positive peritoneal lavage criteria—red blood cells (RBCs) over 20,000 (in penetrating injury), or RBCs over 100,000 (in blunt injury).

► Treatment Steps

Intubation and positive pressure ventilation.

4. Perforation or Rupture of Viscus

► Description

Traumatic abdominal injury may cause rupture of a solid viscus or perforation of a hollow viscus.

► Symptoms

Pain, abdominal rigidity, peritoneal irritation, reduced/absent bowel sounds. Symptoms often delayed with perforation of hollow viscus.

► Diagnosis

History and physical examination (peritoneal irritation, shoulder pain, reduced/absent bowel sounds). Observation with serial exams, x-rays, CT scan, diagnostic peritoneal lavage, exploratory laparotomy.

► Treatment Steps

Laparotomy and surgical repair. May hospitalize, observe minor injury with serial exams and studies.

F. Drowning/Near Drowning

► Description

Asphyxia from water aspiration or water-induced laryngospasm.

► Symptoms

Wheezing, tachypnea, vomiting, **pulmonary edema,** or **unconsciousness, shock,** and **cardiac arrest.**

► Pathology

Dry (laryngospasm) or water-induced asphyxia results in hypoxia and brain damage.

► Treatment Steps

Aggressive supportive care, monitoring, and **100% oxygen.** Remember to continue cardiopulmonary resuscitation (CPR) in hypothermic/prolonged cold-water submersion victims.

G. Insect and Snake Bites

► Description/Diagnosis

Bites may have only local or local and systemic effects. Insects can cause systemic sepsis with anaphylaxis, especially *Hymenoptera* species. Snakes that are venomous cause systemic signs only when envenomation occurs with the bite. Diagnose clinically.

► Symptoms

Insect Bite—**Local erythema, itching, and swelling to anaphylaxis/hypotension.**

Snake Bite—Local signs to systemic signs with hemorrhage, weakness, disseminated intravascular coagulation (DIC), lethargy, vomiting, shock (see Fig. 8–3).

► Pathology

Insect venom can cause true immunoglobulin E (IgE)-mediated anaphylaxis with skin, respiratory, gastrointestinal (GI), or cardiovascular manifestations. Poisonous snake venom causes hemopathic, neu-

cram facts

- Black widow spider—red hourglass design on abdomen; diffuse muscle spasm/cramping typical.
- Brown recluse spider—violin design on back; possible skin necrosis.

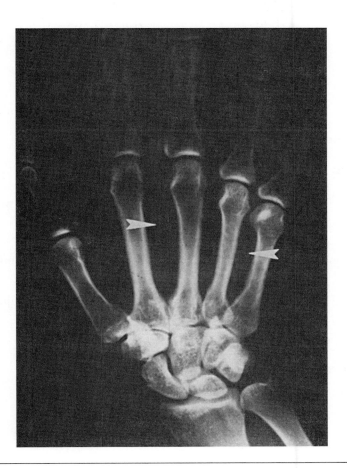

Figure 8–3. Significant local morbidity developed after the bite of a 6-foot boa constrictor. The patient had extensive soft tissue swelling and developed a gas-forming bacterial infection (note gas in interdigital spaces). Subcutaneous gas and/or crepitus following a snakebite does not always indicate a serious infection. Benign ambient air can be injected during the bite. Peroxide use and mouth suction can also introduce air into the wound. There was no fracture, but the force of the bite could have broken a metacarpal. (Reprinted, with permission, from Goldfrank's *Toxicologic Emergencies,* 6th ed., by Lewis R. Goldfrank. Copyright 1998 by Appleton & Lange.)

rotoxic, and general systemic symptoms and can be neutralized with antivenin.

▶ Treatment Steps

Insects—local care is ice and elevation (remove stinger). For cardiovascular collapse:

1. Epinephrine.
2. Fluids.
3. Corticosteroids.
4. Antihistamines.

If wheezing is present: inhaled bronchodilators.

Snakes—rest, immobilization in dependent position, determination of envenomation, and treatment with antivenin.

H. Motion Sickness

▶ Description

Aberrant reaction to motion. **Diaphoresis, nausea, vomiting, vertigo.** Diagnosed clinically.

▶ Pathology

Etiology in **vestibular–visual mismatch.**

► Treatment Steps

1. Antihistamines or scopolamine patch—apply to skin every 72 hours.
2. Avoid inciting etiology.
3. Vestibular training.

I. Head, Eye, and Ear Injury

1. Concussion

► Description

Head injury, with transient alteration of consciousness without physical brain damage.

► Symptoms

Brief altered consciousness, headache, nausea, and vomiting.

► Diagnosis

History and physical, CT scan to rule out acute brain injury.

► Treatment Steps

Observation with serial neurological exams.

2. Subdural Hematoma

See Chapter 11.

3. Epidural Hematoma

See Chapter 11.

4. Ocular Injury

► Symptoms

May have **pain, vision loss,** subconjunctival hemorrhage. If light flashes noted, rule out retinal detachment.

► Diagnosis

History and physical examination, ophthalmoscopic and slit-lamp examination.

► Pathology

Chemicals—Chemical conjunctivitis, blindness.

Trauma—Hyphema, laceration, abrasion.

► Treatment Steps

Hyphema—Anterior chamber hemorrhage (ophthalmologist's evaluation needed as soon as possible).

Chemicals—Irrigation with normal saline.

Corneal Abrasion—Antibiotic, pain control.

Corneal Laceration—**Eye shield, refer to ophthalmologist.**

5. Auditory Injury

► Description

Pinna, external ear canal, and tympanic membrane injury.

► Symptoms

Swelling, pain, hearing loss, vertigo, and hemorrhage.

► Diagnosis

History and physical examination, and audiometric exam, x-ray skull/temporal bone (rule out associated fracture).

► Treatment Steps

Tympanic Membrane Perforation—If small, supportive treatment (cotton earplug, systemic antibiotic for infection); if large, surgical treatment.

Noise-Induced Hearing Loss—No treatment (except hearing aid), but stress prevention of further damage.

J. Industrial and Occupational Dermatitis

► Description

Pathology/dermatitis secondary to industrial/occupational chemical, physical, thermal, and toxin exposure.

► Symptoms

Pruritus, inflammation, erythema, blisters.

► Diagnosis

History and physical examination, skin biopsy, allergic patch test.

► Pathology

Skin contact with foreign agent resulting in dermatitis. **Contact dermatitis most frequent.**

► Treatment Steps

Remove from source, antihistamines, topical/systemic corticosteroids.

K. Anaphylactic Shock

► Description

Systemic severe immune system allergic reaction with cardiovascular collapse. Anaphylactoid reaction is clinically similar but nonimmunologically mediated.

► Symptoms

Shock/cardiovascular collapse is manifested by hypotension, tachycardia, hypoperfused skin with decreased mentation as a late sign. Anaphylaxis can also be manifested in other organ systems: skin (urticaria, angioedema, erythema), airway (stridor, bronchospasm), GI (nausea, vomiting, diarrhea).

► Diagnosis

History, physical exam, and identification of potential allergen.

► Pathology

Hypersensitivity is an exaggerated immune system response to presented antigens, mediated mostly by IgE. Antigen binds to IgE on mast cells and basophils, triggering mediators responsible for local and systemic allergic manifestations. Mediators include histamine, bradykinins, platelet-activating factor (PAF), leukotrienes, etc.

► Treatment Steps
1. Epinephrine is the cornerstone therapy for anaphylactic shock. It can be given slowly IV up to 0.5 mg in 1:10,000 concentration or via endotracheal tube, and IM or SQ in 1:1,000 concentration (0.3–0.5 mL).
2. Large volumes of crystalloid should also be given.

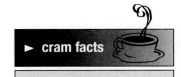

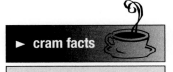

3. IV steroids and antihistamines.
4. Inhaled bronchodilators should be given for bronchospasm.

L. Poisoning

1. General Management

▶ Symptoms

Toxic syndromes, or *toxidromes,* are symptom complexes that allow rapid identification and grouping of numerous poisonings with similar characteristics. Some of these include sympathomimetic, sedative/narcotic/hypnotic, anticholinergic, cholinergic, extrapyramidal, etc.

▶ Diagnosis

History and physical exam identify toxidromes with some additional limited information available from serum and urine drug screens.

▶ Treatment Steps

1. *GI decontamination* limits further absorption and is accomplished with activated charcoal; gastric lavage and cathartics may also be used.
2. *Supportive care and monitoring* prevents or limits complications of poisoning and includes airway protection, breathing control, and circulatory support when needed.
3. *Definitive care* can be used only in a minority of poisonings; this includes enhanced elimination (hemodialysis, multiple doses every 2–4 hours of activated charcoal, alkalinization of the urine) and specific antidotes, which are available for only a handful of poisonings.

2. Acetaminophen

▶ Symptoms

Divided into four stages, beginning with nausea and vomiting, which may be mild or even absent during the first 24 hours. Progresses to hepatic injury and failure.

▶ Diagnosis

Draw plasma acetaminophen level at 4 hours postingestion and compare to nomogram; 140 mg/kg is a potentially serious ingestion.

▶Treatment Steps

1. GI decontamination.
2. Use of the specific antidote *N*-acetylcysteine (Mucomyst).

3. Cyclic Antidepressants

▶ Symptoms

Anticholinergic toxidrome, CNS signs (depression, myoclonus, seizures), cardiac conduction abnormalities (from sinus tachycardia with widened QRS to lethal arrhythmias), and contractile depression with hypotension.

▶ Diagnosis

History and physical and ECG.

▶ Treatment Steps

1. GI decontamination.
2. Multiple-dose charcoal.
3. Supportive care and monitoring.
4. Treat cardiovascular toxicity with alkalinization of the blood with bicarbonate.

▶ **differential diagnosis**

INCREASED ANION GAP METABOLIC ACIDOSIS (MUDPILES)

- **M**ethanol intoxication
- **U**remia
- **D**KA (diabetic ketoacidosis)
- **P**araldehyde intoxication
- **I**ntoxications (e.g., salicylates)
- **L**actic acidosis
- **E**thylene glycol
- **S**tarvation

INCREASED OSMOLAR GAP

- Severe dehydration
- Hyperproteinemia
- Sorbitol
- Glycerol
- Mannitol
- Ethanol
- Isopropyl alcohol
- Methanol
- Acetone
- Ether
- Paraldehyde
- Ethylene glycol

cram facts

SPECIFIC ANTIDOTES TO POISONINGS
TOXIC SYNDROMES (TOXIDROMES): ANTICHOLINERGICS, CHOLINERGIC,
SEDATIVES/NARCOTICS/HYPNOTIC, SYMPATHOMIMETIC, EXTRAPYRAMIDAL, WITHDRAWAL

Poison	Antidote
Acetaminophen	N-acetylcysteine (Mucomyst)
Atropine	Physostigmine
Benzodiazepines	Flumazenil
Carbon monoxide	Oxygen
Cyanide	Amyl nitrite, sodium nitrite, sodium thiosulfate
Heavy metals (lead, arsenic, mercury)	BAL (British Anti-Lewisite, dimercaprol)
Iron	Deferoxamine
Lead	Calcium disodium edetate
Methyl alcohol (ethylene glycol)	Ethyl alcohol
Nitrites	Methylene blue
Opiates	Naloxone
Organophosphates	Atropine and pralidoxime

4. Sedatives/Narcotics/Hypnotics

► **Symptoms**

Toxidrome manifested by CNS and respiratory depression, hypotension. For narcotics, see pinpoint pupils.

► **Diagnosis**

History and physical exam. Reversal of toxidrome by naloxone is safe and diagnostic for narcotics. Reversal by flumazenil is diagnostic for benzodiazepines but often contraindicated and not routinely recommended in acute setting. Urine and serum drug screens include some of these agents.

► **Treatment Steps**
1. GI decontamination.
2. Supportive care and monitoring.
3. For suspected narcotic overdoses, use naloxone.
4. For long-active barbiturates, use forced alkaline diuresis or dialysis.
5. For benzodiazepines, consider flumazenil in carefully selected cases only.

5. Amphetamines/Cocaine

► **Symptoms**
Sympathomimetic toxidrome with hypertension, tachycardia, CNS excitation, seizures.

► **Diagnosis**
History and physical examination.

► **Treatment Steps**
1. GI decontamination.
2. Supportive care and monitoring including core temperature.
3. Sedation may be required using benzodiazepines.
4. Aggressive cooling if indicated.

6. Phencyclidine (PCP)

► **Symptoms**

An hallucinogen, which may show either cholinergic or anticholinergic toxidromes, but most often nystagmus, hypertension, tachycardia, and bizarre behavior (either regressive or excitatory). Vertical nystagmus is characteristic of PCP intoxication and may accompany horizontal or rotational nystagmus.

► **Diagnosis**

History, physical examination, vertical nystagmus, and urine drug level.

► **Treatment Steps**

GI decontamination, supportive therapy and monitoring, sedation.

7. Alcohols (Ethanol, Methanol)

► **Symptoms**
- Ethanol: CNS depression.
- Methanol: CNS depression, visual abnormalities (photophobia, blurred vision, "snowstorm"), abdominal pain with nausea and vomiting.

► **Diagnosis**
- Ethanol: serum alcohol level, rule out other causes of CNS depression (hypoglycemia, trauma, etc.).
- Methanol: osmolal gap, metabolic acidosis, serum alcohol and methanol levels.

► **Treatment Steps**
- Ethanol: thiamine, supportive care.
- Methanol: IV bicarbonate for acidosis, ethanol infusion (prevents conversion of methanol to formate), hemodialysis.

8. Solvent Abuse

► **Symptoms**

CNS euphoria and depression, skin rash (dermatitis) especially on face ("huffer's" rash), cardiac arrhythmias, renal tubular acidosis, hypokalemia.

► **Diagnosis**

History of inhaling toluene (glue, paints) or halogenated hydrocarbons (typewriter correction fluid), nonanion-gap metabolic acidosis, serum potassium.

► **Treatment Steps**

Supportive care and monitoring.

9. Heavy Metals (Lead, Arsenic, Mercury)

► **Symptoms**
- **Lead**—CNS (acute/chronic), peripheral nervous system (acute/chronic), renal (acute/chronic), anemia.
- **Arsenic**—severe gastroenteritis, garlicky breath, metallic taste, CNS symptoms, peripheral neuropathy.
- **Mercury**—neurologic, GI, and renal systems affected depending on form and route of ingestion.

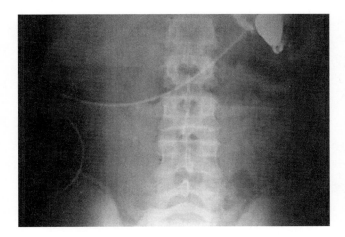
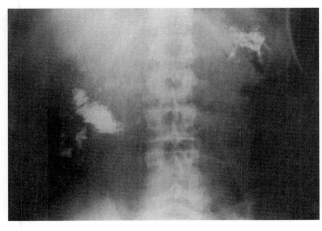

A   B

Figure 8–4. A chemist ingested mercuric oxide in a suicide attempt. **A:** Initial plain abdominal radiograph reveals the radiopaque liquid in the stomach. **B:** A second radiograph shows progression of the toxin through the bowel. The patient was followed radiographically as the substance was eventually expelled into the feces. (Reprinted, with permission, from Goldfrank's *Toxicologic Emergencies,* 6th ed., by Lewis R. Goldfrank. Copyright 1998 by Appleton & Lange.)

▶ Diagnosis

- **Lead**—anemia and peripheral smear, "lead bands" on pediatric x-rays, elevated serum polybrominated biphenyl (PBB), or positive provocation test.
- **Arsenic**—history with severe gastroenteritis followed by shock, 24-hour urine arsenic levels, KUB (kidney, ureter, bladder) with radiopaque materials.
- **Mercury**—history and physical, 24-hour urine mercury level (see Fig. 8–4).

▶ Treatment Steps

- **Lead**—GI decontamination, chelation therapy with dimercaprol (BAL) and ethylenediaminetetraacetic acid (EDTA).
- **Arsenic**—GI decontamination, aggressive supportive care and monitoring, chelation therapy with BAL.
- **Mercury**—GI decontamination with milk or egg whites to bind mercury, chelation therapy with BAL (see Fig. 8–4).

10. Carbon Monoxide

▶ Symptoms

Headache, dizziness, weakness, nausea at low levels. Progression to confusion, syncope, seizures, coma, hypotension.

▶ Diagnosis

History of fire exposure with CO symptoms, and physical examination, elevated blood carboxyhemoglobin.

▶ Treatment Steps

Remove from source, 100% oxygen, hyperbaric oxygen for severe cases and pregnancy.

Additional Poisonings

- **Iron—gastric lavage, parenteral deferoxamine (see Fig. 8–5).**
- **Aspirin—causes respiratory alkalosis and metabolic acidosis.**
- **Drugs visible on x-ray—heavy metals, phenothiazines, iodides, and chloral hydrate.**

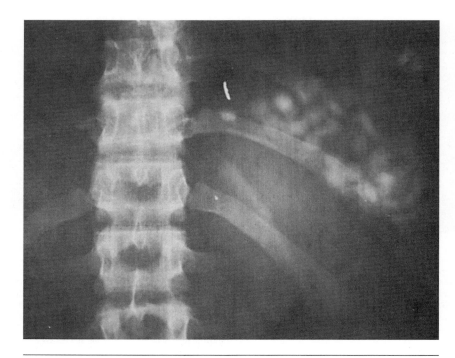

Figure 8–5. This radiograph was taken 12 hours after admission and following emesis, 40 L of lavage fluid, and endoscopy. These adherent fragments of iron, which were the remnants of several hundred ingested iron tablets, give the appearance of a concretion. Endoscopy and laparotomy with gastrotomy demonstrated the absence of a concretion. (Reprinted, with permission, from Goldfrank's *Toxicologic Emergencies,* 6th ed., by Lewis R. Goldfrank. Copyright 1998 by Appleton & Lange.)

► **differential diagnosis**

SHOCK

1. Hypovolemia: hemorrhage, dehydration
2. Cardiogenic shock
3. Sepsis
4. Neurogenic (spinal cord injury)
5. Obstructive (cardiac tamponade, tension pneumothorax, pulmonary embolus)

► **differential diagnosis**

TRAUMATIC SHOCK IN ADULTS

1. Internal hemorrhage: thoracic cavity, peritoneal cavity, retroperitoneal space
2. External hemorrhage: massive bleeding from external wound (arterial)
3. Neurogenic: spinal cord injury
4. Obstructive: impaired cardiac filling from cardiac tamponade, tension pneumothorax

III. PRINCIPLES OF MANAGEMENT

A. Traumatic Injury

Complete a primary survey first, then proceed to full secondary survey. If any abnormalities in primary survey, stop and treat, then continue evaluation. Primary survey: (1) airway, (2) breathing, (3) circulation (shock or continuing external hemorrhage), (4) neurologic status. Once primary survey and any necessary interventions are completed, begin the secondary survey from head to toe.

B. Shock

Assess and control airway, breathing. Treat shock with appropriate modality depending on etiology: cardiogenic, hypovolemic, septic, neurogenic, obstructive. Central venous pressure (CVP) or pulmonary artery catheter monitoring may be required to manage fluids and/or vasopressor therapy.

C. Burns

Assess and control airway, breathing, and circulation. Treat inhalation injuries with intubation. Rule out associated traumatic injuries if acutely hypotensive or if CNS depression. Check carboxyhemoglobin level. Determine level and extent of surface burn. Transfer to burn center if indicated using American Burn Association criteria.

D. Poisoning

Assess and control airway breathing and circulation. Identify syndromes (toxidromes). GI decontamination with lavage and/or activated charcoal. General supportive care and monitoring. Specific antidotes for a few specific ingestions.

E. Abuse of Children, Spouses, Elderly; Sexual Abuse

History and physical examination, medical treatment, documentation of evidence and appropriate reporting, psychological evaluation/support, separation from danger (child abuse), and **long-term care plan.**

BIBLIOGRAPHY

Tintinalli J, et al. *Emergency Medicine, A Comprehensive Study Guide,* 6th ed. ACEP. New York: McGraw-Hill, 2004.

Rosen P, et al. *Emergency Medicine: Concepts and Clinical Practice,* 4th ed. St. Louis: Mosby Yearbook, 1997.

Goldfrank LR. *Toxicologic Emergencies,* 7th ed. New York McGraw-Hill, 2002.

Infectious and Parasitic Diseases

9

I. INFECTIOUS DISEASES BY SYSTEM

A. General Aspects

1. Bacteremia and Septicemia

▶ **Description/Diagnosis**
Spread of infection to the bloodstream (bacteremia); septicemia includes symptoms and infections by fungi and microbes other than bacteria. Diagnosis based on clinical scenarios.

▶ **Symptoms**
Fever, chills, hypotension, hypothermia, shock. Rash (ecthyma gangrenosum, with *Pseudomonas* and others).

▶ **Pathology**
Complex. Endotoxin or other microbial elements may cause symptoms/shock.

▶ **Treatment Steps**
Antibiotics, supportive (fluids, pressors).

2. Toxic Shock Syndrome

▶ **Description**
Toxin-producing staphylococcal (or occasionally streptococcal) infection.

▶ **Symptoms**
Fever, rash, hypotension, dermal peeling of palms and soles (skin desquamation).

▶ **Diagnosis**
History and physical, tampon use, culture (vagina/blood).

▶ **Treatment Steps**
Antibiotics (β-lactamase resistant, antistaphylococcal), remove tampon, supportive care for shock.

B. Infectious and Parasitic Diseases

1. Eyes

1–1. Ophthalmia Neonatorum

▶ **Description/Symptoms**
Purulent conjunctivitis before 1 week old.

▶ **Pathology**
Etiology in *Neisseria gonorrhoeae, Chlamydia, Haemophilus*.

▶ **Treatment Steps**
Antibiotics. Prevent by 1% silver nitrate or erythromycin topically.

1–2. Bacterial Conjunctivitis

▶ **Description/Symptoms**
Conjunctival inflammation, causing exudate, itching, eyelid edema.

▶ **Diagnosis**
Clinical diagnosis, conjunctival scraping and culture used rarely.

► **Treatment Steps**
Antibiotics. Topical and/or systemic.

1–3. Viral Keratoconjunctivitis

► **Description/Symptoms**
Corneal infection/inflammation, causing red, painful eye, especially in children. Clinical diagnosis.

► **Pathology**
Herpes simplex most common in children, also other viruses including adenovirus (common with adult infections).

► **Treatment Steps**
Trifluridine or acyclovir.

2. Ears

2–1. External Otitis

► **Description**
External auditory canal inflammation; swimmer's ear.

► **Symptoms/Diagnosis**
Pain, drainage, itching. Clinical diagnosis.

► **Pathology**
- *Staphylococcus epidermidis,* other bacteria, fungal. If chronic, suspect *Pseudomonas.*
- Malignant otitis (severe infection with temporal bone invasion), suspect *Pseudomonas* (or occasionally *Proteus*).

► **Treatment Steps**
Topical and (if necessary) systemic antibiotics. Systemic needed for malignant otitis.

2–2. Otitis Media

► **Description/Symptoms**
Middle ear inflammation, causing fever, hearing loss, pain.

► **Diagnosis**
History and physical shows loss of light reflex, possible fluid behind tympanic membrane.

► **Pathology**
Streptococcus pneumoniae common. Multiple other agents possible. Common in children with eustachian tube dysfunction as possible etiology.

► **Treatment Steps**
Antibiotics (amoxicillin). If failure, use second-line antibiotic (e.g., oral cephalosporin or clarithromycin). If fails frequently, consider ear, nose, and throat (ENT) evaluation for tubes.

2–3. Mastoiditis

► **Description/Symptoms**
Mastoid air cell inflammation, causing fever, pain, hearing loss, postauricular swelling/erythema, displaced pinna. Cause is usually bacterial infection that started as otitis media.

▶ **Diagnosis**

History and physical, x-ray studies (computed tomography [CT]).

▶ **Treatment Steps**
1. Antibiotics.
2. Myringotomy.
3. Mastoidectomy.

3. Nervous System

3–1. Meningitis
See also Chapter 11, section VII.A.

▶ **Description**

Brain/spinal cord membrane inflammation. Much more serious and fatal if caused by bacteria rather than virus.

▶ **Symptoms of Bacterial Meningitis**

Fever/nuchal rigidity/headache/vomiting.

▶ **Diagnosis**

History and physical. Examination of cerebrospinal fluid (CSF) (bacteria: low glucose, elevated protein, high white blood count [WBC] with predominant neutrophils, positive Gram stain; viral: normal glucose, slightly elevated protein, low WBC [< 100] with predominant lymphs).

▶ **Prevention of Bacterial Meningitis**

Immunization (*Haemophilus influenzae*, *S. pneumoniae*, and *Neisseria meningitidis*) and treatment/prophylaxis of exposed close contacts.

▶ **Pathology**

Spread of germs to the central nervous system (CNS) via the blood. Common germs: up to 1 month of age, *Escherichia coli*, and group B strep; 1 month to age 6, *H. influenzae* type b, *S. pneumoniae*, and *N. meningitidis;* older than 6, *S. pneumoniae* and *N. meningitidis*.

▶ **Treatment Steps**

Antibiotics given parenterally (at high doses). (See Chapter 11, section VII.A.)

3–2. Brain Abscess

▶ **Symptoms**

Headache, mental changes, nausea/vomiting, focal neurologic findings, seizures.

▶ **Diagnosis**

History and physical examination, CT scan.

▶ **Pathology**

Anaerobic bacteria and oral *Streptococcus* common. May extend from ear/sinuses, follow injury, or be bloodborne from other areas (lung).

▶ **Treatment Steps**
1. Antibiotics IV.
2. Surgical drainage.

3–3. Spinal Epidural Abscess

▶ **Description**

Infrequent disease. Early intervention needed to prevent paraplegia.

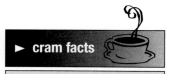

▶ **cram facts**

Brudzinski's sign: Cervical motion elicits pain.
Kernig's sign: Painful hamstring stretch.

► **Symptoms**

Local severe back pain changing to radicular pain, then weakness. Fever and local tenderness also.

► **Diagnosis**

History and physical examination, x-rays, CT, lumbar puncture.

► **Pathology**

Bloodborne spread from skin and IV catheters, usually by *Staphylococcus aureus.*

► **Treatment Steps**

1. Surgical drainage.
2. Antibiotics.

3–4. Poliomyelitis

► **Description**

Poliomyelitis virus can be transmitted by fecal–oral route. Three classes of polio exist:

1. Abortive polio—a febrile illness without CNS involvement.
2. Nonparalytic polio—aseptic meningitis with complete recovery.
3. Paralytic polio—aseptic meningitis followed by development of motor weakness.

► **Symptoms**

Fever, headache, weakness, sore throat. Muscle wasting, lower motor neuron lesion, vomiting.

► **Diagnosis**

History and physical examination. Examination of CSF. Stool/throat/fecal culture. Serologic testing to confirm (polio virus is a type of enterovirus).

► **Treatment Steps**

Supportive treatment. Polio is rare due to vaccination.

3–6. Rabies

► **Description**

Viral encephalitis caused by rabies virus. Very rare in the United States. Only several cases on record of human survival in documented rabies.

► **Symptoms**

Clinically, a prodrome of fever, myalgias, followed by encephalitis with confusion and agitation. Hydrophobia (laryngeal spasm with drinking or just sight of water), paresthesia/pain at bite site. Hyperactivity, ascending paralysis. Excessive salivation can cause classic "foaming at the mouth."

► **Diagnosis**

History and physical, animal bite. Check animal's brain for rabies. Also via state lab: search for rabies virus/antigen by neck skin/cornea biopsy, and serologic screening (for antirabies antibody).

► **Prevention**

Immunize high-risk individuals (veterinarians, cave explorers, animal handlers).

► Treatment Steps

For exposure: Local wound cleaning and postexposure prophylaxis with human rabies immune globulin (HRIG), rabies vaccine. For confirmed rabies: Supportive.

3–6. Herpes Zoster

See Chapter 2.

3–7. Herpes Simplex

See Chapter 2.

3–8. Tetanus

► Description

Neurotoxin-induced muscle spasm disorder.

► Symptoms

Tonic muscle spasms (jaw, trismus/lockjaw), rictus sardonicus: trismus-induced facial sneer. Opisthotonos, tetanospasm.

► Diagnosis

History and physical examination.

► Pathology

Clostridium tetani produces neurotoxin. Several days' to 3 weeks' incubation, after germ entry via wound.

► Treatment Steps

Supportive, tetanus immune globulin, and penicillin G.

3–9. Viral Encephalitis

► Description

CNS inflammation/infection caused by a virus (see Cram Facts).

► Symptoms

Headache, seizures, CNS alterations, fever, vomiting. Symptoms may be subclinical or severe in nature.

► Diagnosis

History and physical, CSF culture/examination (increased protein/pressure), throat/fecal viral cultures, magnetic resonance imaging (MRI), or CT brain.

► Treatment Steps

Supportive.

3–10. Viral Meningitis

► Description

Meningeal inflammation, caused by a virus.

► Symptoms

Severe headache, fever, photophobia.

► Diagnosis

Lumbar puncture with cell count < 100, protein < 100.

► Treatment Steps

Supportive.

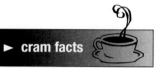

► cram facts

HERPES ENCEPHALITIS

- CT scan of head may show hypodense areas in temporal lobe(s).
- CSF can be tested for herpes simplex using polymerase chain reaction (PCR).
- Acyclovir is often started empirically while results are pending.

3–11. Toxoplasmosis

▶ **Description**

Infection with *Toxoplasma gondii* usually by cyst ingestion (cat litter/soil/undercooked meat, pregnant women must avoid all three). Also, transplacental transmission is possible.

▶ **Symptoms**

Usually asymptomatic; fever, headache, myalgia, adenopathy. Congenital infection (microcephaly, seizures, retinochoroiditis).

▶ **Diagnosis**

Biopsy is definitive for cysts/trophozoites. Serologic testing. Found in people with impaired cell-mediated immunity or children of mothers who acquired toxoplasmosis during pregnancy.

▶ **Treatment Steps**

Pyrimethamine plus sulfadiazine.

4. Nose and Throat

4–1. Common Cold
See Chapter 16.

4–2. Sinusitis
See Chapter 16, section II.A.6.

4–3. Pharyngitis
See Chapter 16, section II.A.2.

4–4. Peritonsillar Abscess
See Chapter 16, section II.A.4.

4–5. Acute Laryngotracheitis
See Chapter 16, section II.A.9.

4–6. Pertussis
See Chapter 16, section II.A.10.

4–7. Diphtheria

▶ **Description**

Upper respiratory tract infection caused by *Corynebacterium diphtheriae*. Prevent via immunization.

▶ **Symptoms**

Purulent nasal discharge, tonsillar membrane, fever, cervical adenopathy, nausea/vomiting.

▶ **Diagnosis**

Clinical, sore throat with green/gray pharyngeal membrane.

▶ **Treatment Steps**
1. Diphtheria antitoxin (DAT) and penicillin or erythromycin.
2. Penicillin or erythromycin for carrier state.

4–8. Epiglottitis
See Chapter 16, section II.A.9–2.

5. Lungs
See Chapter 16.

6. Cardiovascular System

6–1. Endocarditis

See also Chapter 1.

▶ **Description**

Endocardial infection.

▶ **Symptoms**

Fever, murmur, anemia. Multiple other symptoms possible including splinter hemorrhages, Osler nodes (red fingertip bumps), Janeway lesions (red macules on palms/soles), Roth spots on fundoscopic exam, weight loss, petechiae.

▶ **Diagnosis**

History and physical, blood culture, echocardiogram.

▶ **Pathology**

Acute often *S. aureus* (drug use typical). Subacute, often α-hemolytic *Streptococcus viridans* (oral pathology or surgery). Mitral valve most common site, pulmonic least common (in drug users, tricuspid valve more common). Platelets/fibrin form on abnormal area, then bacteria attach.

▶ **Treatment Steps**

1. Consult current literature.
2. *Streptococcus*—penicillin G and gentamicin (or streptomycin).
3. *Staphylococcus*—nafcillin (watch for methicillin-resistant *S. aureus* [MRSA] for which vancomycin is indicated). Also, note association of *Streptococcus bovis* or *Clostridium septicum* and colon cancer.

7. Gastrointestinal System

7–1. Mumps

▶ **Description**

Contagious mumps virus (a paramyxovirus) infection, only in humans. Prevented with vaccination. Most commonly causes parotiditis, but complications can include pancreatitis, orchitis, meningitis, encephalitis, nephritis, or deafness.

▶ **Symptoms**

After 2-week incubation, fever, headache, enlarging parotid (bilateral in 75%).

▶ **Diagnosis**

History and physical, serologic testing/viral isolation.

▶ **Treatment Steps**

No treatment is needed. Prednisone has been used in cases of orchitis.

7–2. Herpetic Gingivostomatitis

▶ **Description/Symptoms**

Common oral infection, usually with herpes simplex type I. Infection may be asymptomatic, or fever, vesicles and ulcers, adenopathy.

▶ **Diagnosis/Treatment**

Clinical diagnosis. Can culture if unsure of herpes vs. bacterial involvement. Often resolves spontaneously. Can use toical pencyclovir or systemic acyclovir.

7–3. Candidiasis

► **Description/Symptoms**

Overgrowth of *Candida* species, which is normally found in the body. Can cause vaginitis (vaginal itch/white thick discharge); diaper erythema and satellite lesions; balanitis; or oral thrush with mucosal disease and esophageal symptoms common.

► **Diagnosis**

Clinical picture, potassium hydroxide (KOH) preparation.

► **Pathology**

Superficial fungal infection, severe mucosal infection (rule out human immunodeficiency virus [HIV]) or fungemia/disseminated disease (rule out neutropenia or intravenous [IV] catheter related).

► **Treatment Steps**

1. Antifungal.
2. Topical and/or oral medication for mild disease.
3. Oral or IV fluconazole or IV amphotericin for moderate to severe disease.

7–4. Thrush

► **Description/Symptoms**

Oral fungal infection, usually caused by *Candida albicans*. Removable white mouth patches, plaque, halitosis. Can progress to esophagitis and cause dysphagia.

► **Diagnosis**

History and physical exam, KOH preparation.

► **Treatment Steps**

Nystatin mouth rinse and/or oral antifungal (fluconazole).

7–5. Retropharyngeal Abscess

► **Description**

Retropharyngeal infection caused by spread of infection from local area (sinus, tooth, etc.).

► **Symptoms/Diagnosis**

Fever, neck extension. Diagnose clinically. May culture abscess.

► **Treatment Steps**

Incision and drainage, antibiotics. Monitor for airway compromise.

7–6. Food Poisoning

► **Description**

Illness from ingestion of contaminated food. Can be due to many bacteria, viruses, or toxins.

► **Symptoms**

Nausea, vomiting, diarrhea, after food ingestion.

► **Diagnosis**

Food/stool culture and toxicologic studies. History and physical exam.

► **Treatment Steps**

Symptomatic, may treat specific bacterial isolate (*Clostridium difficile*—metronidazole or vancomycin by mouth).

7–7. Botulism

▶ Description

Foodborne botulism is caused by ingestion of food containing preformed toxin, most commonly via home-canned food. **Infant botulism** arises from ingesting spores of *Clostridium botulinum,* which produces toxin in the GI tract. **Wound botulism** develops in wounds contaminated by *C. botulinum* (can be wounds contaminated by soil, such as in chronic IV drug users).

▶ Symptoms

Nausea, vomiting, dysphagia, diplopia, progressive paralysis hours to days after ingesting bad fish/meat or canned product. Both myasthenia gravis and Guillain–Barré are usually considered in the differential, as they can all have ascending paralysis.

▶ Diagnosis

History and physical, toxin in serum/stool/food. Differs from myasthenia gravis by negative edrophonium (Tensilon) test. Must have strong clinical suspicion, usually from a thorough history.

▶ Pathology

C. botulinum produces neurotoxin. In infants, the clostridial spores can germinate in the intestine and produce toxin there.

▶ Treatment Steps

1. Trivalent antitoxin (A, B, E) should be given as soon as possible.
2. Supportive treatment including close monitoring of airway, as respiratory failure can develop.
3. Wound botulism—exploration and debridement also needed.

7–8. Viral Gastroenteritis

Vomiting, diarrhea, fever, often due to rotavirus or Norwalk virus. Supportive care.

7–9. Typhoid

▶ Description

Enteric fever, caused by *Salmonella typhi* (a pathogen in humans only). Organism is ingested via contaminated food, water, or milk and is more common in travelers or patients with HIV.

▶ Symptoms

Malaise, delirium, headache, constipation or diarrhea, lethargy, and fever, which could last 4–8 weeks. Exam findings incllude relative bradycardia, hepatosplenomegaly, and rose spots.

▶ Diagnosis

Clinical picture, positive diagnosis by blood culture, presumptive by stool/urine culture, agglutinin titer.

▶ Treatment Steps

Chloramphenicol, ciprofloxacin, amoxicillin. Dexamethasone may be used for severe typhoid.

7–10. Salmonella

▶ Description

Salmonella species are found in contaminated food or drink, commonly eggs or poultry. Can cause mild gastroenteritis or, more seriously, typhoid fever (see above). Immunosuppressed patients are at highest risk.

► Symptoms

Nausea, fever, cramps, bloody diarrhea (gastroenteritis, *S. enteritidis*), bacteremia, or asymptomatic carrier.

► Diagnosis

History and physical, stool culture, negative blood culture with enteritis, may be positive with enteric fever.

► Treatment Steps

No treatment needed for mild disease.

7–11. Shigella

► Description

Bacillary dysentery, caused by *Shigella* species. Fecal–oral and person-to-person transmission exist. At high risk are children and homosexual men, and low socioeconomic status.

► Symptoms

Range from mild watery diarrhea to more severe abdominal pain, tenesmus, bloody stool, cramping, fever.

► Diagnosis

History and physical, stool for WBC and culture.

► Treatment Steps

Resistance to ampicillin now becoming more common. Other antibiotics include ciprofloxacin, trimethoprim–sulfamethoxazole, or ceftriaxone.

7–12. Toxicogenic E. coli (including O157) Infection

► Description

Diarrheal illness (with blood for O157).

► Symptoms

Watery diarrhea, abdominal pain. Enteroinvasive strains present like *Shigella*.

► Diagnosis

Culture, serologic testing.

► Pathology

E. coli producing exotoxin resulting in colon mucosa fluid secretion.

► Treatment Steps

Hydration; try tetracycline or quinolone (no treatment known to be effective for O157). Antibiotics may increase the risk of developing hemolytic–uremic syndrome (HUS).

► Sequelae

HUS in children with O157.

7–13. Clostridial Infection

► Description

Toxin-producing germs.

► Symptoms

Gas gangrene: pain at wound infection, bullae, tissue gas, hypotension.

► Diagnosis

History and physical exam, Gram stain, culture.

► Pathology

Clostridium tetani, see Tetanus section; *C. perfringens,* see Gas gangrene; *C. botulinum,* see Botulism section; *C. difficile,* see Pseudomembranous colitis.

► Treatment Steps

Gas gangrene: debridement, penicillin G.

7–14. Cholera

► Description

Infectious diarrhea caused by a curved gram-negative rod, *Vibrio cholerae.* More common in Asia, Africa. Has occurred sporadically in the United States (Texas, Louisiana).

► Symptoms

Profuse watery diarrhea (rice-water stools), with vomiting, causing dehydration.

► Diagnosis

Culture of stool on special medium.

► Treatment Steps

1. Fluid replacement (lactated Ringer's or other crystalloid).
2. In adults, single-dose tetracyline or ciprofloxacin.
3. Children—erythromycin.

7–15. Pseudomembranous Enterocolitis

► Description

Antibiotic-induced colitis, caused by *C. difficile,* which produces a toxin causing diarrhea and a pseudomembrane in the colon.

► Symptoms

Watery diarrhea, tenesmus, cramps. Diarrhea may have a "characteristic" smell.

► Diagnosis

Clinical scenario, stool for *C. difficile* toxin.

► Treatment Steps

Stop antibiotic; give oral metronidazole, or vancomycin if metronidazole fails.

7–16. Amebiasis

► Description

Infection with *Entamoeba histolytica,* an intestinal protozoan. Highest-risk groups are travelers, recent immigrants, homosexual men, poor socioeconomic status, and residents of institutions. Infection acquired by ingestion of cysts from fecally contaminated water, food, or hands.

► Symptoms

Although asymptomatic passage of cysts can occur, symptomatic amebic colitis develops from 2 to 6 weeks after ingestion. Mild diarrhea, lower abdominal pain, weight loss. Cecal involvement mimics appendicitis. Full-blown dysentery may occur. Stool is almost always heme positive. With fever and right upper quadrant pain, suspect liver abscess.

► Diagnosis

Demonstration of trophozoites or cyst of *E. histolytica* on wet mount, iodine stain of stool, or trichrome stains of stool. Repeated stool exams are needed. Also, differentiate from other types of *Entamoeba* that do not cause disease. Serology may be used.

► Prevention

Water purification, treatment of asymptomatic carriers.

► Treatment Steps

1. Carriers—use one of the following three luminal agents: iodoquinol, diloxanide, and paromomycin.
2. Colitis or liver abscess—a luminal agent plus and metronidazole

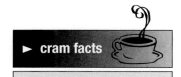

7–17. Giardiasis

► Description

A common parasitic infection caused by digestion of the cyst form of *Giardia lamblia.* Person-to-person transmission can occur, and therefore risks include residents of institutions, children in day care centers, and homosexual men as well as poor socioeconomic status.

► Symptoms

Range from asymptomatic to more fulminant diarrhea and malabsorption. Incubation period 1–3 weeks. Early diarrhea, bloating, and abdominal pain. Also increased flatus and weight loss if infection is chronic. Fever, blood, or mucus in stool is rare.

► Prevention

Hygiene, avoiding water while traveling, treatment of carriers.

► Diagnosis/Treatment Steps

Finding cysts or trophozoites in the feces or small intestine. Repeat exams may be needed. Can also test for parasitic antigen in the stool. Treatment: Metronidazole.

7–18. Hookworm and Pinworm

► Description

Intestinal nematode infection. Hookworm is rare in the United States, while pinworm is common.

► Symptoms

• Hookworm: Cough, anemia, pruritus, weight loss.
• Pinworm: Pruritus ani at night.

► Diagnosis

• Hookworm: Eosinophilia, anemia (microcytic/hypochromic), low albumin, stool exam.
• Pinworm: Scotch tape test, no eosinophilia.

► Pathology

• Hookworm: *Ancylostoma duodenale* or *Necator americanus.* Cycle: eggs in feces reach soil; larvae form; larvae enter skin/blood/ then lungs; larvae swallowed reach intestine.
• Pinworm: *Enterobius vermicularis.* Most frequent worm infection in the United States.

► Treatment Steps

• Hookworm: mild infection, none; severe, mebendazole (Vermox), or pyrantel pamoate.
• Pinworm: same meds.

7–19. Appendicitis (Fig. 9–1)
See Chapter 18.

7–20. Diverticulitis

▶ **Description**
Diverticular inflammation and perforation.

▶ **Symptoms**
Left lower quadrant (LLQ) pain and/or mass, constipation, chills/fever.

▶ **Treatment Steps**
If mild, medical (nothing by mouth [NPO], antibiotics), otherwise surgical resection.

7–21. Intra-abdominal Abscess, Hepatic/ Subphrenic

▶ **Description**
Hepatic abscess: local collection of pus in liver. Intra-abdominal abscess includes subphrenic abscess.

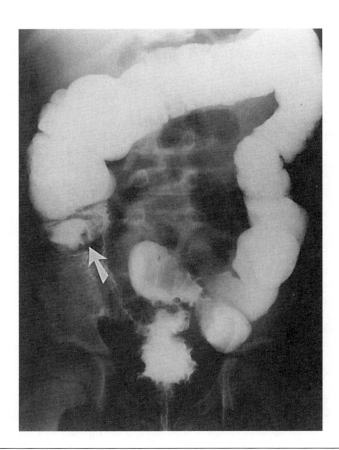

Figure 9–1. Acute appendicitis in a 5-year-old female presenting with fever, diarrhea, and abdominal pain of several days' duration. A frontal view from a barium enema demonstrates "sawtooth" irregularity of the rectosigmoid colon as well as spasm of the cecum and distal small bowel. A filling defect at the base of the cecum (arrow) is noted along with absent appendiceal filling. At surgery the appendix had perforated and generalized inflammation of the adjacent pelvic organs but no discrete abscess had occurred. (From *Pediatric Infectious Diseases Principles and Practice,* Appleton & Lange, 1995.)

► **Symptoms**

Hepatic abscess: fever, right upper quadrant (RUQ) pain, jaundice. Intra-abdominal abscess: fever, elevated diaphragm, leukocytosis, pain.

► **Diagnosis**

History and physical, ultrasound, CT, gallium scan, positive Hoover's sign (x-ray sternochondral widening).

► **Pathology**

E. coli common. Amebic liver abscess in high-risk individual (due to *Entamoeba histolytica*).

► **Treatment Steps**

Surgery and antibiotics.

7–22. Viral Hepatitis

See Chapter 3.

7–23. Strongyloidiasis

► **Description**

A relatively uncommon condition in the United States, caused by infection with *Strongyloides stercoralis*. Endemic areas—tropics. Can be serious infection in an immunocompromised patient.

► **Symptoms**

Can cause cutaneous symptoms (usually pruritus and a mild rash) at the area where the organism penetrated the skin, usually the feet. Pulmonary involvement can cause cough, fever, dyspnea. GI disease can cause nausea, vomiting, and diarrhea.

► **Diagnosis**

Finding worm in feces or other body specimens; serology.

► **Treatment Steps**

Thiabendazole; ivermectin. Prevention: wearing shoes.

8. Urinary Tract and Reproductive System

See OB-GYN (Chapter 13) for discussion of gonorrhea, chlamydia, syphilis, chancroid, urethritis, vulvovaginitis, Bartholin's gland abscess, salpingitis/pelvic inflammatory disease (PID), endometritis.

8–1. Prostatitis

See Chapter 17, section II.A.1.

8–2. Epididymitis

See Chapter 17, section II.A.2.

8–3. Orchitis

See Chapter 17, section II.A.3.

8–4. Pyelonephritis

See Chapter 17, section II.C.

8–5. Abscess: Renal, Pelvic, Perinephric

- **Renal and perinephric abscess**—often sequela from a urinary tract infection or nephrolithiasis. Nonspecific symptoms such as back, flank, or abdominal pain and fever. Organisms include *S. aureus* and *E. coli*. Abscess usually seen on ultrasound or CT scan. Systemic antibiotics and drainage needed.

- **Pelvic abscess**—in females often related to reproductive tract, including septic abortion, endometritis, postoperative infection after hysterectomy, or with pelvic inflammatory disease (tubo-ovarian abscess). A multitude of organisms can cause the abscess. Antibiotics with potent anaerobic coverage should be used with possible surgical exploration/drainage.

9. Skin; Musculoskeletal System

Chickenpox, rubella, measles, Rocky Mountain spotted fever, cellulitis, carbuncle, dermatophytosis, viral warts (see Chapter 2).

9-1. Lymphangitis

▶ Description/Symptoms
Bacterial infection spread into lymph nodes. Exam reveals red streak extending from wound; fever, adenopathy.

▶ Diagnosis/Pathology
Clinical diagnosis. Common cause hemolytic strep; rule out cat scratch fever.

▶ Treatment Steps
Antibiotics.

9-2. Necrotizing Fasciitis and Gangrene
See Chapter 2, section II.J.

9-3. Osteomyelitis
See Chapter 10, section II.A.1.

9-4. Septic Arthritis
See Chapter 10, section II.A.2.

C. Other Important Infectious Disorders

1. Lyme Disease

▶ Description
Multisystem disorder caused by the spirochete *Borrelia burgdorferi*. Usually transmitted by the deer tick *Ixodes dammini*. Three stages of the disease exist.

▶ Symptoms
- **Stage I—early infection.** Classic erythema chronicum migrans rash: a flat to slightly raised erythematous rash with central clearing. Usually occurs at area of tick bite, but many persons do not recall the bite or the tick.
- **Stage II—disseminated infection.** Secondary skin lesions can appear. Complaints include headache, stiff neck, fever, myalgias, arthralgias, and fatigue. Neurologic complaints can include cranial neuritis (particularly cranial nerve VII), myelitis, or subtle encephalitis. CSF may show lymphocytes, elevated protein, and normal to low protein. Cardiac abnormalities can include arteriovenus (AV) block.
- **Stage III—persistent infection.** Intermittent oligoarticular arthritis in large joints, particularly knees.

▶ Diagnosis
Clinical setting, but it can be difficult to diagnose. If the rash is noted in a patient who lives in or has visited an area with a high incidence of Lyme disease (particularly the Northeast United States), empiric treatment should be started. Serologic testing not needed,

as it may come back as a false negative early in the infection. Later in the disease course, serologies can confirm infection. PCR of the CSF or joint fluid can be done to look for presence of the organism.

▶ Treatment Steps

Depends on the stage and the clinical manifestations.

Skin lesions:
• Doxycycline 100 mg bid for 14–21 days.
• Amoxicillin (used in pregnant women and children) for 14–21 days.
• Arthritis.
• Doxycycline or amoxicillin for 30–60 days.

Neurologic or cardiac involvement:
• Often requires intravenous treatment (with ceftriaxone or cefotaxime). Total duration of treatment usually at least 30 days.

2. Malaria

▶ Description

The most important parasitic infection in humans, causing up to 3 million deaths per year worldwide. Infection with one of the following four *Plasmodium* species: *P. vivax, P. ovale, P. malariae,* and *P. falciparum*. Disease found in the tropics and transmitted via mosquitoes. Prevention with antimalarial drugs is of utmost importance in travelers, and is guided by the resistance patterns of the *Plasmodium* species in the particular area they are visiting.

▶ Symptoms

Initially nonspecific: Malaise, headache, fatigue, myalgias, abdominal pain, followed by fevers. Classic malaria paroxysms where fever spikes and chills occur at regular intervals suggests infection with *P. vivax* or *P. ovale*.

▶ Diagnosis

Thick and thin smears of the blood should be done. The parasite can be visualized on these smears. Repeated smears should be examined on successive days before the diagnosis is excluded. Infection with *P. falciparum* versus other species should be defined.

▶ Treatment Steps

1. Antimalarials include chloroquine, sulfadoxin/pyrimethamine, mefloquine, quinine, quinidine.
2. Prophylactic medications include chloroquine (where resistance is not a problem), mefloquine, doxycycline.

3. HIV/AIDS (Human Immunodeficiency Virus/ Acquired Immune Deficiency Syndrome)

▶ Description

(See Chapter 7, section I.B, for epidemiology, impact, and screening.) Infection with the retrovirus HIV is the cause of AIDS. The primary target for HIV is the CD4 T lymphocyte. HIV infection causes CD4 counts to decrease, resulting in a strong inverse relationship between CD4 count and the risk of opportunistic infections (OIs). Patients can be infected with HIV but not have AIDS. AIDS occurs in an HIV-positive patient whose CD4 count is < 200, has had one of many AIDS-defining illnesses (including *Pneumocystis carinii* pneumonia [PCP], disseminated or Kaposi's sarcoma, extrapulmonary histoplasmosis, cerebral toxoplasmosis, esophageal candidiasis).

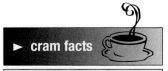
▶ cram facts

RISK FACTORS FOR HIV

• Use of injection drugs or sharing needles
• Unprotected sex with multiple partners, anonymous partners, or men who have sex with men, or exchanging sex for drugs or money
• Prior infection with a sexually transmitted disease
• Blood transfusion received between 1978 and 1985
• Unprotected sex with an individual with the above risk factors
• Child born to a mother who has HIV

▶ **Diagnosis**

Patient consent must be obtained prior to testing for HIV. Screening for HIV antibody is done first with enzyme-linked immunosorbent assay (ELISA). If the first ELISA screen is positive, the test is repeated. If positive a second time, confirmatory testing is done with Western blot. If HIV diagnosed, patient's total CD4 count and viral load (using PCR for HIV RNA) should be obtained.

▶ **Symptoms**

Variable depending on stage of disease and OIs. Primary infection with HIV is often asymptomatic; but a viral illness occurring with acute HIV infection has been described. Symptoms are nonspecific (fever, fatigue, rash, lymphadenopathy, night sweats) but if suspected clinically, HIV can be diagnosed if blood is sent for HIV RNA via PCR.

▶ **Treatment Steps**

1. Antiretroviral treatment. There are multiple drugs used in the treatment of HIV/AIDS, and their management should be by an infectious disease/HIV specialist. Drugs are given in combination. Drug resistance patterns can be identified. Goals of therapy are to raise the CD4 count and suppress the HIV viral load (to undetectable levels, if possible).
   - **Nucleoside analog reverse transcriptase inhibitors:**
     - AZT (zidovudine, Retrovir). Not used with d4T. Side effects: Headaches, stomach upset, anemia, neutropenia, myopathy.
     - ddI (didanosine, Videx). Side effects: Pancreatitis, fat redistribution, peripheral neuropathy.
     - ddC (zalcitabine Hivid). Side effects: Pancreatitis and peripheral neuropathy.
     - d4T (stavudine, Zerit). Side effects: Pancreatitis, fat redistribution, peripheral neuropathy. Not be used with AZT.
     - 3TC (lamivudine, Epivir). Side effects: Headaches and insomnia; pancreatitis, particularly in pediatric patients.
     - Abacavir (Ziagen, Epzicom). A potentially serious hypersensitivity reaction occurs in about 3% of patients; begins days to 4 weeks after starting the drug, and resolves without further problem if the drug is stopped and not restarted. Symptoms include fever, nausea, malaise, and possibly rash. If hypersensitivity is suspected, Abacavir should **never** be restarted, since restarting can cause a more serious and possibly fatal reaction.
     - Emtricitabine (Truvada). Side effects: Gastrointestinal (GI) upset, hyperpigmentation of palms or soles.
     - Tenofovir (Viread). Bioavailability enhanced by a high-fat meal. Side effects: GI upset, fat redistribution, lactic acidosis.
   - **Non-nucleoside reverse transcriptase inhibitors:**
     - Nevirapine (Viramune). Side effects: Severe hepatotoxicity or Stevens–Johnson syndrome.
     - Delavirdine (Rescriptor). Side effects: Rash, GI upset, abnormal liver function tests.
     - Efavirenz (Sustiva). Side effects: CNS and psychiatric side effects, fat redistribution.
   - **Protease inhibitors:**
     - Saquinavir (Fortovase, Invirase). Works well with ritonavir, lowering doses of both drugs. Side effects: stomach upset, elevated liver enzymes.

- Ritonavir (Norvir). Multiple drug interactions. Side effects: GI upset, generalized discomfort, tingling or numbness around the mouth.
- Indinavir (Crixivan). Avoid dehydration, as drug can precipitate and cause nephrolithiasis.
- Nelfinavir (Viracept). Side effects: Fat redistribution, stomach upset, diarrhea.
- Atazanavir (Reyataz). Side effects: GI upset, hyperglycemia, fat redistribution.
- **Fusion inhibitor:**
  - Enfuvirtide (Fuzeon). Subcutaneous injection. Side effects: Peripheral neuropathy, pancreatitis, elevated liver enzymes.
- **Combination pills:**
  - Combivir—AZT and 3TC
  - Kaletra—lopinavir and ritonavir
  - Trizivir—abacavir, zidovudine, lamivudine
2. Prevention of opportunistic infections. Prophylaxis for certain conditions is based on CD4 count.
   - **CD4 < 200:**
     - *P. carinii* pneumonia—regimen of choice is trimethoprim–sulfamethoxazole (alternative regimens include dapsone, pentamidine).
   - **CD4 < 100:**
     - *Toxoplasma gondii*—in patients with serum anti-*Toxoplasma* antibodies, regimen of choice is trimethoprim–sulfamethoxazole (alternative regimens include dapsone/pyramethamine/leukovorin, atovaquone).
   - **CD4 < 50:**
     - *M. avium* complex—azithromycin weekly or clarithromycin daily.
   - **Other considerations:**
     - *M. tuberculosis*—primary prophylaxis indicated for patients with a positive purified protein derivative (PPD) (induration > 5 mm) who have never been treated for tuberculosis, and patients with recent exposure to someone with active tuberculosis, regardless of CD4 count. Depending on drug resistance patterns, regimens vary.
     - Primary prophylaxis is not routinely recommended against herpesviruses (cytomegalovirus [CMV], herpes simplex virus, and varicella–zoster virus) or fungi (*Candida* species, *Cryptococcus neoformans, Histoplasma capsulatum,* and *Coccidioides immitis*).
3. Treatment of opportunistic infections as appropriate. Examples:
   - Bactrim/pentamidine for PCP
   - Pyrimethamine for toxoplasmosis
   - Amphotericin for cryptococcal meningitis
   - Ganciclovir for CMV

4. Syphilis

▶ Description

Infection with the spirochete *Treponema pallidum,* transmitted sexually (or from mother to fetus). Four stages of disease—primary, secondary, latent, and tertiary. An infected, untreated person is contagious during the first two stages, which usually last 1–2 years.

▶ Symptoms

- **Primary syphilis:** Painless chancre generally appears within 2–6 weeks of infection, most commonly on the penis, vulva, or vagina, but can develop on the cervix, tongue, lips, or other parts of the body. Associated with lymphadenopathy. Chancre heals within 4–6 weeks even without treatment, but lymphadenopathy can be persistent. If not treated during the primary stage, about one-third of people will go on to the chronic stages.

- **Secondary syphilis:** Includes rash, lymphadenopathy, and constitutional symptoms. A skin rash begins as pale, pink to red macules which can progress to papules or pustules. Rash can occur anywhere, but almost always on the palms and soles. Papules can enlarge, usually in intertriginous areas, to form moist pint-gray lesions called condylomata lata, which are highly infectious. Rash usually heals within several weeks or months. Constitutional symptoms can occur (mild fever, fatigue, headache, sore throat), may be very mild, and, like primary syphilis, will disappear without treatment. The signs of secondary syphilis may come and go over the next 1–2 years of the disease.
- **Latent syphilis:** Positive lab testing for syphilis in a patient with no clinical manifestations of syphilis and a normal CSF exam indicate latent syphilis. Two designations:
  - **Early latent**—latency within the first year after infection
  - **Late latent**—latency after 1 year of infection
- **Tertiary syphilis:** One-third of people who have had secondary syphilis develop tertiary syphilis (includes neurosyphilis, cardiovascular syphilis, and gummas).
  - **Neurosyphilis**—meningeal involvement (usually within the first year of infection), general paresis (after about 20 years), and tabes dorsalis (after 25–30 years).
  - **Cardiovascular syphilis**—includes aortitis, aortic regurgitation, saccular aneurysm.
  - **Gummas**—granulomatous inflammatory lesions; involves skin, bones, mouth, upper respiratory tract, larynx, liver, stomach.

▶ Diagnosis

Serologic testing most often used for diagnosis. Nontreponemal tests (Venereal Disease Research Laboratory [VDRL] and rapid plasma reagin [RPR]) are used as initial screening test and become negative with treatment. Specific treponemal tests (fluorescent treponemal antibody absorption test [FTA-ABS]) are more specific and confirm syphilis when positive, and remain positive even after therapy. Darkfield examination can be used to evaluate suspicious moist cutaneous lesions. All patients with syphilis should undergo HIV testing.

▶ Treatment Steps

1. Primary, secondary, or early latent—penicillin G (2.4 million units IM, once).
2. Late latent (or latent of uncertain duration), cardiovascular, or benign tertiary)—penicillin G (2.4 million units IM weekly for 3 weeks) (lumbar puncture should be done in these cases, and if abnormal, treat as neurosyphilis even if asymptomatic).
3. Neurosyphilis—penicillin G 12–24 million units daily given intravenously in divided doses q4h for 10–14 days.

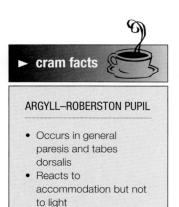

▶ **cram facts**

ARGYLL–ROBERSTON PUPIL

- Occurs in general paresis and tabes dorsalis
- Reacts to accommodation but not to light

BIBLIOGRAPHY

Bass JB, et al. Treatment of tuberculosis infection in adults and children. *Am Rev Resp Dis,* May 1994;1359–1374.

Beaver PC. *Clinical Parasitology,* 9th ed. Philadelphia: Lea & Febiger, 1984.

Braude AI. *Infectious Disease and Medical Microbiology,* 2nd ed. Philadelphia: W.B. Saunders, 1986.

Civetta JM. *Critical Care,* 3rd ed. Philadelphia: J.B. Lippincott, 1997.

Fauci AS, et al. *Harrison's Principles of Internal Medicine,* 14th ed. New York: McGraw-Hill, 1998.

Kovacs JA. Prophylaxis against opportunitistic infections in patients with human immunodeficiency virus infection. *N Engl J Med* May 11, 2000;342:1416–1429.

Mandell GL. *Principles and Practice of Infectious Disease,* 5th ed. New York: Churchill Livingstone, 2000.

Schillinger D. *Infections in Emergency Medicine,* Vol. 2. New York: Churchill Livingstone, 1997.

Schroeder SA. *Current Medical Diagnosis and Treatment,* 31st ed. Norwalk, CT: Appleton & Lange, 1992.

Thoene JG. *Physicians Guide to Rare Diseases.* Montvale, NJ: Dowden Publishing Company, 1992.

www.niaid.nih.gov/factsheets/stasyph.htm.

Musculoskeletal and Connective Tissue Disease

10

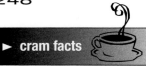

► cram facts

SIGN OR SYMPTOM: BACK PAIN

Think of: Musculoskeletal, DJD, arthritis, pancreatitis, peptic ulcer disease (PUD), pyelonephritis, renal infarct, kidney stones, sometimes renal vein thrombosis as well as cholecystitis, dissecting aortic aneurysms, ectopic pregnancy, spinal canal stenosis, radiculopathies (disk problems), pelvic or abdominal tumors, and others.

► cram facts

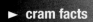

DIAGNOSIS OF OSTEOMYELITIS

Diagnosis can be difficult and often an opinion of an infectious disease specialist is helpful.
- Lab findings can include elevated white blood cell (WBC) count, ESR, and C-reactive protein.
- Radiologic studies have pluses and minuses.
- X-ray (Fig. 10–1) can miss very early osteomyelitis.
- Bone scan will pick up bony abnormalities but is very nonspecific and often picks up noninfectious lesions.
- MRI is the most sensitive and specific but also costly.
- Bone biopsy may be done surgically to confirm infection and organism causing infection, but results are sometimes negative if antibiotic treatment started prior to biopsy.

I. HEALTH AND HEALTH MAINTENANCE

A. Exercise, Fitness, and Conditioning

► **Description**

Benefits of exercise include stress reduction; prevention of osteoporosis; maintaining and/or increasing strength; improving cardiovascular fitness, joint mobility, and flexibility. High-repetition exercise with low weight resistance builds endurance and tones. Low repetition with heavy weights improves strength/muscle size.

B. Prevention of Disability Due to Osteoporosis

► **Description**
- **Impact** as a significant health concern with vast numbers of affected individuals at increased fracture risk; resulting morbidity/mortality (15% of hip fractures result in death); and tremendous financial/medical resource costs.
- **Prevention** is optimal treatment. See section II.E.1 for more discussion.

C. Degenerative Joint and Disk Disease

Epidemiology may relate to **aging, genetics,** and/or **injury.** Degenerative joint disease (DJD) is **common.**

- **Impact** in chronic pain and disability is significant. May be asymptomatic in many individuals.
- **Prevention** includes maintenance of flexibility, weight reduction, education regarding proper body mechanics for exercise/weight lifting and work. Avoiding occupational overuse/trauma and early treatment of associated metabolic/systemic disorders (hyperparathyroidism) are other considerations.

D. Prosthetic and Orthotic Devices

Orthotic devices reduce joint stress, provide patient mobility where previous joint weakness/injury prevented ambulation, and may prevent/correct joint deformity (juvenile rheumatoid arthritis [JRA]). Prosthetic devices for use by amputees provide physical and emotional benefits.

In early surgically implanted prosthesis infections, *Staphylococcus aureus* is the most common pathogen.

II. MECHANISMS OF DISEASE, DIAGNOSIS, AND TREATMENT

A. Infections

1. Osteomyelitis (Infection of Bone)

► **Symptoms**

Pain in area of infection (e.g., persistent backache in vertebral osteomyelitis). Also, fever/chills/malaise, history of prior infection, refusal to walk (infant).

► **Diagnosis**

See Cram Facts.

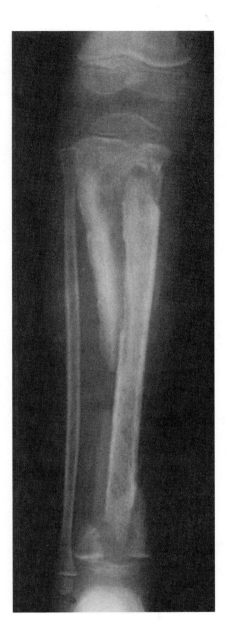

Figure 10–1. Chronic osteomyelitis of the tibia of a 4-year-old child with long-standing pain and swelling of the lower leg. A frontal radiograph shows extensive destruction and reactive bone formation of the tibial shaft. The "moth-eaten" sclerotic central fragment represents the dead sequestrum. The surrounding partially reconstituted bone is the involucrum. Note that the adjacent fibula is unaffected. (From *Pediatric Infectious Diseases Principles and Practice,* Appleton & Lange, 1995.)

► **Pathology**

Etiology by **hematogenous spread** (*S. aureus* **most common**), and direct bone infection (open fracture, trauma). Direct infection extension is possible, as in postoperative infection.

► **Treatment Steps**

1. Antibiotics.
2. Surgical debridement may be needed.

2. Septic Arthritis

► **Description**

Joint infection, usually in patient with coexisting illness or debilitated state.

► **Symptoms**

Joint pain/swelling/motion limitation, fever/chills, redness.

► **differential diagnosis**

INFECTIONS

- **Osteomyelitis:** bone infection, fever, metaphyseal area of bone tender, elevated CBC and sed rate, bone aspiration, *S. aureus* most common all ages.
- **Septic arthritis:** joint infection, fever, pain with joint motion, elevated CBC and sed rate, joint aspiration, *S. aureus* children and elderly, gonococcus young adult females.

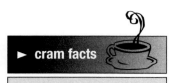

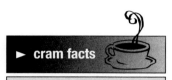

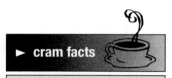

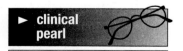

► Diagnosis

History and physical exam, **blood culture, joint fluid culture, lab (complete blood count** [CBC], erythrocyte sedimentation rate [ESR], C-reactive protein [CRP]), x-ray.

► Pathology

May be bacterial (**S. aureus most frequent in older adult** and childhood, with gonococcus [GC] most common in ages 20 to 50), viral, fungal; **most frequently by hematogenous spread; risk factors include** drug abuse (*Pseudomonas*), chronic disease/cancer, and prior joint pathology.

► Treatment Steps
1. Antibiotics.
2. Surgical drainage (arthroscopic vs. open) or repeated arthrocentesis.

3. Lyme Disease

See Chapter 9, section I.C.1.

4. Gonococcal Tenosynovitis

► Description

Tendon sheath inflammation. A common manifestation of disseminated GC infection.

► Symptoms

Tenosynovitis, pain, inflamed/red joint, fever, migratory polyarthritis, and wrist/knee/ankle arthritis.

► Diagnosis

History and physical exam, culture of joint fluid.

► Treatment Steps

Penicillin G or ceftriaxone.

B. Degenerative Disorders

1. Osteoarthritis (OA)

► Description/Symptoms

Chronic inflammatory joint disorder. Presents with joint pain and stiffness. A significant problem as the population ages.

► Diagnosis

Clinical, x-ray (narrowed joint cartilage, osteophytes, and sclerosis) (see Fig. 10–2).

► Pathology

Cartilage damage/erosion, with bone cyst/osteophyte lesions, and bone sclerosis.

► Treatment Steps
1. Nonsteroidal anti-inflammatory drugs (NSAIDs), rest, weight reduction, physical therapy modalities.
2. Corticosteroid injection.
3. Hyaluronate viscosupplementation.
4. Joint replacement.

2. Degenerative Disk Disease and Low Back Pain

► Description

Disk-space narrowing, with resulting signs and symptoms.

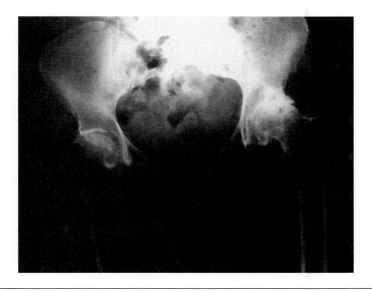

Figure 10–2. Degenerative joint disease. Note the changes of osteoarthritis in the right hip as manifested by joint space narrowing, subchondral cysts, and sclerosis.

► Symptoms
Back pain, loss of full motion, stiffness, referred pain, muscle spasm.

► Diagnosis
History and physical exam, x-ray (including computed tomography (CT)/magnetic resonance imaging (MRI) for disk and cord-compression evaluation), bone scan.

► Treatment Steps
1. NSAIDs, physical therapy, back support, weight reduction, rest.
2. Corticosteroid injection.
3. Surgery—rarely.

C. Neurologic Disorders

1. Carpal Tunnel Syndrome

► Symptoms
Fingertip and/or **hand numbness/weakness,** and **pain.** Most commonly due to entrapment of the median nerve at the wrist.

► Diagnosis
History and physical (Tinel's [wrist percussion] and Phalen's [wrist flexion] signs), electromyogram (EMG), and nerve conduction velocity (NCV) study.

► Pathology
Median nerve compression. Most commonly noted with overuse. Also seen with myxedema, rheumatoid arthritis (RA), pregnancy, injuries, amyloid disease, and others.

► Treatment Steps
1. Rest, wrist splint, workplace modifications.
2. NSAIDs to decrease inflammation.
3. Corticosteroid injection.
4. Surgery (nerve release).

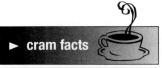

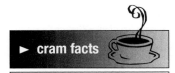

► cram facts

MEDICAL TREATMENT OF OA

- NSAIDs have been problematic, as long-term use can cause GI ulcers and bleeding.
- COX-2 inhibitors (celecoxib, valdecoxib) have been promising but questions have arisen regarding cardiovascular risks since Merck withdrew its drug Vioxx (rofecoxib) from the market.
- Intra-articular steroid injections can control symptoms without systemic side effects.

► cram facts

Herniated disk: Most at L4–5 (weak big toe) and L5–S1 (reduced Achilles reflex).

► cram facts

TESTS FOR CARPAL TUNNEL SYNDROME

Tinel's = tapping
Phalen's = "phlexing"

2. Charcot Joint

► Description

Charcot joint is actually a neuropathic osteoarthropathy, or neuropathic joint. Although exact pathology is debated, basically a patient first has peripheral neuropathy (commonly due to diabetes, but can also include amyloidosis, spinal cord injury, others). As the patient cannot sense pain or position, the joint is repeatedly injured and deformed.

► Symptoms

Joint swelling, deformity, mild pain, warmth, and erythema. Characteristic changes are seen on x-ray.

► Treatment Steps

1. Joint immobilization (acute stage).
2. Shoes, braces (chronic stage).
3. Surgery for unbraceable deformity.

3. Poliomyelitis (Infantile Paralysis)

► Symptoms

Fever, gastrointestinal (GI) and central nervous system (CNS) symptoms (meningeal irritation, muscle weakness/spasm, encephalitis), respiratory paralysis.

► Diagnosis

History and physical exam, spinal fluid examination.

► Pathology

Poliovirus infection resulting in CNS injury (anterior horn motor cells of spinal cord).

► Treatment Steps

1. Supportive treatment, bedrest, physical therapy (acute stage).
2. Physical therapy, braces, surgery (chronic stage).

4. Cerebral Palsy

See Chapter 11, section XVII.A.

D. Congenital and Inherited Disorders

1. Developmental Dysplasia of the Hip

See Chapter 14, section VII.B.

2. Phocomelia

► Description

A congenital malformation in which the hand or foot is directly connected to the trunk.

► Pathology

Classically noted with thalidomide, but can be inherited (genetically transmitted).

3. Osgood–Schlatter's Disease

► Description

Inflammation of the tibial tubercle. Usually affects preteen/teenage boys. Common in a fast-growing child.

► Symptoms

Anterior knee pain and lump. Clinical diagnosis.

► Treatment Steps
1. Rest.
2. Immobilization.

4. Osteochondritis Dissecans

► Description
Disorder in which portion of articular cartilage and subchondral bone separates from normal location in skeletally immature individual.

► Symptoms
Knee pain, effusion, locking. Ankle or elbow pain.

► Diagnosis
History and physical exam, x-ray (joint mouse), MRI (see Fig. 10–3).

► Pathology
Ischemia or trauma, usually of **medial femoral condyle,** in teenage males.

► Treatment Steps
1. Casting.
2. Surgery.

5. Slipped Capital Femoral Epiphysis

► Description
Adolescent hip disorder, more common in overweight/obese children/adolescents.

► Symptoms
Groin/thigh or knee pain, and **limp** in adolescent. Bilateral involvement in approximately one-third of cases.

► Diagnosis
History and physical exam, **x-ray evaluation** (see Figs. 10–4 and 10–5).

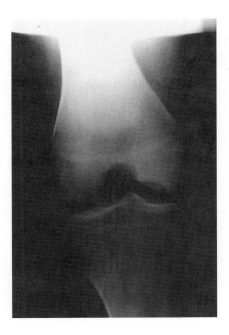

Figure 10–3. Osteochondritis dissecans. The lateral aspect of the medial femoral condyle is the usual location of osteochondritis dissecans. Note the subchondral fragment of bone surrounded by a radiolucent line in this 18-year-old male.

Figure 10–4. Slipped capital femoral epiphysis. The epiphysis of the proximal femur has been displaced posteriorly and inferiorly in this skeletally immature individual.

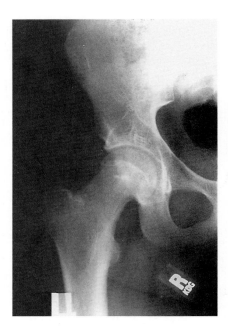

▶ Pathology

Displacement of femoral epiphysis at hip.

▶ Treatment Steps

Surgical (pinning).

6. Legg–Calvé–Perthes Disease

▶ Description

Avascular necrosis of the hip in children. More common in males. **"Osteochondritis deformans."**

▶ Symptoms

Hip or knee pain and **limp.**

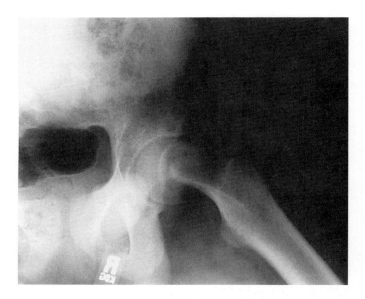

Figure 10–5. Slipped capital femoral epiphysis. The epiphysis of the proximal femur has been displaced posteriorly and inferiorly.

► Diagnosis
History and physical exam, x-ray.

► Treatment Steps
1. Observation, pain relief.
2. **Bracing in abduction.**
3. **Surgery may be necessary.**

7. Transient Synovitis

► Description
Most common cause of childhood hip pain. Occurs in young children, ages 3–10. Etiology unknown.

► Symptoms
Hip pain, **low-grade** fever possible, limp.

► Diagnosis
History and physical, x-ray, joint aspiration (to rule out septic arthritis), sedimentation rate, CBC.

► Treatment Steps
Bed rest (at least 7–10 days).

8. In-Toeing

► Symptoms
In-toeing gait (neutral position to 20° out-toeing is normal).

► Pathology

Metatarsus Adductus Deformity—forefoot adduction (front of foot turns in), passively correctable, treat with foot stretching (casting if not passively correctable).

Tibial Torsion—inward tibia rotation with knee straight but whole foot pointing inward (thigh–foot angle normally neutral to 30° outward), no treatment.

Femoral Anteversion—internal hip rotation over 65°, no treatment.

► Treatment Steps
As in pathology.

9. Clubfoot
See Chapter 14, section VII.C.

E. Metabolic and Nutritional Disorders

1. Osteoporosis

► Description
Decreased bone mass. Risk factors iclude early menopause (medical or surgical), alcohol use, Caucasian, thin body habitus, tobacco use.

► Symptoms
Pain, fractures (vertebral compression common).

► Diagnosis
Dual-energy x-ray absorptiometry (DEXA) scan is definitive for bone mass (see Clinical Pearl). Labs include calcium, phosphate, thyroid-stimulating hormone (TSH).

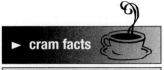

► cram facts

If temperature high, or elevated WBCs/sed rate: consider patient to have a septic joint and aspirate.

► clinical pearl

DIAGNOSIS OF OSTEOPOROSIS

The World Health Organization (WHO) has defined osteoporosis on the basis measurements of bone density on DEXA scanning (T-scores).

- Normal: > –1
- Osteopenia: –1 to –2.5
- Osteoporosis: > –2.5

It is important to note that these scores are based on the DEXA scan. A patient may be diagnosed with osteoporosis if the DEXA scan shows osteopenia but she has fractures.

It is also important to rule out secondary causes of osteoporosis, such as hyperthyroidism, multiple myeloma.

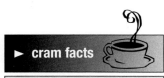

► cram facts

Rule out multiple myeloma (serum protein electrophoresis, bone marrow study, etc.), **which may present like osteoporosis.**

Osteomalacia: inadequate bone mineralization; a result of renal disease or malabsorption; **bones are soft, with low serum calcium and elevated alkaline phosphatase.**

► differential diagnosis

METABOLIC DISORDERS

• **Gout:** Monarticular—first metatarsal phalangeal joint common, often elevated serum uric acid; x-ray—possible articular erosions; aspirate—intracellular sodium urate crystals (negative birefringence).

• **Pseudogout:** Monarticular—knee joint common, serologic studies normal; x-ray—cartilage calcification; aspirate—extracellular calcium pyrophosphate crystals (positive birefringence).

► Pathology

May be primary (postmenopausal), or secondary (drugs/alcohol, nutritional, and endocrine).

► Treatment Steps

1. Weight-bearing exercise.
2. Correct secondary cause (stop alcohol, smoking, etc.).
3. Calcium and vitamin D.
4. Estrogen–progesterone (somewhat controversial).
5. Biphosphonates (inhibit osteoclastic bone resorption).
6. Calcitonin (effectiveness may wane after 2 years).
7. Estrogen-modifying drugs.

2. Gout

► Description

Monarticular arthritis. Extremely painful. Caused by monosodium urate crystals.

► Symptoms

Pain, redness, swelling, and **warm joint.**

► Diagnosis

Clinical, **positive joint aspiration for rodlike negative birefringent intracellular urate crystals,** serum uric acid.

► Pathology

Hyperuricemia with crystal deposition in joints; **first metatarsal phalangeal (MTP) joint most often affected.**

► Treatment Steps

Acute—Indomethacin or colchicine.

Chronic—Allopurinol and probenecid.

3. Pseudogout

► Description

Arthritis caused by deposition of calcium pyrophosphate crystals.

► Symptoms

Acute joint inflammation, similar to gout.

► Diagnosis

History and physical exam, x-ray **(chondrocalcinosis–cartilage calcification), extracellular calcium pyrophosphate crystals in aspirate.**

► Treatment Steps

1. NSAIDs.
2. Intra-articular corticosteroids.

4. Rickets

► Description

Inadequate bone mineralization, in growing bone.

► Symptoms

Craniotabes (soft skull), frontal bossing, lethargy, rachitic rosary (large costochondral junction bumps), bow-legs, potbelly.

► Diagnosis

History and physical examination, **x-ray (frayed/widened growth plates, pseudofractures),** elevated alkaline phosphatase.

► Pathology
Due to vitamin D deficiency (poor intake, malabsorption) **or vitamin D resistance; growing plates affected,** so a **disease of children.**

► Treatment Steps
Vitamin D and light.

F. Inflammatory and Immunologic Disorders

1. Polymyalgia Rheumatica (PMR)

► Description
Inflammatory disorder of elderly.

► Symptoms
Hip and **shoulder muscle pain/stiffness in elderly patient.**

► Diagnosis
History and physical exam, **elevated sed rate. Both x-rays** and **muscle biopsy are normal.**

► Pathology
Inflammatory disorder. Human leukocyte antigen (HLA) associated.

► Treatment Steps
1. **Corticosteroids give rapid relief.**
2. NSAIDs—mild cases.

2. Fibromyalgia

► Description
Nonarticular, noninflammatory muscular pain. Etiology unknown.

► Symptoms
Multiple trigger points, irregular sleep pattern, anxiety/depression/hysteria, widespread achiness, fatigue.

► Diagnosis
History and physical exam, classic trigger points (**superior** or **inferior medial scapula border are common** points) and widespread pain.

► Treatment Steps
1. Patient education.
2. Cyclobenzaprine, amitriptyline.
3. Stretching, aerobic exercise.
4. Trigger-point injection.

3. Lupus Arthritis

► Description
Polyarthritis, without destructive joint disease. Autoimmune disease.

► Symptoms
Arthralgias (hip joints and hands typically), **Raynaud's phenomenon,** morning stiffness, myalgias.

► Diagnosis
History and physical exam, serologic testing (**antibody to native deoxyribonucleic acid [DNA], antinuclear antibodies** [ANA]).

► Pathology
More common in young women.

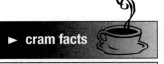

► cram facts

Phenytoin sodium (**Dilantin**) and phenobarbital affect vitamin D metabolism, and may predispose to rickets. Other causes: liver and renal disease. Harrison's groove sign: indentation of lower ribs at diaphragm insertion site; typical of rickets.

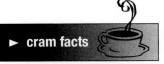

► cram facts

INFLAMMATION AND IMMUNOLOGIC DISORDERS

• **Rheumatoid arthritis:** systemic polyarthritis, rheumatoid nodules, pleural effusion, joint deformity, elevated sed rate and rheumatoid factor.
• **Lupus arthritis:** polyarthritis, arthralgias, myalgias, and Raynaud's phenomenon, joint preserved, antibody to native DNA and antinuclear.
• **Ankylosing spondylitis:** back pain and stiffness, joint arthralgias, sacroiliitis, reduced chest expansion, positive HLA-B27 antibody.
• **Juvenile rheumatoid arthritis:** fever, joint deformity, iridocyclitis, rash, splenomegaly, negative rheumatoid factor and ANA possible.

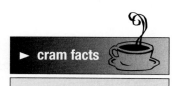

► **cram facts**

Complications of PMR include temporal arteritis (may result in blindness). Fibromyalgia: normal sed rate

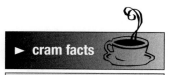

► **cram facts**

- Psoriatic arthritis: joint damage and opera glass deformity on x-ray.
- Gouty arthritis: proximal great toe joint and hands.

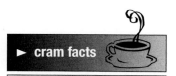

► **cram facts**

- Dermatomyositis is polymyositis plus a rash.
- Coexisting malignancy may be present with both **polymyositis** and **dermatomyositis.**
- No ocular muscle problems with polymyositis or dermatomyositis (unlike myasthenia gravis).

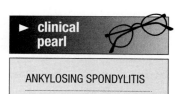

► **clinical pearl**

ANKYLOSING SPONDYLITIS

Classic x-ray finding: "bamboo spine"

► Treatment Steps
1. **Rest.**
2. **NSAIDs.**
3. **Corticosteroids.**
4. Hydroxycholoroquine

4. **Polymyositis, Dermatomyositis**

► Description
Skeletal muscle inflammatory disorder. Autoimmune disorder.

► Symptoms
Weak muscles proximally, arthralgias, **heliotrope** (eyelid) **rash,** dysphagia.

► Diagnosis
History and physical examination, **elevated muscle enzymes, muscle/skin biopsy,** abnormal EMG study.

► Pathology
Abnormal muscle biopsy (degenerated/regenerated muscle fibers).

► Treatment Steps
1. **Rest.**
2. Physical therapy.
3. **Corticosteroids.**
4. Methotrexate if corticosteroids fail.

5. **Rheumatoid Arthritis**
See Chapter 7, section II.H.3.

6. **Juvenile Rheumatoid Arthritis (Still's Disease)**
See Chapter 7, section II.H.2.

7. **Ankylosing Spondylitis**

► Description
A chronic inflammatory condition commonly causing inflammation of the sacroiliac joint. Common in young males.

► Symptoms
Back pain and **stiffness,** joint pains and swelling.

► Diagnosis
History and physical exam (reduced chest expansion), **positive human lymphocyte antigen (HLA)-B27, elevated ESR, x-ray (sacroiliitis).**

► Treatment Steps
1. **NSAIDs.**
2. Physical therapy.
3. Sulfasalazine, methotrexate.

8. **Bursitis**

► Symptoms
Nontender swelling (prepatellar) or pain (hip). Other common sites include elbow and shoulder. Clinical diagnosis.

► Pathology
Bursa inflammation from overuse, abnormal joint motion, trauma.

► Treatment Steps
1. Rest.
2. NSAIDs.
3. Physical therapy.
4. Aspiration (with/without corticosteroid injection).
5. Surgery.

9. Tendinitis—General Information

► Description/Symptoms
Inflammation of the tendon, causing pain at tendon insertion, or along tendon.

► Diagnosis
History and physical exam, MRI.

► Pathology
Inflammation secondary to overuse or abnormal mechanics.

► Treatment Steps
1. Rest.
2. NSAIDs.
3. Physical therapy.
4. Corticosteroid injection.
5. Surgery.

10. Tendinitis—Iliotibial Band Syndrome

► Symptoms
Distal thigh and **lateral knee pain.**

► Diagnosis
Pain with stretching leg/hip on affected side (Ober's sign). Pain worse with stairs.

► Treatment Steps
1. NSAIDs.
2. Adjust mechanical factors (shoes, terrain, activity level, etc.).
3. Physical therapy (stretching).
4. Corticosteroid injection.

11. Achilles Tendinitis

► Symptoms
Pain along heel/Achilles tendon (see Fig. 10–6).

► Treatment Steps
1. NSAIDs.
2. Heel lift.
3. Correct mechanical dysfunction.
4. Therapy (stretching).
5. Immobilization.
6. Surgery.

12. Patellar Tendinitis (Jumper's Knee)

► Symptoms/Diagnosis
Patellar tendon tenderness.

► Pathology
Overuse and **jumping sports** resulting in quadriceps contraction and tendon inflammation.

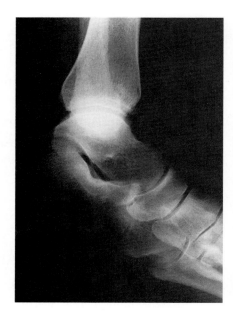

Figure 10–6. Achilles tendinitis. There is extensive calcification in the area of attachment of the Achilles tendon into the posterior calcaneus. This is commonly seen in cases of Achilles tendinitis.

► **Treatment Steps**
1. Rest.
2. NSAIDs.
3. Physical therapy (stretching).
4. Surgery.

13. Rotator Cuff Tendinitis

► **Symptoms**
Lateral shoulder pain, worse with overhead activity.

► **Diagnosis**
History and physical exam (tender anterior acromion, **pain with resisted shoulder abduction**), x-ray, MRI.

► **Pathology**
Overuse, repetitive activity with arm overhead, trauma, and anterior acromial osteophytes.

► **Treatment Steps**
1. Rest.
2. NSAIDs.
3. Physical therapy.
4. Corticosteroid injection.
5. Surgery.

G. Neoplasms

1. Osteosarcoma

► **Description**
Most frequent primary bone cancer.

► **Symptoms**
Pain, mass, limping, metastatic signs (usually lungs).

► **Diagnosis**
History and physical exam, **x-ray (long bone metaphysis destruction), biopsy,** elevated alkaline phosphatase, bone scan, CT scan, MRI.

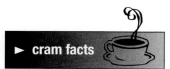

► **cram facts**

NEOPLASMS

- **Osteosarcoma:** most common primary bone malignancy, bone pain and lethargy, long bone metaphyseal destruction, elevated serum phosphatase, common near knee.
- **Osteochondroma:** most common benign bone tumor, asymptomatic or localized tenderness, pedunculated metaphyseal tumor, common distal femur.
- **Ewing's sarcoma:** malignant round cell bone tumor, children frequently, fever and bone tenderness, destruction of any portion of long bone.

► Pathology

Osteoid production by the tumor, which is **usually near knee joint; in 10- to 25-year-old age group.**

► Treatment Steps

Surgery (limb-sparing usually), **plus chemotherapy** (preoperative and postoperative)

2. Osteoid Osteoma

► Description

Benign bone tumor.

► Symptoms

Pain (worse at night).

► Diagnosis

History and physical examination, **pain relieved by NSAID, x-ray (sclerotic area with central lysis), biopsy, bone scan, CT scan.**

► Pathology

Affects young individuals.

► Treatment Steps

1. Observation and NSAID.
2. Surgical removal.

3. Osteochondroma

► Description/Symptoms

Most frequent benign bone tumor. Can be asymptomatic or present with pain.

► Diagnosis

History and physical examination, **x-ray (pedunculated metaphyseal tumor),** biopsy (see Fig. 10–7).

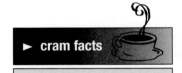

► cram facts

The most common site for osteochondroma is the distal femur.

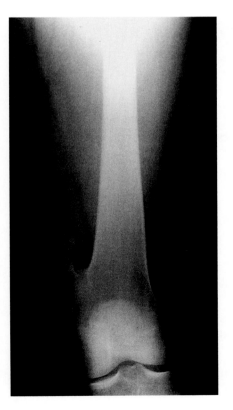

Figure 10–7. Osteochondroma. A large pedunculated lesion in the metaphyseal region of the distal femur.

► Treatment Steps
1. Observation.
2. **Surgical removal.**

4. Ewing's Sarcoma

► Description
Malignant round-cell **bone tumor;** frequently children.

► Symptoms
Pain, fever, swelling, and tenderness.

► Diagnosis
History and physical exam, **x-ray (any portion of long bone), bone biopsy.**

► Pathology
Pelvis and femur most often.

► Treatment Steps
Radiation, chemotherapy, and surgery.

5. Hypertrophic Osteoarthropathy

► Description
Pulmonary and **arthritis syndrome.**

► Symptoms
Arthritis, clubbing, diaphoresis.

► Diagnosis
History and physical examination, **x-ray (periostitis).**

► Pathology
Etiology unknown; lung cancer/chronic obstructive pulmonary disease (COPD) often present.

► Treatment Steps
1. Treat primary condition.
2. NSAIDs.
3. Therapy.
4. Corticosteroids.

H. Other Disorders

1. Frozen Shoulder Syndrome (Adhesive Capsulitis)

► Symptoms
Pain, reduced glenohumeral motion.

► Pathology
Adhesions and shoulder capsule fibrosis.

► Treatment Steps
1. Range-of-motion exercise.
2. NSAIDs.
3. Manipulation.
4. Surgery.

2. Reflex Sympathetic Dystrophy (Sudeck's Atrophy)

► Symptoms
Burning pain, skin changes (temperature/color), **edema** in a patient with a prior injury to that area. Clinical diagnosis.

► Pathology

Posttraumatic sympathetic nerve disorder, with reflex vasospasm-induced symptoms.

► Treatment Steps

Can be difficult to treat.
1. NSAIDs, amitriptyline, gabapentin.
2. Physical therapy.
3. Sympathetic block.

3. Dupuytren's Contracture

► Description/Symptoms

Lump in the hand; contracture of fourth or fifth fingers, in flexion. Clinical diagnosis.

► Pathology

Thick palmar fascia, of unknown etiology. Genetic component.

► Treatment Steps

Surgical.

4. Carpal Tunnel Syndrome

See section II.C.1 earlier in this chapter.

5. Patellofemoral Pain Syndrome

► Symptoms

Anterior knee pain; worse with hills/steps, and distance running.

► Diagnosis

History and physical exam (crepitus), x-ray, arthroscopic examination.

► Pathology

Chondromalacia patella. Increased softening and roughness of cartilage under patella.

► Treatment Steps

1. Rest.
2. NSAIDs.
3. Physical therapy including quadriceps strengthening.
4. Knee brace.
5. Surgery.

6. Paget's Disease of Bone

► Description

Bone disorder; more common in elderly; **osteitis deformans.**

► Symptoms

Symptoms depend on area of bone affected. May be asymptomatic or pain, bone deformity, arthritis, and fractures.

► Diagnosis

History and physical exam, **elevated alkaline phosphatase, bone scan, x-ray.**

► Pathology

Excessive/overactive osteoclasts.

► Treatment Steps

1. NSAIDs.
2. **Antiresorptive agents (calcitonin, bisphosphates, and plicamycin).**

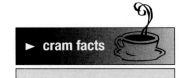

► cram facts

DUPUYTREN'S CONTRACTURE

Positive association with cirrhosis, diabetes, and epilepsy.

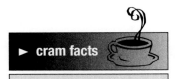

► cram facts

Complications of Paget's—osteogenic sarcoma, spinal cord compression, and high-output congestive heart failure (CHF) (affected bone has higher blood flow).

3. Physical therapy.
4. Surgery.

7. Histiocytosis (Eosinophilic Granuloma)

▶ Description
Reticuloendothelial proliferative disorder (histiocytosis).

▶ Symptoms
Vertebral collapse, **pain.**

▶ Diagnosis
History and physical examination (tenderness, swelling), **x-ray,** biopsy.

▶ Pathology
Destructive eosinophilic/histiocytic infiltrate in bone; most often childhood disorder.

▶ Treatment Steps
Rest and bracing, low-dose radiation, surgery, and corticosteroids have been tried.

8. Shin Splints

▶ Description
Painful lower leg disorder in athletes (posterior tibialis periostitis).

▶ Symptoms
Exercise-induced lower leg **pain,** medial location. Clinical diagnosis.

▶ Treatment Steps
1. Rest.
2. NSAIDs.
3. Physical therapy (stretching).
4. Control mechanical dysfunctions.

9. Cervical Sprain (Whiplash)

▶ Symptoms
Patient initially relates neck pain (then relates his attorney's name and telephone number).

▶ Diagnosis
History and physical examination, x-ray, and CT/MRI to rule out disk disease (if indicated).

▶ Pathology
Hyperextension and flexion injury.

▶ Treatment Steps
1. Rest.
2. Cervical collar.
3. NSAIDs.
4. Physical therapy.

10. Thoracic Outlet Syndrome

▶ Description/Symptoms
Arm pain from compression of nerve/vascular structures. Hand/arm/back numbness and pain; may be positional.

▶ Diagnosis
History and physical exam **(positive Adson's test), Doppler study,** x-ray.

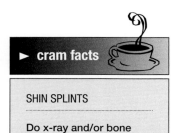

▶ cram facts

SHIN SPLINTS

Do x-ray and/or bone scan to rule out stress fracture.

► Pathology

Anatomic neurovascular compression.

► Treatment Steps

1. Exercises.
2. Physical therapy.
3. Surgical rib/muscle resection.

11. Nursemaid's Elbow

► Symptoms

Elbow pain, arm held flexed. Child will not use arm.

► Diagnosis

History **(child pulled by arm),** and physical. No fracture on x-ray.

► Pathology

Subluxed radial head.

► Treatment Steps

Push back head of radius with arm supinated and flexed.

12. Metatarsalgia

► Description

Forefoot pain disorder.

► Symptoms/Diagnosis

On history and exam, **area under metatarsal head(s) is tender.**

► Pathology

Overuse or faulty mechanics.

► Treatment Steps

1. NSAIDs.
2. Shoe padding.
3. Arch support.
4. Achilles tendon stretching.
5. Surgery.

13. Acromioclavicular (AC) Separation

► Description/Symptoms

Shoulder pain disorder, after fall/injury.

► Diagnosis

History and physical **(AC tenderness),** x-ray **(elevated end of clavicle possible).**

► Treatment Steps

1. **Sling prn if mild** (first-degree without separation on x-ray), sling **7 to 14** days **for second-degree injury** (second-degree, separation not greater than clavicle width), and **conservative or internal fixation for third-degree** (greater AC separation).
2. Physical therapy after sling.
3. Surgery for residual symptoms.

14. Lateral Epicondylitis (Tennis Elbow)

► Symptoms

Elbow pain, increasing with activity.

► Diagnosis

History, physical (lateral epicondyle tender, and pain on resisting patient's attempts on hand/middle finger dorsiflexion).

10-1

LOWER EXTEMITY NEUROLOGIC EXAMS				
Nerve Root	Disk Level	Motor	Sensation	Reflex
L4	L3–4	Tibialis anterior	Medial leg	Patella
L5	L4–5	Extensor hallucis longus	Dorsum foot	
S1	L5–S1	Gastroenemius	Lateral foot	Achilles

► Pathology

Overuse of forearm muscles creates inflammation at tendon insertion.

► Treatment Steps

1. Rest/brace/NSAIDs.
2. Physical therapy.
3. Corticosteroid injection.
4. Surgery.

I. Neurologic Exams

1. Lower Extremity (See Table 10-1)

► Description

L3—Quadriceps muscle.

L4—Patella reflex.

L5—Great toe dorsiflexion, sensation at web of great and first toes.

S1—Achilles reflex, gastrocnemius muscle, and plantar flexors.

2. Cervical Region (See Table 10-2)

► Description

C5—Deltoid muscle, biceps tendon reflex.

C6—Biceps/thumb muscle, brachioradialis tendon reflex.

C7—Affects triceps muscle, triceps reflex, sensation middle finger.

C8—Grip strength.

T1—Intrinsic hand muscles.

10-2

CERVICAL REGION NEUROLOGIC EXAMS				
Nerve Root	Disk Level	Motor	Sensation	Reflex
C5	C4–5	Biceps	Lateral arm	Biceps
C6	C5–6	Wrist estensor	Lateral forearm	Brachioradialis
C7	C6–7	Triceps	Middle finger	Triceps
C8	C7–8	Finger flexors	Medial forearm	
T1	C8–T1	Hand intrinsics	Medial arm	

BIBLIOGRAPHY

Aboulafia A, Kennon R, Jelinek J. Benign bone tumors of childhood. *J Am Acad Orthop Surg* 1999;7:377–388.

Gibbs CP Jr., Weber K, Scarborough MT. Malignant bone tumors. *J Bone Joint Surg Am* 2001;83:1728–1745.

Kelly WN, Ruddy S, Harris ED Jr., Sledge C. *Textbook of Rheumatology,* 5th ed. Philadelphia: W.B. Saunders, 1997.

Snider RK. *Essentials of Musculoskeletal Care.* Rosemont, IL: American Academy of Orthopedic Surgeons, 1997.

Tachdjian MO. *Pediatric Orthopaedics,* 2nd ed. Philadelphia: W.B. Saunders, 1998.

Weinstein SL, Buckwalter JA. *Turek's Orthopaedics—Principles and Their Application,* 5th ed. Philadelphia: J.B. Lippincott, 1994.

Neurology | 11

I. HEADACHE

A. Migraine

▶ Description
- **Classic** migraine—**unilateral throbbing headache with aura.**
- Common migraine—subtle onset, no aura, represents 80% of cases.

▶ Symptoms
Unilateral, throbbing, visual and autonomic disturbances, nausea. **Basilar** migraine may present with ataxia, vertigo, dysarthria.

▶ Diagnosis
Typical symptoms in young adult, **positive family history** often, 75% of cases are women. Increased incidence of motion sickness and infantile colic.

▶ Pathophysiology
Serotonergic neurons in brain stem raphe involved. Vasomotor changes. Spreading depression of Leao (neuronal depression). Cortical oligemia, extracranial vasodilation.

▶ Treatment Steps
1. Pharmacotherapy—**acute headache: ergot alkaloids,** serotonin (5-HT) agonists, prochlorperazine, metoclopramide.
2. Preventive treatment: β-blockers, **sodium valproate,** topiramate, gabapentin, lamotrigine, **methysergide** (potential for retroperitoneal fibrosis with long-term use), calcium channel blockers, antidepressants, nonsteroidal anti-inflammatory drugs (NSAIDs), cyproheptadine.
3. Avoid alcohol, tyramine (cheese), chocolate, citrus, onions, and nitrite.

B. Cluster Headache

▶ Description
Vascular headache, also known as **histamine cephalalgia, Horton's headache, migrainous neuralgia.**

▶ Symptoms
Severe pain in short episodes without aura, for weeks to months, then remits, ipsilateral lacrimation, nasal congestion, conjunctival injection, nasal congestion, dilated superficial temporal artery.

▶ Diagnosis
Typical symptoms, **men more often** (95%), **worse with alcohol** and sleep.

▶ Treatment Steps
1. Similar to migraine.
2. Also prednisone, oxygen, lithium.

C. Temporal Arteritis (Giant Cell)

▶ Description
Inflammatory systemic illness in elderly. Medical emergency.

► Symptoms

Temporal headache, focal tenderness superficial temporal/occipital arteries, vision loss, malaise. Can be associated with **polymyalgia rheumatica.**

► Diagnosis

Clinical suspicion, elevated erythrocyte sedimentation rate (ESR), biopsy of temporal artery.

► Pathology

Mononuclear cell and **giant-cell infiltrates** in cranial arteries. Skip lesions.

► Treatment Steps

Corticosteroids (see Cram Facts).

D. Benign Intracranial Hypertension (Pseudotumor Cerebri)

► Symptoms

Those of increased intracranial pressure without tumor, **headache,** visual disturbances, nausea, vomiting, dizziness.

► Diagnosis

Clinical seting (headache, papilledema, no focal neurologic findings, obese female). Magnetic resonance imaging (MRI) more sensitive to look for hydrocephalus, rule out tumor or dural sinus vein thrombosis. Lumbar puncture shows elevated opening pressure.

► Pathology

Decreased cerebrospinal fluid outflow conductance.

► Treatment Steps

1. Acetazolamide, diuretics.
2. Prednisone.
3. Serial lumbar punctures.
4. Optic nerve sheath incision, lumboperitoneal shunts.

E. Trigeminal Neuralgia (Tic Douloureux)

► Symptoms

Brief episodes of **pain in fifth cranial nerve distribution,** third and second divisions.

► Diagnosis

Onset after 40, more often in women, may coexist with multiple sclerosis (MS); history is diagnostic, may have facial trigger points but no sensory impairment.

► Pathology

Degenerative changes gasserian ganglion. **Compression of trigeminal nerve** by vascular loops causing demyelination. **MS;** demyelination of root entry zone.

► Treatment Steps

1. **Phenytoin, carbamazepine,** baclofen, gabapentin, amitriptyline, lamotrigine.
2. Alcohol nerve block.
3. Microvascular decompression.
4. Percutaneous radiofrequency nerve thermocoagulation.

► cram facts

TEMPORAL ARTERITIS

- Medical emergency.
- Must have a high clinical suspicion in a patient over age 50 (but often much older) who presents with unilateral headache in temporal region, or eye pain.
- Treatment with steroids must be started immediately to prevent loss of vision.
- Surgical biopsy is definitive for diagnosis, and although starting steroids empirically may alter biopsy results, it is often done to prevent blindness.

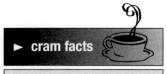

II. DIZZINESS

A. Syncope and Presyncope

Impending loss of consciousness secondary to **inadequate cerebral perfusion. Etiology vascular** or **cardiac,** not neurologic. May be due to hyperventilation, orthostatic hypotension, vasovagal, micturition.

B. Dysequilibrium

Disorder of **balance** system, dizziness when standing and walking, multiple possible central nervous system (CNS) causes. Chronic and common in elderly.

C. Vertigo

Sensation of movement, due to **abnormality** of the **peripheral** or **central vestibular system** pathways. **Nystagmus** may be present. **Peripheral nystagmus** is **unidirectional** and **suppressed by fixation. Central nystagmus** may be **multidirectional** and is **never suppressed by fixation.**

   Ménière's disease: **hearing loss, tinnitus,** and **vertigo. Perilymph fistula: oval window tear** resulting in vertigo aggravated by change in head position, sneezing, noises. Other disorders resulting in vertigo include vestibular neuronitis, labyrinthitis, posttraumatic brain stem transient ischemic attack (TIA), MS, posterior fossa tumor, and basilar artery migraine.

III. EPILEPSY

A. Generalized Epileptic Seizures

1. **Tonic and/or clonic**—premonitory phase followed by immediate loss of consciousness, tonic, clonic, and postictal (confusion) phases. Electroencephalogram (EEG) hallmark is immediate bihemispheric discharges.
2. **Absence seizures**—brief loss of consciousness (5–10 seconds), sudden blank stare, abrupt cessation of activity; clonic movements, automatisms such as lip smacking. **EEG three per second spike-and-wave pattern. Drug of choice: ethosuximide.**
3. **Myoclonic**—sudden generalized or focal muscle jerk, EEG discharge concurrent with jerk.
4. **Atonic seizures**—1 to 2 sec. Drop attacks limited or generalized, secondary to diffuse brain disease.
5. **West syndrome**—infantile spasms (sudden extensor/flexor trunk movements) psychomotor retardation and EEG hyparrhythmia (disorganized high-voltage slow waves, spikes, and sharp waves); pre- and postnatal causes including genetic disorders, injuries, infections, metabolic disorders.
6. **Atypical absence**—less abrupt onset, longer, loss of postural tone, associated with other seizure types; EEG background abnormal, ictal 0.5- to 2.5-Hz spike-and-wave discharges.

B. Focal Epilepsy

1. **Simple partial sezures**—no impairment of consciousness.
   a. Motor, start in one motor cortical area—may spread with progressive jerking (jacksonian seizures).
   b. Sensory—parietal, occipital, temporal.
      Parietal: tingling, numbness, sensation of movement or absence of body part.

Occipital: flashes of light, hemianopsia, scotomata. Visual association cortex, complex images—micropsia, macropsia, distortions.

Temporal: auditory, olfactory hallucinations, emotional or psychic phenomena, memory or cognitive distortions (déjà vu), time distortions, detachment, affective (fear, depression).

2. Complex partial seizures—impaired level of awareness and consciousness, amnesia for event, automatisms may occur.

3. **Partial epileptic syndromes:**

   a. Benign childhood epilepsy with centrotemporal spikes; stops in adolescence—somatosensory, tonic/tonic–clonic activity involving face to arm, generalized with nocturnal seizures.

   b. Childhood epilepsy with occipital paroxysms (spikes)—visual seizures while awake, motor seizures during sleep.

C. Status Epilepticus

Continued or recurrent seizures of any type with unconsciousness for 20 or more minutes. Treat as medical emergency, intravenous (IV) lorazepam (binds γ-aminobutyric acid [GABA]$_A$ receptor) followed by IV phenytoin.

D. Seizure Medication

1. **Treatment of generalized tonic–clonic** seizures.

   a. **Diphenylhydantoin (Dilantin).** Metabolized through hepatic p450 mixed oxidases. **Ataxia, nystagmus, and sedation with high levels. Side effects** include **hirsutism, gingival hypertrophy,** allergic skin reactions, **Stevens–Johnson** syndrome, hypocalcemia, megaloblastic anemia.

   b. **Carbamazepine (Tegretol).** Diplopia, ataxia, dizziness, rash; may induce bone marrow suppression. Oxcarbamazepine (keto homologue of carbamazepine) monohydroxylated in liver. No induction of metabolism or drug interactions. Similar side effects to carbamazepine.

   c. **Phenobarbital.** Sedation. Long half-life. Induces hepatic enzymes.

   d. **Valproic acid.** Sedation, tremor, hair loss, weight gain, edema. Possible **liver failure, fatal pancreatitis,** and **bone marrow suppression,** may help **atypical absence** spells.

   e. **Primidone (Mysoline).** Metabolized to phenobarbital and phenylethylmalonic acid. May cause sedation, **ataxia.**

   f. **Ethosuximide (Zarontin). Drug of choice** for **absence spells.**

   g. **Adrenocorticotropic hormone (ACTH).** Used for **infantile spasms,** as is valproic acid and clonazepam.

2. **Treatment of focal seizures**—similar to that for generalized seizures; however, multiple medications may be needed.

   a. **Gabapentin.** GABA analog. Does not bind receptor. Second drug for partial, secondary generalized seizures. Possible fatigue, somnolence, unsteady gait.

   b. **Lamotrigine.** Partial and primary generalized seizures. Drowsiness, unsteady gait, dizziness, tremor.

   c. **Vigabatrin.** Inhibits GABA-transaminase, increases GABA inhibition. Drowsiness, confusion, weight gain, and psychosis are side effects.

   d. **Topiramate.** Refractory partial seizures. Dizziness, fatigue, drowsiness, abnormal thinking, and ataxia are side effects.

   e. **Levetiracetam.** Exact mechanism of action unknown. Adjunctive therapy for partial seizures. Somnolence, asthenia, dizziness.

   f. **Zonisamide.** Sulfonamide. Blocks sodium channels, inward calcium currents. Adjunctive therapy for partial seizures. Stevens–Johnson syndrome, toxic epidermal necrolysis, blood dyscrasias.

IV. COMA

▶ Description
Patient cannot be aroused, total unresponsiveness. Light coma may demonstrate response to noxious stimuli, whereas there is no response in deep coma.

Locked-in syndrome: quadriplegia and lower cranial nerve paralysis, but conscious with higher mental activity intact. **Akinetic mutism (coma vigile):** patient in coma, but appears awake.

▶ Diagnosis
Clinical. On physical exam, may have Battle's sign: blue mastoid area, suggesting basal skull fracture or temporal bone fracture. Breath odor fruity or acetone in ketoacidosis, musty in hepatic coma. **Cheyne–Stokes** respiration (hyperpnea alternating with apnea) noted with bilateral cerebral hemisphere damage. **Apneustic** respiration (long inspiration then pause): lower pontine lesions, as does **ataxic** (chaotic) breathing.
- *Decerebrate posture.* Midbrain lesion, extension/adduction of arms and legs.
- *Decorticate posture.* Lower diencephalon lesion, flexion arms, wrists, and fingers.

▶ Pathology
Diffuse cerebral hemisphere dysfunction and/or involvement of the brain stem ascending reticular activating system.
- *Trauma.* History of injury. Epidural hematoma: lucid interval. Subdural: depressed consciousness, then focal findings.
- *Vascular disease.* Sudden onset, nuchal rigidity, bloody cerebrospinal fluid (CSF).
- *Neoplasm.* Focal signs, papilledema.
- *Infection.* Cerebrospinal fluid increased protein normal or low CSF glucose.
- *Metabolic.* Abnormal labs.

▶ Treatment Steps
1. **Establish airway,** and IV line.
2. **Determine cardiovascular status, history, and physical.**
3. Obtain full lab, skull x-ray, computed tomography (CT), and/or MRI.
4. May need lumbar puncture.
5. Give thiamine, dextrose, and possibly naloxone.
6. If **cerebral edema** or increased intracranial pressure, restrict fluids, hyperventilate, **mannitol,** and **steroids.**

V. CEREBROVASCULAR DISEASE

▶ Description
- Stroke—sudden onset of a focal neurologic deficit due to cerebrovascular disease, lasting more than 24 hours.
- **TIA**—focal, abrupt in onset, usually lasts less than 1 hour; resolve within 24 hours. Greatest risk for stroke in days to weeks.
- Two major types—**ischemic** (embolic and thrombotic) and **hemorrhagic** (intraparenchymal and subarachnoid). **Stroke** is the third leading cause of death in the United States.

► Diagnosis

Cerebral Embolism—**abrupt onset while active;** most common source of embolism is the heart; less common peripheral arterial embolization. Patients rarely lose consciousness.

Subarachnoid Hemorrhage—**abrupt onset while active** from aneurysm at circle of Willis; may lose consciousness.

Intraparenchymatous Hemorrhage—**abrupt onset while active,** may lose consciousness; CT positive for hematoma.

Thrombotic—**10% preceded by TIA,** often **during sleep;** rarely lose consciousness. May have normal CT and lumbar puncture early; rarely have headache.

A. Ischemic Stroke (80%)

► Risk Factors
- **Nonmodifiable**—race, age, gender, family history prior TIA or cerebrovascular accident (CVA).
- **Modifiable**—hypertension, diabetes mellitus, smoking, alcohol abuse, oral contraceptives, cardiac disease, prior stroke, lipoprotein abnormalities, elevated homocysteine and C-reactive protein, coagulopathies.

► Symptoms

Symptoms are based on blood vessel and subsequent area of brain involved.
1. **Middle cerebral artery**—contralateral hemiplegia/paresis. Dominant hemisphere—**nonfluent** or **Broca's aphasia** from upper-division occlusion. **Wernicke's (fluent)** aphasia from lower-division lesions.
2. **Anterior cerebral artery**—contralateral leg paralysis, abulia, akinetic mutism, sphincter incontinence.
3. **Carotid artery**—contralateral weakness or sensory loss, speech disturbance, ipsilateral visual loss.
4. **Posterior cerebral**—contralateral homonymous hemianopia, cortical blindness, prosopagnosia, alexia without agraphia.
5. **Vertebrobasilar**—ataxia, hemiplegia, horizontal gaze, palsy, nystagmus vertigo, deafness, dizziness.
6. **Cerebellar**—ataxia, dizziness, nausea, vomiting.
7. **Lacunar infarct**—due to **lipohyalinosis,** may present with pure motor or sensory strokes, clumsy hand syndrome may be seen.

► Treatment Steps
1. Prevention—treat modifiable risk factors (above).
2. TIA—antiplatelet aggregating drugs (aspirin, ticlopidine, clopidogrel).
3. Acute ischemic infarction—protect airway, prevent aspiration, avoid aggressive blood pressure (BP) control. Treat **BP** slowly if over 170/100 mm Hg. Treat hyperglycemia, reduce fever. Thrombolysis in infarcts less than 3 hours old with tissue plasminogen activator. Cerebral edema peaks in 2 to 7 days; treat with modest fluid restriction, intubation and hyperventilation, mannitol.
4. Elective carotid endarterectomy if carotid stenosis present.

B. Hemorrhagic Stroke (20%)

► Symptoms
1. **Hypertensive intracerebral hemorrhage**—the most common sites are putamen, thalamus, cerebellum, pons, lobar. Due to lipohyalinosis of small intraparenchymal arteries. Presentation reflects in-

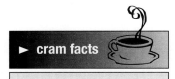

► **cram facts**

The most common site for ischemic/embolic stroke is the middle cerebral artery.

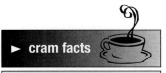

► **cram facts**

DIAGNOSIS OF STROKE

- Clinical signs and symptoms.
- CT scan will not usually show an early acute ischemic stroke, but it is often the first test done in the emergency department to rule out hemorrhage.
- MRI is much more sensitive for ischemia.
- CT or MR angiography of the head and neck may pinpoint the vascular lesion.

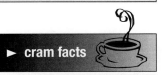

► **cram facts**

WORKUP OF STROKE

To identify cause of stroke, the following tests are usually completed:
- Carotid ultrasound.
- Echocardiogram (transesophageal echocardiogram done in certain settings).
- Fasting lipid panel.
- Hypercoagulability workup may be indicated in certain cases, particularly young individuals with no other source of stroke.

creased intracranial pressure (headache, vomiting, decreased level of consciousness) and location. **Unusual eye signs** may indicate **thalamic** hemorrhage. **Pontine** hemorrhage results in pinpoint reactive pupils, coma, quadriplegia, ophthalmoplegia, decerebrate posturing. **Cerebellar bleed** results in vertigo, headache, vomiting, and ataxia. Ventricular extension results in hydrocephalus and is associated with poor prognosis.

2. **Subarachnoid hemorrhage**—caused by saccular aneurysm or vascular malformation. Sudden severe headache, meningeal irritation; exam may be normal.

3. **Other causes** of bleeding include arteriovenous malformation, tumor, anticoagulant therapy, cocaine abuse, cerebral amyloid angiitis.

4. **Initial test of choice—CT scan. Do lumbar puncture only if CT not available, and check for papilledema before doing lumbar puncture.**

▶ Treatment Steps
1. Control BP.
2. Treat seizures.
3. Control raised intracranial pressure (ICP).
4. Surgery in selected cases—ventriculostomy to decrease ICP and remove blood, hemorrhage removal in some instances (cerebellum, putamen, lobar).

VI. DEMYELINATING DISEASE

A. Multiple Sclerosis

▶ Description
Multiple areas of neurologic deficits, peak age 20 to 24. **Increased incidence** in **women** and north temperate latitudes, etiology unknown, possibly autoimmune. Fewer exacerbations during pregnancy.

▶ Symptoms
Optic neuritis, vertigo, paresthesias, sensory loss, pain, **incoordination,** bladder dysfunction, nystagmus, weakness in 50%, trigeminal neuralgia, diplopia, **internuclear ophthalmoplegia, characteristically bilateral.**

▶ Diagnosis
See Cram Facts.

▶ Pathology
Plaques—areas of myelin destruction associated with lymphocytic and macrophage infiltrates. Gliosis and axonal loss in chronic lesions.

▶ Treatment Steps
1. Acute exacerbations: Intravenous or oral steroids.
2. Prophylaxis: Interferon-β (Avonex, Betaseron, Rebif), interferon-α (Intron A), or glatiramer acetate (Copaxone).
3. Symptomatic treatment: Spasticity—Lioresal, Tizanidine, Dantrium; bladder—oxybutinin, hyoscyamine, antiseptics (vitamin C, methenamine); pain—carbamazepine, gabapentin, amitriptyline, lamotrigine.

B. Optic Neuritis

▶ Description
Inflammation of the optic nerve, often from **optic nerve demyelination.** Episode of optic neuritis may precede MS. Papillitis, swelling of

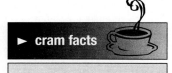

▶ **cram facts**

DIAGNOSIS OF MS

- No one single test will diagnose MS.
- Signs and symptoms typical of the disease are needed and must be present at two different points in time.
- Testing will help confirm the diagnosis.
- Demyelinating plaques seen on MRI of brain/spinal cord.
- CSF often reveals oligoclonal bands.
- Increased latency in visual evoked response (VER), brain stem auditory evoked response (BAER), or somatosensory evoked potential (SSEP)

the optic nerve head may occur. May cause acute visual loss (see Cram Facts).

► Diagnosis

Decreased visual acuity and color vision, scotomata, ocular pain. Abnormal VER, visual fields, and contrast sensitivity. MRI may demonstrate T2-weighted and gadolinium-enhancing lesions of optic nerve. Brain or spinal cord MRI abnormalities—greater risk of MS with two or more.

► Treatment Steps

Intravenous methylprednisolone (Solu-Medrol). Interferon-β prohylaxis with two or more MRI lesions.

C. Acute Disseminated Encephalomyelitis

► Description

Monophasic, mostly postinfectious and postvaccinal.

► Symptoms

Headache, stiff neck, confusion, seizures, fever, coma. Focal and multifocal signs. Mortality 10–30%.

► Treatment Steps

Corticosteroids.

D. Guillain–Barré Syndrome—A Peripheral Neuropathy

► Description

Acute inflammatory polyradiculoneuropathy in young to middle-aged adults. Frequently preceded by upper respiratory or gastrointestinal (GI) infection (*Campylobacter jejuni*), surgery, immunization. Linked to Epstein–Barr virus (EBV), cytomegalovirus (CMV), human immunodeficiency virus (HIV).

► Symptoms

Progressive ascending weakness, areflexia.

► Diagnosis

High CSF protein, with few cells, short duration of progression; nerve conduction studies. With HIV infection, CSF pleocytosis is found.

► Pathology

Endoneurial perivascular mononuclear cell infiltration; multifocal root and nerve demyelination.

► Treatment Steps

Spontaneous recovery may occur, plasmapheresis, or intravenous immunoglobulin.

VII. CNS INFECTIONS

A. Acute Meningitis

► Symptoms

Headache, fever, stiff neck. Minimal neurologic signs in viral meningitis, which is a benign self-limited disorder and also termed *aseptic meningitis.* Positive **Kernig's** and **Brudzinski's signs.**

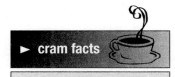

► cram facts

OPTIC NEURITIS AND MS

- 15–20% of patients with MS initially present with optic neuritis.
- 70% of patients with MS have at least one episode of optic neuritis at some point during their illness.

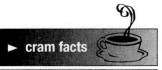

► cram facts

GUILLAIN–BARRÉ SYNDROME

- Patients must be followed closely to avoid respiratory compromise as paralysis ascends.
- Can monitor with serial measurements of negative inspiratory force (NIF). If NIF shows progressive reduction elective intubation may be needed.

► Diagnosis

Gram stain and culture of CSF. CSF protein **over 50,** viral; in **bacterial** or **fungal** up to 400. **Hypoglycorrhachia** (CSF glucose less than 40% of serum level) **suggests bacterial** cause. **Tuberculous** (characteristically lymphocytic meningitis) active pulmonary disease in one third, positive purified protein derivative (PPD) in 50% (see Fig. 11–1).

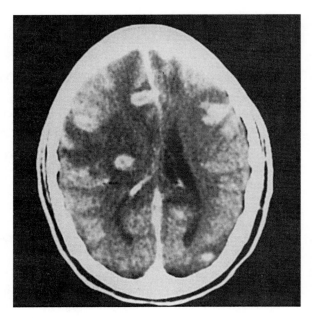

A

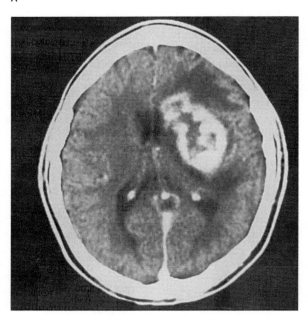

B

Figure 11–1. Two patients with ring-enhancing intracerebral lesions complicating intravenous drug use. These patients presented with headache, fever, altered mental status, or focal neurological deficits. **A:** Multiple foci of toxoplasmosis in a patient with AIDS. **B:** Primary CNS lymphoma in another patient with AIDS. The patient did not respond to initial empiric therapy with antitoxoplasmosis antibiotics. The lesion was then treated with radiation therapy with partial regression.

▶ Pathology
1. **Neonatal**—group B **streptococcus,** *Escherichia coli.*
2. **Early childhood**—*Haemophilus influenzae, Streptococcus pneumoniae,* and *Neisseria meningitidis.*
3. **Young adults**—*Neisseria meningitidis* (petechial or ecchymotic rash often), *S. pneumoniae, H. influenzae.*
4. **Nosocomial**—Gram-negative bacteria and *Staphylococcus aureus.*
5. **Immunosuppressed**—*Listeria monocytogenes, S. pneumoniae, H. influenzae, Nocardia, Mycobacterium tuberculosis, Cryptococcus neoformans.*
6. **HIV patients**—acute aseptic meningitis.
7. **Viral meningitis**—most common agent is mumps; enterovirus is most common viral group.

▶ Treatment Steps
1. *Toxoplasma*—pyrimethamine plus sulfadiazine.
2. *Brucella*—tetracycline and aminoglycoside. Chronic neurobrucellosis—rifampin, trimethoprim–sulfamethoxazole, doxycycline.
3. **Neonatal**—ampicillin and gentamicin.
4. **Adults**—ceftriaxone or ampicillin.
5. **Tuberculous**—isoniazid, ethambutol, rifampin, pyrazinamide.
6. **Fungal**—amphotericin B.

B. Neurosyphilis

▶ Symptoms

Tabes dorsalis, general paresis, gumma, optic atrophy, cerebrovascular disease from invasion of leptomeninges with *Treponema pallidum.* Neurosyphilis most often is asymptomatic.

▶ Treatment Steps

High-dose parenteral penicillin. **Jarisch–Herxheimer** reaction: hypotension, fever, headache, chills, and tachycardia in first 24 hours of treatment from release of treponemal products; not a penicillin reaction.

C. Empyema (Subdural)

Infection spread from paranasal sinuses and middle ear, *Streptococcus* most often, marked peripheral leukocytosis.

D. Viral Encephalitis

▶ Description
Mortality of 10%.

▶ Symptoms
Focal signs and **acute febrile** illness, **seizures** and **coma,** or depressed state of consciousness. Headache, fever, and nuchal rigidity.

▶ Diagnosis
Aseptic CSF, lymphocytic CSF with normal glucose.

▶ Pathology
Caused by mumps, herpes simplex type 1, lymphocytic choriomeningitis, arboviruses, EBV. Mouse and hamster exposure linked to lymphocytic choriomeningitis.

▶ Treatment Steps
Treat edema and seizures.

▶ **clinical pearl**

- Newer studies have suggested dexamethasone may be useful in acute bacterial meningitis if given before or with first dose of antibiotics.
- Prophylaxis (rifampin or ciprofloxacin) is given to close contacts of patients with meningitis due to *N. meningitidis*, rifampin, or ciprofloxacin.

E. Other CNS Infections

1. **Rabies**—brain stem encephalitis, incubation 30 to 60 days or more, respiratory spasms, dysphagia–hydrophobia, fatal in acute stage in 95%.
2. **Polio**—etiology: enteroviruses that damage anterior horn cells of spinal cord, an acute febrile illness with evidence of lower motor neuron paralysis.
3. **Toxoplasmosis**—intracellular parasite, **most common opportunistic CNS pathogen in acquired immune deficiency syndrome (AIDS)** (cryptococcal is second most common).
4. **Slow viruses:**
   a. **Creutzfeldt–Jakob, kuru.** Ataxia and myoclonus, dementia.
   b. **Subacute sclerosing panencephalitis.** In childhood, mostly from measles infection. Elevated gamma globulin and measles antibodies in CSF.
   c. **Progressive multifocal leukoencephalopathy (PML).** Due to SV40-PML.
5. **AIDS.**
6. **Herpes simplex encephalitis**—treat with acyclovir. Diagnosis may be suggested by temporal lobe localization.

VIII. NEUROMUSCULAR DISEASE

A. Disorders of Muscle—Muscular Dystrophy

1. **Duchenne**—sex-linked recessive trait, **progressive muscle weakness** and **atrophy,** due to mutation on X chromosome (dystrophin gene; Xp21 locus), diagnosis by family history, weakness, muscle biopsy, probable death by age 20. Elevated creatine kinase (CK).
2. **Limb–girdle**—autosomal recessive and dominant forms.
3. **Myotonic**—thinning face muscles, electromyogram (EMG) shows a decremental pattern, and irregular after potentials. Autosomal dominant (chromosome 19q. Expanded CTG repeats in myotonin protein kinase). Treat with phenytoin sodium (Dilantin).
4. **Fascioscapulohumeral**—autosomal dominant. No carriers.

B. Disorders of Neuromuscular Junction

1. Myasthenia Gravis

▶ Description
Autoantibodies against acetylcholine receptor. Associated with thymic hyperplasia and thymoma. Women more than men.

▶ Symptoms
Weak with activity, fatigue, ocular symptoms; facial muscles, voice, limb muscles, and respiration can be affected.

▶ Diagnosis
Tensilon test, electromyogram—repetitive nerve stimulation, positive antibodies to acetylcholine receptor.

▶ Treatment Steps
1. Cholinesterase inhibitors.
2. Steroids.
3. Plasmapheresis.
4. Thymectomy.
5. Immunosuppressants, IV immunoglobulin.

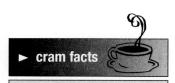

▶ cram facts

Thymectomy may offer a cure to patients with myasthenia gravis (MG). Thymectomy is offered to all patients with a thymoma and patients aged 10–55 without a thymoma but with generalized MG.

2. Eaton–Lambert Syndrome

▶ Description

Facilitating neuromuscular transmission disorder due to autoantibodies against presynaptic neuromuscular voltage-gated calcium channels.

▶ Symptoms

Limb weakness without cranial muscle weakness and absence of deep tendon reflexes. Found with **small cell lung cancer** or as autoimmune disease.

▶ Diagnosis

Response to repetitive stimulation (**increasing action potential**).

▶ Treatment Steps

Guanidine. Calcium channel antagonists are contraindicated.

3. Botulism

▶ Description

Toxin of *Clostridium botulinum* blocks acetylcholine release.

▶ Symptoms

Begin 12–36 hours after ingestion of exotoxin in contaminated food. Blurred vision, dilated fixed pupil, flaccid quadriplegia, dysphagia, dysarthria, respiratory paralysis, dry mouth.

▶ Diagnosis

Isolate toxin from stool, stomach, or food. **Spores** also found in **honey.** EMG—decreased compound muscle action potentials; post-tetanic facilitation.

▶ Treatment Steps

1. **Cathartics.**
2. **Trivalent antitoxin** (A, B, E).
3. Quinidine.
4. Supportive therapy.

C. Myotonia

1. **Myotonia congenita**—dominant and recessive mutations of chloride channel. Impaired muscle relaxation, treat with phenytoin.
2. **Myotonic dystrophy—predominantly distal weakness,** cardiac conduction problems, cataracts, testicular atrophy, endocrine dysfunction, increased sensitivity to medications which depress respiratory drive, ptosis, temporalis and masseter muscle wasting.

D. Trichinosis

▶ Description

Nematode *Trichinella spiralis* infection, undercooked pork most common source. Causes eosinophilia, weakness, myalgia.

▶ Treatment Steps

Thiabendazole, mebendazole.

E. Tetanus

▶ Description

Lockjaw, intense motor neuron activity.

▶ Symptoms/Diagnosi

Muscle spasms, trismus (lockjaw), facial muscle spasm (risus sardonicus), opisthotonos, autonomic dysfunction. Clinical diagnosis.

▶ Pathology

Caused by neurotoxin (tetanospasmin) from *Clostridium tetani,* a gram-positive coccus, which inhibits spinal inhibitory interneurons.

▶ Treatment Steps

1. Cleaning and debridement of infected site.
2. **Antibiotics.**
3. **Antitoxin** (human hyperimmune globulin).
4. Skeletal muscle relaxants (diazepam).

F. Bell's Palsy

▶ Symptoms

Idiopathic, acute, peripheral facial weakness; may have ipsilateral hyperacusis and decreased taste.

▶ Diagnosis

Inexcitable facial nerve, denervation of facial muscles after 2–3 weeks.

▶ Treatment Steps

Supportive treatment Artificial tears to prevent corneal drying. Often self-limited. If patients present early, steroids and/or antiviral medications may be helpful.

G. Motor Neuron Disease

1. **Amyotrophic lateral sclerosis (ALS)—middle-age** rapid progression of **weakness.** Combination of upper (spasticity, hyperreflexia, emotional lability) and lower (atrophy, weakness, cramps, fasciculations) neuron involvement. Bulbar and respiratory weakness in 50%. Is most common motor system disease. Familial ALS has mutation for superoxide dysmutase gene. Treated with riluzole.
2. **Type 1 proximal spinal muscular atrophy (Werdnig–Hoffmann)—** floppy infant, delayed milestones, progressive atrophy, respiratory and swallowing problems. Autosomal recessive, deletions in neuronal apoptosis inhibitory gene in two-thirds.
3. **Bulbospinal muscular atrophy (Kennedy's disease)—**X-linked recessive, increased CAG repeats in androgen receptor gene. Weakness, onset age 20–40, muscle cramps, gynecomastia, dysphagia, dysarthria.

IX. MOVEMENT DISORDERS

A. Huntington's Disease

▶ Description

Chorea, personality change, psychiatric syndromes, progressive dementia. Autosomal dominant with expanded CAG repeat sequence in huntingtin gene.

▶ Symptoms

Progressive emotional or **intellectual decline** associated with chorea, abnormalities in gait, ocular motor function, and dexterity. Onset in fourth or fifth decades in most. Patients live an average of 15 years after diagnosis.

► Diagnosis

Exam, family history.

► Pathology

Caudate nucleus and cerebral cortex atrophy, neuronal loss and gliosis, and decreased GABA and acetylcholine have been noted along with spared somatostatin–neuropeptide Y neurons.

► Treatment Steps

No cure but dopaminergic antagonists: presynaptic—tetrabenazine, reserpine; postsynaptic—haloperidol (Haldol).

B. Wilson's Disease (Hepatolenticular Degeneration)

See also Chapter 4.

► Description

Chromosome 13 autosomal recessive disorder of copper metabolism (mutations in copper-transporting P-type ATPase), characterized by **deficient ceruloplasmin,** elevated urinary copper excretion. Presents in adolescence or early adulthood.

► Symptoms

Neurologic—tremor, incoordination, ataxia, akinesia, dysarthria, dysphagia, dystonia.

Hepatic—hepatitis, which may be acute or chronic; cirrhosis.

Ocular—Kayser–Fleischer ring in Descemet's membrane of cornea noted (rusty brown ring at limbus).

Psychiatric—variable presentation.

► Diagnosis

High serum copper and high urine copper. Slit lamp exam, low serum ceruloplasmin, and elevated 24-hour urine copper; liver biopsy and copper quantitation are also helpful. Abnormal liver function tests. Aminoaciduria. MRI—cerebral atrophy, putaminal, thalamic, and brain stem hypodensities. Pathology—excess copper deposits in liver and brain.

► Treatment Steps

D-penicillamine. Adverse effects of therapy include hypersensitivity, fever, nephrotic syndrome, myasthenia gravis, Goodpasture syndrome, bone marrow suppression (agranulocytosis and thrombocytopenia), and collagen vascular disorders.

C. Parkinson's Disease

► Description

An idiopathic **extrapyramidal movement disorder** affecting the elderly. Reduced activity complex I mitochondrial electron transport chain. Mutation in α-synuclein gene in familial Parkinson's disease.

► Symptoms

Characterized by **resting tremor (pill-rolling—5–7 Hz), cogwheel rigidity, bradykinesia,** impaired postural reflexes, masked facies, flexed posture, hypophonia.

► Diagnosis

Clinical exam. Reduced 6-[^{18}F]-fluorolevodopa in striata with positron-emission tomography (PET).

► Pathology

Depigmentation, neuronal loss and gliosis in substantia nigra and pigmented nuclei. Cytoplasmic inclusion (Lewy) bodies. Results in reduced striatal dopamine. Associated decreased activity complex I mitochondrial electron transport chain.

► Treatment Steps

1. **Levodopa/carbidopa** (Sinemet), toxicity with levodopa: dyskinesias, hallucinations, confusion.
2. Anticholinergics, amantadine.
3. Dopamine agonists (bromocriptine, pergolide, pramipexole, ropinirole) particularly late.
4. Catechol-*O*-methyltransferase (COMT) inhibitors prolong L-dopa availability.
5. Pallidotomy and deep brain stimulation for end-stage disease.

D. Iatrogenic Dyskinesias

1. **Drug-induced parkinsonism**—methylphenyltetrahydropyridine (MPTP); neuroleptics block striatal dopamine receptor sites.
2. **Tardive dyskinesia**—linguofasciobuccal, choreiform.
3. **Dopamine agonist-induced chorea**—levodopa.
4. **Neuroleptic dystonia.**

E. Noniatrogenic Dykinesias

1. **Dystonia**—inappropriate cocontraction of antagonistic muscles, resulting in repetitive twisting movements. Focal dystonias treated with botulinum toxin injection: generalized with trihexiphenidyl (Artane).
2. **Chorea**—random twitching or jerking, excessive, involuntary, purposeless movements.

► **cram facts**

MOVEMENT DISORDERS

- **Huntington's disease:** adult, insidious onset of chorea, autosomal dominant.
- **Parkinson's disease:** resting tremor (5–7 Hz), cogwheel rigidity, bradykinesia, impaired postural reflexes. Dopa responsive.
- **Wilson's disease:** tremors, incoordination, ataxia, akinesia, dysarthria, dystonia. Kayser–Fleischer ring, hepatitis, cirrhosis.

DEMENTIA

- **Alzheimer's disease:** global cognitive decline in elderly. Amnesia, language, visuospatial impairments, personality and behavioral change.
- **Pick's disease:** frontotemporal atrophy. Personality change, apathy, abulia, aphasia.
- **Multi-infarct dementia:** recurrent strokes. Features of dementia secondary to cortical/subcortical locations.
- **Normal pressure hydrocephalus:** progressive dementia, urinary incontinence, gait disorder. Hydrocephalus without cortical atrophy.

3. **Blepharospasm**—oromandibular dystonia (Meige syndrome).
4. **Spasmodic torticollis**—most frequent focal dystonia, involving neck muscles. Intermittent or sustained head deviation.

F. Tremor (Essential)

Involves the distal upper extremity, postural or action tremor; is often progressive. May be familial (autosomal dominant with variable penetrance). Treatment includes propranolol, primidone, topiramate. Alcohol responsive.

G. Myoclonus

Rapid jerking movement, treat primary cause when known. Clonazepam, 5-hydroxytryptophan (5-HTP) and valproic acid often used.

H. Asterixis

Sudden loss of postural tone. Occurs in metabolic encephalopathies (uremic, hepatic), drug intoxications, and structural brain lesions. Classically described as a "flap." Patient has arms outstretched, palms out, but cannot keep hands still.

X. DEMENTIA

A. Alzheimer's Disease

► Description

A progressive dementia (global cognitive decline) of middle and late life.

► Symptoms

Memory loss, language and visuospatial impairments, mood disturbance, delusions, hallucinations, changes in personality and behavior. Generalized seizures (10–20%).

► Diagnosis

No one test is diagnostic. It is a clinical diagnosis/diagnosis of exclusion. Clinical, abnormal mental status exam and exclusion of other illnesses (e.g., normal pressure, hydrocephalus, metabolic disease, multi-infarct dementia, tumor, and infections). Etiology is unknown, but frequency increases with age. Familial associations with amyloid precursor protein and presenilin protein mutations; inheritance of E4 allele apolipoprotein E. MRI demonstrates cortical atrophy. Single photon-emission computed tomography (SPECT), PET scans have bilateral temporoparietal hypometabolism.

► Pathology

Senile plaques (dystrophic neurites surrounding an amyloid core) **and neurofibrillary tangles** are prominent, associated with cerebral atrophy and ventricular dilatation.

► Treatment Steps

Symptoms such as agitation and depression are treatable. Acetylcholinesterase inhibitors (tacrine, donepezil, rivastigmine, galantamine). Newer medications include memantine (Namenda).

B. Pick's Disease

► Description

Dementia with lobar atrophy.

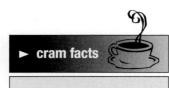

► Symptoms

Prominent, early personality change, apathy, abulia, disordered speech, aphasia.

► Diagnosis

Occasionally familial. CT/MRI—prominent symmetric/asymmetric frontotemporal atrophy.

► Pathology

Frontotemporal lobar atrophy. Argyrophilic neuronal (Pick) inclusion bodies in frontal and temporal lobes. Frontal and temporal atrophy sparing superior temporal gyrus.

► Treatment Steps

Supportive treatment for dementia.

C. Multi-infarct Dementia

► Description

Episodic neurologic dysfunction secondary to infarcts of the cerebral hemispheres leading to dementia.

► Symptoms

Dementia. Clinical features determined by location of infarctions. Subcortical infarcts lead to psychomotor slowing, decreased attention, concentration and memory deficits, gait disorder (lower half parkinsonism). Cortical infarcts produce aphasia, apraxia, visuospatial defects, amnesia.

► Diagnosis

Progressive intellectual decline. Associated stroke risk factors and multiple infarctions, ventricular dilatation. Multifocal decreases in cerebral blood flow on PET/SPECT.

► Treatment Steps

1. Aspirin, ticlopidine, clopidogrel.
2. Treat hypertension.

D. Hydrocephalus (Normal Pressure)

► Description

Progressive dementia usually occurring in the elderly.

► Symptoms

Urinary incontinence, dementia, gait disturbance (slow, short steps; unstable).

► Diagnosis

Normal CSF pressure. Enlarged cerebral ventricles, relatively normal cortical gyri on CT/MRI. Subependymal CSF resorption on MRI.

► Pathology

Increased resistance to arachnoid villus absorption of CSF. Associated with subarachnoid hemorrhage, trauma, tumor, infection.

► Treatment Steps

Ventriculoperitoneal shunt. Significant improvement with CSF removal.

E. Creutzfeldt–Jakob Disease

► Description

Progressive dementia, due to abnormal isoform of prion protein (PrP^{Sc}). Disease may be infectious, inherited, or sporadic.

► Symptoms
Subacute progressive dementia, myoclonus.

► Diagnosis
Clinical, EEG high-voltage, triphasic periodic complexes on depressed background.

► Pathology
Spongiform change (vacuolar dilatation of neurons), amyloid plaques, loss of neurons, and gliosis.

► Treatment Steps
None.

XI. NEUROLOGIC EYE SIGNS

A. Horner Syndrome

► Symptoms
Ptosis, **miosis, anhidrosis, enophthalmos,** narrowing palpebral fissure, flushing on affected side of face.

► Pathology
Interruption of the unilateral sympathetic system due to trauma, **lung apex tumor,** CNS lesions, vascular headache.

► Diagnosis
Cocaine and *para*-**OH-amphetamine** tests.

B. Adie's Pupil

► Symptoms
Unilaterally dilated pupil with **slow response to light** and accommodation; areflexia may be present.

► Pathology
Postganglionic parasympathetic lesion.

► Diagnosis
Weak pilocarpine solution results in Adie's pupil contraction.

C. Argyll–Robertson Pupil

► Symptoms
Very small pupils that **fail to constrict to light** with **accommodation preserved.** One or both eyes affected.

► Diagnosis
Argyll–Robertson pupil is a sign of neurosyphilis. Rule out CNS structural lesions.

D. Uncal Herniation Syndrome

► Symptoms
Pupils fixed and **dilated,** ophthalmoplegia and contralateral hemiparesis.

E. Marcus Gunn Pupil

► Symptoms
Defective direct light reflex with intact consensual reflex on "swinging flashlight test."

F. Third Cranial Nerve Lesion

▶ Symptoms

Affects medial rectus, superior rectus, inferior rectus, inferior oblique, and levator of eyelid. Eye "down and out."

G. Fourth Cranial Nerve Lesion

▶ Symptoms

Superior oblique muscle affected; vertical diplopia.

H. Sixth Cranial Nerve Lesion

▶ Symptoms

Weak lateral rectus, poor abduction.

I. Pupil Signs in Examination

Unreactive, Midposition—Midbrain lesion.

Pinpoint Pupils—Pontine lesion.

Unilaterally Dilated and Unreactive—Possible third nerve lesion.

XII. SLEEP DISORDERS

See also Chapter 15.

A. General Information

Adults spend 20% of sleep in rapid eye movement **(REM)** sleep. Non–rapid eye movement sleep **(NREM) has four stages.** Three major disorders include **insomnia, hypersomnia,** and **parasomnia. Early morning awakening** is a **symptom of depression.**

*Narcolepsy—***Daytime** sleep attacks accompanied by cataplexy, hypnogogic hallucinations, and sleep paralysis. Rapid onset REM sleep. Treat with amphetamine, pemoline, methylphenidate, dextroamphetamine. Clomipramine for cataplexy.

*Night Terror—***Arousal from NREM sleep.**

*Nightmare—***Awakening from REM sleep.**

*Obstructive Sleep Apnea—***Overweight,** hypertension, arrhythmias. Treat with nasal continuous positive airway pressure (CPAP).

*Central Sleep Apnea—*Older age, not overweight.

XIII. NEOPLASMS

A. Gliomas (60% of CNS Tumors)

1. **Astrocytoma**—most common of all gliomas, and **most common brain tumor in childhood.** Low grade—astrocytoma; high grade—glioblastoma multiforme.
2. **Oligodendroglioma**—usually frontal lobe, slow growing, presents with headache, seizures, and the tumor may bleed.
3. **Medulloblastoma—most common posterior fossa tumor in children.** Fast growing, radiosensitive.
4. **Ependymoma**—ependymal surface location. Infratentorial more than supratentorial and filum terminale.

B. Meningiomas

Usually benign, **associated** with type 2 **neurofibromatosis.**

C. Craniopharyngiomas

Suprasellar, visual field defects often (bitemporal hemianopsia), endocrinopathies, diabetes insipidus.

D. Pituitary Tumors

Secretory in 75%, **nonsecretory** in 25%. **Endocrine** and visual symptoms.

E. Acoustic Schwannoma

Unilateral hearing loss, tinnitus. May compress cranial nerves V, VII, and brain stem. Bilateral in neurofibromatosis type 2.

XIV. TRAUMA AND EMERGENCIES

A. Epidural Hematoma

► Symptoms

Lucid interval after brief unconsciousness followed by increasing obtundation. Sometimes no lucid interval present. **Extreme headache, contralateral hemiparesis.**

► Diagnosis

History and physical, CT scan.

► Treatment Steps
1. Neurosurgical evaluation for possible drainage.
2. Empiric anticonvulsants.
3. May use mannitol to control intracranial pressure/swelling.

B. Subdural Hematoma

► Symptoms

Acute, subacute, and **chronic** from cortical vein tear.

Acute—From high speed trauma, coma from impact; CT useful (see Fig. 11–2).

Subacute—Several days of lethargy, then deterioration; MRI.

Chronic—Minor trauma may cause gradual deterioration; MRI.

C. Subarachnoid Hemorrhage

► Symptoms

Sudden-onset severe headache, may have **sentinel bleed** with minor symptoms. May have stiff neck, photophobia, nausea, and focal signs (see Fig. 11–3).

► Treatment Steps
1. Supportive care.
2. Bed rest, analgesics.
3. Prophylactic anticonvulsants.
4. Carefully control blood pressure.

D. Neuroleptic Malignant Syndrome (NMS)

► Symptoms

High fever, muscular rigidity, akinesia, decreased consciousness, autonomic dysfunction all as a complication of major tranquilizers, tricyclic antidepressants, or withdrawal from dopaminergic agents.

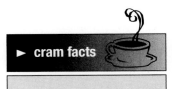

► cram facts

Only 1–2% of all patients exposed to neuroleptics develop NMS.

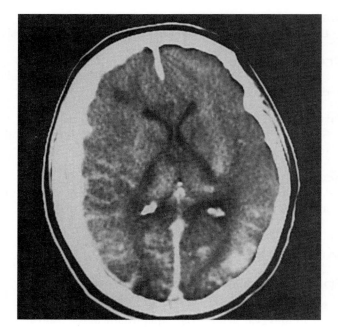

A

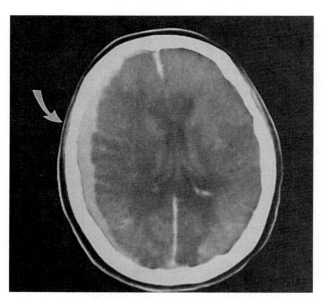

B

Figure 11–2. Acute subdural hematoma in an alcoholic patient following an alcohol binge. The patient's mental status did not steadily improve during several hours of observation. There were no external signs of head trauma. **A:** A narrow "brain window" view displays subtle soft tissue radiodensity differences within the brain, but the acute hematoma is not radiographically distinct from the adjacent bone. **B:** A wider "subdural window" better demonstrates the crescent-shaped blood collection between the right cerebral convexity and the inner table of the skull (arrow). (Reprinted, with permission, from Goldfrank's *Toxicologic Emergencies,* 6th ed., by Louis R. Goldfrank. Copyright 1998 by Appleton & Lange.)

► Treatment Steps
1. Withdraw neuroleptics.
2. Bromocriptine or dantrolene.
3. Supportive care.

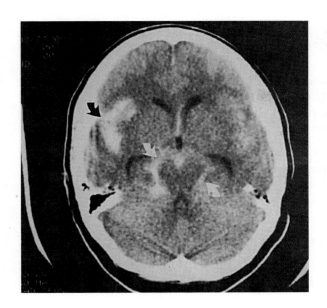

Figure 11–3. Subarachnoid hemorrhage following intravenous cocaine use. The patient had a sudden severe headache followed by a generalized seizure. Extensive hemorrhage is seen surrounding the midbrain at the level of the cerebral peduncles (white arrows) and in the right sylvian fissure (black arrow). Angiography revealed an aneurysm at the origin of the right middle cerebral artery. The aneurysm rupture was presumably provoked by the acute elevation of blood pressure following a cocaine-induced catecholamine surge.

E. Myasthenic Crisis

▶ Symptoms

Acute respiratory failure in a patient with myasthenia gravis.

▶ Treatment Steps
1. Discontinue cholinesterase (ChE) inhibitors.
2. Ventilate patient in intensive care unit (ICU).
3. Slowly reintroduce ChE inhibitors.

XV. TOXIC/METABOLIC DISEASE

A. Uremic Encephalopathy

▶ Symptoms

Depression of level of consciousness with myoclonus, asterixis, tremor, seizures. EEG abnormal; may have triphasic waves. Treat renal disease.

B. Hyponatremia

▶ Symptoms

Confusion, lethargy, headache, **seizures.** The more rapid the sodium drop, the more severe the symptoms. **Syndrome of inappropriate antidiuretic hormone (SIADH): treat with water restriction; demeclocycline if chronic.**

C. Acute Intermittent Porphyria

▶ Symptoms

Abdominal pain, vomiting, constipation or diarrhea, confusion, seizures, neuropathy.

▶ Diagnosis

Watson–Schwartz test for **elevated aminolevulinic acid.**

▶ Pathology

Deficiency of porphobilinogen deaminase.

▶ Treatment Steps
1. Hematin and high-carbohydrate diet.
2. Carbamazepine for seizures.

D. Lead Toxicity

See also Chapter 8.

► Symptoms

Acute exposure—abdominal colic, headache, behavioral change, encephalopathy, seizures. Chronic exposure—gastrointestinal disturbances, anemia, weight loss, behavioral disturbances, cognitive impairment. Peripheral neuropathy (wrist drop) in adults.

► Diagnosis

Basophilic stippling, lead line on x-ray. **Lead colic is most frequent sign in adults.** Screen with lead level, ethylenediaminetetraacetic acid (EDTA) test if lead level not over 80.

► Pathology

Neuropathy from segmental demyelination.

► Treatment Steps

Chelation with Ca-EDTA or penicillamine.

E. Liver Disease—Hepatic Encephalopathy

► Symptoms

Asterixis, slow EEG, depressed mental status, elevated blood ammonia. Give protein-free diet, neomycin, or lactulose.

F. Arsenic Toxicity

See also Chapter 8.

► Symptoms

Nausea, vomiting, abdominal pain, renal failure, neuropathy, encephalopathy.

► Diagnosis

History, exam, Mees' lines (**transverse lines in nails**).

► Treatment Steps

Use dimercaprol (BAL) or penicillamine.

G. Carbon Monoxide Toxicity

See Chapter 8.

H. Vitamin Disorders

1. **Thiamine (B_1) deficiency**—*Wernicke's encephalopathy,* nystagmus, ataxia, confusion, amnesia.
2. **Cobalamin (B_{12}) deficiency**—*Pernicious anemia,* megaloblastic anemia, subacute combined spinal cord degeneration.
3. **Pyridoxine (B_6)**—*Excess can produce sensory neuropathy.*

I. Salicylate Toxicity

► Symptoms

Tinnitus, hearing loss, delirium, coma, seizures.

► Diagnosis

History, respiratory alkalosis, serum salicylate level, rapid screen: **ferric chloride test.**

► Treatment Steps

1. Treat shock.
2. Protect airway.
3. Routine drug intoxication measures.

J. Reye's Syndrome

▶ **Symptoms**

Vomiting, lethargy, and delirium due to brain edema after a viral illness that was treated with aspirin, with abnormal liver functions, hypoglycemia, and respiratory alkalosis. Liver shows **microvesicular fatty infiltration.**

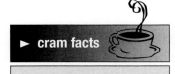

REYE'S SYNDROME

- A potentially fatal condition.
- The incidence has declined markedly since aspirin is no longer recommended for use in children.

XVI. GENETIC DISORDERS

A. Gaucher's Disease

▶ **Description**

Glucocerebroside lipidosis.

▶ **Symptoms**

Type I—visceromegaly. Type II/III—gaze palsies, trismus, spasticity, dementia, seizures, and visceromegaly.

▶ **Diagnosis**

Clinical. Bone marrow may contain Gaucher cells (lipid-laden macrophages). Enzymatic analysis.

▶ **Pathology**

Deficiency of lysosomal glucocerebrosidase. Autosomal recessive.

B. Fabry's Disease

▶ **Description**

Sphingolipidosis. Inborn error of metabolism.

▶ **Symptoms**

Polyneuropathy with neuralgia, cerebrovascular disease in middle age, vasculopathy with renal and cardiac disease, cutaneous angiokeratoma and telangectasias.

▶ **Diagnosis**

Clinical exam. Enzymatic analysis.

▶ **Pathology**

Deficiency of lysosomal α-galactosidase A. Sex-linked recessive. Glycosphingolipid deposition in tissues (eyes, kidney, heart, CNS).

▶ **Treatment Steps**

Carbamazepine, phenytoin for pain. Renal transplantation.

C. Tay–Sachs Disease

▶ **Description**

Infantile cerebromacular degeneration caused by mutations of α-subunit of the lysosomal β-hexosaminidase A gene.

▶ **Symptoms**

Progressive dementia and visual impairment, irritability, muscle weakness, spasticity, seizures.

▶ **Diagnosis**

Cherry-red spot in the fovea. Abnormal electroretinogram (ERG) and visual evoked potential (VEP).

▶ **Pathology**

Accumulation of gangliosides in retina and CNS neurons. Autosomal recessive.

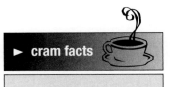

TAY–SACHS DISEASE

- More common in persons of Ashkenazi Jewish descent.
- Prenatal genetic testing may be offered.

D. McArdle's Disease

► Description

A glycogen-storage disorder due to a mutation in the myophosphorylase gene.

► Symptoms

Pain, fatigue, and stiffness on exertion.

► Diagnosis

Forearm exercise test—low/absent lactate production. Elevated muscle glycogen on biopsy.

► Pathology

Deficient muscle phosphorylase.

► Treatment Steps

Glucose and reduce exercise.

E. Pompe's Disease

Acid α-glycosidase (acid maltase) deficiency. Progressive weakness, hypotonia, heart failure.

F. Episodic Muscle Weakness

1. **Familial hypokalemic periodic paralysis**—autosomal dominant, due to mutation of DHP-sensitive calcium channel; weakness, low potassium.
2. **Familial hyperkalemic periodic paralysis—autosomal dominant (mutation of the human muscle sodium channel), shorter weakness attacks, elevated potassium.**

G. Pick's Disease

See section X, Dementia.

H. Huntington's Disease

See section IX, Movement Disorders.

I. Laurence–Moon–Biedl Syndrome

Obesity, mental retardation, retinitis pigmentosa, hypogonadism, polydactyly, diabetes insipidus, autosomal recessive.

J. Shy–Drager Syndrome

Multisystem atrophy with orthostatic hypotension and CNS degeneration (parkinsonism; cerebellar, pyramidal features). Neuronal loss intermediolateral cell column.

K. Friedreich's Ataxia

Most common spinocerebellar degeneration, onset childhood. Mutation in GAA repeat frataxin (X25) gene.

L. Charcot–Marie–Tooth Disease

Demyelinating polyneuropathy, slowly progressive, peroneal muscle atrophy. Mutation in peripheral myelin protein-22 gene.

M. Amino Acid Metabolism Disorders

Maple syrup urine. Hartnup disease.

N. Neurofibromatosis

Autosomal dominant disorders. **Neurofibromatosis 1**—due to mutation in NF-1 neurofibromin gene. Café au lait spots (more than six of 1.5-cm size), neurofibromas, schwannomas, optic nerve gliomas, Lisch nodules iris. **Neurofibromatosis 2**—due to mutation in NF-2 (MERLIN protein) gene. Bilateral vestibular schwannomas, meningiomas, astrocytomas, posterior lens opacities.

O. Tuberous Sclerosis

Autosomal dominant, mental retardation, epilepsy, cutaneous facial lesions, and organ hamartomas.

P. von Hippel–Lindau Disease

Autosomal disorder with retinal and cerebral hemangioblastomas; renal, pancreatic, and epididymal cysts; and renal carcinomas.

Q. Ataxia–Telangiectasia

Progressive cerebellar ataxia (Purkinje cell degeneration), oculocutaneous telangiectasia, radiosensitivity, immunodeficiency and lymphoid malignancies. Due to mutated ATM gene with phosphoinositol-3′kinase activity.

XVII. OTHER DISORDERS

A. Cerebral Palsy

▶ Description
Static encephalopathy with abnormal motor function from birth. Antepartum events cause 90%; also associated with prematurity and low birth weight.

▶ Symptoms
- **Spastic diplegia**—associated with prematurity. Either periventricular leukomalacia or periventricular hemorrhage (greater involvement of intellectual function).
- **Spastic quadriplegia**—associated with congenital malformations and intrauterine infections. Severe disability associated with mental retardation and seizures (Lennox–Gastaut syndrome).
- **Spastic hemiplegia**—caused by developmental malformations, stroke, trauma. Seizures associated.
- **Athetosis**—bilirubin encephalopathy (rare) and causes of spastic quadriplegia.

▶ Diagnosis
History and physical examination, skull x-ray, CT/MRI of the head, EEG, and psychological testing, evaluation of developmental milestones.

▶ Pathology
Includes periventricular leukomalacia, periventricular/intraventricular hemorrhages, infarction.

▶ Treatment Steps
1. Multidisciplinary support.
2. Orthopedic intervention.
3. Physical/occupational therapy.
4. Control seizures.
5. Social services.

B. Attention Deficit Disorder

See Chapter 15.

C. Febrile Seizures

▶ Description

Seizure in child age 3 months to 5 years, associated with fever/infection.

▶ Symptoms

Febrile seizure (short seizure without focal features).

▶ Diagnosis

History and physical exam; rule out meningitis, septicemia. Hospital admission, including routine lab, lumbar tap.

▶ Pathology

Unknown.

▶ Treatment Steps

1. Temperature reduction (tub bath, acetaminophen [Tylenol]).
2. Medication (diazepam [Valium] 0.2 mg/kg rectally or IV).

XVIII. OPHTHALMIC DISORDERS

A. Glaucoma

▶ Description

Ophthalmic disorder of elevated intraocular pressure, which is etiology of 10% of blindness in the United States.

▶ Symptoms

Asymptomatic, or may demonstrate **pain, red eye,** and **vision loss. May note halos around lights.**

▶ Diagnosis

On exam, elevated intraocular pressure (**over 22 mm Hg** by Schiøtz' tonometry).

▶ Pathology

Types include **primary angle-closure, open-angle, secondary, and congenital.** May be of sudden obstructive (primary angle-closure) etiology, or chronic obstruction (open-angle).

▶ Treatment Steps

Primary Angle-Closure—Surgical iridectomy, with acetazolamide (Diamox) and β-blockers preop.

Primary Open-Angle—Treatment includes topical (eyedrops):
- β-Blockers—Timoptic (timolol).
- Carbonic anhydrase inhibitors—Trusopt(clorzolamide), Diamox (acetazolamide).
- Prostaglandin analogs—Xalatan (latanoprost).

B. Papilledema

▶ Description

Elevation/swelling of optic nerve head.

▶ Symptoms

Narrowed visual field; larger blind spot, vision may be normal or impaired. Papilledema may cause optic atrophy.

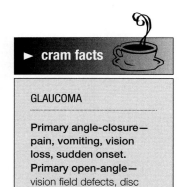

▶ **cram facts**

GLAUCOMA

Primary angle-closure—pain, vomiting, vision loss, sudden onset. Primary open-angle—vision field defects, disc cupping, no pain!

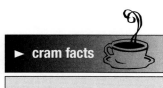

▶ **cram facts**

Consider optic atrophy, if disc is pale. Etiology of optic atrophy: demyelinating disease, drugs, glaucoma, familial.

► Diagnosis

Fundoscopic exam (disc swollen, associated hemorrhages/exudates).

► Pathology

Secondary to elevated CSF pressure, and a result of infection, optic neuritis, metabolic disease, CNS lesions.

► Treatment Steps

Treat primary cause.

C. Cataract

► Description

Lens opacity (nuclear, cortical, and subcapsular).

► Symptoms/Diagnosis

Progressive painless visual loss, or asymptomatic. Diagnose via ophthalmoscopic examination.

► Pathology

Age related; ultraviolet light exposure association, and may also relate to trauma, corticosteroids, and diabetes.

► Treatment Steps

Cataract removal and intraocular lens implantation.

► **cram facts**

HEADACHE

- **Migraine:** classic, unilateral throbbing headache with aura. Common, no aura. Positive family history, nausea, vomiting.
- **Cluster headache:** recurrent orbital stabbing/throbbing headache. Ipsilateral lachrymation, nasal congestion.
- **Temporal arteritis:** focal tenderness, superficial temporal artery; visual loss, increased sedimentation rate.

EPILEPSY

- **Generalized:** immediate loss of consciousness. Tonic–clonic, absence, myoclonic, atonic.
- **Focal:** Simple partial—motor, sensory, special sensory. Complex partial—impaired level of awareness and consciousness, automatisms, amnesia.
- **Status epilepticus:** continued or recurrent seizures lasting 30 min or more. Medical emergency.
- **Therapy:** Generalized—diphenylhydantoin, carbamazapine, valproic acid, ethosuccimide. Focal—above and gabapentin, lamotrigine, vigabatrin, topiramate, levetiracetam, zonisamide.

STROKE

- **Risk factors:** race, age, gender, family history, hypertension, diabetes mellitus, smoking, alcohol abuse, cardiac disease, lipoprotein abnormalities.
- **TIA:** focal neurologic signs, usually last < 1 hr. Evaluate CT/MRI, echocardiogram, ultrasound intra- and extracranial vessels.
- **Hemorrhagic:** sites include putamen, thalamus, pons. CT scan.

► **cram facts**

DEMYELINATING DISEASE

- **Multiple sclerosis:** optic neuritis, vertigo, weakness, incoordination, nystagmus, diplopia, neurogenic bladder.
- **Optic neuritis:** sudden visual loss, scotomata, decreased color vision, ocular pain. Risk for multiple sclerosis increases with MRI abnormalities.
- **Guillain–Barré syndrome:** acute inflammatory polyradiculoneuropathy. Ascending weakness, areflexia, autonomic dysfunction. Albuminocytologic dissociation in CSF.

CNS INFECTIONS

- **Meningitis:** headache, fever, stiff neck, Kernig and Brudzinski signs.
- **Encephalitis:** decreased level of consciousness, fever, focal neurologic signs. May have meningeal signs.

NEUROMUSCULAR DISEASE

- **Dystrophy:** inherited disorder of muscle. Includes Duchenne, limb–girdle, myotonic, and facioscapulohumeral dystrophies.
- **Myasthenia:** muscle fatigue. Myasthenia gravis—exercise-induced fatigue. Ocular, respiratory, and limb involvement.

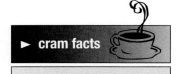

► **cram facts**

Corticosteriods—induce posterior subcapsular cataracts.

D. Other Items of Interest

1. **Retinal detachment—light flashes, retinal degeneration** or **trauma induced.**
2. **Constricted pupil**—iritis, drugs, Horner's.
3. **Dilated pupil**—Adie's, glaucoma, drugs, third nerve lesion.
4. **Pinguecula—thickened conjunctiva.**
5. **Pterygium—pinguecula encroaching on cornea.**
6. **Most frequent etiology of bacterial conjunctivitis—** *Staphylococcus aureus.*

► **differential diagnosis**

- **Raised intracranial pressure:** evaluate fundi (papilledema) pupils, cranial nerves, limbs. Obtain CT/MRI.
- **Coma:** unresponsive. Evaluate response to noxious stimuli, pupils, eye movements, cranial nerves, gag reflex, respiration. Decerebrate posture—midbrain lesion. Decorticate posture—lower diencephalon.
- **Stroke:** ischemic, embolic, hemorrhagic (parenchymal, subarachnoid). Localize vascular territory clinically.
- **Loss of consciousness:** coma, encephalopathy, seizures, sleep disorder, hysteria.
- **Paralysis:** upper motor neuron—weakness, increased tone, hyperreflexia, atrophy late. Lower motor neuron—weakness, atrophy, hypotonia, hypo/areflexia, fasciculations.
- **Encephalopathy:** metabolic—uremia, hepatic failure, porphyria, hypoxia–anoxia, electrolyte imbalance. Toxic—drugs, metals, carbon monoxide.
- **Hypotonia:** cerebral, spinal, muscular atrophies, polyneuropathies, dystrophies, myopathies.
- **Vertigo:** peripheral—trauma, perilymph fistula, benign paroxysmal vertigo, Ménière's syndrome. Central—vertebrobasilar ischemia, migraine, complex partial seizure, familial ataxia, drugs, posterior fossa lesions, multiple sclerosis.

7. **Iritis—small pupil, ciliary injection (treat with cycloplegics and steroids); glaucoma: large pupil, diffuse injection (treat with pilocarpine, acetazolamide** [Diamox], etc.).

8. **Hyphema—trauma induced, anterior chamber blood.**

9. **Chalazion—blocked meibomian gland duct.**

10. **Sudden vision loss—rule out artery** (secondary to emboli, retina white) **or vein occlusion.**

BIBLIOGRAPHY

Adams RD, Victor M, Ropper AH. *Principles of Neurology,* 7th ed. New York: McGraw-Hill, 2000.

Bradley WG, Daroff RB, Fenichel GM, Marsden CD. *Neurology in Clinical Practice,* 3rd ed. Boston: Butterworth Heinemann, 2000.

Bogousslavsky J, Fisher M. *Textbook of Neurology.* Boston: Butterworth Heinemann, 1998.

Haere AF. *DeJong's The Neurologic Examination.* Philadelphia: Lippincott-Raven, 1992.

Goetz CG, Pappert EJ. *Textbook of Clinical Neurology,* 2nd ed. Philadelphia: W.B. Saunders, 2003.

Joynt RJ, Griggs RC (eds.). *Baker's Clinical Neurology.* Philadelphia: Lippincott Williams & Wilkins, 2001.

Mayo Clinic Department of Neurology. *Mayo Clinic Examinations in Neurology,* 7th ed. St. Louis: Mosby, 1998.

Samuels MA (ed.). *Hospitalist Neurology.* Boston: Butterworth Heinemann, 1999.

Normal Growth and Development and General Principles of Care | 12

I. REPRODUCTION—PHYSIOLOGIC AND ENDOCRINE ASPECTS

A. Reproductive Anatomy

► Description

1. **Male**—**sperm** are **formed** in the **seminiferous** tubules of the testis, then travel to the **epididymis,** and then to the **vas deferens.** The **vas enters the prostate gland,** via the ejaculatory duct, on the way to the urethra. The **seminal vesicle** also empties into the ampulla of the vas, and ejaculatory duct.

2. **Female**—midcycle release of ovum, which travels via the fallopian tube to the uterus. Ovarian function depends on **anterior pituitary** release of follicle-stimulating hormone (FSH) and luteinizing hormone (LH).

Genetics—Ovum and spermatozoon nuclei divide (meiosis), reducing the 46 chromosomes in each to 23. Fertilization brings the number back to 46. Core to heredity and present on chromosomes are genes. Alleles (genes from one parent) are dominant or recessive.

Heterozygous—Having two different alleles for a given gene.

Homozygous—Having two of the same alleles for a given gene.

Dominant Inheritance—Parent-to-child transmission with 50% of male or female offspring affected. Trait on dominant allele is always displayed in the carrier.

Recessive Inheritance—Need both genes at locus to produce trait. Offspring have 25% chance of being affected (see Fig. 12–1).

Sex-linked—Sex chromosome (XX female, XY male) transmit trait. Single gene will produce trait. Female carrier will result in 50% of male offspring having trait (hemophilia: sex-linked recessive).

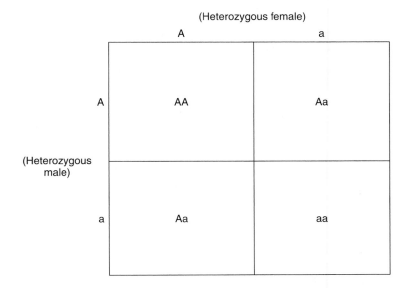

Figure 12–1. Punnett square.

B. Menstruation

► Description

Cyclic monthly flow.

1. **Follicular phase**—lasts 14 days, with **primordial follicle** enlarging. **Graafian** follicle is the resulting maturing follicle. **Main estrogen source is the theca interna cells of this follicle. Follicular phase ends with ovulation.**
   a. **Corpus luteum** is formed from ruptured ovarian follicle directly after ovulation.
   b. **Corpus hemorrhagicum** is the blood-filled ruptured follicle.
   c. **Mittelschmerz** is midcycle abdominal pain secondary to peritoneal irritation from release of small amounts of this blood in the abdomen.
   d. **Ovulation** is preceded by an **LH surge** following an estradiol surge, and the mature follicle becomes the **corpus luteum.**
   e. **At ovulation, positive ferning and greatest spinnbarkeit** is noted.
   f. **Ferning—palm-leaf cervical mucus pattern.**
   g. **Spinnbarkeit—elastic cervical mucus.**
2. **Luteal phase**—from ovulation to menses, lasting 14 days. **Progesterone is produced by the corpus luteum,** resulting in increased tortuosity and coiled gland appearance. **Cervical mucus is thick without ferning or spinnbarkeit.**

C. Intercourse and Conception

► Description

Ovum will survive 72 hours after release from the follicle. **Sperm will survive 48 hours.** Autonomically controlled contractions of the vaginal wall and bulbocavernosus muscles (orgasm) is not necessary for fertilization.

Sexual response cycle includes four phases: excitement, plateau, orgasm, and resolution (Masters and Johnson).

D. Pregnancy—Physiologic Changes

► Description

Increased cardiac output, heart rate, blood volume (50%), appetite, salivation, and gum fragility, glomerular filtration rate (GFR) (50%). *Decreased* gastrointestinal (GI) motility.

Pregnancy Testing—Detects elevated β-human chorionic gonadotropin (hCG) levels produced by the placenta.

Physical Changes—Include breast tenderness, purple cervical color (**Chadwick's** sign), softening uterine isthmus (Hegar's sign), urinary frequency.

Gestational age—Fundus palpable above the pubic symphysis (14 weeks), umbilicus (20 weeks), xiphoid process (38 weeks). Sensation of fetal movements noted by the mother at 16–18 weeks is termed *quickening.*

E. Labor and Delivery

► Description

Exact physiologic triggers are unknown, but prostaglandin release may stimulate uterine contractions, and oxytocin levels increase during labor.

Cervical Dilatation—For the head of the fetus to pass through the cervix, the cervix must dilate to a diameter of 10 cm (fully dilated).

► **cram facts**

RULES OF THUMB

• Gestational age—fundus at symphysis pubis at 8 weeks, above symphysis at 14 weeks, umbilicus at 20 weeks, and at xiphoid at 38 weeks' gestation.
• Estimated delivery date (Naegele's rule)—the date of the last known menstrual period minus 3 months plus 7 days.
• Infant size—gains back birth weight by 2 weeks of age, doubles birth weight by 6 months, and triples by 12 months.

Cervical Effacement—Cervical muscle fibers are pulled upward resulting in "thinning" of the cervix.

First Stage—From start of labor to full dilation, lasting 8–12 hours in a primigravida, 6–8 hours in a multipara, includes latent and active phases.

Second Stage—Includes full dilation to infant delivery, primigravida duration 1 hour, multipara one-half hour.

Third Stage—Includes infant birth to placenta delivery.

F. The Puerperium

Puerperium means postpartum. Most common postpartal time of maternal hemorrhage is shortly after placenta delivery, due to uterine relaxation. Later hemorrhage may result from infection (number one cause) or a retained placenta (number two cause). Physiologic changes include **uterine involution** with **lochia rubra** (bloody tissue discharge), **lochia serosa** (lighter color), and **lochia alba** (thicker yellow for several weeks postpartum). Water loss is associated with elevated serum sodium and diminished progesterone levels.

G. Lactation and Breast-Feeding

▶ Description

Estrogen produces **mammary duct tissue growth. Progesterone** stimulates **alveolar glands.** Postpartum, estrogen/progesterone levels drop, and **prolactin increase** is needed for milk formation. **Oxytocin is responsible for "milk letdown." Nipple stimulation** results in **oxytocin release** and increased prolactin secretion by the anterior pituitary.

Prolactin inhibits ovulation but is an unrealiable form of contraception (breast-feeding).

H. Fetus, Placenta, and Newborn

See also Chapter 13.

▶ Definitions

- **Fetal–placental** unit secretes hCG, progesterone, estriol, thyroid hormone, and adrenocorticotropic hormone (ACTH). Placenta utilizes oxygen and glucose to supply nutrition to the fetus and remove byproducts.
- **Umbilical cord** contains two **umbilical arteries** and one **vein.**
- **Wharton's jelly** is **umbilical** cord **connective tissue.**
- **Large placenta** noted in diabetes, erythroblastosis, and syphilis.
- **Small placenta** with hypertension.
- **Nuchal cord** found at delivery in 25%, without consequence.
- **Absence** of an **umbilical artery** may reflect multiple anomalies.
- **Hydatidiform mole** (molar pregnancy)—abnormality of chorionic villi that appears as grapelike vesicles. Secrete hCG and have potential for malignancy. Complete mole has absence of fetus. Partial mole has fetus or embryo present.
- **Short cord** may result from reduced amniotic fluid in early pregnancy.
- **Velamentous insertion—umbilical vessels separate before the placental margin and travel in placental membranes.**
- **Vasa praevia** describes membranes with fetal vessels appearing at the cervical os. Baby at risk for rupture of vessel and exsanguination.
- **Placenta previa**—placenta located at the cervical os.

- **Placenta accreta**—abnormal placental attachment to the uterine wall.
- **Placental abruption**—premature separation of the placenta.
    Check painless vaginal bleeding for fetal hemoglobin to detect **hemoglobin F,** which is the **major fetal hemoglobin.**

I. Obstetric Care
See also Chapter 13.

▶ Description
1. Pregnancy diagnosis:
    a. Presumptive signs and symptoms—nausea, amenorrhea, urinary frequency, **chloasma** (mask of pregnancy, increased facial pigmentation), **linea nigra** (nipples and linea alba darkening), **quickening** (fetal movement).
    b. Probable signs—**Chadwick's** (blue cervix), **Hegar's** (enlarged soft isthmus), **Braxton Hicks** (false) **contractions,** uterine souffle (auscultated blood-flowing sound from the placenta), **Ladin's** sign (anterior midline uterine softening).
    c. Positive signs—ultrasound, fetal heart tones, palpated fetal movement.
2. Pregnancy age:
    a. *Gestational age* by ultrasound. Uterus at 8 weeks is at the pubic symphysis; 20 weeks, at the umbilicus. Fetal maturation best determined by amniocentesis.
    b. *Quickening* at 17 to 18 weeks.
    c. *Nägele's rule*—estimated date of confinement (EDC) = last normal menstrual period (LNMP) month minus 3, then add 7 to the first day of the LNMP.
3. Prenatal care:
    a. *Prenatal care* will identify the high-risk patient, address nutrition and the need to avoid drugs, alcohol, smoking, and toxin exposure.
    b. *Contractions* are effective when regular and strong and produce cervical effacement and dilation.
    c. *False labor* contractions are irregular without cervical change; discomfort is abdominal.
    d. *Bloody show* is the passage of a **bloody cervical mucous plug** from cervical dilation.
4. **Fetal position:**
    a. *Fetal presentation.* Vertex, 95%; breech, 5%. Palpate abdomen **(Leopold maneuver).**
5. **Fetal station:**
    a. *Presenting part* at ischial spines is **zero,** above the spines in centimeters is minus, below the spines in centimeters is plus.
    b. *Pelvic inlet* should be 12 cm or greater; **midpelvis,** 9 cm or longer.
    c. *Pelvic types*—android, gynecoid, anthropoid, and platypelloid (see Fig. 12–2).
    d. *Midpelvis* is smallest pelvic measurement.
6. **Monitoring of labor**—frequent exam, fetal internal or external monitoring. Observe fetal **rate, variability,** and **effect under contractions. Normal fetal rate** 110 to 150, some beat-to-beat variability is normal. Small dips that recover with end of contraction are okay; if severe, get scalp pH (from vagal response of uterine pres-

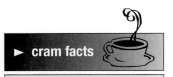

▶ cram facts

- Quickening is the term used to describe the initial movements of the fetus appreciated by the mother.
- **Lightening** occurs several weeks before birth. It is the settling of the infant's head down in the pelvis.

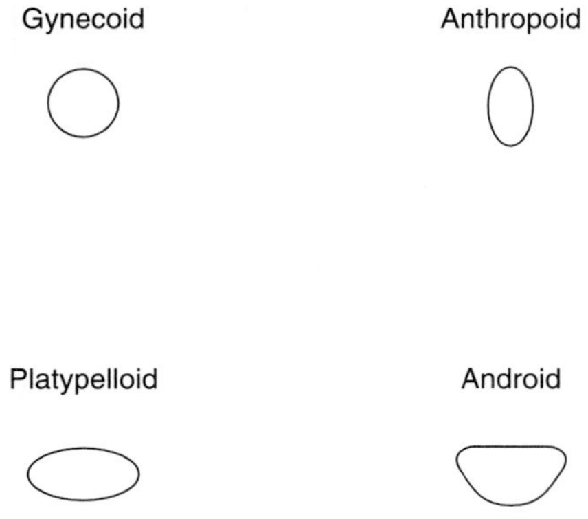

Gynecoid

Anthropoid

Figure 12–2. Caldwell–Mallory classification of pelvic shapes.

Platypelloid

Android

sure on baby's head). **Late decelerations** after uterine relaxation may indicate fetal distress. **Fetal scalp** pH 7.25 to 7.45 is okay.

7. **Puerperium**—check for blood loss, infection, mastitis (breast infection, usually *Staphylococcus aureus*), endometritis (bleeding, fever), anesthetic complications, cardiomyopathy, psychosis.

8. **Breast-feeding** should be encouraged in almost all cases. Contraindicated when mother with cytomegalovirus (CMV), human immunodeficiency virus (HIV), or on certain medications. Advantages include: immunoglobulin A (IgA) providing local gut immunity, psychosocial benefits, economical, convenient, and possibly decreases allergies. Mother needs to be relaxed and rested. To stop lactation, discontinue nursing, bind breasts, ice if needed.

9. **Newborn care**—clear and suction airway, dry and warm infant, apply antibiotic eye drops or ointment (GC prophylaxis), give vitamin K, 1 mg, intramuscularly (IM), check hemoglobin and glucose if indicated, check **Apgar** score. **Newborn examination notes:**

- *Caput succedaneum* is scalp edema, trauma, or vacuum extractor use, **which will cross the suture line.**
- *Cephalhematoma* is scalp hematoma not crossing suture line.
- *Mongolian spot* is a bluish discoloration from pigment deep within the dermis. Commonly over sacrum, always benign.
- *Vernix caseosa* is waxy material covering newborn.
- *Omphalocele* is intestine or abdominal contents protruding through umbilicus (versus gastroschisis, or abdominal wall absence/fissure).
- *Acrocyanosis* is bluish color of hands and feet, normal if lasting short time.
- *Moro reflex* is embracing/startle reaction to slightly lifting infant's upper torso by the hands, and suddenly releasing.
- *Rooting reflex* (stroke infant's cheek and infant turns toward your finger), **sucking** reflex and **grasp** reflex present, upward Babinski reflex is normal.

Also check for red reflex in eye (rule out retinoblastoma, congenital cataracts), Ortolani and Barlow maneuvers (to recognize developmental dysplasia of the hips), and abdomen for masses (polycystic kidneys, Wilms' tumor, neuroblastoma, hernia, etc.).

II. INFANCY AND CHILDHOOD

A. Physical Growth and Development

▶ Description

Evaluate growth and development at each visit. Monitor blood pressure (BP) and advise dental evaluation after age of 3 years. Discuss accident prevention, drowning, fire, and automobile safety.

1. **Development:**
   One month—positive head lag, prone may lift head above surface.
   Three months—some head lag, prone may raise head/chest.
   Six months—rolls over both ways, sits alone.
   Nine months—creeps or crawls, may take steps if hands held, says ba-ba, da-da.
   Twelve months—walks if one hand held, speech of three words.
   Fifteen months—walks, builds two-block tower.
   Twenty-four months—six-cube tower, talks, checks everything out. Poison-proof home!
2. **Infant size**—infants double weight by 6 months and triple weight by 1 year. **Anterior fontanel** closes 9 to 18 months. **Posterior** by 3 to 4 months.
3. **Teeth**—**lower central incisors** are **first** at 6 to 9 months, followed by upper central incisors. **Six or more teeth** present **by age 1.**

B. Psychosocial Development

▶ Description

Social smile at 3 to 5 weeks. Laughs at 4 months, possible stranger anxiety at 6 months, less dependent on mother at 12 months. **Second-year** play is solitary, third-year involves other children.

C. Well-Baby Care

▶ Description

Monitor physical development, orthopedic development, dental, hearing and vision screening, hemoglobin and tuberculosis (TB) screening. Provide routine immunizations and lead screening. **Child abuse** may present as failure to thrive, emotional or physical deprivation. High frequency of parents having been abused.

III. ADOLESCENCE

A. Puberty

▶ Symptoms

Onset of secondary sexual characteristics (growth spurt, genital development, pubic hair, menarche).

▶ Diagnosis

Tanner stages 1 to 5: 1 = preadolescent, 5 = maturity.

▶ Physiology

1. **Females**—estrogen secreted by the ovary in response to FSH results in breast development. Adrenal androgens produced result in axillary and pubic hair. **Female sequence: ovary growth, breast bud, growth spurt, then pubic hair.**
2. **Males**—testicular enlargement from testosterone. Adrenal androgens for pubic and axillary hair also. **Male sequence: testicular**

growth, followed by growth spurt, **then pubic hair,** then facial hair and voice change.

B. Nutrition and Growth

► Description

Rapid growth at a time of increased activity is present. Poor dietary planning is common. Anemia and/or iron deficiency may be present, as well as dental caries and obesity.

C. Emotional and Cultural Adaptations

► Description

Quest for independence and concern with peer group, self-image anxiety, and possible conflicts may take place. Increasing interest in peer group and attempt at separation from parental control. Increasing interest in sex, and reduced impulse control may be noted. Dangers of risk-taking behavior may be of concern. Acceptance of body, parents, needs, and trials of adolescence are noted in later stages of adolescence.

D. Adolescent Sexuality

► Description

Increasing sexual energy and interest. Guilt over masturbation or sexual fantasies may be present. Peer and media pressure may play a role. Sex education for sexually transmitted disease (STD) prevention and guidance, as lack of knowledge is common.

E. Physician–Parent–Patient Communication

► Description

Need to recognize both parental concerns and adolescent's privacy. Need to discuss with adolescent concerns regarding confidentiality and privacy. Importance of discussion regarding **drugs, alcohol, birth control,** and **prevention of STDs.**

IV. ADULTHOOD

A. General Checkups

► Description

Routine evaluation to include review of systems, physical examination, preventive care and instruction, and screening testing and/or procedures where indicated. Key aspects may include alcohol and smoking cessation, cancer screening (breast, colon/rectal, prostate), immunization review, and cholesterol/lipid evaluation. Additional evaluations indicated in high-risk individuals may include glucose, TB testing, HIV testing, STD screening, dermatologic and audiometric examination.

B. Contraception

► Description
- *Abstinence* remains difficult; peer pressure not helpful.
- *Vaginal spermicides* are safe and more effective if a condom is used in addition.
- *Condoms* are safe and effective if correctly used. Help prevent STDs.
- *Diaphragms* are safe, but preparation may inhibit use.

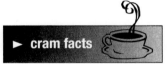

► cram facts

COMMON CONTRACEPTION CHOICES

- **Barrier method**—condoms (help prevent STDs) and diaphragm (preparation might inhibit use).
- **Hormonal contraceptives**—combination oral estrogen/progestins (safe and effective), "minipill" (more pregnancy and more bleeding problems), or injectable and implanted progestins (long lasting).
- **Other methods**—vaginal spermicides (more effective if used with a barrier method), IUD, and surgical sterilization (essentially irreversible).

- *Combination oral contraceptives* (estrogen/progestins) are safe and effective with proper instruction and medical follow-up. May aggravate migraine. Contraindicated with prior thromboembolic disease, coronary artery disease, pregnancy, liver tumors, breast malignancy, vaginal bleeding of unknown etiology, or hypertension.
- *Estrogen excess*—nausea, headache, hypermenorrhea, bloating.
- *Estrogen shortage*—amenorrhea, reduced libido, early-cycle spotting.
- *Oral contraceptive use and cancer*—reduced endometrial and ovarian cancer.
- *Oral progestins* (without estrogen)—"minipill"—higher pregnancy rate and abnormal bleeding more common.
- *Injectable progestin contraceptives*—injections of medroxyprogesterone (Depo-Provera) required 4 to 6 times per year.
- *Implanted contraceptives*—silastic containers of levonorgestrel implanted subdermally (Norplant). Lasts 5 years.
- *Intrauterine device (IUD)*—will not protect against STDs, and infertility complication is present.

C. Stress Management

▶ Description
Increasing and **frequent stress** may result in **increased illness. Most stressful event is death of a spouse. Holmes and Rahe** scale of life stress events **ranks divorce** number two.

▶ Treatment Steps
Support of family and friends, exercise, hobbies, biofeedback, counseling, medication when indicated, remove source of stress, relaxation techniques.

D. Menopause

▶ Symptoms
Increasing irregularity of menstrual cycle, average age 51. Anxiety, depression, hot flushes (or flashes, due to estrogen withdrawal), dyspareunia, bone loss. Eventual cessation of menses.

▶ Diagnosis
Elevated FSH and **LH,** amenorrhea, negative pregnancy test.

▶ Pathology
Decreasing ovarian function.

▶ Treatment Steps
Consider estrogen replacement.

E. Osteoporosis
See Chapter 10, section II.E.

F. Male and Female Climacteric

▶ Description
Female—menopause.
Male—diminished sexual activity.

▶ Symptoms
Reduced sexual frequency and/or reduced libido.

▶ Diagnosis
Sexual history, physical examination, rule out other physical disorders.

► Pathology
• Female—lack of estrogen.
• Male—reduced testosterone.

► Treatment Steps
Hormone replacement(?), office discussion/counseling.

V. SENESCENCE

A. Physical/Mental Aging Changes

► Description
1. **Cardiac**—decreased output.
2. **Musculoskeletal**—reduced bone mass.
3. **Pulmonary**—decreased muscle strength and chest wall compliance.
4. **Immune system**—thymus involution.
5. **Senses**—decreased visual, auditory, tactile, and taste sensation.
6. **Endocrine**—reduced insulin-secreting cells, glucose intolerance.
7. **Mental**—reduced memory, learning ability, and calculation speed.

► Treatment Steps
Adequate nutrition, exercise, mental stimulation, preventive medical evaluations.

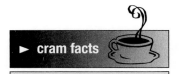

► **cram facts**

New medications for erectile dysfunction (ED) (approved for use in males only):
• Viagra (sildenafil)
• Cialis (tadalafil)
• Levitra (vardenafil)
Do not give if patient takes nitroglycerin—will precipitate hypotension.

B. Nutrition in the Elderly

► Description
Often inadequate; psychosocial problems may exist.

► Symptoms
Inadequate diet may present with **weight loss, cognitive impairment** from vitamin deficiency.
    Protein-calorie malnutrition—depression, mental changes, anorexia, and weight loss.

► Diagnosis
Patient examination and physician–patient, physician–family discussion. Careful history.

► Treatment Steps
Encourage family support and psychosocial health. Periodic evaluations to prevent potential problems. Treat other medical problems (poor dentition, depression), monitor medications for side effects and discuss nutrition. Evaluate for alcohol abuse.

C. Social Adaptation

► Description
Ability to accept aging process and cope with physical and mental changes and illness. Sleep disturbances and depression are common.

D. Death and Dying

► Description
Honest physician–patient discussion is essential. Common patient reaction is **denial.**

► Treatment Steps

Importance of support system for patients and their ability to maintain control must be stressed. Pain medication to effect comfort is essential. Hospice to support patient and family.

VI. GENERAL PRINCIPLES OF MEDICAL CARE

A. Informed Consent

► Description

Acceptance of a medical intervention after full disclosure of the intervention, its risks, and its benefits as well as disclosure of the alternatives and their risks and benefits.

1. Assumes that the physician is competent, the information is standard in the community, and the information is properly conveyed and understood by the patient.
2. Exceptions: emergency care, incompetent patients, minors.

B. Competence and Mental Capacity

► Description

Patients are competent when they are able to understand and make choices about their health care. Mental capacity, which may be compromised by anxiety, pain, illness, or hospitalization, occasionally impairs the ability to participate in these decisions. A surrogate decision maker is necessary when the patient is incompetent.

C. Minors

► Description

Children (under the statutory age of consent, as determined by a state) require parental consent for care except in a few situations, including emergency care and sensitive issues (e.g., contraception).

D. Confidentiality

► Description

Physician is obligated to maintain patient confidentiality (found in the Hippocratic Oath). Family members of competent adult patients may receive information only on the patient's approval.

VII. QUANTITATIVE METHODS

A. Concepts of Measurement

1. Measurement of Central Tendency

► Description

A measure of the center of the distribution.

- *Mean* is the sum of the data divided by their numbers.
- *Median* is the middle number when the measurements are arranged in order of magnitude; 50th percentile.
- *Mode* is the value that occurs most often.

2. Measurement of Deviations From the Center

▶ Description

- *Variability* provides the range of the most frequent values and their relation to the center (dispersion of the data). It also refers to inconsistency found in or among studies.
- *Range* is the difference between the largest and smallest measurement.
- *Standard deviation* is the average distance of the events or observations from the mean.
- *Frequency distribution* is a way of organizing a collection of measurements (graphic or tabular form), so that common and rare events can be identified.

3. Measurement of a Disease

▶ Description

- *Probability* is the likelihood of an event to occur. It is defined as the number of times an event occurs divided by the total number of times the event can occur.
- *Incidence rate* measures the number of *new* cases of a disease in a population during a specified period of time (i.e., the rate people develop the disease over a period of time).
- *Prevalence rate* measures the number of *all* cases of a disease at a given point in time. It is the product of the incidence and a specified time period.

4. Measurement of Risk

▶ Description

- *Relative risk* measures the strength of an association between a particular factor and a certain outcome. It does not measure the probability of developing the disease if the person is exposed to the factor (see Table 12–1).
- *Attributable risk* measures the incidence of a disease that can be attributed to one certain factor.
- *Odds ratio* is a close estimation of the relative risk. Useful for retrospective studies if there is a low incidence of the disease in the population and the control group reflects the general population with respect to the frequency of the specific factor.
- *Attack rate* measures the proportion of the population who develops a disease among those who were exposed to a specific risk factor.

12-1

MEASUREMENT OF RISK FOR EPIDEMIOLOGIC STUDIES

$$\text{Relative risk} = \frac{a/a+b}{c/c+d}$$

$$\text{Attributable risk} = \frac{a}{a+b} - \frac{b}{c+d}$$

$$\text{Odds ratio} = \frac{ad}{bc}$$

$$\text{Attack rate} = \frac{a+c}{a+b}$$

5. Measurement of Mortality

► Description
- *Crude death rate* measures the number of deaths in a population under study. It reflects age-specific death rates and age compositions of a population.
- *Case fatality rate* provides the probability of death for a specific disease.
- *Age-adjusted death rate* is used when a comparison is necessary among a group with different age distributions.

B. Statistics and Significance

1. Null Hypothesis

► Description
Assumes that there are no differences in population parameters among groups; the observed difference is the result of random variation in the data.

2. Statistical Significance

► Description
When a critical value is exceeded and the null hypothesis is rejected.

3. *P* Value

► Description
Lowest significant level at which the null hypothesis can be rejected. *P* value 0.05 has been arbitrarily chosen as the level for statistical significance.

4. Type I Error

► Description
The rejection of the null hypothesis when it is true.

5. Type II Error

► Description
The acceptance of the null hypothesis when it is false.

6. Confidence Interval

► Description
A device that estimates the likelihood of probability that a population parameter is included.

C. Study Design

1. Experimental Studies

► Description
Clinical trials, community intervention trials, controlled and non-controlled trials (see Table 12–2).

2. Observational Studies

► Description
Case-control, case-series, cross-sectional, and cohort.
1. Case-control—**start with outcome, then check backwards to evaluate risk or cause. Retrospective design.**
2. Case-series—**features noted in a group of patients are reviewed.**
3. Cross-sectional—**evaluate data on a group of patients at one point in time.**

12-2

STUDY DESIGN FOR EPIDEMIOLOGIC STUDIES

		Disease/Outcome	
		Present	Absent
Exposure	Present	a	b
	Absent	c	d

4. Cohort—**a group with a common factor observed over a defined period of time. Prospective design.**

3. Exposure Allocation

► Description

Allocation on the basis of randomization, self-selection, and systematic assignment.

4. Advantages and Disadvantages of Different Designs

► Description

1. **Case-control**—elements of bias and difficulty establishing causality, but less expensive and quicker to perform. Good for conditions that develop over long periods and for rare diseases.
2. **Case-series**—simple but **subject to bias.**
3. **Cross-sectional**—quick and inexpensive. Good for evaluation of a condition in a population base. Disadvantage is that the study observes conditions only at one instant. Determines prevalence, not incidence. Provides distribution of a disease rather than its etiology.
4. **Cohort**—establishes hypothesis, but causation difficult to prove. More costly. Requires more time (see Table 12–3).

► **cram facts**

COMPARISON OF PROSPECTIVE AND RETROSPECTIVE STUDIES

	ADVANTAGES	DISADVANTAGES
Prospective	Incidence determined Accurate relative risk Less control group bias	Long duration Costly Attrition problem Large sample size Ethical problem risk
Retrospective	Short duration Relatively inexpensive No attrition problem Small sample size Minimal ethical risk	Incidence not determined Relative risk approximated Control group bias in selection

12-3

STUDY DESIGN FOR A SCREENING TOOL		
	True Diagnosis	
Test Result	Disease	No Disease
Positive	a	b
Negative	c	d

VIII. EPIDEMIOLOGY OF HEALTH AND DISEASE

A. Patterns of Disease Occurrence

1. Demographic Characteristics

▶ Description
Age, race, gender, socioeconomic features. Different socioeconomic environments result in very different disease patterns.

2. Geographic Distribution

▶ Description
Consider national, international, and regional variations.

3. Temporal Trends

▶ Description
Consider sporadic, seasonal, secular, and birth cohort patterns.

4. Disease Surveillance

▶ Description
Observe and compare frequency of events.

5. Excess Disease Occurrence

▶ Description
1. Epidemic—significantly more cases of a disease than predicted from past experience at that time, for that place, among that population.
2. **Endemic**—disease in small numbers in a given area or group.
3. **Pandemic**—disease in many numbers in many areas at once.

6. Outbreak Investigation

▶ Description
Key concerns are evaluation of the source, host, and environment. Necessary next step is a plan to control the outbreak.

7. Etiology of Death and Disability

▶ Description
Epidemiologic study obtained from death certificates, where the cause of death and the contributing causes are listed.

B. Natural History and Prognosis

1. Modes of Disease Transmission

▶ Description
Primary, person-to-person; secondary via vectors.

2. Incubation Periods

▶ Description

Longer incubation period may allow increased disease transmission by infected, but still asymptomatic individuals (as in HIV infection).

3. Early-Detection Methods

▶ Description

Patient education and screening.

4. Disease Manifestation

▶ Description

Disease produced when an **agent** (bacteria, virus, etc.), via a **transmission vehicle** (insect, food, etc.), finds a **reservoir** (person or animal) who is a **susceptible host.**

5. Treatment Efficacy Evaluation

▶ Description

Perform an experimental study to compare outcome in both treated and control group.

6. Disease Progression Determination

▶ Description

Measure rate of disease in terms of incidence and prevalence (defined earlier).

C. Risk Factors for Disease Occurrence

1. Hereditary/Genetic Traits

▶ Description

Genetic disorders resulting in reduced defense mechanisms (neuromuscular disorder resulting in poor cough reflex, for example).

2. Personal Characteristics

▶ Description

Age, race, gender, socioeconomic status, heredity, immunization programs, habits (cleanliness, food selection), and customs.

3. Lifestyle and Behavioral Aspects

▶ Description

Habits including alcohol and tobacco use, drug abuse, exercise, sexual behavior, religion (avoiding blood transfusions for reduced hepatitis and HIV exposure, for example).

4. Occupational Exposure

▶ Description
- **Chemical** agents including chemicals, pollution.
- **Infectious** or biologic agents such as bacteria, fungi, viruses, protozoa, insects.
- **Mechanical** agents as in equipment at work.

5. Environmental Aspects

▶ Description

Food, air, and water purity. Exposure to hazardous materials. Temperature, humidity, and sanitation conditions. Bioterrorism.

6. Nutritional Aspects

► Description
Vitamin, mineral, and nutritional excess and deficiency in adults, children, and pregnant women.

7. Iatrogenic Exposure

► Description
Medications, risky behavior, toxins.

8. Prenatal Exposure

► Description
Tobacco, alcohol, drugs, chemicals, toxins.

9. Abnormal Physiologic or Metabolic States

► Description
Multiple medical conditions (hypertension, diabetes, hyperlipidemia, etc.).

IX. HEALTH SERVICES—ORGANIZATION AND DELIVERY

A. Health Care Policy and Planning

► Description
Quality assurance is often judged by medical audits and peer review process, and may help to determine health care policy.

B. General Aspects of Health Care System Structure

► Description
Be aware of programs available including USMLE-listed community preventive medicine service programs, health education, community nursing, chronic and infectious disease control, consulting services, immunization, school and occupational health programs, and programs for the elderly and industry.

C. Health Care Financing and Programs

► Description
Health care costs have risen dramatically, partly due to new and costly technology, and the practice of defensive medicine. Increase in illness rises with advancing age and poor socioeconomic class (groups often unable to pay for health care). Insurance may be traditional or prepaid health maintenance organizations (HMOs). Taxes support state health departments.

- *Social Security Act* of 1935 brought the government into health care, to help states develop public health services.
- *Medicare Act* of 1965 provided hospital/health insurance for those older than 65.
- *Hill Burton Act* helped supply funds for hospital construction and renovation.
- *Kerr–Mills Bill* developed the **Medicaid** program for indigent persons.
- *Sheppard–Tower Act* supplied funds for maternal and child health concerns.

X. COMMUNITY DIMENSIONS OF MEDICAL PRACTICE

A. General Aspects of Community Organization

► Description

Population health assessment. Health surveys and vital statistics are produced by the State Health Department. Disease reporting systems allow monitoring of reportable diseases, which may result in earlier detection and treatment.

B. Public Health Issues

► Description

Public health programs need to be available to all, and comprehensive in scope.

C. Environmental and Occupational Health

► Description

1. **Environmental control**—multiple aspects including providing community education (e.g., to prevent lead poisoning) and accidents. Insect vector education and control (mosquito: encephalitis).
2. **Air and water quality**—impure water may result in cholera, typhoid, and *Salmonella* transmission. Air pollution could predispose to chronic obstructive lung disease, allergic reactions.
3. **Occupational health**—caution with machinery, radiation, toxin exposure, noise exposure, and accident prevention. Exposure to inhalants (silicosis, asbestosis, etc.). Occupational health also includes treatment and rehabilitation of employees injured at work, and acute emergency care.

D. Prevention in Primary Care

► Description

An intervention that decreases morbidity in a person's future life.

► Types

1. **Primary prevention**—targets a disorder that has not occurred (e.g., polio vaccine).
2. **Secondary prevention**—identifies a disease in its asymptomatic stage (e.g., breast cancer screening).
3. **Tertiary prevention**—halts the progressing of a disease (e.g., insulin for insulin-dependent diabetes).

► **cram facts**

PREVENTION IN PRIMARY CARE

TYPE	TARGET	EXAMPLE
Primary	Identify future disease	Polio vaccine
Secondary	Identify asymptomatic disease	Breast cancer screen
Tertiary	Halt disease progression	Insulin for diabetes

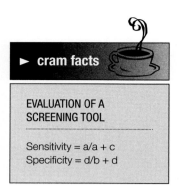

EVALUATION OF A SCREENING TOOL

Sensitivity = a/a + c
Specificity = d/b + d

► Implementation

1. Law mandate (e.g., seat belts, water fluoridation).
2. Periodic health examination (e.g., prostate exam).
3. Mass screening (e.g., glaucoma, hypertension).

► Screening Test

Identifies a person with a high probability of having the disease from a large group of apparently well persons.

1. **Sensitivity**—ability of a screening test to correctly identify a disease (good sensitivity implies few false negatives).
2. **Specificity**—ability of a screening test to be negative when the person is truly free of disease (good specificity implies few false positives).

Injuries

► Description

Recognized as the leading cause of death in childhood. Fall, suffocation, burns, drowning, sports, bicycles, firearms, and motor vehicle injuries are among the most common causes of morbidity or mortality.

► Treatment Steps

Identifing children at increased rick for recurrent injury. Anticipatory guidance.

- Falls: gates and window guards, no walkers, never leave child unattended.
- Drowning: supervison of children under 4 in bathtub, fence should be used around pools.
- Burns: pot handles should be turned to side, water heaters should be set below 120°F.
- Firearms: lock ammunition and weapon separately.
- Bicycle: wear helmets.
- It is currently advised that children stay in appropriate car seats through age 8 years, 80 pounds, or 49 inches. Children under age 12 should remain in the back seat.

BIBLIOGRAPHY

Cunningham FG, Gant NF, Leveno KJ, et al. *Williams Obstetrics,* 21st ed. New York: McGraw-Hill, 2001.
Dawson-Saunders BK. *Basic and Clinical Biostatistics,* 3rd ed. New York: McGraw-Hill, 2000.
Gilbert SF. *Developmental Biology,* 6th ed. Sunderland, MA: Sinauer Associates, 2000.

Obstetrics and Gynecology | 13

I. HEALTH AND HEALTH MAINTENANCE— OBSTETRICS

A. Prenatal Care

▶ Description

The objective of prenatal care is to ensure that every wanted pregnancy culminates in the delivery of a healthy baby without impairing the health of the mother. A full history and physical examination is performed in order to determine the health condition of both mother and fetus, evaluate and monitor risk factors, determine pelvic measurements, lab screening. Ensure **adequate nutrition,** and **prevent vitamin and/or iron deficiency.** Increased protein and calcium are needed and special prenatal vitamins are prescribed, as well as iron supplements.

▶ **clinical pearl**

Fundal height (a measure from the top of the pubic bone to the top of the uterus) at 20 weeks should correlate to the level of the umbilicus.

1. General Prenatal Care

- Preexisting illnesses should be addressed (i.e., diabetes, asthma, epilepsy). Ideally, these conditions were under optimal conditions and treatment prior to conception but this is not always the case.
- Identify medications (prescription, over-the-counter, and herbal) that the woman is taking and eliminate those that are not safe in pregnancy.
- History will concentrate not only on the health of the mother, but also on preexisting conditions in the families of the mother and the father of the baby.
- Physical exam may be unremarkable early in pregnancy. May see Chadwick's sign (blue cervix). Some physicians use early transvaginal ultrasound to document that an intrauterine embryo is present (versus an ectopic or molar pregnancy). Also, a beating heart should be seen, and twin/multiple embryos may be seen.
- Lab workup includes a urine or serum β-human chorionic gonadotropin (β-hCG). Routine screening labs can include complete blood count, blood typing, urinalysis, rapid plasma reagin (RPR), and testing for immunity against hepatitis B and rubella. Later (weeks 35–37) the woman is tested for colonization with group B streptococcus (see Cram Facts).
- Most states utilize voluntary testing of mother and child for human immunodeficiency virus (HIV). As of 2002, four states require HIV testing of the mother unless she refuses. Only two states, Connecticut and New York, mandate HIV testing of all newborns.

2. Other Prenatal Issues

There are a multitude of tests which may be done to diagnose certain conditions prenatally.

- *Triple or quad screen.* Triple screen includes testing the maternal serum for levels of α-fetoprotein (AFP), hCG, and unconjugated estriol. Inhibin-A is added for quad screen (see Cram Facts).
- *Screening for cystic fibrosis and Tay-Sachs disease* may be desired, depending on risk factors in the parents of the child.
- *Obstetrical (also known as level II) ultrasound.* Includes information on gestational age, fetal measurements, amniotic fluid volume, and structural abnormalities of the fetus.
- *Amniocentesis.* A procedure in which a sample of amniotic fluid is obtained and analyzed to detect genetic abnormalities in the fetus, usually done between weeks 15 and 18.

- *Chorionic villus sampling (CVS).* This will also detect genetic abnormalities in the fetus. One advantage is that it is performed earlier than amniocentesis, between weeks 10 and 12.

3. Teratogens

Certain medications that are used to treat medical conditions cannot be used in pregnancy. Under ideal conditions, patients who are trying to conceive a child will have discussed this with their health care provider prior to conception and medications can be adjusted to minimize risk to the fetus.

Examples:
- A woman with diabetes should not only try and optimize her glucose control prior to conception, but if she is taking an angiotensin-converting enzyme (ACE) inhibitor for blood pressure or proteinuria, this should be changed to a safer drug.
- Thalidomide is sometimes given for multiple myeloma and is well known for causing birth defects (i.e., phocomelia). Thankfully, most patients with myeloma are older and women are not often of childbearing age. However, consideration must be taken if the father is older and taking thalidomide.
- Isotretinoin (Accutane) should never be given to any woman who may conceive a child. Due to the high risk of fetal deformities, the

► **clinical pearl**

A woman who is Rh negative and undergoes CVS should receive Rhogam following the procedure.

U.S. Food and Drug Administration (FDA) requires extensive written disclosure to the patient. It requires that she is not pregnant or breast-feeding, has taken two negative pregnancy tests prior to her first prescription, has monthly pregnancy tests, and uses two forms of contraception. (See www.fda.gov for more information.)

- Other medications (see Cram Facts).

B. Assessment of the At-Risk Pregnancy

▶ Description

In certain scenarios, one of the following can be used:

1. *Nonstress test* (NST) if nonreactive, indicates a problem. Should have two accelerations (every 20 minutes) of 15 seconds or longer, at 15 beats above baseline.
2. *Stress test* involves testing uteroplacental/fetal well-being by inducing uterine contractions with oxytocin or nipple stimulation.
3. *Pulmonary maturity evaluation* performed by amniotic fluid analysis for **lecithin/sphingomyelin ratio.** Ratio of > 2:1 is preferred.
4. *Ultrasound*—amniotic fluid volume, biophysical profile. Biophysical profile (BPP) consists of (a) NST that is *reactive,* (b) one episode of *fetal breathing* lasting 30 seconds over 30 minutes, (c) three or more *fetal movements* over 30 minutes, (d) adequate *fetal tone,* (e) adequate *amnotic fluid volume.*

See also Chapter 14, section X.C.

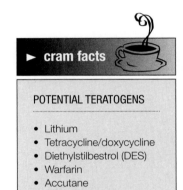

▶ cram facts

POTENTIAL TERATOGENS

- Lithium
- Tetracycline/doxycycline
- Diethylstilbestrol (DES)
- Warfarin
- Accutane
- ACE inhibitors
- Thalidomide
- Certain anticonvulsants
- Alcohol and tobacco

C. Intrapartum Care

▶ Description

Monitor mother, fetus, and stages of labor (see Fig. 13–1). Fetal monitoring to identify problems early.

D. Newborn Care

▶ Description

Suctioning, laryngoscopic exam if meconium is thick, clamp cord, dry, and position infant in Trendelenberg position in warmer. Mother–infant bonding if infant stable. Physical examination, Apgar scores, *Neisseria gonorrheae* conjunctivitis prophylaxis, and vitamin K. Hepatitis B vaccine now indicated for newborn. Phenylketonuria (PKU) test.

E. Postpartum Mother Care

▶ Description

Relieve episiotomy pain, observe for infection, hemorrhage, anesthetic complications. Consider family planning and options for birth control and sexually transmitted disease (STD) prevention.

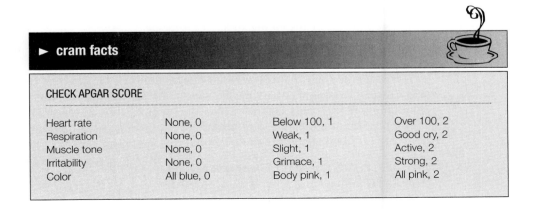

▶ cram facts

CHECK APGAR SCORE			
Heart rate	None, 0	Below 100, 1	Over 100, 2
Respiration	None, 0	Weak, 1	Good cry, 2
Muscle tone	None, 0	Slight, 1	Active, 2
Irritability	None, 0	Grimace, 1	Strong, 2
Color	All blue, 0	Body pink, 1	All pink, 2

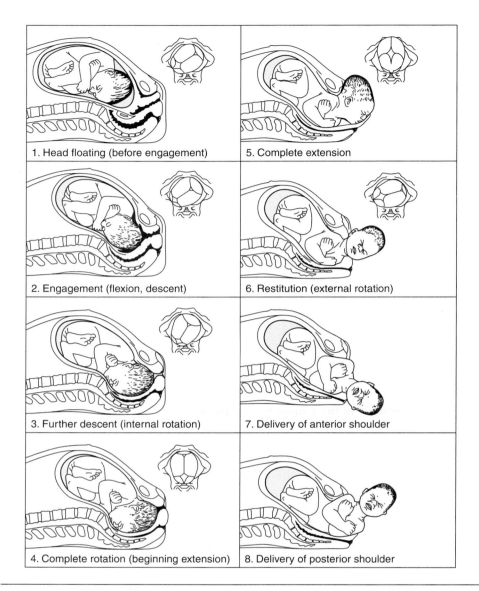

1. Head floating (before engagement)

2. Engagement (flexion, descent)

3. Further descent (internal rotation)

4. Complete rotation (beginning extension)

5. Complete extension

6. Restitution (external rotation)

7. Delivery of anterior shoulder

8. Delivery of posterior shoulder

Figure 13–1. Cardinal movements in the mechanism of labor and delivery, left occiput anterior position. (Reproduced, with permission, from Gant NF, Cunningham FG. *Basic Gynecology and Obstetrics.* Norwalk, CT: Appleton & Lange, 1993.)

F. Community and Social Dimensions

▶ Description

- *Maternal mortality* most commonly is due to hemorrhage. Mortality is greater with advancing age.
- *Neonatal mortality* and morbidity **most often** is **due to low birth weight secondary to prematurity.**

Teenage pregnancy has increased due to multiple factors including increased adolescent sexual activity, poor availability of family planning services, and lack of education in the schools. Maternal mortality, infant mortality, and frequency of low birth weight are all increased in teenage pregnancy.

G. Contraception and Sterilization

See also Chapter 12, section IV.B.

► **cram facts**

FAMILY PLANNING

Method	IFR (%)	AFR (%)	Comments
Injectable progestins	0.25	0.25	Irregular bleeding, but convenient
Oral contraceptives	0.5	2	Most used, daily compliance required
IUD	1.5	5	Risk of PID, ectopic; not for nullips
Condoms	2	10	Use with foam; best STD protection
Diaphragm (and jelly)	2	19	Messy, left in 6 hr postcoitus
Sponge (and jelly)	9–11	10–20	Not as effective
Foams, creams, jellies	3–5	18	Better in combination with condom
Withdrawal	16	23	Unreliable
Rhythm	2–20	24	Cannot be used with irregular cycles
Douching	—	40	Unreliable
Abstinence	0	—	Not realistic
No contraception	90	90	No comment

IFR = ideal failure rate

AFR = actual failure rate

► Description

The oral contraceptive (OC) is the most popular method of birth control in the United States. The failure rate in typical users is 2.0%. Only injectable progestins have a lower failure rate (0.25%). The problem with OCs is that they do *not* protect against STDs. Thus, they are recommended in combination with barrier methods (condoms) in a high-risk population.

Other methods include diaphragm, rhythm, cervical cap, intrauterine device (IUD), spermicides, sponge, and vaginal condom. Abstinence is certainly effective, but not always realistic.

Sterilization—Tubal ligation is effective; has a < 0.3% failure rate. Vasectomy is effective (but not 100% effective); semen analysis should be performed to confirm sperm absence.

Oral Contraceptives—Carry an increased risk of deep vein thrombosis (DVT) and myocardial infarction (MI), decreased risk of endometrial and ovarian cancer. Absolute contraindications include liver tumor, pregnancy, breast cancer, heart disease, thromboembolism, cerebrovascular disease, genital bleeding of unknown cause, estrogen-dependent tumor.

II. MECHANISMS OF DISEASE AND DIAGNOSIS—OBSTETRICS

A. Obstetric Complications of Pregnancy

1. Ectopic Pregnancy

► Description

Implantation of the fertilized ovum outside of the endometrial cavity. **Most common site of ectopic—ampullary portion of tube.** Increasing incidence (1 in 70 pregnancies) due to increasing incidence of STDs.

► differential diagnosis

ACUTE PELVIC PAIN

- **Ectopic pregnancy:** unilateral lower quadrant pain; amenorrhea × 6 weeks with recent spotting/bleeding; +hCG; no fever; no nausea and vomiting; ultrasound shows no intrauterine sac; normal white blood count (WBC).
- **Pelvic inflammatory disease:** bilateral lower quadrant pain; –hCG; no change in menses from the usual pattern; fever; may have slight nausea and vomiting; ultrasound may show bilateral tubo-ovarian complex masses (abscesses); elevated WBC.
- **Endometriosis:** unilateral or bilateral pain; –hCG; no change in menses from the usual pattern; no fever; no nausea and vomiting; ultrasound not usually helpful; normal WBC.
- **Ruptured follicular cyst:** unilateral pain; –hCG; late for anticipated menses; no fever; no nausea and vomiting; ultrasound may show ovarian cyst ± fluid in cul-de-sac; normal WBC.
- **Appendicitis:** right lower quadrant pain; –hCG; no change in menstrual flow; fever; nausea and vomiting; ultrasound not helpful; elevated WBC.
- **Threatened abortion:** midline cramping; +hGC; amenorrhea × 7–8 weeks with recent onset of bleeding; no fever (unless septic abortion); may have nausea and vomiting; ultrasound shows intrauterine pregnancy (or remains thereof); normal WBC.

► Symptoms

Symptom triad of **abdominal/pelvic pain, adnexal mass, missed period/spotting.** Also syncope or shoulder pain (late sign of ruptured ectopic) and symptoms of early pregnancy (usually are not as significant as in a normal intrauterine pregnancy).

► Diagnosis

Ultrasound absent intrauterine sac, fluid in cul-de-sac, poorly rising titers of serum, β-hCG, progesterone levels < 10 ng/mL.

► Treatment Options

1. Surgery—laparoscopic salpingostomy or salpingectomy.
2. Medical—methotrexate IM followed by serial β-hCG levels.

2. Abortion

► Description

Pregnancy termination, either elective or spontaneous, before 20 weeks. In missed abortion, the fetus usually dies in the first trimester but may be retained in the uterus for 2–4 weeks or longer.

If postabortal infection occurs, a **septic abortion** may occur with abnormal vaginal discharge, pain, fever, and possible peritonitis; treat with antibiotics, dilatation and curettage (D&C), and possibly hysterectomy.

► Symptoms

Vaginal bleeding and cramping, loss of symptoms of pregnancy (decreased breast tenderness, decreased morning sickness).

► Diagnosis

Physical examination, poorly rising titers of β-hGC, ultrasound (no heart motion seen). Differential diagnosis includes ectopic pregnancy, molar pregancy, or other causes of first-trimester bleeding (e.g., cervicitis, abnormal dysplasia, vaginitis, etc.).

► Pathology

Uterine contractions expel detached products of conception, usually without incident. Chorionic villi seen in curettings. Fetal parts may be identified.

► Treatment Steps
1. Expectant management.
2. Dilatation and evacuation.
3. Monitoring serial β-hCG titers until they are < 5 mIU/mL.

3. Pregnancy-Induced Hypertension (PIH)

► Description

PIH can be divided into four categories:
1. Preeclampsia (see Cram Facts).
2. Chronic hypertension that existed prior to the patient's pregnancy and is not associated with any end-organ damage.
3. Chronic hypertension and superimposed preeclampsia.
4. Transient hypertension (> 140/90) without proteinuria or end-organ damage, occurring late in pregnancy or during delivery, with a return to normal blood pressures within 10 days of delivery.

► Symptoms

May be asymptomatic, or headache, abdominal pain (right upper quadrant), dyspnea, nausea, vomiting, change in vision, edema of face and hands, oliguria.

► Diagnosis

• **Mild preeclampsia**—increase in systolic pressure of 30 mm Hg, diastolic 15 mm Hg, or a reading 140/90 with minimal proteinuria and edema.
• **Severe preeclampsia**—systolic pressure 160 mm Hg or greater, diastolic 110 mm Hg or greater, with significant proteinuria and evidence of end-organ damage. Lab workup includes complete blood count (CBC), liver function tests (LFTs), prothrombin time/partial thromboplastin time (PT/PTT), and urinalysis.

► Treatment Steps

1. Bed rest/admission to the hospital for monitoring and treatment.
2. Drug treatment consists of seizure prophylaxis and antihypertensives.
   • Magnesium sulfate to prevent and treat seizures.
   • Hydralazine is the drug of choice to control blood pressure.

► **cram facts**

PREECLAMPSIA

• Defined as hypertension, edema, and proteinuria after 20 weeks' gestation.
• Sometimes referred to as *toxemia*.
• *Eclampsia* refers to seizures in the setting of preeclampsia.
• Severe preeclampsia can progress to the HELLP syndrome (hemolysis, liver abnormalities, low platelets).
• Etiology unknown.
• Increased risk of PIH in primigravidas, extremes of maternal age, multiple gestation, molar pregnancy, diabetes, renal disease, heart disease, and patients with personal or family history of hypertension, PIH, or eclampsia.
• Patients may be asymptomatic and exhibit only elevated blood pressures and proteinuria. Severe preeclampsia is characterized by end-organ damage.
• Fetus may exhibit intrauterine growth retardation (IUGR).

- Labetalol can be used if hydralazine is unavailable.
- Diuretics should be avoided, as patients are relatively intravascularly volume depleted.

3. The definitive treatment is delivery of the fetus.

4. **Third-Trimester Bleeding**

The three major causes are placenta previa, abruptio placentae, and bloody show. The first two are serious and potentially dangerous conditions; the third condition is a normal process (see Cram Facts).

► Symptoms

Abruptio placentae presents with **painful** vaginal bleeding **(hemorrhage may be concealed),** shock, poor fetal heart tones, tetanic uterine contractions, pain, expanding uterus. It may be associated with disseminated intravascular coagulation (DIC) and severe hemorrhage, even resulting in fetal death.

Placenta previa presents with painless bleeding usually in the third trimester (ultrasound may not show a small abruption); CBC/diff, platelets, LFTs.

► Diagnosis

Ultrasound, coagulation studies (PT, PTT, fibrinogen, fibrin split products [FSPs]).

► Pathology

Abruptio placentae results in hemorrhage between uterine wall and placenta. "Currant jelly" clots on placental surface.

► Treatment Steps

1. **Above all, stabilize mother *first*!**
2. May observe in mild cases of abruption and previa and allow labor to progress. Labor is often precipitous in cases of abruption.
3. Fluids, transfusion, plasma expanders; in severe cases, hysterectomy.

- **Abruptio placentae**—delivery, treat shock and possible coagulopathy (see Fig. 13–2).

► **cram facts**

THIRD-TRIMESTER BLEEDING

Placenta previa: Painless bleeding; associated with abnormally low implantation of the placenta over the cervix. May be (1) complete, (2) partial, (3) marginal, or (4) low lying. The diagnosis is usually made by ultrasound. Complete previa usually requires cesarean section. Partial (< 30%) previa may be delivered vaginally, while being ready for stat section. Marginal and low-lying placentas usually present no problems at vaginal delivery.

Abruptio placentae: Painful bleeding; associated with premature separation of the placenta from the uterus. Hypertonic uterine contractions and irritability noted often with fetal tachycardia secondary to anemia. Ultrasound usually confirms the diagnosis, but the area of retroplacental clot must be large enough to be seen on ultrasound. If the blood does not escape externally, it is a concealed abruption, but with pain nonetheless. In severe cases, abruption can result in fetal demise, maternal hemorrhage associated with DIC, and even maternal death.

Bloody show: Painless bleeding associated with expulsion of the cervical mucous plug, heralding the start of labor. It is usually associated with only a few drops of blood; anything more may be suggestive of pathology.

- **Placenta previa**—delivery if possible in a "double" setup, (i.e., vaginal delivery in an operating room [OR] that is ready for C-section).

5. Preterm Labor

▶ Description
Onset of labor prior to 37 weeks' estimated gestational age (EGA), includes regular, painful contractions. Membranes may be ruptured (preterm rupture of membranes [ROM]) or unruptured.

▶ Symptoms
Include usual symptoms of term labor: Cervical dilation and effacement with regular contractions, with or without ROM.

▶ Diagnosis
History and physical exam, electronic fetal monitoring (EFM). If ROM is suspected, do ferning and nitrazine testing (see Clinical Pearl).

▶ Pathology
PGF_2-α(?) and PGE_2 prostaglandin release, resulting in increased uterine muscle contractility. Other etiologies include maternal dehydration, exhaustion, sexual activity (nipple stimulation), maternal infection, overdistention of uterine cavity (multiple gestation, polyhydramnios, macrosomia).

▶ Treatment Steps
1. **Fluids and bed rest in the left lateral decubitus position are the *first* line of therapy.**
2. Tocolytic medications.
3. Magnesium sulfate and terbutaline, only if fluids and bed rest fail.

With **ROM,** perform cervical cultures. **Check for fetal lung maturity** (see Clinical Pearl). Watch for signs of **amnionitis** (fever, uterine tenderness, elevated white blood count [WBC]).

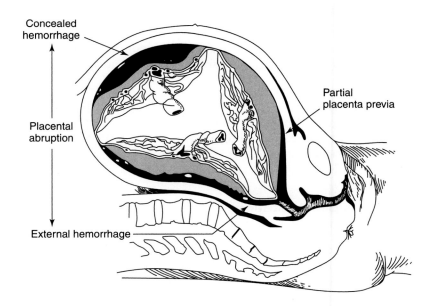

Figure 13–2. Hemorrhage from premature placental separation. Upper left: Extensive placental abruption but with the periphery of the placenta and the membranes still adherent, resulting in completely concealed hemorrhage. **Lower:** Placental abruption with the placenta detached peripherally and with the membranes between the placenta and cervical canal stripped from underlying decidua, allowing external hemorrhage. **Right:** Partial placenta previa with placental separation and external hemorrhage. (Reproduced, with permission, from Cunningham FG, MacDonald PC, Gant NF, Leveno KJ, Gilstrap LC (eds): *Williams Obstetrics,* 19th ed. Appleton & Lange, 1993.)

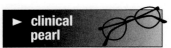

► **clinical pearl**

TESTS FOR FETAL LUNG MATURITY

- Lecithin/sphingomyelin (L/S) ratio
- Phosphatidylglycerol (PG)
- Phosphatidylinositol (PI)

---

6. **Polyhydramnios**

   ► **Description**
   Increased amniotic fluid over 2,000 mL.

   ► **Symptoms**
   Excessive uterine size, preterm labor.

   ► **Diagnosis**
   Physical exam reveals size greater than dates discrepancy. Ultrasound can be done to measure fluid.

   ► **Pathology**
   Cause unknown. Associated with fetal anomalies, gestational diabetes, esophageal atresia, open neural tube defects, multiple gestation.

   ► **Treatment Steps**
   1. Bed rest and observe, amniocentesis if necessary.
   2. Delivery if maternal respiration is compromised.
   3. Overdistention of the uterus may result in preterm labor (which should be stopped if possible).

7. **Rh Isoimmunization**

   ► **Description**
   Erythroblastosis fetalis is fetal red blood cell hemolysis from maternal antibodies produced in response to fetal cells getting into maternal blood (where the fetus may have a different blood group from the mother). Incompatibility of Rh or ABO.

   ► **Symptoms**
   Fetal hemolytic anemia, heart failure, acidosis.

   ► **Diagnosis**
   History, elevated bilirubin (jaundice).

   ► **Pathology**
   Kernicterus—elevated bilirubin deposition in the brain; antibodies cause hemolysis, high-output failure, edema, ascites.

   ► **Treatment Steps**
   1. **Prevention**—give Rh-negative mother an injection of Rh immune globulin (RhoGAM, which is IgG to the Rh factor) at 28 weeks, or any episode of bleeding, CVS, amniocentesis, or trauma.
   2. Transfusion.
   3. Delivery.

8. **Multiple Gestation**
   See also Chapter 14, section XIII.

   ► **Description**
   More than one fetus. Increasing incidence due to fertility drugs. Native incidence of identical twins is 1/88 pregnancies. Increased incidence of gestational diabetes, preterm labor, PIH

   ► **Symptoms**
   Uterine size greater than dates discrepancy, two or more heartbeats, increased weight gain.

▶ Diagnosis

Physical exam reveals uterine fundus greater than dates. Doppler shows two fetal heart tones (FHTs). Ultrasound confirms the diagnosis.

▶ Pathology

Familial tendency, race, medication (fertility drugs).

▶ Treatment Steps

Prenatal monitoring for maternal diabetes, PIH, and preterm labor are essential. Complex management protocol depending on fetal weight and position. All multiple gestations greater than twins are delivered by cesarean section.

9. Intrapartum Fetal Distress/Death

▶ Description

Pattern of failing fetal response to stress usually refers to pregnancy after 20 weeks' gestation. Prior to 20 weeks is an abortion.

▶ Symptoms

Abnormal stress test or NST, abnormal fetal monitor pattern or scalp pH. Decreasing variability, prolonged/late decelerations (see section I.B).

▶ Diagnosis

Ultrasound, BPP, and NST (see section I.B).

▶ Pathology

Uteroplacental insufficiency of fetal or maternal etiology. Drug or alcohol use, or smoking. Postdates pregnancy may result in placental calcification and uteroplacental insufficiency.

▶ Treatment Steps

Delivery, usually by stat cesarean section. If infant is preterm, have neonatal staff in attendance for advanced resuscitation.

10. Anxiety/Depression

▶ Description

Postpartum depression may be mild to severe in intensity. Temporary "baby blues" may occur and require only supportive treatment. With more severe depression, antidepressant medication and psychologic evaluation may be necessary.

Postpartum psychosis is less common and may require both medication and inpatient management.

Anxiety disorders are treated with counseling and medication as necessary.

11. Maternal Mortality

▶ Description

Maternal mortality has been decreasing over the past century. In 1985, there were 7.8 maternal deaths/100,000 live births. Maternal mortality is four times higher in women of color.

▶ Pathology

Hemorrhage, infection, and hypertension. Often may be due to socioeconomic factors (e.g., nutritional status, drug use, etc.).

► **differential diagnosis**

SIZE GREATER THAN DATES DISCREPANCY

- **Incorrect calculation of dates:** Serial ultrasounds should show normal interval growth.
- **Maternal diabetes:** Diagnosed by abnormal glucose tolerance test.
- **Maternal obesity:** Based on 20% above nonpregnant ideal body weight.
- **Posdatism:** > 42 weeks' gestation.
- **Multiparity:** Causes laxity and diastasis recti, leading to larger-than-expected fundal height.
- **Multiple gestation:** Twins or greater gestation; diagnosed by ultrasound.
- **Advanced maternal age:** Predisposes to gestational diabetes.
- **Large maternal stature:** Large mothers have large babies.
- **Polyhdramnios:** Excess amniotic fluid seen on ultrasound.
- **Fetal anomalies:** Such as sacrococcygeal teratomas, open neural tube defects—polyhydramnios.
- **Macrosomia:** Large baby, based on ultrasound estimated fetal weight.
- **Uterine fibroids:** Diagnosed on ultrasound, make the uterus appear larger than expected.

SIZE LESS THAN DATES DISCREPANCY

- **Incorrect calculation of dates:** Serial ultrasounds show normal interval growth.
- **Oligohydramnios:** Abnormally low amount of amniotic fluid seen on ultrasound.
- **Intrauterine growth retardation (IUGR):** Abnormal fetal growth, asymmetric (head sparing), symmetric (non–head sparing).
- **Advanced maternal diabetes:** Associated with placental insufficiency.
- **Nutritional factors:** Maternal inadequate diet—IUGR.
- **Maternal substance abuse:** Tobacco, alcohol, drugs, cocaine, etc.
- **Small maternal stature:** Small mothers have small babies.
- **Trisomies 13, 18, 21:** Diagnosed by chorionic villous sampling or amniocentesis.
- **Congenital infections:** TORCH (toxoplasmosis, rubella, cytomegalovirus, herpes) titers; associated with IUGR.

---

12. Fetal Growth and Congenital Abnormalities

► Description

See Chapter 14.

Screen with amniocentesis if mother is older than 35, or has prior history of giving birth to child with neural tube defect or chromosome abnormality. Consider targeted level II ultrasound, triple or quad screen. May also screen when positive history for multiple miscarriages and if the mother is diabetic.

13. Gestational Trophoblastic Disease

► Description

Gestational trophoblastic disease (GTD) is a term describing abnormal growth of cells inside a woman's uterus. Incidence of GTD is about 1 in 2,000 pregnancies. They are rare but curable tumors that arise in tissue that develops immediately after conception. However, they are not normal pregnancies and do not end with the birth of a neonate.

The three diseases of GTD are:

1. Hydatidiform mole (also known as a molar pregnancy) (90%)
2. Invasive mole (5–8%)
3. Choriocarcinoma (1–2%)

► Symptoms

Uterine size large for dates, first-trimester bleeding, hyperemesis gravidarum, abnormally elevated β-hCG, passage of grapelike vesicles per vagina, and severe eclampsia.

► Diagnosis

Clinical setting. Ultrasound examination shows an enlarged uterus but no fetal parts, classically described as "snowstorm" pattern on ultrasound.

► Pathology

1. **Hydatidiform mole**—villous stroma edema, avascular villi, syncytiotrophoblastic groups near the villi.
2. **Invasive mole**—invades myometrium.
3. **Choriocarcinoma**—epithelial tumor.
4. Distant metastases may involve lung, brain, etc.

► Treatment Steps

1. **Cure rate 90%,** so obtain β-hCG and ultrasound to diagnose.
2. Hydatidiform mole. **Suction curettage is method of choice.** Invasive mole and choriocarcinoma: chemotherapy.
3. Most highly sensitive neoplasm to chemotherapy (specifically methotrexate), if distant mets exist.

14. Hyperemesis Gravidarum

► Description

Severe, intractable nausea and vomiting in a pregant female. Etiology unclear. Peak incidence 8–12 weeks. Usually resolves by week 16.

► Treatment Steps

IV rehydration and correction of electrolyte abnormalities, psychological support, hospital care, and hyperalimentation if necessary; medication (antiemetics), vitamin B_6.

B. Nonobstetric Complications of Pregnancy

1. Major Medical Complications

► Description

Most important nonobstetric complication is cardiovascular disease. Most important postanesthetic cause of death is gastric aspiration.

2. Surgical Complications

► Description

Appendicitis is the **most common surgical condition** during pregnancy. Cholecystitis is the second. During surgery, need to ensure adequate fetal oxygenation, and be aware of fetal risk with anesthesia. Nonetheless, maternal health and well-being comes before that of the fetus.

C. Abnormal Labor

► Description

Abnormal labor or dystocia may occur secondary to abnormal presentations. Anything other than occiput anterior may cause dystocia. Transverse lie, as well as variable lies, often need to be treated with version, external or internal (depending on the situation). Breech presentations may also be subject to version. Breech presentations may be complete or incomplete. Only complete breech (specifically frank breech) may be delivered vaginally. All others by cesarean section.

Uterine dysfunction is another cause of dystocia; including prolonged latent and second stages, secondary arrest, and protraction disorder. Treat prolonged latent phase with sedation. Protraction and arrest disorders: oxytocin (possibly), ambulation, amniotomy, cesarean section.

Shoulder Dystocia

- This is an obstetrical emergency. Occurs more commonly in women with gestational diabetes, postdates pregnancy, abnormal pelvic anatomy, prior history of dystocia, and fetal macrosomia.
- Emergent treatment can include episiotomy, suprapubic pressure, internal rotation, delivery of the posterior arm, altered positioning of the mother (including McRoberts maneuver and moving onto all fours).
- Maneuvers of a last resort may include deliberate fracture of the infant's clavicle, or Zavanelli maneuver (replacing the head into the birth canal followed by cesarean delivery).

Cephalopelvic disproportion (CPD)—Perform cesarean section.

Use of Forceps

- Outlet scalp at introitus.
- *Low forceps:* Skull +2 or more.
- *Midforceps* (almost never used): Head engaged but skull above +2.

D. Abnormal Fetal Positioning

1. Breech Presentation

Of all deliveries 3–4% incidence **(incidence inversely proportional to gestational age).** Higher neonatal **morbidity and mortality** than with cephalic presentation at all gestational ages and birth weight. Delivery problems result from umbilical cord prolapse, cephalopelvic disproportion, trauma. Management includes early diagnosis, preparation, external version maneuver, vaginal delivery (assuming frank breech position, fetal weight 2,000–3,800 g, normal gynecoid pelvis), and/or cesarean section.

2. Transverse Lie (Shoulder Presentation)

One in 300 deliveries. Associated with **prematurity, increased parity,** premature rupture of membrane, placenta previa. Management depends on fetal size, gestational age, and placental position. External version attempts if gestational age > 37 weeks, membranes intact, no cephalopelvic disproportion (CPD), no placenta previa. Cesarean section unless no chance of fetal survival.

3. Deflexion Abnormality (Brow and Face Presentation)

One in 500 deliveries. **Spontaneous correction** often results as labor progresses. Associated with CPD, increased parity, prematurity, premature rupture of membranes, fetal anomaly (anencephaly). Higher perinatal mortality related to fetal abnormality, prematurity, trauma, asphyxia.

E. Complications of the Puerperium

1. Breast-Feeding and Mastitis

▶ Description

Mastitis is most often due to *Staphylococcus aureus.* Occurs after several weeks, often from infant's germs. Breast is red and tender; patient has chills or fever. Treat with warm soaks and antibiotics. Prevent by good hygiene and infant care.

- *Galactocele* is milk excess from blocked duct.
- *Painful nipples* often during early days of breast-feeding. Treat with local measures.
- *Engorgement* treated with analgesics, breast-feeding, cool compress.

2. Postpartum Hemorrhage (PPH)

▶ Description

- Blood loss > 500 cc after vaginal delivery.
- Blood loss > 1,000 cc after cesarean section.

▶ Symptoms

Bleeding, hypotension, shock, may have boggy uterus. Severe hemorrhage/hypotension may result in Sheehan syndrome (postpartum pituitary necrosis), resulting in panhypopituitarism: amenorrhea, hypothyroidism, and addisonian crisis.

▶ Diagnosis

Physical examination, estimation of blood loss, inspection of placenta for completeness.

▶ Pathology

1. Early PPH
   a. Retained products of conception.
   b. Abnormal placentation (e.g., placenta accreta, increta, percreta), succenturiate lobe.
   c. Laceration of birth canal (e.g., vagina, cervix) (especially common in precipitous labors (< 30 minutes), periurethral tear, etc.
   d. Uterine atony: associated with long labors, long oxytocin induction of labor, large overdistended uterine cavity (multiple gestation, polyhydramnios, macrosomia), uterine fibroids, halogenated anesthetics; most common etiology is atony.
   e. Coagulopathy, DIC (severe PIH, HELLP syndrome [hemolysis, elevated liver enzymes, and low platelet count]).
2. Late PPH may be due to retained products of conception, molar pregnancy, uterine atony.

▶ Treatment Steps

1. Find source of bleeding.
2. Stabilize patient.
3. IV fluids, blood replacement if necessary.
4. If uterine atony: Uterine massage, administer ergot alkaloids/oxytocics.
5. If retained products, remove retained products of conception, may need to do postpartum curettage, uterine packing.
6. If severe continued bleeding, surgical intervention: uterine artery ligation, hypogastric ligation, ultimately hysterectomy if all else fails.

3. Postpartum Sepsis

▶ Description

Endometritis most common. Infection of the endometrium and myometrium usually following operative delivery.

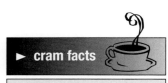

POSTPARTUM SEPSIS

- Caused by bacteria normally present in the urogenital tract.
- Increased risk with more frequent exams, prolonged premature rupture of membranes, use of scalp monitor, obesity, C-section, prior infections.

► **Symptoms**

Presents with fever, uterine tenderness, discharge may be foul, elevated WBC.

► **Diagnosis**

Elevated WBC, fever, uterine tenderness, foul-smelling discharge, positive uterine cultures.

► **Treatment Steps**

Give IV antibiotics. Other potential infections include wound, urinary tract, mastitis (see section II.D.1), and septic thrombophlebitis.

4. Postpartum Depression and Psychosis

► **Description**

See section II.A.10.

III. PRINCIPLES OF MANAGEMENT—OBSTETRICS

A. Intrapartum Care

1. Assessment of Labor

► **Description**

History and physical examination, need to determine if rupture of membranes has occurred (ferning and nitrazine tests), bloody show (expulsion of bloody mucoid cervical plug). Differentiation of true versus false labor (Braxton Hicks contractions); patient is monitored via EFM.

False labor: Irregular, infrequent contractions of varying intensity and **no progress or cervical change occurs.** Patient sent home for observation.

If cervical change occurs, patient admitted. PROM is defined as ROM **prior** to the onset of labor (contractions). If ROM or PROM, patient must be watched for infection (i.e., chorioamnionitis), may be monitored at home. If signs of infection, induce labor immediately, may need cesarean section if severe infection.

2. Electronic Fetal Monitoring (EFM)

► **Description**

May be done outside the abdomen (external) or intrauterine (internal). External monitoring is done prior to ROM or PROM. External is less accurate than internal. EFM measures the fetal heart rate and the uterine contractions. Fetal heart rate (FHR) is further analyzed in five ways: (1) rate (normal: 120–160 bpm); (2) short-term beat-to-beat variability; (3) long-term beat-to-beat variability; (4) reactivity: accelerations of the FHR of 15 bpm for at least 15 seconds, occurring at least twice during a 20-minute period; and (5) decelerations in the FHR. Decelerations (onset with respect to uterine contractions can be (1) early (head compression), (2) late (ominous sign due to fetal hypoxia, uteroplacental insufficiency), and (3) variable (cord compression) (see Fig. 13–3).

3. Anesthesia and Analgesia

► **Description**

See Cram Facts. Nitrous oxide is infrequently used and will provide analgesia but **not true anesthesia.** If general anesthesia used, pre-

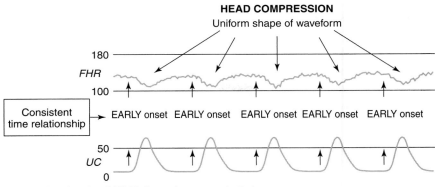

HEAD COMPRESSION
Uniform shape of waveform

A. Early deceleration (HC) Uniform shape – early timing

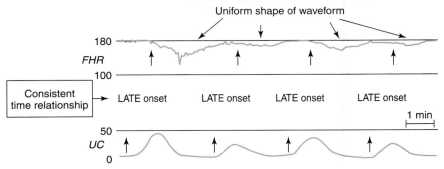

UTEROPLACENTAL INSUFFICIENCY
Uniform shape of waveform

B. Late deceleration (UPI) Uniform shape – late timing

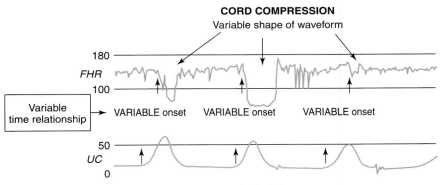

CORD COMPRESSION
Variable shape of waveform

C. Variable deceleration (CC) Variable shape – variable timing

Figure 13–3. Fetal heart rate decelerations in relation to the time of onset of uterine contractions. HC. head compression; UPI, uteroplacental insufficiency; CC, cord compression. (Reproduced, with permission, from Hon EH: *An Atlas of Fetal Heart Rate Patterns.* Harty, 1968.)

cautions must be taken against aspiration (number one cause of anesthetic death), including fasting, intubation with cricoid pressure, antacids. Other methods include pudendal block (second-stage labor), paracervical block (for first-stage labor, complications include fetal bradycardia), spinal and epidural blocks, and saddle block. Complications of spinal/epidural block include hypotension. **Most commonly used second-stage method is epidural.** Spinal may be used for cesarean sections or operative deliveries (e.g., forceps).

Early labor: uterine pain. Advanced labor: lower tract pain via **pudendal** nerve. Pudendal block may also be used in vacuum or forceps deliveries.

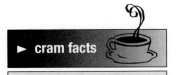

► **cram facts**

MEDICATIONS USED DURING ACTIVE LABOR

- Meperidine HCl (Demerol)
- Morphine
- Nalbuphine HCl (Nubain)
- Butorphanol tartrate (Stadol)

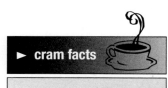

CONTRAINDICATIONS TO SPINAL OR EPIDURAL BLOCK

- Hypertension (relative contraindication)
- Bleeding disorder, low platelets, or recent use of anticoagulant
- Infection near site

4. Induction of Labor

▶ Description

Use of medication or other means to stimulate uterine contraction and bring on labor. **Oxytocin** commonly used. Also **amniotomy** (artificial rupture of membranes) will hasten onset of labor. PGE_2 and $PGF_{2\alpha}$ in the form of cervical gels also help ripen and soften the cervix.

1. **Indications**—preeclampsia, PROM, prolonged pregnancy, diabetes, and others.
2. **Contraindications**—CPD is a relative contraindication, placenta previa, multiple gestations, and abnormal presentations.
3. **Complications**—uterine rupture, hemorrhage (due to uterine atony), infection, amniotic fluid embolism (extremely rare).

5. Episiotomy

A surgical incision of the perineum made to facilitate delivery and reduce possible perineal tearing.

▶ Description

- *Median* is simple to repair and less bloody/painful. However, it may extend to fourth-degree laceration.
- *Mediolateral* results in increased problems, more pain, does not extend to fourth-degree tear.

All are repaired usually under local anesthesia.

6. Forceps Delivery

▶ Description

Each forceps consists of a blade, shank, lock, and handle. May be fenestrated or nonfenestrated. Low forceps (outlet) are applied with the fetal head at the perineal/pelvic floor. If head is higher, it is termed *midforceps* (almost never done).

- *Indications*—any problem affecting mother or fetus that would ßbe resolved by delivery. This includes uterine inertia, maternal illness/exhaustion, prophylactic infection hemorrhage. **High forceps is almost never performed.**
- *Conditions required*—membrane rupture, empty bladder, known position, anesthesia, cervical dilation, no CPD present, head vertex occiput anterior preferable (or face with anterior chin) and engaged. Occiput posterior more difficult to extract and may need to be rotated first.

Tucker–McLane for outlet forceps where little or no traction needed. **Simpson** for molded heads.

7. Emergency Problems and Cesarean Delivery

▶ Description

Indications for cesarean include CPD (most common reason for primary cesarean section), placentia previa, abruptio placenta, failure to progress, fetal distress, preeclampsia/eclampsia, cord prolapse, maternal distress, hemorrhage, shock. Most common reason for repeat cesarean section is previous cesarean section.

8. Vaginal Birth After Cesarean Delivery

▶ Description

Vaginal birth after cesarean (VBAC) is possible in about 75% of patients if given a trial of labor.

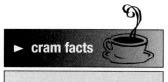

CLASSIC C-SECTION INCISION

- Refers to a vertical incision
- Usually reserved for cases in which the transverse incision is too small to deliver the fetus (i.e., transverse lie)

May be indicated with a noncomplicated pregnancy and one or more prior cesarean sections with a low transverse incision.

Contraindications include **classic C-section incision** previously. Complications include uterine rupture and hemorrhage.

9. Vacuum-Assisted Delivery

▶ Description

Traction is applied to a suction cup attached to the baby's head. Pull is maintained during contractions. Cephalhematoma is not uncommon and usually resolves spontaneously.

B. Postpartum/Immediate Newborn Care

1. Immediate Action Situations

▶ Description

Hemorrhage, thromboembolism, **amniotic fluid embolism** (extremely rare) (hypotension, cardiorespiratory collapse, treat with cardiopulmonary resuscitation [CPR], pressors, fluids, oxygen), newborn resuscitation if indicated.

Routine newborn care see section I.D in this chapter.

2. Postpartum Contraception

▶ Description

Lactational amenorrhea is *not* a reliable form of contraception. If the patient is breast-feeding, barrier methods are best. Progesterone-only ("mini-pill") is safe in breast-feeding. Also see section I.G.

Sterilization (e.g., postpartum tubal ligation) may be done immediately following delivery. It has a higher failure rate than interval tubal ligation.

C. Abortion: Elective and Therapeutic Indications

▶ Description

Therapeutic abortion is medically necessary pregnancy termination.

Indications—**Breast** and **cervical cancer, severe hypertensive and cardiovascular disease,** and other medical disorders affecting the life of the mother.

Methods—Dilatation and evacuation (D&E) via suction curettage generally performed up to 16 weeks. Intra-amniotic saline has been used at 14–24 weeks, but complications include DIC, renal failure, seizures, and hypernatremia. Hyperosmotic urea and prostaglandins have been used.

Elective abortion is usually performed in the first trimester per the mother's choice.

IV. HEALTH AND HEALTH MAINTENANCE— GYNECOLOGY

A. Annual Pelvic Examination

▶ Description

Important for patient screening, education, and disease prevention/treatment. Must include **breast, abdomen, pelvic,** and **rectal ex-**

amination. All women should have their first pelvic exam and Papanicolaou (Pap) smear by age 18, or sooner if sexually active prior to that time.

B. Sexually Transmitted Diseases

► Description

Epidemiology/transmission involves close contact and/or intercourse. **Impact** may mean death from HIV, infertility (gonorrhea or chlamydia), increased cancer risk human papillomavirus (HPV). Additionally, serotyping of HPV may guide clinician as to future risk of cervical cancer. **Screening/prevention** should involve evaluation of high-risk patients and their partners. Role of patient/community education to be noted.

C. Gynecologic Cancer Screening

► Description

- **Cervical cancer: Screening** by the Pap test has reduced the frequency of invasive cancer of the cervix. **Epidemiology** (see Cram Facts).
- **Uterine cancer:** Risk elevated with infertile, nulliparous, obese patients, and higher levels of estrogen increase risk.

D. Breast Cancer

► Description

Epidemiologic evidence demonstrates higher incidence in patients with family history of breast cancer, and those who had children later in life. One of the leading causes of cancer and cancer death in

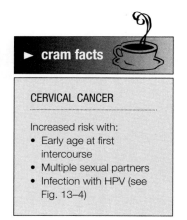

► cram facts

CERVICAL CANCER

Increased risk with:
- Early age at first intercourse
- Multiple sexual partners
- Infection with HPV (see Fig. 13–4)

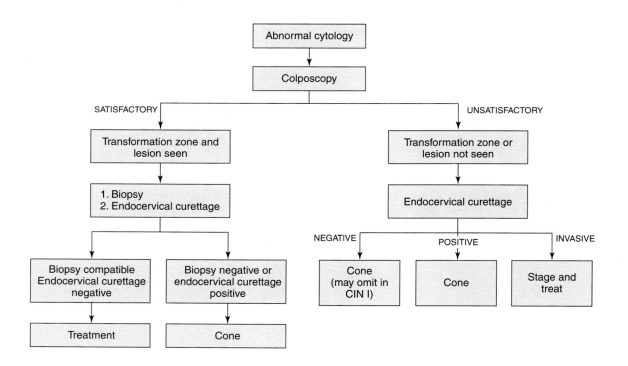

Figure 13–4. Diagnostic evaluation of a suspicious Papanicolaou smear. (Reproduced, with permission, from Gant NF, Cunningham FG. *Basic Gynecology and Obstetrics.* Norwalk, CT: Appleton & Lange, 1993.)

women. Importance of mammography **screening** and patient education should be noted. Initially at age 35 and then yearly after age 40.

BSE (breast self-examination) should be stressed at every annual and/or semiannual visit. Patient should do SBE monthly after menses are finished.

E. Osteoporosis

▶ Description

Epidemiology—increased incidence in fair, thin smokers of Northern European origin. Other risk factors include lack of exercise, early menopause (medical or surgical), and steroids. Significant impact in multiple areas including hip fractures and increased morbidity/mortality. **Prevention** via screening (dual-energy x-ray absorptiometry [DEXA]), patient education, diet, exercise, calcium and institution of calcium/estrogen replacement. (See also Chapter 10, section II.E.)

V. MECHANISMS OF DISEASE AND DIAGNOSIS—GYNECOLOGY

A. Infections

1. Vulvovaginitis

▶ Description

Vulvar/vaginal irritation and/or infection/inflammation.

▶ Symptoms

Itching, discharge (leukorrhea), burning, swelling, dysuria.

▶ Diagnosis

Physical and microscopic specimen examination including potassium hydroxide (KOH) and saline wet mount slides, culture.
1. *Candida*—thick white discharge, **itching, hyphae** on wet mount exam, no odor.
2. *Trichomonas*—**may be asymptomatic,** irritating gray discharge, **punctate cervical hemorrhages (strawberry cervix),** trichomonads on microscopic exam with odor.
3. *Gardnerella*—previously termed *nonspecific* or *Hemophilus*, thin discharge with characteristic fishy odor (especially on 10% KOH slide prep), **clue cells on microscopic exam.**

▶ Pathology

Organisms as described. May include foreign body, atrophic, viral (herpes, condylomata), chemical, and others.

▶ Treatment Steps

Candida—Clotrimazole, miconazole, terconazole, oral fluconazole (diflucan).

Trichomonas—Metronidazole or Metrogel.

Gardnerella—Metronidazole, Cleocin vaginal cream, or Metrogel.

2. Salpingitis, Pelvic Inflammatory Disease, and Toxic Shock

▶ Description

Salpingitis—Infection/inflammation of fallopian tubes.

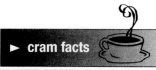

► cram facts

- *Behçet's syndrome*—oral and **genital ulcers**.
- *Molluscum contagiosum*—viral **umbilicated lesions,** curette, or try tretinoin (Retin-A).
- *Lichen sclerosus et atrophicus*—vulvar **atrophic dystrophy,** unknown cause.
- *Hidradenitis suppurativa*—apocrine **sweat gland infection.**

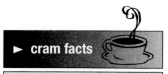

► cram facts

Fitz-Hugh–Curtis syndrome may be **seen in PID,** as **perihepatitis** (abnormal liver functions, abdominal, shoulder pain). **Complications of PID: infertility, tubo-ovarian abscess,** elevated ectopic pregnancy risk.

Endometritis—Endometrial infection/inflammation, usually postabortal or postpartum.

Pelvic Inflammatory Disease (PID)—Consists of salpingitis and/or endometritis of polymicrobial origin, usually related to sexually transmitted disease.

Toxic Shock Syndrome—Acute multisystem failure illness.

► Symptoms

PID—Pelvic pain and fever. In severe cases, peritoneal signs, cervical motion tenderness, vomiting, and even shock.

Toxic Shock—Fever, rash, hypotension, vomiting.

► Diagnosis

PID—Tender abdominal and adnexal/cervical discharge and pain with motion, fever, leukocytosis, ultrasound (looking for tubo-ovarian abscesses), cervical cultures.

Toxic Shock—Presentation, cultures.

► Pathology

PID—Pelvic spread of infection, **Chlamydia** (most common pathogen) and **Neisseria gonorrhoeae** often.

Toxic Shock—**Staphylococcus aureus.**

► Treatment Steps
Antibiotics as per culture and degree of infection:

1. Doxycycline for *Chlamydia.*
2. Usually broad-spectrum cephalosporin (e.g., Rocephin) and coverage of gram-negative anaerobes below the disphragm (metronidazole, clindamycin).

3. **Sexually Transmitted Diseases**

► Description
Viral, bacterial, spirochetal, or other illnesses spread by sexual contact.

► Symptoms

Herpes—Inguinal nodes, fever, crop of tender vesicles.

Gonorrhea—Discharge, abdominal pain, or asymptomatic.

Syphilis—Painless chancre, fever, secondary skin rash, condyloma lata—tertiary syphilis.

Chlamydia—Endocervicitis with grayish mucopurulent discharge or asymptomatic.

Chancroid—Soft painful ulcer.

HPV—Multiple fleshy warts or abnormal Pap smear.

Lymphogranuloma venereum (LGV)—Groove sign (line between lymph nodes), buboes.

Granuloma inguinale—Painless ulcer (a rare cause of ulcers in the United States).

► Diagnosis

Herpes—Clinical, viral culture.

Gonorrhea—Culture on Thayer–Martin media ("chocolate agar").

Syphilis—Rapid plasma reagin (RPR), Venereal Disease Research Laboratory (VDRL), fluorescent treponexral antibody absorption (FTA-ABS).

Chlamydia—Culture. (Also, *Chalamydia* antibody titers may be diagnostic of prior infection, even when cervical cultures are negative.)

Chancroid—Biopsy.

HPV—Diagnose clinically from genital wart. Can test cervical biopsy specimens for polymerase chain reaction (PCR) to HPV.

LGV—Serologic testing.

Granuloma Inguinale—Donovan bodies (rounded coccobacilli seen on biopsy of ulcer).

▶ Pathology

Herpes—Herpesvirus, usually herpes simplex type II.

Gonorrheae—*Neisseria gonorrhoeae.*

Syphilis—*Treponema pallidum.*

Chlamydia—*Chlamydia trachomatis.*

Chancroid—*Hemophilus ducreyi.*

HPV—Human papillomavirus.

LGV—*Chlamydia trachomatis.*

Granuloma Inguinale—*Calymmatobacterium granulomatis.*

▶ Treatment Steps

Herpes—Acyclovir.

Gonorrhea—Tetracycline, amoxicillin/probenecid, cefoxitin, ceftriaxone, azithromycin, ciprofloxacin, and others.

Syphilis—Intramuscular (IM) benzathine penicillin.

Chlamydia, LGV, and Granuloma Inguinale—Tetracycline or doxycycline.

Chancroid—Trimethoprim–sulfamethoxazole (Bactrim) or erythromycin.

HPV—No actual treatment for virus, but follow abnormal Pap smears closely. May use 5-fluorouracil (5-FU) or cryosurgery on cervical lesions.

4. Endometritis

▶ Description/Symptoms

Endometrial infection with **fever, tender uterus,** pain, discharge possible.

▶ Diagnosis

History and physical, elevated WBC, ultrasound to rule out retained products of conception.

▶ Pathology

Enterococci and streptococci. Bacteroides.

► Treatment Steps

Antibiotics IV, may also need D&C to remove remaining products of conception.

5. Urethritis

► Symptoms

Dysuria, frequency, and urgency, if severe—back pain may be a symptom of pyelonephritis.

► Diagnosis

Clinical diagnosis. Urine dipstick, certain cases urinalysis and culture.

► Treatment Steps

Antibiotics. Can treat empirically for the most common causes (*Escherichia coli*) using 3 days of trimethoprim–sulfamethoxazole or 5 days of a fluoroquinolone (levofloxacin).

6. Bartholin's Gland Abscess

► Description

Bartholin's gland duct obstruction, resulting in cyst, which becomes infected; often associated with gonorrhea.

► Symptoms

Enlarging mass, pain, dyspareunia, fever.

► Diagnosis

Tender mass at posterior fourchette, to the side.

► Treatment Steps
1. Incision and drainage (I&D).
2. Ward catheter, marsupialization.
3. Antibiotics as appropriate.

7. Breast Abscess/Mastitis

► Description

Mastitis—See section II.D.1 in this chapter.

Breast Abscess—Local infection.

► Symptoms/Diagnosis
Pain, erythema, fever, induration. Clinical diagnosis.

► Treatment Steps
1. Antibiotics.
2. Drain local abscess.

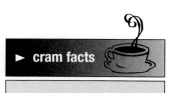
► cram facts

If mastitis occurs in a nonlactating woman, rule out breast cancer.

B. Urinary Incontinence: Infection

► Description
See section V.A.5. May be a sign of urethritis.

C. Uterovaginal Prolapse

► Description
Different types:

Cystocele—Bladder wall/trigone drops into the vagina.

Rectocele—Rectum prolapse into vagina.

Enterocele—Rectouterine pouch of Douglas herniation.

Urethrocele—Urethral wall protrusion.

► Symptoms
Stress incontinence, difficulty with defecation, vaginal fullness sensation, and mass.

► Diagnosis
History and physical, cystoscopy (cystocele), barium enema (rectocele).

► Treatment Steps
1. Cystocele treated by observation if minimal symptoms.
2. Otherwise pessary.
3. Kegel exercises, estrogen if postmenopausal, surgery. Rectocele treated by a pessary, surgery.

D. Endometriosis and Adenomyosis

► Description

Endometriosis—Functioning endometrial tissue located outside of the uterine cavity.

Adenomyosis—Endometrial tissue in the myometrium, also called "endometriosis interna."

► Symptoms

Endometriosis—Symptoms include **dysmenorrhea,** infertility, **pelvic/low back pain,** and **dyspareunia.**

Adenomyosis—Symptoms include menorrhagia and **dysmenorrhea.**

► Diagnosis

Endometriosis—History and physical. Uterosacral nodules. **Fixed retroverted uterus. Laparoscopy is the only way this disease can be 100% diagnosed.**

Adenomyosis—Tender, boggy uterus; microscopic diagnosis. Rule out leiomyomas, cancer, and pelvic congestion syndrome.

► Pathology

Endometriosis—Cause unknown but most probably due to retrograde menstruation. Other theories include hematogenous or lymphogenous dissemination, and/or coelomic metaplasia.

Adenomyosis—**Stroma and glands in muscular wall.**

► Treatment Steps

Endometriosis—Leuprolide acetate (Lupron) and other gonadotropin-releasing hormone (GnRH) agonists are the medical treatments of choice. Surgery may be needed to treat stage 3–4 disease. Danazol not used anymore because of androgenic side effects. Progestins are also used, although they may not be as effective GnRH agonists. Will regress with **menopause.** Observation if minimal symptoms.

Adenomyosis—See above.

E. Neoplasms

1. Cervical Dysplasia and Cancer

▶ Description

Dysplasia is cells of disordered growth, which, if untreated, may turn into cancer in situ, then invasive.

▶ Symptoms

Postcoital bleeding, vaginal discharge, or asymptomatic.

▶ Diagnosis

Pap Smear—If abnormal Pap smear with dysplasia, colposcopic exam.

Colposcopic-Directed Biopsy—In abnormally appearing areas (e.g., punctation, mosaicism, leukoplakia).

▶ Pathology

HPV 16 and 18, herpesvirus 2 all increase the risk of cancer.

▶ Treatment Steps

- Mild dysplasia (cervical intraepithelial neoplasia [CIN] 1), colposcopy, biopsy, and treat topically, or cryosurgery.
- Moderate (CIN 2), colposcopy with biopsy, cryosurgery, loop electrosurgical excision procedure (LEEP).
- Severe (CIN 3, carcinoma in situ), conization with biopsy, laser cone, or simple hysterectomy.

Cervical cancer is third most common female cancer. **Most common metastasis site: liver. Most common type: squamous cell.** Treatments include radiation and surgery. In cervical cancer, spread occurs by local extension and through the lymphatics. Death most commonly due to ureteral obstruction causing uremia.

2. Uterine Myoma

▶ Description

Benign uterine smooth muscle growth. **Most frequent gynecologic pelvic neoplasm.**

▶ Symptoms

Enlarging uterus, menorrhagia, pain, irregular menses. Very common in women in their 30s and 40s; more common in black women. Growth is estrogen dependent. Regression after menopause. Etiology unknown.

▶ Diagnosis

History and physical, ultrasound (may also show hydronephrosis), intravenous pyelogram (IVP).

▶ Pathology

Benign smooth muscle submucous, intramural, or subserous tumors, originating from one myometrial cell.

▶ Treatment Steps

1. Observation—serial ultrasound monitoring.
2. Medical—Lupron or other GnRH agonists may shrink tumors.
3. Surgical—hysteroscopic resection, myomectomy by laparotomy, hysterectomy.

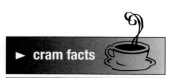

▶ cram facts

Abnormal colposcopic findings include mosaicism and white epithelium. Normal findings include original squamous and columnar epithelium. If entire lesion and transformation zone not seen, perform conization.

3. Cancer of the Endometrium

▶ Description

Endometrial cancer. May be preceded by endometrial hyperplasia. Usually occurs in women between ages 55 and 69. Fourth most common cancer in women after breast, colorectal, and lung.

▶ Symptoms

Abnormal postmenopausal vaginal bleeding. Risk factors include obesity, diabetes, hypertension, early menarche, late menopause, chronic anovulation, estrogen usage, primary infertility.

▶ Diagnosis

History and physical exam. **Ultrasound** shows thickened endometrium (> 13 mm). Endometrial biopsy done to confirm diagnosis. Fractional D&C. Computed tomography (CT) or magnetic resonance imaging (MRI) in advanced cases.

▶ Pathology

Usually **adenocarcinoma.**

Cancer limited to endometrium/myometrium (stage 1), cervix (stage 2), still in true pelvis (stage 3), or vaginal metastases/pelvic nodes bladder/rectum or out of pelvis (stage 4) with distant metastases.

▶ Treatment Steps

Total abdominal hysterectomy (TAH) and bilateral salpingo-oophorectomy (BSO; ovaries/tubes removed) for stage 1. Adjuvant radiation when there is lymph node involvement.

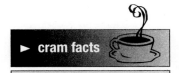

▶ **cram facts**

Most tumors are stage 1 at time of diagnosis. Three types: adenocarcinoma, adenoacanthoma, adenosquamous carcinoma. For stage IV— may add chemotherapy.

4. Ovarian Carcinoma

▶ Description

Ovarian cancer—second most common gynecologic malignancy in United States.

▶ Symptoms

Pain, weight loss, abdominal distention, early satiety, shortness of breath, or may be asymptomatic. Oral contraceptives are thought to be protective.

▶ Diagnosis

Diagnosis is difficult. Most are diagnosed at stage 3 after spread has occurred beyond ovaries and pelvis. Marker CA-125 of limited use. Ultrasound, Doppler flow, barium enema (BE), IVP, CT, MRI.

▶ Pathology

Children: germ cell tumors are most common. Adults: epithelial, 80% of all ovarian cancers.

Most common site of metastases through direct abdominal distention. Death occurs by bowel obstruction and chronic malnutrition. Stage 1, limited to ovaries; stage 2, pelvic extension; stage 3, outside pelvis; stage 4, distant metastases.

Peritoneum and **omentum** are **most common** epithelial **metastatic sites.**

Five-year survival rate overall 30%.

▶ Treatment Steps

Total hysterectomy, BSO, and omentectomy. Adjunctive chemotherapy.

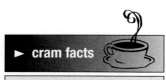

5. Neoplastic Breast Disorders

See Chapter 6, section VII.F.9.

6. Vulvar Neoplasms

► **Description**

Malignant vulvar neoplasms, often preceded by vulvar intraepithelial neoplasia (VIN). Most commonly seen in women between 60 and 70.

► **Symptoms**

Discharge, mass, dysuria, pruritus, bleeding.

► **Diagnosis**

History and physical, punch biopsy, and fine-needle aspiration of suspicious nodes.

► **Pathology**

Squamous cell, Paget's, adenocarcinoma, sarcoma, melanoma. **More common in the aged. Spreads to Cloquet's** (deep femoral) **node. Epidermoid cancer most common.**

Staged with TNM (tumor, node, metastasis) system. Lymph node status is most important prognostic factor.

► **Treatment Steps**

1. Wide local excision for microinvasive cancer.
2. Stage 1 invasive—radical vulvectomy and bilateral inguinal femoral node removal.
3. Stage 4—may add radiotherapy.

F. Fibrocystic Breast Disease

► **Description**

Common benign cystic breast disorder.

► **Symptoms**

Multiple lumps of changing size, tender, may or may not be cyclic in nature.

► **Diagnosis**

History and physical, biopsy, mammography, and ultrasound. Aspiration via fine needle may be both diagnostic and therapeutic. Solid masses require histologic analysis.

► **Pathology**

Fibroadenoma is the most common benign neoplasm of the breast. Benign papillomatosis, fibrosis, cysts. Ductal and fibrous tissue hyperplasia.

► **Treatment Steps**

1. Biopsy.
2. Cyst aspiration.
3. Support bra.
4. Danazol, low-dose oral contraceptives (first choice); avoid caffeine and chocolate.

G. Menstrual and Endocrinologic Disorders

1. Amenorrhea

▶ **Description**
- *Primary* is defined as **no menses by age 16.**
- *Secondary* is 3 months or longer amenorrhea in a normal-cycle individual.
- Causes—see Cram Facts.

▶ **Symptoms**

Except for complaints of amenorrhea, patients may be asymptomatic. Look for symptoms of pregnancy (nausea, vomiting, tender breasts, fatigue). Look for signs of PCOS (hirsutism, obesity); see next section.

▶ **Diagnosis**

Primary Amenorrhea—History and physical. Physical exam may reveal absence of vagina, imperforate hymen, transverse vaginal septae, or cervical stenosis. If gonadal dysgenesis is suspected, karyotyping can be done. If cause is still unclear, can also proceed with labs and testing as in secondary amenorrhea.

Secondary Amenorrhea—**Pregnancy test.** (It should be assumed a woman with secondary amenorrhea is pregnant until proven otherwise.) Progesterone withdrawal testing can be done. (see Cram Facts) Lab workup can include thyroid-stimulating hormone (TSH), follicle-stimulating hormone (FSH),

▶ **cram facts**

PROGESTERONE WITHDRAWAL TESTING

Progesterone can be given orally (for 5 days) or IM (once). If estrogen levels are adequate and no abnormality exists in the outflow tract, menses should occur within 1 week of ending progesterone.

- If bleeding occurs (which means adequate estrogen is present), causes include anovulatory cycles, obesity, hypothyroidism, or PCOS.
- If no bleeding occurs (hypoestrogenism), causes include anorexia, stress, gonadal dysgenesis, or premature ovarian failure.

▶ **cram facts**

AMENORRHEA

- **Pregnancy:** Most common cause of secondary amenorrhea.
- **Imperforate hymen:** 46XX; female phenotype, cyclic menstrual pain from menarche, bulging hymen, predisposition to endometriosis, surgically corrected.
- **Müllerian agenesis:** 46XX; female phenotype, absence of any or all of müllerian tract; sterile, does not need estrogen replacement therapy.
- **Gonadal dysgenesis:** 45XO; abnormal female phenotype; stigmata of Turner syndrome: short stature, webbed neck, shield chest, premature ovarian failure; sterile, needs estrogen replacement.
- **Androgen insensitivity:** 46XY; female phenotype, sparse sexual hair; remove gonads (testes) because of malignant transformation, raise as female on estrogen replacement.
- **Asherman syndrome:** 46XX; female phenotype; intrauterine scarring secondary to D&E. Surgically removed via hysteroscopy, then high-dose estrogen for 1 month to regenerate lining.
- **Polycystic ovarian syndrome (PCOS):** 46XX; female phenotype: often associated with obesity, hirsutism, acne, and infertility; needs ovulation induction for fertility; metformin may also be efficacious; otherwise, cycle with OCs or progestins.
- **Hypothalamic amenorrhea:** 46XX; female phenotype: may be associated with Kallman syndrome (anosmia, amenorrhea), anorexia (thin habitus), exercise; needs DEXA bone density scan to look for osteoporosis, needs estrogen replacement, dietary counseling, and lifestyle alteration.
- **Prolactinoma:** 46XX; female phenotype; galactorrhea, bitemporal hemianopsia, secondary amenorrhea; treated with bromocriptine mesylate (Parlodel).

luteinizing hormone (LH), dehydroepiandrosterone (DHEA), prolactin, and testosterone.

► Pathology
- Elevated prolactin—rule out hypothyroidism. If TSH is normal, check MRI of pituitary to rule out prolactinoma.
- Elevated FSH—consider genetic or autoimmune ovarian failure
- Elevated testosterone—look for hyperandrogenism, adrenal hyperplasia, PCOS.
- Kallman's syndrome—congenital isolated gonadotropin deficiency. Often associated with anosmia and midline anatomic defects.

► Treatment Steps
- If hypoestrogenism—replacement of estrogen, calcium, etc.
- If hyperestrogenism—treat cause of elevated estrogens, e.g., lose weight in cases of obesity.
- If PCO and patient desires fertility—consider metformin or ovulation induction.
- If no fertility desired—cycle with OCs or progestin therapy.
- If thyroid is abnormal—treat appropriately.
- If hyperprolactinemia—Parlodel.
- If Asherman syndrome—hysteroscopic surgical resection.
- If Kallman syndrome—estrogen replacement therapy.

2. PCOS

► Description

A syndrome occurring in young females. Also known as Stein–Leventhal syndrome, the classic triad consists of hirsutism, obesity, amenorrhea/infertility. Criteria from the National Institutes of Health (NIH) outline hyperandrogenism, menstrual dysfunction, and exclusion of other causes of hyperandrogenism. Polycystic ovaries are not needed for the diagnosis.

► Symptoms

Irregular menses have usually been present since menarche. Signs of hyperandrogenism can include hirsutism, acne, obesity, acanthosis nigricans, and male pattern baldness.

► Diagnosis

Clinical picture. Other sources of hyperandrogenism should be ruled out (congenital adrenal hyperplasia, androgen-secreting tumors, and hyperprolactinemia). Labs include TSH, FSH, LH, prolactin, total and free testosterone, DHEA. In PCOS the LH/FSH ration is usually > 3 and DHEA is often mildly elevated.

► Complications

Due to insulin resistance that is independent of body weight, women are at increased risk of diabetes. Because of prolonged unopposed estrogen stimulation of the endometrium, patients have an increased risk of endometrial cancer. Patients often seek treatment when they are trying to conceive and have trouble with infertility.

► Treatment Steps
- Oral contraceptives are often prescribed to regulate menstrual cycles and decrease the risk of endometrial cancer.

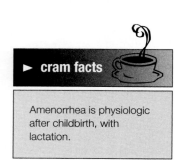

► cram facts

Amenorrhea is physiologic after childbirth, with lactation.

- Metformin has been used in trials and it can help with insulin resistance and in some reports infertility.
- Spironolactone is also used as an antiandrogen.

3. Abnormal Uterine Bleeding

▶ **Description**

Menorrhagia—Increased amount of flow.

Oligomenorrhea—Increased length of time between menses (35–90 days between cycles).

Metrorrhagia—Bleeding outside of normal menses.

Menometrorrhagia—Bleeding excessively and irregularly.

▶ **Symptoms**
Abnormal bleeding as described, anemia, pelvic pain (fibroids).

▶ **Diagnosis**
History and physical. CBC/diff. FSH, LH, DHEAS, TSH, testosterone, prolactin (PRL), β-hCG, endometrial biopsy (over age 35 to rule out hyperplasia). Also pelvic ultrasound to rule out fibroids, PCOS, etc.

▶ **Pathology**
Most common cause is dysfunctional uterine bleeding, usually secondary to anovulatory cycles. Infrequent etiology is organic (trauma, foreign body, tumor, hormonal, coagulopathy, etc.). In child, usually due to foreign body; in teenager, usually anovulatory cycle.

▶ **Treatment Steps**
1. If no fertility is desired: Fibroids: GnRH analog to shrink tumors, or surgery. PCOS: Cycle with oral contraceptives or progestins.
2. If fertility is desired: Monitor cycle with ovulation-induction medicines.

4. Dysmenorrhea

▶ **Description**
Painful menstruation. Further divided into primary and secondary dysmenorrhea.
- Primary is without pathology.
- Secondary is due to pathology (multiple etiologies such as endometriosis, fibroids, infection, cancer).

▶ **Symptoms**
Pain, cramping, nausea, bloating, may also have dysuria, dyschezia, diarrhea, constipation, or other gastrointestinal or genitourinary symptoms.

▶ **Diagnosis**
Clinical, laparoscopy to rule out secondary cause.

▶ **Pathology**
- Primary dysmenorrhea is prostaglandin mediated—causes smooth muscle contractions.
- Secondary dysmenorrhea depends on the organic pathology present in the pelvis.

► **cram facts**

HORMONE REPLACEMENT THERAPY

The estrogen and progesterone arm of the Women's Health Initiative was stopped prematurely and subsequently raised many questions and concerns about the use of hormone replacement therapy. The combination of estrogen and progesterone was found to:

- Increase risk of coronary events
- Increase risk of invasive breast cancer
- Increase risk of stroke
- Increase risk of pulmonary embolism
- Decreased risk of hip fracture and colon cancer

As a general rule, women need to discuss the risk and benefits of hormone replacement therapy before being started on or continuing the medication.

► **Treatment Steps**
1. Primary is treated with prostaglandin synthetase inhibitor as are the nonsteroidal anti-inflammatory drugs (NSAIDs). Also birth control pills may help.
2. Secondary treatment as per individual etiology.

5. Menopause

► **Description**

Menopause is the normal cessation of menses in females. It correlates with low levels of estrogen and progesterone, and elevated FSH and LH.

Some women tolerate these changes without many symptoms. However, most women will experience at least one of the following: atrophic vaginitis, hot flashes, changes in skin collagen content, osteoporosis, abnormal lipid profile, and others.

Postmenopausal women have an increased risk of osteoporosis and atherosclerosis/coronary artery disease compared with menstruating females.

► **Treatment Steps**

Calcium, exercise, dietary changes, and lubricants for sexual activity. If poor libido, may add low-dose testosterone. Hormone replacement therapy is controversial (see Cram Facts).

6. Premenstrual Syndrome (PMS)

► **Description**

Multiple symptoms prior to menses.

► **Symptoms/Diagnosis**

Anxiety, bloating, headache, depression, acne, breast tenderness, aggression. Clinical diagnosis.

Four subtypes have been described, including A, C, H, D (anxiety, carbohydrate, H_2O [edema], and depression).

► **Pathology**

Despite multiple studies, etiology *remains* unknown. Low progesterone levels seem to be the most accepted hypothesis.

► Treatment Steps

Counseling, exercise, diet (reduce sugar, salt, alcohol, caffeine), vitamin B_6, progesterone, diuretics. None have been proven to be effective in double-blind placebo-controlled studies.

7. Virilization and Hirsutism

► Description

- *Hirsutism* is **excessive sexual hair.**
- *Virilization* is **excessive androgenic influence** (acne, balding, deep voice, increased strength, clitoromegaly, amenorrhea in severe cases, etc.).
- *Hypertrichosis* is **excessive nonsexual hair,** may be drug or hereditary etiology.

► Diagnosis

History and physical. Serum testosterone, 17-OH progesterone levels, DHEAS level, and other testing including **dexamethasone-suppression test** to rule out **Cushing's disease,** ultrasound. Adrenocorticotropic hormone (ACTH) stimulation test rules out congenital adrenal hyperplasia.

► Pathology

1. Ovarian (PCOS)—increased testosterone production by the theca in chronic anovulatory women.
2. Adrenal (especially congenital adrenal hyperplasia). Enzymatic defect in adrenal steroid pathways leads to build-up of androgen precursor products.
3. Metabolic—peripheral metabolism of testosterone.

► Treatment Steps

1. Ovarian source—OCs, GnRH analogs, ovarian wedge resection.
2. Adrenal source—dexamethasone suppression.
3. Metabolic source—spironolactone, flutamide.

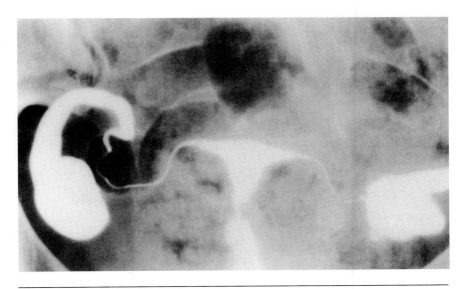

Figure 13–5. Hysterosalpingogram revealing severe bilateral hydrosalpinx. (Reproduced, with permission, from Gant NF, Cunningham FG. *Basic Gynecology and Obstetrics.* Norwalk, CT: Appleton & Lange,) 1993.

8. Infertility

► Description

Inability to conceive after 1 year of unprotected intercourse.
- Primary infertility—never pregnant (G_0P_0).
- Secondary infertility—pregnant at least once ($\geq G_1$).
- About 15% of all couples in the United States are infertile.

► Diagnosis

History and physical (both partners). Complex protocol for workup including semen analysis, basal body temperature, hysterosalpingogram (see Fig. 13–5), endometrial biopsy, postcoital test, antisperm antibodies, luteal progesterone levels; if all above is negative—screening laparoscopy.

► Pathology

- 40% male factors (low sperm count, low motility).
- 40% female factors (anovulation, tubal blockage).
- 10–20% idiopathic.
- Other causes: endometriosis, luteal phase defect, antisperm antibodies, STD, pelvic adhesions, intrauterine adhesions.

► Treatment Steps

1. Male factor: intrauterine insemination, donor insemination, in vitro fertilization (IVF).
2. Female factor: ovulation induction, tubal surgery, IVF, uterine surgery, GnRH analogs (for fibroids or endometriosis).
3. Unexplained: injectable gonadotropins with insemination, IVF.

BIBLIOGRAPHY

Beckmann CR, Ling FW, et al. *Obstetrics and Gynecology,* 4th ed. Baltimore: Lippincott Wiliams & Wilkins, 2002.

Cunningham FG, MacDonald PC, et al. *Williams Obstetrics,* 22nd ed. Norwalk, CT: Appleton-Century-Crofts, 2005.

DeChenney AH, Pernoll ML. *Current Obstetric and Gynecologic Diagnosis and Treatment,* 9th ed. Norwalk, CT: Appleton & Lange, 2002.

Gant NF, Cunningham FG. *Basic Gynecology and Obstetrics.* Norwalk, CT: Appleton & Lange, 1993.

Congenital Anomalies and Perinatal Medicine | 14

I. MALFORMATIONS—GENETIC FACTORS

Malformations are primary structural defects of development affecting 5% (**2% major**) of all newborns, causing 9% of perinatal deaths and 20–50% of spontaneous abortions. Causes include genetic, environmental, and unknown.

A. Down Syndrome (Trisomy 21)

► **Description**

Most common autosomal chromosome abnormality with a characteristic appearance. A common cause of **mental retardation** (1/700 live births).

► **Symptoms**

Newborn hypotonia, simian creases (50%), flat occiput, upslanting palpebral fissures, 40% with cardiac anomalies (ventricular septal defect [VSD], atrioventricular [AV] canal), duodenal atresia (4–7%), small stature, ocular problems, thyroid disease, chronic otitis media/hearing problems, atlantoaxial instability (12%), male sterility, obesity, leukemia (1%), premature senescence, life span typically to fourth or fifth decade.

► **Diagnosis**

Clinical with chromosome confirmation: classic trisomy 95% (sporadic), 4% translocation, 1% mosaic (see Fig. 14–1).

► **Treatment Steps**

1. Prenatal considerations—identification of increased risk profile: advanced maternal age, first-trimester serum α-fetoprotein (AFP), human chorionic gonadotropin (hCG), estriols.
2. Definitive prenatal diagnosis—amniocentesis, chorionic villus sampling if indicated.
3. Neonatal echocardiogram.
4. Genetic counseling (especially translocations).
5. Family support groups—optimal potential in home setting/special education.

► **cram facts**

CHROMOSOMAL ABNORMALITIES

- **Trisomy 21:** Down syndrome; 1/700 births; mental retardation, cardiac (AV canal), duodenal atresia, simian creases, epicanthal folds.
- **Trisomy 13:** poor prognosis; 1/10,000 births; cleft lip/palate, CNS malformations (holoprosencephaly), renal and ocular malformations.
- **Trisomy 18:** poor prognosis; 1/5,000 births; IUGR, clenched hands, rocker-bottom feet, cardiac (VSD, PDA).
- **5p:** cri du chat; cat-like cry, mental retardation, microcephaly.
- **45,XO:** Turner syndrome; 1/2,000 newborn girls; short webbed neck, horseshoe kidney, coarctation of aorta, primary amenorrhea.
- **47,XXY:** Klinefelter syndrome; 1/1,000 boys, seminiferous tubule dysgenesis, hypogonadism, tall stature, gynecomastia, infertility.

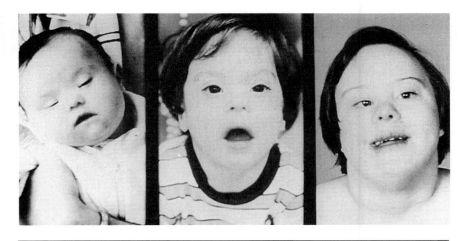

Figure 14–1. Typical phenotype in Down syndrome.

B. Trisomy 18 (Edwards' Syndrome)

▶ Description

Second most frequent autosomal disorder (1/5,000) with severe malformations.

▶ Symptoms

Intrauterine growth retardation (IUGR), micrognathia, **clenched hand,** overlapping fingers, **rocker-bottom feet, congenital heart disease** (VSD, patent ductus arteriosus [PDA]), mental retardation, central nervous system (CNS) malformation.

▶ Diagnosis

Clinical with chromosome confirmation. Translocations rare.

▶ Treatment Steps

1. Aggressive treatment usually not indicated; 50% die by 1 week, 5–10% survive 1 year.
2. Grief and genetic counseling.
3. Recurrence < 1% if no translocation.

C. Trisomy 13 (Patau's Syndrome)

▶ Description

Third most common autosomal disorder (1/10,000) with severe malformations.

▶ Symptoms

Cleft lip and/or **palate** (60–80%), CNS malformation **(holoprosencephaly),** microcephaly, **urinary tract** malformations, **ocular** malformations, polydactyly.

▶ Diagnosis

Clinical with chromosome confirmation.

▶ Treatment Steps

1. Aggressive treatment usually not indicated; 80% die by 1 month, 5% survive 6 months.
2. Grief and genetic counseling.
3. Recurrence < 1% if no translocation.

► **cram facts**

MATERNAL SERUM α-FETOPROTEIN (MSAFP)	
ELEVATED	**DECREASED**
Neural tube defect	Chromosomal anomaly
Intrauterine fetal demise	(Trisomy 21, 13, 18; Turner syndrome)
Multiple gestation	Missed abortion
Omphalocele defect	Hydatidiform mole
Normal pregnancy	Normal pregnancy

D. 5p Syndrome (Cri du Chat Syndrome)

► Description

Chromosome deletion syndrome named for the characteristic **cat-like cry.**

► Symptoms

Mental retardation, microcephaly, congenital heart disease.

► Diagnosis

Clinical, chromosome confirmation; 15% parental translocation.

► Treatment Steps

1. Supportive environment, special schooling.
2. Family and genetic counseling.
3. May function at 5- to 6-year-old level.

E. Gonadal Dysgenesis 45,XO (Turner's Syndrome)

► Description

Most common female sex chromosome disorder in which there is only one X chromosome (1/2,500 newborn girls).

► Symptoms

Most are spontaneously aborted in early pregnancy (95%). **Transient lymphedema** feet and hands at birth (80–90%), **short webbed neck,** short fourth metacarpal, renal anomalies **(horseshoe kidney),** cardiac defects **(coarctation of aorta), short stature,** lack of secondary sex characteristics with **primary amenorrhea** (due to **gonadal dysgenesis), normal intelligence.**

► Diagnosis

Clinical with chromosome confirmation (60% chromatin negative 45,XO, 40% mosaic).

► Treatment Steps

1. Identify any associated anomalies.
2. Family and genetic counseling.
3. Estrogen replacement at puberty.
4. Consider growth hormone therapy.

F. Seminiferous Tubule Dysgenesis 47,XXY (Klinefelter's Syndrome)

► Description

Male sex chromosome abnormality with extra X chromosome (1/1,000 newborn boys).

► Symptoms

Hypogonadism (number one cause in males), infertility, gynecomastia, tall stature, behavior problems. Mean intelligence quotient (IQ) 80–90 with great variability.

► Diagnosis

Chromosomes.

► Treatment Steps

1. Testosterone replacement at 12 years old, if indicated.
2. School support in reading, spelling.

G. Fragile X Syndrome

► Description

Abnormality of X chromosome and common cause of mental retardation in males (1/1,000); can also affect females.

► Symptoms

Prominent ears, long face, **macro-orchidism, mental retardation,** seizures, hyperactivity.

► Diagnosis

Chromosomes with fragile X study.

► Treatment Steps

1. Family and genetic counseling.
2. Special education.

H. Achondroplasia

► Description

The most common genetic skeletal dysplasia (1/15,000), with characteristic features. **Autosomal dominant,** 90% new mutations in gene for fibroblast growth factor receptor 3.

► Symptoms/Diagnosis

Short limbs (especially proximally), low nasal bridge, large head and forehead, small foramen magnum, kyphosis, **hydrocephalus,** severe otitis media (see Fig. 14–2). Usually normal intelligence and life span. Clinical diagnosis.

► Treatment Steps

1. Family and genetic counseling.
2. Follow closely for hydrocephalus.
3. Careful head support—spinal cord injury risk due to small forumen magnum.
4. Treat spine complications.

I. Xeroderma Pigmentosa

► Description

Defect in deoxyribonucleic acid (DNA) repair mechanism of ultraviolet radiation–induced lesions, causing **skin scarring** and **malignancy** (1/250,000 individuals).

► Features

Sunlight sensitivity (from first exposure), skin atrophy, **basal** and squamous cell carcinomas, melanomas, conjunctivitis leading to scarring and **blindness.** Seizures, developmental delay.

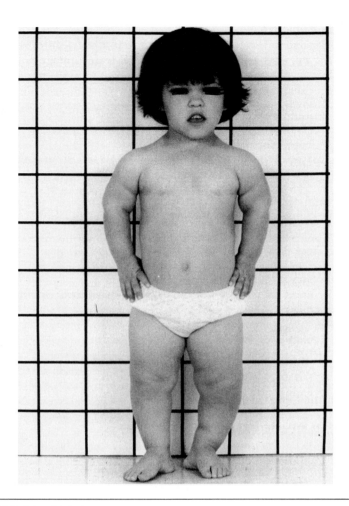

Figure 14–2. Achondroplasia.

▶ Diagnosis

Autosomal recessive. Clinical diagnosis plus characteristic biopsy. May be fatal before adulthood due to malignancies. Seventy percent survival to age 40.

▶ Treatment Steps

1. Strict avoidance of sun exposure.
2. Close dermatologic and neurologic monitoring.

II. MALFORMATIONS—MATERNAL/ENVIRONMENTAL FACTORS

A. Fetal Alcohol Effects/Syndrome

▶ Description

Results from fetal exposure through maternal alcohol use. Fetal alcohol exposure is **the most common teratogen** and a leading cause of mental retardation.

▶ Symptoms

Intrauterine growth retardation, **mental retardation** (mean IQ 63), microcephaly, flattened philtrum, thin upper lip, upturned nose, cardiac defects (septal). Early failure to thrive, hyperactivity.

► Diagnosis
Clinical.

► Treatment Steps
1. Counseling and prenatal care.
2. Most damaging in first trimester but alcohol use during pregnancy is never safe.
3. Special education programs.

B. Tobacco
Considered a common cause of intrauterine **growth retardation.**

C. Cocaine
Maternal use during pregnancy can cause CNS damage, low birth weight, urinary tract abnormalities in newborns. Placental abruption. Also, dependence in the neonate.

D. Coumadin Derivatives
Fetal warfarin syndrome: typical facial features, auditory and ocular defects, CNS malformations, mental retardation, perinatal hemorrhage.

E. Thalidomide
A popular antiemetic for pregnant women in the 1960s, caused **phocomelia** (absence of long bones in extremities). Recently approved in the United States to treat leprosy.

F. Fetal Hydantoin Syndrome
Maternal use of this antiseizure medication causes congenital heart defects, nail hypoplasia, growth retardation, mental retardation.

G. Tetracycline
Maternal use in second and third trimester causes **tooth enamel** hypoplasia and staining.

H. Maternal Diabetes (Infant of Diabetic Mother)
Increases risk of congenital anomalies **threefold:** congenital heart defects, sacral agenesis, anencephaly, small left colon, and caudal regression syndrome.

I. Maternal Phenylketonuria
If mother **not** controlled with diet, infant with increased risk for **mental retardation,** microcephaly, heart defects.

J. Congenital Syphilis

► Description
Congenital infection caused by **spirochete** *(Treponema pallidum)* with multiorgan involvement and variable severity, usually transmitted in later pregnancy.

► Symptoms

Early—(Only 40% of infected newborns are symptomatic at birth) rash **(palms and soles), snuffles** (blood-tinged nasal discharge), hepatosplenomegaly, jaundice, pseudoparalysis of Parrot (periostitis), anemia, often asymptomatic early.

Late—Frontal bossing, saber shins, Hutchinson (peg) teeth, **saddle nose.**

► Diagnosis

Serology (rapid plasma reagin [RPR], fluorescent treponemal antibody absorption [FTA-ABS]), dark-field examination. Cerebrospinal fluid (CSF), Veneral Disease Research Laboratory (VDRL).

► Treatment Steps

1. Screen all pregnant women for syphilis.
2. Treat all mothers/infants with positive maternal serology without *documented* adequate treatment with IV penicillin (Jarisch–Herxheimer reaction common).

K. Congenital Cytomegalovirus Infection

► Description

A herpesvirus, the most common cause of congenital infection in the United States. Most severe if transmitted in early pregnancy. Ubiquitous virus. Transmitted during both primary and secondary maternal infection.

► Symptoms

Majority (93%) are asymptomatic at birth. Hepatosplenomegaly, jaundice, chorioretinitis, **deafness, microcephaly,** petechial rash, developmental delay, periventricular **CNS calcifications.**

► Diagnosis

Urine isolation, serology.

► Treatment Steps

1. Antiviral therapy for congenital cytomegalovirus (CMV) is not proven.
2. Symptomatic treatment.

L. Congenital Toxoplasmosis Infection

► Description

Intracellular protozoan parasite *(Toxoplasma gondii),* which can affect fetus in all trimesters (usually the third).

► Symptoms

Hydrocephalus, chorioretinitis (99%), microcephaly, scattered CNS calcifications, developmental delay.

► **cram facts**

CONGENITAL INFECTIONS (STORCH)

- **S**yphilis: *Treponena pallidum;* snuffles, palm and sole rash, anemia, hepatosplenomegaly, periostitis, peg teeth, saddle nose; Rx penicillin.
- **T**oxoplasmosis: *Toxoplasma gondii;* oocysts from cat litter and meat; hydrocephalus, chorioretinitis, scattered CNS calcifications; Rx pyrimethamine.
- **O**ther: HIV, hepatis B, varicella.
- **R**ubella: blueberry muffin lesions, hepatosplenomegaly, anemia, cardiac lesions, deafness, cataracts.
- **C**ytomegalovirus: most common congenital infection; usually asymptomatic; hepatosplenomegaly, jaundice, deafness, microcephaly, perventricular CNS calcifications.
- **H**erpes simplex: usually acquired at birth; seizures (temporal lobe); encephalitis, vesicles, overwhelming sepsis, hepatitis; Rx acyclovir.

► Diagnosis

Serology, parasites in CSF.

► Treatment Steps

1. Prevention: Counsel pregnant women to avoid cat litter, infected meat (sources of *Toxoplasma* oocysts).
2. Shunt for hydrocephalus.
3. Pyrimethamine, sulfadiazine, and leukovorin for 1 year.
4. Multidisciplinary medical management.

M. Congenital Rubella Infection (German Measles)

► Description

Virus occurring in epidemics that causes multiple congenital anomalies, especially in first-trimester exposure. Incidence greatly decreased with immunizations, obstetric serology screening.

► Symptoms

Hepatosplenomegaly, **"blueberry muffin"** lesions, anemia with extramedullary hematopoiesis, thrombocytopenia, **cardiac lesions** (PDA, VSD), **cataracts,** mental retardation, **deafness.**

► Diagnosis

Serology, virus isolation (pharyngeal, urine, CSF).

N. Herpes Simplex Virus (HSV)

► Description

Neonatal HSV infection affects 1 of 5,000 deliveries, occasionally by in utero transmission (10%) but usually at delivery. Most common HSV-2 (70%), highest transmission during **primary maternal infection.**

► Symptoms

- Intrauterine—**seizures,** microcephaly, chorioretinitis, CNS calcifications.
- Neonatal acquired—**encephalitis seizures, skin vesicular lesions** (also eye and mouth). Overwhelming sepsis with disseminated infection.

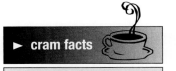

► **cram facts**

A woman with a herpes outbreak at the time of delivery should have a C-section to avoid transmission of herpes to the newborn.

► Diagnosis

Symptoms at birth of scarring, chorioretinitis, and hydranencephaly may have intrauterine growth retardation, microcephaly, strabismus.

► Treatment Steps

1. Antiviral therapy (acyclovir or vidarabine).
2. Pediatric infectious disease consult.

O. Human Immunodeficiency Virus (HIV)

► Description

Ninety percent of pediatric HIV infection in the United States is from vertical transmission from HIV+ mother. Untreated newborns usually develop full-blown acquired immune deficiency syndrome (AIDS) by 5–8 years of age.

► Symptoms

Infected newborns usually asymptomatic but usually show first symptoms by 6 months. Generalized lymphadenopathy, multiple bacterial infections, hepatosplenomegaly, chronic diarrhea, persistent thrush, poor growth, respiratory distress (lymphoid interstitial pneumonitis, *Pneumocystis carinii* pneumonia [PCP]), pancytopenia.

► Diagnosis

Early newborn serology limited—reflects maternal state. Polymerase chain reaction (PCR)-DNA most sensitive (50% at newborn, 94% at 0–4 months), HIV culture, p24 antigen. Can completely rule out vertical HIV by 2 years of age.

► Treatment Steps

1. Intrapartum maternal treatment (oral zidovudine [azidothymidine, AZT] last 2 trimesters plus IV AZT during labor) plus 6 weeks oral AZT for newborns decreases vertical transmission from 28% to only 8%.
2. Close clinical and lab monitoring of at-risk newborns.
3. Inactivated polio vaccine, annual influenza vaccine, pneumococcal vaccine, annual purified protein derivative (PPD) tuberculosis (TB) test, trimethoprim–sulfamethoxazole PCP prophylaxis.
4. Antiretroviral therapy including reverse transcriptase inhibitors and protease inhibitors for proven HIV infection.

III. RENAL AND URINARY SYSTEM DISORDERS

Of all newborn abdominal masses, 60% are renal in origin, and ultrasound is the imaging modality of choice.

A. Hypospadias

► Description/Diagnosis

Anomaly of penile urethra that opens on ventral glans, shaft, or perineum. Clinical diagnosis.

► Symptoms

Hooded prepuce, chordee (ventral curving of penis), undescended testis (10%); **if severe,** consider ambiguous genitalia.

► Treatment Steps

1. Avoid circumcision—save foreskin for reconstruction.
2. Surgical reconstruction in first year.

B. Bladder Exstrophy

► Description

Uncommon (1/20,000 births) congenital absence of anterior wall of bladder and abdomen, with exposure of bladder mucosa.

► Symptoms

Pubic rami and rectus muscles widely separated, males with **epispadias** (urethra opens on dorsum of penis), undescended testes, inguinal hernia, severe genitourinary (GU) reflux.

► Treatment Steps

1. Cover exposed bladder with plastic wrap.
2. Surgical closure within 24 hours.
3. Family counseling, multidisciplinary approach.
4. Urinary control, ambulation, and sexual function usually preserved.

C. Prune-Belly Syndrome (Eagle–Barrett Syndrome)

Triad of **deficient abdominal muscles, undescended testes,** and **urinary tract abnormalities.** Prognosis based on degree of renal and pulmonary dysplasia (1/30,000 live births).

D. Posterior Urethral Valves

▶ Description

Congenitally abnormal sail-like valves in male posterior urethra causing variable degrees of obstruction.

▶ Symptoms

If severe, may be stillborn with **Potter syndrome** due to severe oligohydramnios (lung hypoplasia, fetal compression: **flat nose, recessed chin, low-set ears**). Milder cases may present with abdominal masses (hydronephrosis), urinary tract infections (UTIs), or a **weak urinary stream.**

▶ Diagnosis

Voiding cystourethrography.

▶ Treatment Steps

1. Transurethral endoscopic valve ablation.
2. Prognosis based on renal and pulmonary damage.

E. Ureteropelvic Junction (UPJ) Obstruction

Common cause of congenital renal obstruction, usually unilateral (80%).

F. Unilateral Renal Agenesis

Usually seen on left, often with single umbilical artery (1/1,000 births).

G. Multicystic Kidney

Nonfunctioning, unilateral cystic flank mass with little or no identifiable renal tissue. Usually excised due to possible risk of later malignancy or infection.

H. Polycystic Diseases of the Kidney

1. Infantile

Autosomal recessive inheritance presenting at birth with severe oligohydramnios/Potter syndrome or bilateral flank masses and hypertension. Multiple small renal cysts. Congenital hepatic fibrosis. Poor prognosis.

2. Adult

Autosomal dominant, cause of **renal failure** in adults, usually presents in the fourth or fifth decade. Variable number of renal cysts, **may** have some cysts beginning in childhood.

I. Undescended Testicle (Cryptorchidism)

▶ Description

Failure of location of testes in scrotum. Location may be intra-abdominal, inguinal canal, ectopic, or absent. Bilateral 25%. Incidence in preterm infants 17%, newborns 3%, children/adults 0.7%. Testis rarely spontaneously descends after 1 year of life. Often associated indirect inguinal hernia.

► Diagnosis

Clinical, must differentiate from **retractable testis.** Ultrasound, magnetic resonance imaging (MRI), or laparoscopy may be helpful if testis not palpable.

► Treatment Steps

1. Testis palpable: watch for descent. Orchiopexy after 1 year.
2. Testes not palpable: consider hCG trial if bilateral.
3. Orchiectomy for atrophied testis due to risk of malignancy and infertility for contralateral testis.

J. Pseudohermaphroditism

► Description

A state in which an individual is distinctly one sex or another with somatic characteristics of both sexes.

1. Female

Genotype XX, ovaries and uterus with virilized genitalia due to androgen exposure.

    a. **Congenital adrenal hyperplasia (adrenogenital syndrome [CAH])**—disorder of steroidogenesis, 95% caused by **21 hydroxylase deficiency** with **ambiguous genitalia,** 50–75% **salt losing** with severe life-threatening **hyperkalemia.**

    b. **Maternal use of androgens in pregnancy.**

► Diagnosis

Elevated serum 17-OH progesterone. **Newborn screening** program in some states.

► Treatment Steps

1. Treat severe hyperkalemia with calcium, alkalinization, insulin/glucose, kayexalate.
2. Glucocorticoid and mineralocorticoid replacement.

2. Male

Genotype XY, lack of virilization. Testicular feminization: phenotypic female with blind vaginal pouch due to **lack of testosterone receptors;** X-linked recessive. Typically presents in later childhood with inguinal masses (testes) or amenorrhea. Careful psychosocial counseling and education to determine gender assignment.

IV. RESPIRATORY SYSTEM DISORDERS

A. Pierre Robin Anomaly

Severe **micrognathia** (hypoplastic mandible) plus glossoptosis (displacement of tongue downward), causing variable degrees of respiratory distress. Airway problems usually resolve as child grows.

B. Choanal Atresia

► Description

Unilateral or bilateral bony (90%) or membranous (10%) septum between nose and pharynx.

► Symptoms

Respiratory distress/cyanosis **relieved by crying** (bilateral); unilateral discharge (unilateral). Up to 50% with associated anomalies. **CHARGE**

syndrome (**c**oloboma of eye, **h**eart defects, **a**tresia of choanae, **r**etardation, **g**enital hypoplasia/cryptorchidism, **e**ar anomalies).

► Diagnosis

Inability to pass catheter through nostril to pharynx, confirm with computed tomographic (CT) scan.

► Treatment Steps

1. Respiratory support, oral airway if bilateral.
2. Bilateral repaired in infancy.
3. Unilateral repaired electively at 2–5 years.

C. Congenital Laryngeal Stridor (Laryngomalacia)

► Description

Most common congenital laryngeal abnormality. Increased flexibility of larynx with intermittent collapse and airway obstruction on inspiration (crowing respirations). Worst in early infancy, exacerbated with crying or prone position. Diagnose clinically by fluoroscopy or direct laryngoscopy. Visually self-limited but may need airway support if severe, failure to thrive. Also consider vocal cord paralysis, true airway lesions (hemangiomas, papillomas, webs).

D. Vascular Rings and Slings

Anomalous thoracic vessels compressing the airway causing wheezing or stridor. Examples include double aortic arch, right aortic arch with either aberrant subclavian artery or ligamentum arterosum (PDA remnant). Barium swallow, airway fluoroscopy, echocardiograms, and MRI helpful for diagnosis.

E. Congenital Lobar Emphysema

► Description

Number one congenital lung lesion, usually unilateral lobar hyperinflation (often left upper lobe) due to early in utero bronchial obstruction with **normal alveolar** histology.

► Symptoms

Newborn respiratory distress, mediastinal shift.

► Diagnosis

Chest radiograph with hyperinflation (must distinguish from pneumothorax).

► Treatment Steps

Surgical resection.

F. Cystic Adenomatoid Malformation

► Description

Number two congenital lung lesion, single enlarged lobe due to early **embryonic** insult with **little normal lung tissue** seen in the cystic structures.

► Symptoms

Newborn respiratory distress, mediastinal shift.

► Diagnosis

Chest radiographic variable with opaque or multiple cystic areas (must distinguish from diaphragmatic hernia).

► Treatment Steps
Surgical resection.

G. Pulmonary Sequestration

► Description
Segments of embryonic lung tissue that is nonfunctional and nourished by anomalous systemic vessels. May present with infection, respiratory distress.

1. **Intralobar**—within normal visceral pleura, 2/3 left-sided; arterial supply, aorta. Venous drainage, pulmonary veins.
2. **Extralobar**—separate visceral pleural covering, 90% left-sided, arterial supply, pulmonary artery or systemic artery. Venous drainage, azygos or portal vein.

► Diagnosis
Chest x-ray (CXR), chest CT/MRI, arteriogram.

► Treatment Steps
Surgery as indicated.

H. Diaphragmatic Hernia

► Description
Disorder of fetal diaphragm development with intrusion of abdominal contents into the thorax (1/2,000 births).

► Symptoms
• **Foramen of Bochdalek** hernia—left-sided 90%, severe newborn respiratory distress, scaphoid abdomen, mediastinal shift, pulmonary hypoplasia.
• **Foramen of Morgagni** hernia—often presents later as a bowel obstruction.

► Diagnosis
Clinical, CXR shows bowel in thorax. Often diagnosed at prenatal ultrasound.

► Treatment Steps
1. Aggressive newborn resuscitation.
2. Consider extracorporeal membrane oxygenation (ECMO) or high-frequency ventilation if deteriorates.
3. Surgical correction when stable.
4. Prognosis depends on degree of pulmonary hypoplasia.

V. CARDIOVASCULAR SYSTEM DISORDERS

Congenital heart disease (CHD) is present in 8 of 1,000 live births; 50% present in first month, most multifactorial inheritance.

• Cyanotic lesions—right (R)-to-left (L) shunt.
• Acyanotic lesions—obstructive or L-to-R shunt.
• **Eisenmenger syndrome**—long-standing L-to-R shunt causing pulmonary hypertension and reversal to R-to-L (cyanotic) flow.

Common presentations of congestive heart failure (CHF) in infants include **feeding difficulties, sweating, failure to thrive, tachycardia, hepatomegaly, respiratory distress.**

▶ differential diagnosis

CONGENITAL HEART DISEASE

Cyanotic
- **Tetralogy of Fallot:** RV outflow obstruction/VSD/overriding aorta/RVH: most common cyanotic CHD; "tet spells," boot-shaped heart.
- **Transposition of the great vessels:** aorta arises RV, pulmonary artery arises LV; "egg on a string" heart; balloon atrial septostomy, then arterial switch.
- **Total anomalous pulmonary venous return:** pulmonary veins drain into systemic venous circulation (total or partial); "snowman" heart.
- **Truncus arteriosus:** single great artery is origin of aorta and pulmonary artery and coronary artery; truncal valve click.

Noncyanotic
- **Ventricular septal defect:** most common CHD, holosystolic murmur, usually presents first 1–2 months, subacute bacterial endocarditis (SBE) prophylaxis.
- **Coarctation of aorta:** pressure gradient upper extremity (UE) > lower extremity (LE), poor femoral pulses, Turner syndrome; rib notching CXR, balloon angioplasty.
- **Atrial septal defect:** pulmonary ejection murmur plus wide split S2. No SBE prophylaxis, usually presents after infancy.
- **Patent ductus arteriosus:** premature babies; congenital rubella; continuous machinery murmur, wide pulse pressure.
- **Hypoplastic left heart:** underdeveloped LV and aorta; vascular collapse in first week; ductus dependent, prostaglandin E treatment initially; Norwood or transplant.

A. Coarctation of the Aorta

See Chapter 1, section VII.D.

B. Patent Ductus Arteriosus (PDA)

See Chapter 1, section VII.C.

C. Ventricular Septal Defect (VSD)

See Chapter 1, section VII.A.

D. Atrial Septal Defect (ASD)

See Chapter 1, section VII.B.

E. Endocardial Cushion Defect/Ostium Primum (AV Canal)

See Chapter 1, section VII.F.

F. Hypoplastic Left Heart Syndrome

▶ **Description**
Underdeveloped left ventricle and ascending aorta often with mitral valve abnormalities or AV canal. Responsible for up to 20% CHD neonatal deaths.

▶ **Symptoms**
Ductal-dependent lesion: when PDA closes in first 2 weeks, get sudden cyanosis, respiratory distress, **acidosis,** and CHF with **vascular collapse.**

▶ **Diagnosis**
Echocardiogram diagnostic.

► Treatment Steps
1. Immediate prostaglandin E to keep ductus open.
2. Correction by heart transplant or staged cardiac reconstruction (Norwood procedure).

G. Tetralogy of Fallot (Fig. 14–3)

See Chapter 1, section VII.E.

H. Transposition of the Great Vessels (TGV)

► Description

Defect in which the aorta arises from right ventricle (RV) and pulmonary artery from left ventricle (LV), usually with mixing through VSD, ASD, or PDA (5% of all CHD).

► Symptoms

Cyanosis from birth, CHF. Later clubbing.

► Diagnosis

Clinical—RV heave with loud S2.

CXR—**Narrow cardiac waist, "egg on a string."**

ECG—Normal as newborn.

Echocardiogram—Diagnostic.

► Treatment Steps
1. Balloon atrial septostomy (Rashkind procedure) to increase atrial level mixing.

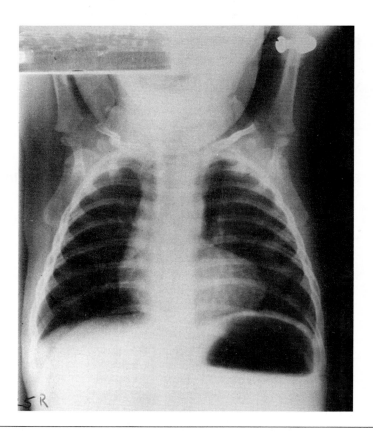

Figure 14–3. "Boot-shaped" heart in tetralogy of Fallot.

2. Definitive arterial switch repair has mostly replaced mustard (atrial baffle) procedure.

I. Truncus Arteriosus

▶ **Description**
A single great artery arising from the base of the heart giving origin to the coronary, pulmonary, and systemic arteries, usually with VSD (2% of all CHD).

▶ **Symptoms**
Presentation dependent on the specific anatomy and degree of pulmonary flow. May be increased flow with CHF or decreased flow with cyanosis.

▶ **Diagnosis**
May hear ejection click of truncal valve.

CXR—Right aortic arch 33%.

Electrocardiogram (ECG)—Right ventricular hypertrophy (RVH).

Echocardiogram—Cardiac catheterization.

▶ **Treatment Steps**
1. Treat CHF.
2. Surgical repair to avoid persistent pulmonary hypertension.

J. Total Anomalous Pulmonary Venous Return

Anomalous pulmonary veins drain **partially** or **totally** into systemic venous circulation (right atrium [RA], superior vena cava [SVC], inferior vena cava [IVC], portal veins) instead of left atrium. May have **cyanosis,** often with ASD. Heart may have "snowman" appearance on CXR.

▶ **Treatment Steps**
1. Medical management.
2. Definitive surgical repair.

VI. NERVOUS SYSTEM AND SPECIAL SENSES

A. Hydrocephalus

▶ **Description**
Condition of impaired circulation, absorption, or overproduction of CSF leading to **increased intracranial pressure (ICP)** and risk of brain herniation.

1. Communicating Hydrocephalus
Blockage of CSF outside the ventricular system or its exit foramina or an overproduction of CSF. Commonly from subarachnoid and intraventricular hemorrhage as seen in premature infants and postmeningitis, causing obstruction of arachnoid villi with decreased CSF resorption.

2. Noncommunicating Hydrocephalus
Ventricular system obstruction including:

a. **Aqueductal stenosis**—congenital, postinfectious.

b. **Chiari malformation**—low cerebellar tonsils.

c. Dandy–Walker cyst of fourth ventricle.

► Symptoms

Rapid increase in head circumference, split sutures, bulging anterior fontanelle, setting-sun sign (of eyes), irritability, lethargy, vomiting, *sixth nerve palsy, papilledema, long tract signs.*

► Diagnosis

Clinical plus head CT scan. **Avoid lumbar puncture: risk of herniation.**

► Treatment Steps

1. Emergency management for signs of severe increased ICP including hyperventilation, osmotherapy (mannitol).
2. Emergency ventriculoperitoneal (VP) shunt usually indicated.

B. Congenital Cataract

► Description

Any opacity of the lens—requires early intervention to prevent permanent visual impairment.

► Pathology

Hereditary (autosomal dominant/recessive, X-linked), chromosomal abnormalities (trisomies), congenital infection (**rubella,** CMV, toxoplasmosis), metabolic (**galactosemia,** hypocalcemia), prematurity (usually resolves spontaneously).

► Treatment Steps

1. Surgical removal of lens material.
2. Correction of resultant retractive errors with spectacles.
3. Correction of sensory deprivation amblyopia.

C. Congenital Glaucoma

► Description

Abnormal elevation of intraocular pressure, causing eye damage and visual impairment. May present with **tearing,** photophobia, **corneal clouding,** eye enlargement, conjunctivitis. Seen in Sturge–Weber syndrome (facial port-wine stain, seizures, CNS calcifications), neurofibromatosis, congenital rubella, and retinopathy of prematurity. Treatment is surgical.

D. Congenital Deafness

► Description

Conductive (abnormal sound transmission up to middle ear) or **sensorineural** (disorder of inner ear or auditory nerve) hearing disorder. Hearing loss often manifested by delay in language skills.

► Pathology

Syndromes:

- *Waardenburg* (autosomal dominant, **white forelock**).
- *Alport* (X-linked dominant, **nephritis**).
- *Familial* (70% recessive).
- *Craniofacial anomaly/syndrome* (Pierre Robin, Treacher–Collins, Crouzon's).
- *Isolated ear malformations.*
- *Congenital infection* (CMV, rubella).
- *Maternal ototoxic drugs.*
- *Prematurity.*

► Diagnosis

Clinical suspicion (especially by caretaker). Screen high-risk newborns (family history, ear anomalies, congenital infections, prematurity) with auditory-evoked brain stem response test, audiology assessment. Universal screening at birth identifies congenital causes.

► Treatment Steps

1. Evaluate for early amplification device.
2. Consider surgical implant if indicated.
3. Counseling, family support. Consider sign language, lip reading.

E. Neural Tube Defects

► Description

Failure of neural tube closure in utero (normally closes by day 26). Degrees of severity include: *spina bifida occulta* (incomplete closure of the posterior lumbosacral spinal cord) (see Fig. 14–4), *meningocele* (herniation of the meninges through the spinal canal defect without neural tissue), *encephalocele* (herniation of the meninges and brain substance through a skull defect, *myelomeningocele* (severe herniation of the meninges and spinal cord), and *anencephaly* (congenital absence of the cerebral hemisphere and cranial vault). Associated with hydrocephalus, Arnold–Chiari malformation, and tethered cord syndrome.

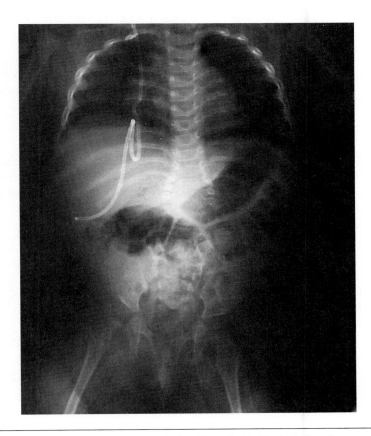

Figure 14–4. Spina bifida. Radiographic study of an 11-month-old with a lumbothoracic myelomeningocele who had undergone a surgical repair as a neonate. A right ventriculoperitoneal shunt was placed for the associated hydrocephalus.

► Symptoms

Signs and symptoms depend on the region of spinal cord involved and the extent of the lesion. Clues to diagnosis are **sacral dimple, tuft of hair, or birthmark** over the spine. Asymptomatic or disturbances of bowel, bladder, and motor function. Seventy-five percent of anencephalics are stillborn. Majority have normal intelligence.

► Diagnosis

Prenatal ultrasonography. **MSAFP.** Maternal acetylcholinesterase (ACHE). Clinical exam, MRI.

► Treatment Steps

1. Prevention by **maternal folate supplementation** during pregnancy.
2. Cover lesion with sterile saline-soaked dressing.
3. Surgical resection and closure, unless vital neurologic or vascular structures involved.
4. Orthopedic and urologic investigation and intervention.
5. Monitor for subsequent hydrocephalus.

VII. MUSCULOSKELETAL AND SKIN DISORDERS

A. Osteogenesis Imperfecta (Brittle Bone Disease)

► Description

Inherited disorder of collagen characterized by variable bone fragility.

► Symptoms

There are four types with variable severity. Severe form (type II) = early death. **Blue sclera,** hearing loss, **osteoporosis, multiple fractures,** teeth deformities, growth retardation. Autosomal dominant or recessive.

► Diagnosis

Child abuse a common differential diagnosis when multiple fractures. Triad of positive family history, frequent fractures, or blue sclera not 100% sensitive. Need skin biopsy for definitive diagnosis.

► Treatment Steps

1. Genetic classification.
2. Orthopedic and dental care.
3. Genetic counseling.

B. Developmental (Congenital) Dysplasia of the Hip (DDH)

► Description

Spectrum of hip dysplasia ranging from mild subluxation to total dislocation of the femoral head from the acetabulum, due to multifactorial genetic plus environmental factors (1–2/1,000 births). Left hip most common. Leads to avascular necrosis.

► Symptoms

Risk factors include **female, breech** presentation, positive family history, neonatal positioning (excessive hip extension). Associated with torticollis, metatarsus varus, calcaneovalgus, talipes equinovarus (clubfoot).

► Diagnosis

Clinical exam: Asymmetric thigh creases or leg lengths, positive Ortolani sign (hip reducibility), positive Barlow sign (hip dislocatability), limitation of hip abduction (late sign). Hip ultrasonography. Hip radiograms (age 2–3 months).

► Treatment Steps

Management depends on degree of hip dysplasia.

1. Pavlik harness.
2. Closed reduction (traction).
3. Open surgical reduction (over age 6 months, failed above treatment).

C. Talipes Equinovarus (Clubfoot)

► Description

Complex foot deformity with plantar flexion, medial rotation, varus angulation, metatarsal adduction (1/1,000 births). Fifty percent bilateral.

► Symptoms

Severity varies. Increased risk of DDH.

► Diagnosis

Clinical exam. Foot small compared with opposite foot, deep medial foot crease, forefoot adducted, heel in equinovarus.

► Treatment Steps

1. Manipulation and serial corrective casting.
2. Surgical correction.

D. Congenital Torticollis (Wryneck)

► Description

Head tilts to affected side and chin rotates to opposite side. Usually due to sternocleidomastoid (SCM) fibrosis.

► Symptoms

Head tilt. Usually palpable subcutaneous mass over muscle.

► Diagnosis

Clinical exam.

► Treatment Steps

1. Resolution in 2–6 months with stretching exercises.
2. Differentiate from **Klippel–Feil syndrome** (cervical spine, renal, genital, cardiac, nervous system anomalies), isolated hemivertebra, unilateral absence of SCM.
3. Surgery if persists for over a year, facial asymmetry, limitation of neck movement by 30°.

E. Cerebral Palsy

See Chapter 11.

F. Albinism

Defect in the formation of the pigment melanin. Multiple variants, tyrosinase + or −. Autosomal recessive oculocutaneous forms common with numerous ocular abnormalities.

► Treatment Steps

1. Sun protection.
2. Ophthalmologic care.

3. Psychosocial support.
4. Genetic counseling.

G. Epidermolysis Bullosa

Heterogeneous group of congenital hereditary blistering disorders with lesions often produced by mechanical trauma. Range from mild simplex form to life-threatening fetalis form. Characteristic **mitten hand** deformities in severe cases. Autosomal dominant or recessive. Infection causes most morbidity/mortality.

▶ Treatment Steps
1. Multidisciplinary approach.
2. Prevention of infection and dehydration.
3. Dental and nutritional support.

VIII. GASTROINTESTINAL SYSTEM DISORDERS

A. Cleft Lip/Palate

▶ Description
Failure of primary (lip) and secondary (cleft) palate closure. Common (1/1,000 live births). **Multifactorial inheritance** (3–5% recurrence with affected parent or sibling; 10% if two parents or siblings).

▶ Symptoms
Associated with **feeding problems, otitis media, speech problems.** Linked with many syndromic disorders.

▶ Diagnosis
Clinical exam.

▶ Treatment Steps
1. Airway protection as needed.
2. Modified feeding nipple.
3. Surgical repair.
4. Multidisciplinary approach.

B. Tracheoesophageal Fistula (TEF)

▶ Description
Failure of trachea and esophagus to separate during embryogenesis. Tracheal-to-distal esophageal fistula with proximal esophageal atresia is most common type (85%). Survival dependent on birth weight and presence of major cardiac defects.

▶ Symptoms
Maternal polyhydramnios, excessive oral secretions, respiratory distress, signs or symptoms of aspiration pneumonia.

▶ Diagnosis
Failure to pass nasal catheter to stomach, air-distended proximal esophageal pouch on radiograph. Barium studies rarely needed. Surgical exploration.

▶ Treatment Steps
1. Usually initial gastrostomy tube.
2. Search for VATER or VACTERL association: **V**ertebral defects, **A**nal atresia, **C**ardiac anomalies, **T**racheo**E**sophageal fistula, **Re**nal anomalies, **L**imb malformations.
3. Surgical repair.

C. Duodenal Atresia

► Description
Complete obstruction of duodenal lumen. Associated with midgut malrotation, CHD, esophageal atresia.

► Symptoms
Maternal polyhydramnios. Bilious projectile emesis. Abdominal distention.

► Diagnosis
Double bubble on abdominal radiograph (air-distended stomach and proximal duodenum) (see Fig. 14–5). Barium study.

► Treatment Steps
1. Correct fluid and electrolyte imbalance.
2. Evaluate for associated congenital anomalies.
3. Surgical repair.

D. Pyloric Stenosis

► Description
Mechanical gastric outlet obstruction due to hypertrophied pylorus, increased in **males/firstborn** (1/250 births).

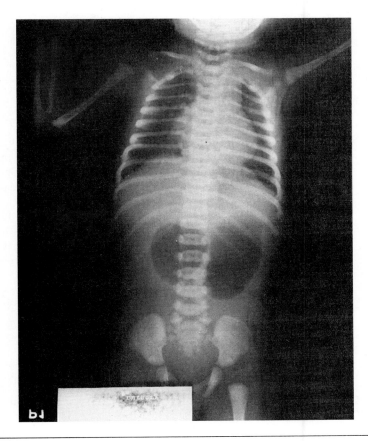

Figure 14–5. Duodenal atresia. Radiographic study of a 1-day-old infant with bilious emesis and features suggestive of Down syndrome. The "double-bubble sign" reflects the absence of distal bowel gas with two large gas bubbles in the stomach and proximal duodenum. Congenital heart disease is also noted.

► Symptoms

Progressive **nonbilious emesis (projectile).** Palpable right upper quadrant (RUQ) mass (olive). Peristaltic abdominal waves in epigastrium. Dehydration with hypochloremic alkalosis.

► Diagnosis

Clinical. Can confirm with ultrasound or barium study if necessary.

► Treatment Steps

Correction of fluid and electrolyte abnormality, then **pyloromyotomy.**

E. Malrotation of Small Intestine

► Description

Potentially life-threatening gastrointestinal (GI) malformation due to incomplete rotation of bowel. Mechanical obstruction from either poor fixation of cecum to abdominal wall (midgut volvulus or twisting) or extrinsic bands (Ladd's bands). Fifty percent present under age 1 month. Volvulus has 15–20% mortality rate.

► Symptoms

Neonatal bilious emesis **(think malrotation with volvulus),** abdominal distention, bloody stools (secondary to intestinal ischemia), signs or symptoms of peritonitis or perforation. Malrotation may be asymptomatic, found incidentally.

► Diagnosis

Clinical. Barium study: locate ligament of Treitz and cecum.

► Treatment Steps

1. Correct fluid and electrolyte imbalances.
2. Surgery.

F. Meckel's Diverticulum

► Description

Anomalous outpouching in distal ileum (proximal to ileocecal sphincter) 50–100 cm from ileocecal junction in 2% of population. Two types of ectopic tissue (pancreatic, gastric). Associated with other congenital anomalies (cardiac, Hirschsprung's disease, duodenal atresia, Down syndrome, omphalocele).

► Symptoms

Most common presentation is **painless rectal bleeding** (peak at 2 years). Also can present as abdominal pain, intussusception.

► Diagnosis

Clinical plus technetium-labeled nuclear scan, barium study.

► Treatment Steps

1. Correct life-threatening anemia.
2. Surgical excision.
3. Evaluate for associated congenital anomalies.

G. Congenital Megacolon (Hirschsprung's Disease)

Functional obstruction of colon due to absence of normal innervation (aganglionosis) of distal colon. (Auerbach's and Meissner's plexus). Increased mortality with enterocolitis.

► Symptoms

Presents as intestinal obstruction (with risk of enterocolitis), failure to pass meconium in first week, emesis, long-term constipation, abdominal distention. Presentation can simulate sepsis or necrotizing enterocolitis.

► Diagnosis

Clinical. Barium enema with **transition zone** (not always reliable) (see Fig. 14–6). **Rectal biopsy** to detect absence of ganglion cells for definitive diagnosis (80% involves rectum only; 20%, longer segment).

► Treatment Steps

1. Correct fluid and electrolyte imbalances.
2. Broad-spectrum antibiotics if enterocolitis suspected.
3. Surgical excision of a ganglionic segment.

H. Imperforate Anus

Failure of anal development. Fistulas associated with high lesions (above puborectal component of levator ani complex). Associated with **VACTERL anomalies.**

► Symptoms/Diagnosis

Absence of stool. Signs or symptoms of tethered cord or neurogenic bladder. Clinical diagnosis.

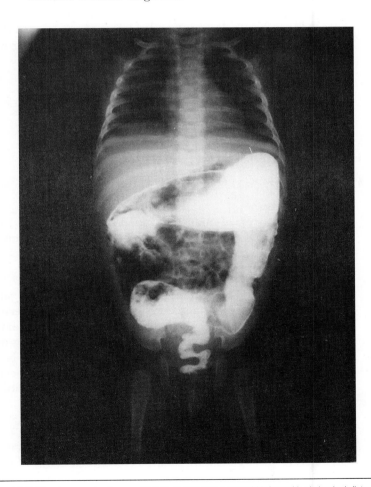

Figure 14–6. Hirschsprung's disease. Barium enema of a 4-day-old infant with abdominal distention, green emesis, a tight rectum, and an explosive liquid stool following the rectal examination. The lumen of the rectum is contracted with proximal colonic dilatation, suggesting congenital aganglionosis. The diagnosis was confirmed with a rectal biopsy.

▶ Treatment Steps
1. Evaluate for associated congenital anomalies.
2. Surgical repair.
3. Orthopedic and urologic care.

IX. HEMORRHAGIC AND HEMOLYTIC DISEASES

A. Hemorrhagic Disease of Newborn

▶ Description

Vitamin K deficiency causing decreased production of clotting factors II, VII, IX, X. Usually presents in first week of life. A delayed form due to malabsorption of vitamin K can occur at 4–12 weeks (i.e., liver disease, prolonged antibiotic use, cystic fibrosis).

▶ Symptoms

Bleeding from **GI tract,** nose, intracranium, or **circumcision site.** Increased risk with **prematurity,** breast feeding (poor source of vitamin K), or prenatal maternal drug use (**phenytoin,** phenobarbital, **salicylates,** Coumadin).

▶ Diagnosis

Suspect with bleeding in infants who have not received vitamin K. **Prolonged** prothrombin time (PT)/partial thromboplastin time (PTT), low serum clotting factors, presence of serum PIVKA (protein produced in vitamin K absence). **Normal bleeding time. Normal platelet count. Hemophilia usually presents later.**

▶ Treatment Steps
1. Prevention by vitamin K injection, intramuscular (IM) for all newborns.
2. Vitamin K and fresh frozen plasma for acute bleeding.

B. Hemolytic Disease

1. Rh Incompatibility

▶ Description

Hemolytic process of infant red blood cells (RBCs) due to transplacental passage of maternal antibody against Rh D antigen from Rh-negative mother to Rh-positive infant.

▶ Symptoms

Wide spectrum of presentation from mild anemia and jaundice to profound anemia, extreme jaundice leading to **kernicterus** (neurotoxicity), **hydrops fetalis (hepatosplenomegaly, respiratory distress, massive anasarca,** and **circulatory collapse)** often causing death. Hemolysis worsens with each subsequent pregnancy or fetal blood exposure. Thus, previously affected infant, stillborn, transplacental hemorrhage (abortion), or previous maternal blood transfusions are risk factors.

▶ Diagnosis

Clinical picture, blood typing, **positive direct Coombs' test,** high maternal anti-D antibodies, smear (nucleated RBCs, cells of hemolysis), reticulocytosis, indirect hyperbilirubinemia. Prenatal ultrasound diagnosis of hydrops shows skin/scalp edema, ascites, pleural/pericordial effusions. Prenatal confirmation by spectophotometric **analysis of amniotic fluid.**

▶ Treatment Steps

1. Prevent sensitization by RhoGAM (anti-D gamma globulin) injection to all Rh-negative women with possible fetal blood exposure within 72 hours.
2. In utero transfusion (intraperitoneal or umbilical vein) and/or early delivery (32–34 weeks) if severe.
3. Cardiopulmonary resuscitation if necessary.
4. Correct severe anemia and reduce toxic bilirubin concentration (consider exchange transfusion).

2. ABO Incompatibility

▶ Description

Infant hemolytic process due to major blood group incompatibility between mother (type O) and infant (type A or B). Milder than Rh incompatibility.

▶ Presentation

Usually mild with **jaundice** as only manifestation. Rarely severe anemia, hydrops.

▶ Diagnosis

Suspect with type O mother and jaundice. **Positive direct Coombs',** indirect hyperbilirubinemia, mild anemia, and spherocytosis and hemolysis on blood smear.

▶ Treatment Steps

1. Phototherapy for jaundice.
2. Exchange transfusion for anemia or hyperbilirubinemia rare (bilirubin level for exchange is controversial).

X. FETAL GROWTH AND MONITORING

A. Fetal Growth

▶ Description

Minimal growth in first half of pregnancy (5 g/day at week 14–15 gestation). Peak growth rate at week 33–36 gestation (30–35 g/day).

▶ **cram facts**

INTRAUTERINE GROWTH RETARDATION: DIFFERENTIAL		
	SYMMETRIC	ASYMMETRIC
Head:body size	Proportional	Increased
Onset	Early (< 28 weeks)	Late (> 28 weeks)
Perinatal asphyxia	+/–	+++
Hypoglycemia	+/–	+++
Causes	Chromosomal abnormality	Maternal disease
	Congenital malformation	(preeclampsia, diabetes)
	Congenital infection	Poor maternal nutrition
		Uteroplacental insufficiency

B. Categories of Intrauterine Growth Retardation (IUGR)

1. Early Onset (Symmetric)

Fetal insult in early pregnancy (< 28 weeks' gestation). **Proportional head:body size.** Causes include maternal vascular disease (hypertension [HTN], renal disease), congenital malformation, chromosome abnormalities (trisomies). Low risk for perinatal asphyxia and hypoglycemia.

2. Late Onset (Asymmetric, Head Sparing)

Fetal insult in later pregnancy (> 28 weeks' gestation). Head size relatively large for body size. Causes include milder maternal diseases (including HTN), poor maternal weight gain/nutrition. Increased risk for perinatal asphyxia and hypoglycemia.

C. Fetal Monitoring

1. Nonstress Test (NST)

Monitors fetus by skin surface electrodes or Doppler ultrasonic device on maternal abdomen. Reliable and harmless. At 32 weeks' gestation, **reflex acceleration** of fetal heart rate (FHR) normally occurs with fetal activity. If a repeated NST is nonreactive, contraction stress test or delivery is indicated.

2. Contraction Stress Test (CST)

Monitors uterine contraction in relation to fetal heart rate (FHR—usually increases 15–30 seconds after onset of maternal contractions). Abnormal study is associated with higher mortality (88/1,000 deaths versus 0.4/1,000 deaths if normal response).

3. Intrapartum Continuous

Electronic monitor (FHR and uterine activity during labor).

a. **Baseline pattern (normally 120–160 beats/min)**—bradycardia may suggest congenital heart block (fetal congenital heart defect, maternal systemic lupus erythematosus [SLE]). Tachycardia reflects maternal fever, chorioamnionitis, fetal dysrhythmia.

b. **Beat-to-beat variability (usually 5–10 beats/min fluctuation in FHR)**—loss of variability is associated with autonomic nervous system, fetal sleep, fetal immaturity, maternal narcotic or sedative use, fetal CNS depression.

c. **Deceleration pattern**
(1) **Type I (early deceleration, head compression)—asymmetric** fetal heart pattern that closely mirrors uterine contraction. Benign pattern—often due to fetal head compression against maternal bony pelvis.
(2) **Type II (late decelerations, uteroplacental** insufficiency)—**asymmetric** fetal heart pattern associated with a prolonged deceleration phase and shorter return to baseline. Suggestive of **fetal hypoxia.** Management consists of mother repositioning, intravenous fluids, oxygen, and/or prompt delivery.
(3) **Type III (variable, cord patterns)—variable** shape and timing of FHR in relation to uterine contraction. Associated with **cord compression.** Worrisome if severe pattern (<< 60 beats/min, lasting > 60 seconds) or if associated with late

decelerations or poor beat-to-beat variability. Management includes maternal and/or fetal repositioning.

4. Fetal Scalp Blood Sample
pH < 7.20 suggests fetal hypoxia and requires prompt attention.

5. Maternal Serum α-Fetoprotein (MSAFP)
Elevated with **neural tube defects** (80–85%), omphalocele defect, multiple gestation, intrauterine fetal demise. Low MSAFP with fetal chromosome anomalies such as Down syndrome, trisomy 13 and 18, and Turner's syndrome.

6. Amniocentesis
Measures karyotype, biochemical or enzyme assays. Performed at **15–16 weeks' gestation.** Procedure associated with small risk of spontaneous abortion.

7. Chorionic Villus Sampling
Placental tissue sampling. Similar study as aminocentesis, but **earlier results** (first trimester).

XI. PERINATAL ASPHYXIA

▶ Description

Inadequate oxygenation and/or perfusion of visceral tissue leading to tissue hypoxia, hypercapnia, and acidosis. Incidence 1.0–1.5% in newborns (related to gestational age and birth weight).

▶ Symptoms

Fetal and/or neonatal distress, depending on the severity as well as the timing of the insult. Often **multiorgan involvement.** The presentation of **hypoxic–ischemic brain injury** depends on which area of the CNS is involved. Diffuse hypoperfusion of the brain results in mental retardation, seizures, motor deficits, and/or spastic diplegias. Hypoxia to the brain stem or thalamus results in cranial nerve palsy, reflex disorders, or problems with breathing and temperature regulation. Watershed infarcts result in auditory/visual deficits or motor weakness. Impaired ventricular function or congestive heart failure usually resolves over 1–3 months. Newborns rarely present with thrombocytopenia, bleeding (secondary to impaired clotting factor production), or disseminated intravascular coagulation (DIC). Risk factors include IUGR, breech presentation, prematurity, placental abnormalities, or systemic maternal insult (diabetes, drugs, infection).

▶ Treatment Steps

Treatment is **supportive.** Mortality 10–20% for full-term infant. Of the survivors 20–45% have **neurologic sequelae.** Preterm newborns have worse mortality and morbidity. Worse outcome associated with prolonged asphyxia, severe encephalopathy, poorly controlled seizures, persistent abnormal CT scan, elevated serum creatine kinase (CK) BB, or absent heartbeat for 5 minutes. Survivors have subsequent epilepsy (20–30%); (50% risk if presence of neurologic deficit). If infant survives, organ systems excluding the nervous system usually resolve spontaneously.

XII. PREMATURITY

► Description

Delivery **prior to 37 weeks' gestation.** Incidence 4–8% in United States. Number one cause of **perinatal death** in nonanomalous newborns.

► Symptoms

Multisystem involvement depending on gestational age, birth weight, and etiology. Acute problems include **respiratory distress,** apnea, **intraventricular hemorrhage,** hypoxic–ischemic encephalopathy, feeding dysfunction, necrotizing enterocolitis (NEC), PDA, cardiovascular compromise, and temperature instability. Long-term problems include CNS dysfunction (intellectual, motor, visual, auditory), chronic lung disease, poor growth, metabolic problems, retinopathy of prematurity (ROP). Marked increase in mortality/morbidity < 26 weeks' gestation and < 500 g.

► Risk Factors

Lower socioeconomic status, black race, maternal age (under age 16 years; over age 35 years), maternal history of preterm labor, pregnancy complications (infections, fetal anomaly, antepartum hemorrhage, preeclampsia, first-trimester bleeding), multiple gestation, maternal smoking, uterine anomalies (incomplete septae, bicollis bicornuate), uterine trauma.

► Treatment Steps

1. Prenatal care/counseling.
2. Tocolytic therapy (ritodrine, terbutaline) delays delivery by 24–48 hours.
3. Consider magnesium sulfate, prostaglandin synthetase inhibitors.
4. Consider steroid administration to mature fetal lung.
5. Treat maternal bacterial vaginosis.

XIII. MULTIPLE GESTATION

► Description

Monozygous: identical twinning. **Dizygous:** fraternal twinning. Twins 1 in 80 incidence (*851* monozygous; *852* dizygous). One in 86 pregnancies is triplets. Incidence is increasing with more patients needing and utilizing fertility assistance (i.e., fertility drugs, in vitro fertilization).

► Complications

Problems include abortions, congenital anomalies, severe pregnancy-induced HTN, preterm delivery, intrauterine growth retardation, fetal malpresentation, cord prolapse, cord entrapment, and **twin–twin tranfusion syndrome** (**donor [arterial] twin** is associated with oligohydramnia, growth retardation, anemia, hypovolemia, and microcardia. **Recipient [venous] twin** is associated with polyhydramnia, large size, polycythemia, hypervolemia, and cardiac hypertrophy).

Mortality rates: 65–120 of 1,000 births (twins) and 250–310 of 1,000 births (triplets). Increased mortality if monozygotic twins (versus dizygotic), under 32 weeks' gestation, under 1,500 g body weight, discordancy of fetal size, late detection of monozygosity, malpresentation, labor outside high-risk center.

▶ Diagnosis

Antepartum **sonogram.** Elevated maternal serum AFP. Zygosity determination is aided by sex (different sex = dizygous), placenta (monochorion = monozygous), blood or tissue typing, DNA fingerprinting. Suspect if family history, fertility hormonal treatment, in vitro fertilization.

▶ Treatment Steps

1. Early detection and careful antepartum monitoring.
2. Early intervention for potential complications.
3. High-risk perinatal center ideal.

XIV. RESPIRATORY DISTRESS SYNDROME (HYALINE MEMBRANE DISEASE)

▶ Description

Pulmonary disease in newborns is responsible for the majority of neonatal deaths. Incidence is inversely proportional to newborn's gestational age and birth weight (60–80% < 28 weeks, 10–15% < 2,500 g).

▶ Symptoms

Early onset (hours after delivery). Present with respiratory distress (tachypnea, grunting, nasal flaring, retractions). **Early problems** include breathing problems/asphyxia, metabolic disturbances, anemia, infection, cardiovascular compromise. **Long-term complications** include **bronchopulmonary dysplasia** (BPD), cor pulmonale, ROP, poor growth, tracheal/glottic damage, persistent PDA. In mild cases, the severity of symptoms peaks by day 2–3. **Risk factors** include prematurity, maternal diabetes, multiple pregnancy, precipitous delivery. Survival rate 95% if birth weight > 2,500 g; 65% survival if birth weight < 1,000 g.

▶ Diagnosis

Clinical presentation. CXR: fine **reticular granularity** of lung fields, air bronchograms. Prenatal lung maturity tests include amniotic fluid's **lecithin/sphingomyelin ratio** > 2:1 and positive **phosphatidyl glycerol.** Must differentiate from sepsis, congenital heart disease, hypothermia, congenital lung anomaly (diaphragmatic eventration, cystic malformation), CNS disorder.

▶ Pathology

Lung immaturity is due to **surfactant deficiency,** incomplete structural development of lung, and highly compliant chest wall. These factors result in atelectasis, hyaline membrane formation, retractions, and pulmonary edema. Surfactant reduces surface tension of alveoli (prevents collapse). Synthesized and stored in **type II pneumocytes** of fetal lung. Composed of phospholipids (77%), protein (11%), cholesterol (8%). **Dipalmitoyl phosphatidylcholine** is major ingredient.

▶ Treatment Steps

1. **Prevention** of prematurity is goal (see Prematurity section).
2. Consider **maternal steroid** administration 48–72 hours prior to delivery to stimulate fetal surfactant production if < 33 weeks' gestation (exception: maternal toxemia, diabetes, renal disease).
3. Neonatal **surfactant** administration (via endotracheal tube) at delivery. Known benefits of early surfactant therapy include im-

proved initial respiratory status, decreased incidence of pneumothorax and pulmonary interstitial emphysema, decreased mortality incidence. Surfactant's theoretical risk is intravascular hemolysis (IVH), pneumonia, sepsis, pulmonary hemorrhage, allergic reaction.

4. Correction of acidosis, hypoxia, hypercapnia, hypotension, hypothermia, anemia.
5. Maximize air exchange.
6. Avoid unnecessary pulmonary barotrauma or oxygen toxicity.

XV. PERINATAL BACTERIAL INFECTIONS

A. Chlamydia

▶ Description

Chlamydia trachomatis. Most common sexually transmitted infection in the United States. Transmission 50% from infected mother.

▶ Symptoms

Conjunctivitis; afebrile pneumonia **(repetitive staccato cough).**

▶ Diagnosis

Organism isolation, monoclonal antibody, enzyme-linked immunoassay.

▶ Treatment Steps

Erythromycin. Appropriate isolation.

B. Gonococcal Infections

▶ Description

Neisseria gonorrhoeae. Concurrent infection with chlamydia is common.

▶ Symptoms

Ophthalmia conjunctivitis, disseminated infection (bacteremia, arthritis, meningitis, endocarditis), scalp abscess.

▶ Diagnosis

Organism isolation (chocolate agar in 10% CO_2; Thayer–Martin media).

▶ Treatment Steps

Parenteral antibiotics (pending sensitivity). Appropriate isolation.

C. Gram-Negative Bacilli (GNB)

▶ Description

Escherichia coli, Klebsiella, Enterobacter, Proteus, Citrobacter, Salmonella. All can cause neonatal sepsis.

▶ Symptoms

Neonatal distress. Increased risk with maternal perinatal infection, low birth weight, prolonged rupture of membranes, traumatic delivery, underlying immunologic or metabolic abnormalities.

▶ Treatment Steps

Broad-spectrum antibiotics pending sensitivity. Isolation for *Salmonella* meningitis.

D. Group B Streptococcal Infection

▶ Description

One to five cases per 1,000 live births. Can cause neonatal sepsis or meningitis.

▶ Symptoms

1. **Early onset** (first 3 days of life)—respiratory distress, apnea, pneumonia, cardiovascular compromise, meningitis.
2. **Late onset** (7 days to 3 months of age)—meningitis, osteomyelitis, septic arthritis, occult bacteremia.

▶ Treatment Steps

1. Prevention—most women are screened for the presence of GBS in the vagina at weeks 35–37. If GBS is present, antibiotics are given to the mother during labor to prevent transmission to neonate. Antibiotics include penicillin, ampicillin, and clindamycin, and are given intravenously.
2. Antibiotics are usually reserved for the neonate if signs of infection are present (fever).

E. Tetanus

▶ Description

Clostridium tetani spores. Contamination of umbilical stump.

▶ Symptoms

Marked dysphagia, respiratory distress, high fever ± seizure, continuous crying. **High mortality** rate.

▶ Diagnosis

Organism isolation, exclusion.

▶ Treatment Steps

Supportive care. **Tetanus immune globulin.** ± Penicillin.

F. Listeriosis

▶ Description

Sepsis due to *Listeria monocytogenes*.

▶ Treatment Steps

Broad-spectrum antibiotics pending sensitivities. **Ampicillin** must be used for empiric treatment of sepsis when *Listeria* is a possibility.

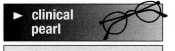

▶ **clinical pearl**

Three groups at high risk for infection with *Listeria*:
- Neonates
- Elderly
- Immunosuppressed

BIBLIOGRAPHY

Behrman RE, Kliegman RM, Nelson WE, et al. *Nelson Textbook of Pediatrics,* 16th ed. Philadelphia: W.B. Saunders, 2000.

Jones KL. *Smith's Recognizable Patterns of Human Malformation,* 5th ed. Philadelphia: W.B. Saunders, 2005.

Spitzer AR. *Intensive Care of the Fetus and Neonate,* 3rd ed. Philadelphia: Mosby-Yearbook, 2005.

Psychiatry | 15

I. DISORDERS USUALLY FIRST DIAGNOSED IN INFANCY, CHILDHOOD, OR ADOLESCENCE

A. Mental Retardation (Axis II)

▶ Description

Intelligence quotient (IQ) of 70 or below with impaired adaptive functioning in two or more: communication, self-care, social skills, academic skills, home living, work, others. Three percent live births, 1% overall prevalence; 90% are mildly retarded (IQ 55–70).

▶ Pathophysiology

- Mild: familial, environmental/perinatal toxicities, deprivation.
- Severe/profound: 75% have known chromosomal/inherited etiology (e.g., Down syndrome, fragile X, phenylketonuria [PKU]).

▶ Diagnosis and Treatment Steps

1. Assess for treatable causes (e.g., thyroid, lead, amino acids, karyotyping); comorbid medical, neurologic (e.g., seizures, sensory impairment), and psychiatric (three to four times general population) disorders.
2. Psychometric testing.
3. Educational placement.
4. Family counseling (increased risk of child abuse), genetic counseling, social service.
5. Psychotherapy, behavior modification, medication as needed for specific behavioral/psychiatric disorders.

B. Pervasive Developmental Disorders

▶ Description

- **Autism:** Impairments in reciprocal social interaction, verbal and nonverbal communication, restricted repertoire of interests, stereotyped behavior. Not psychotic. Associated with mental retardation (70%), seizures.
- **Others: Asperger's** (no language delay); **Rett's,** childhood disintegrative disorders (normal development followed by degenerative course).

▶ Pathophysiology

Genetic component. Associated with multiple neurologic syndromes (e.g., tuberous sclerosis, fragile X, PKU) and biological abnormalities (e.g., dilated ventricles, increased plasma serotonin).

▶ Diagnosis and Treatment Steps

1. Evaluate for sensory function, metabolic disorders, karyotype, electroencephalogram (EEG), IQ testing, neuroimaging.
2. Structured classroom training, behavioral modification, family support.
3. Haloperidol, risperidone for hyperactivity, stereotypies, irritability; selective serotonin reuptake inhibitors (SSRIs) may help with social interaction, compulsive behaviors.

C. Specific Developmental Disorders

▶ Description/Diagnosis

Achievement on standardized tests substantially below expected for age, education, and intelligence.

1. **Learning Disorders**
   1. Reading disorder (80% of learning disorders).
   2. Mathematics disorder.
   3. Disorder of written expression.

   ► **Treatment Steps**
   Educational intervention.

2. **Communication Disorders**

   ► **Description**
   1. Expressive language disorder (developmental or acquired).
   2. Mixed receptive/expressive language disorder (high comorbidity).
   3. Phonological disorder (articulation [e.g., lisping]).
   4. Stuttering (speech dysfluencies). Genetic predisposition.

   ► **Diagnosis and Treatment Steps**
   1. History, neurologic, sensory, psychological evaluations.
   2. Specific language/speech therapies.
   3. Psychological support.

3. **Developmental Coordination Disorder (Motor Skills Disorder)**
   Coordination problem not due to general medical condition.

D. Attention Deficit–Hyperactivity Disorders (ADHD)

► **Description**
Inattention, hyperactivity, impulsivity: distractible, impersistent, disorganized, procrastinates, talks excessively, intrudes, fidgets, loses things, accident-prone, impatient. School failure. Onset < age 7; many continue to have symptoms as adults. Males > females; females more inattentive than hyperactive.

► **Pathophysiology**
Familial aggregation. Decreased frontal cerebral blood flow on positron-emission tomography (PET) scan. Medications increase availability of central nervous system (CNS) dopamine and norepinephrine.

► **Diagnosis**
Clinical diagnosis. Neurologic exam, EEG, sensory evaluation, psychological testing. Rule out thyroid disorder, lead poisoning, iron deficiency, child abuse. Highly comorbid: rule out learning, communication, conduct, mood, anxiety, substance use, tic disorders.

► **Treatment Steps**
1. Individual/family therapy, environmental management, behavior modification.
2. Stimulants (methylphenidate [Ritalin], dextroamphetamine [Dexedrine]). May cause headache, abdominal pain, nausea, insomnia, growth suppression, emergence/exacerbation of tics; tricyclic antidepressants (TCAs), clonidine, bupropion also used.

E. Disruptive Behavior Disorders

1. **Conduct Disorder**

   ► **Description**
   Basic rights of others and age-appropriate societal norms violated: aggression to people and animals, destruction of property, deceitfulness, theft, serious rule violations.

▶ Pathophysiology

Genetic, neurodevelopmental, environmental risk factors contribute.

▶ Diagnosis

Rule out immediate response to social context (e.g., runaway episodes due to abuse).

▶ Treatment Steps

1. **Evaluate suicide and violence potential.**
2. Containment may involve parents, peers, schools, legal system, hospitalization, residential placement.
3. Aggression may respond to SSRI, lithium, clonidine, haloperidol.
4. Individual, group, family therapies, behavioral management.
5. Evaluate and treat comorbid ADHD, mood, substance use disorders.

2. Oppositional Defiant Disorder

▶ Description

Age-inappropriate negativistic, hostile, annoying, angry, defiant behavior toward authority figures.

▶ Pathophysiology

Disrupted, harsh, inconsistent, neglectful parenting; marital discord; difficult early temperament.

▶ Diagnosis

Rule out comorbid ADHD, learning, mood, conduct, substance use disorders, immediate response to social context.

▶ Treatment Steps

Individual/family therapy, behavioral managment.

F. Separation Anxiety Disorder

▶ Description

Excessive anxiety concerning separation from home or from those to whom the child is attached (e.g., refusal to sleep alone or go to school, extreme homesickness, catastrophic fears, depression, somatic symptoms).

▶ Pathophysiology

Familial aggregation; close-knit families, genetic relationship to panic disorder.

▶ Diagnosis

Not diagnosed in presence of pervasive developmental, psychotic, or panic/agoraphobic disorders.

▶ Treatment Steps

1. **School refusal is psychiatric emergency**—prompt evaluation and treatment involving parents, school, peers to reinforce gradually increasing time in school.
2. Individual/family therapy, behavioral management.
3. SSRIs helpful with anxiety and depression.

G. Tic Disorders

1. Tourette's Disorder

▶ Description

Multiple motor and one or more vocal tics. Both types of tics may be simple (e.g., blinking, grimacing) or complex (e.g., grooming, touching, smelling, echopraxia, repeating words or phrases, coprolalia [1/3], echolalia). Anatomic location/complexity/severity of tics varies over time. Persists at least 1 year.

► Pathophysiology

Part of genetic spectrum including other tic disorders, ADHD, obsessive–compulsive disorder (OCD). Dopamine suppression reduces symptoms. Opiates, serotonin may play a role. Exacerbated by anxiety, stress.

► Diagnosis

Rule out neurologic disease (Huntington's, Parkinson's, Sydenham's, Wilson's).

► Treatment Steps

1. Haloperidol improves 80%; watch for extrapyramidal symptoms (EPS), mental dulling, tardive dyskinesia. Pimozide also effective. Clonidine is alternative to antipsychotics.
2. Evaluate for ADHD (50%), OCD (40%), depression; stimulants used to treat ADHD increase dopamine and may precipitate/exacerbate tics.
3. SSRIs helpful for OCD symptoms.

2. Chronic Motor or Vocal Tic Disorder

Similar to, much more common than, Tourette's; either motor or vocal tics; at least 1 year.

3. Transient Tic Disorder

Tics occur 4 weeks to 1 year.

H. Elimination Disorders

1. Functional Encopresis

Voluntary or involuntary repeated passage of feces into inappropriate places (clothing, floor) after age 4, not due to medical condition. May develop psychogeneic megacolon with overflow incontinence. Rule out Hirschsprung's disease. Behavioral, family, individual therapies.

2. Functional Enuresis

Voluntary or involuntary repeated voiding of urine into bed or clothes after age 5. Rule out urinary tract infection (UTI), diabetes, seizures, spina bifida, obstruction. Behavioral techniques (i.e., bell or buzzer apparatus). Bedtime fluid restriction; imipramine used as last resort—may be cardiotoxic; desmopressin nasal spray.

I. Miscellaneous Childhood Issues

1. Child Physical and Sexual Abuse

► Description

Risk factors include prematurity, low birth weight, physical/mental disability, illness, "difficult" temperament; parental history of child abuse, current substance abuse, depression, impulsivity; family isolation, conflict, stress, poverty; current toilet training; perfectionistic parental expectations. Adolescent may run away.

► Diagnosis

History of injury inconsistent with physical findings; multiple injuries of different ages; delay in care-seeking; abdominal, genital, rectal pain/trauma in sexual abuse; signs of disturbed attachment, developmental delay, disturbed play, sexual acting out may be present. Rule out unintentional injury; bleeding diathesis; osteogenica imperfecta; dermatologic conditions through physical exam, skeletal series, serology, bleeding times, complete blood count (CBC), creatine kinase as indicated.

► Treatment Steps
1. Prevention: early indentification of high-risk families with provision of support, education, treatment; licensing, screening of child care professionals.
2. Interview child alone; expert may be required; document findings.
3. All states mandate reporting of suspected abuse (physical, sexual, emotional, severe neglect).
4. Ensure safety of child.
5. Individual/group psychotherapy.

2. Suicide

Increasing incidence in adolescents. Risk factors include conduct disorder, depression, substance/alcohol abuse, aggressive behavior, psychosis, hopelessness, poor problem-solving skills, male sex, previous attempt; access to guns, family history of suicide, family violence, recent suicide of peer. Must question directly if suspicious. Family supervision, cooperation with treatment essential. Safety contract, psychotherapy, pharmacotherapy, family therapy; hospitalization if high risk.

3. Adolescent Risk-Taking Behavior

Related to feelings of omnipotence/invulnerability; peer pressure; fears of inadequacy; rebelliousness. Includes experimentation with drugs, alcohol, tobacco; sexual promiscuity; accident-prone behavior (leading cause of death among teens). Risk decreased with higher education, social class. Education/information helpful (e.g., regarding contraception) but not always effective (e.g., regarding behavior leading to human immunodeficiency virus [HIV] infection). Ask about peers', then teen's, behavior. Emphasize immediate disadvantages of behavior (e.g., smoking costs money, diminishes athletic performance, results in bad breath). Behavioral rehearsal helpful.

II. COGNITIVE DISORDERS

Disordered cognition (memory, attention, abstraction, judgment) that is a direct physiologic consequence of a general medical condition.

A. Delirium

See Chapter 19, section IV.B.

B. Dementia

► Description
Acquired impairment of memory with at least one other cognitive deficit (e.g., executive dysfunction, impaired planning, abstract thinking, judgment); apraxia (inability to carry out motor activities); aphasia (language disturbance); agnosia (inability to identify objects). Accompanied by slow, progressive decline is functioning. Losses often denied. Personality, mood disturbance. Late in course may have psychotic symptoms, severely impaired social judgment, extreme regression. Incidence increases with advancing age.

▶ differential diagnosis

DELIRIUM	VS.	DEMENTIA
Rapid onset		Insidious onset
Fluctuating, clouded consciousness		Clear sensorium until late in course
Often reversible		Most irreversible and progressive
Perceptual disturbances, sleep–wake cycle abnormalities, incoherent speech common		These symptoms uncommon until late in course

▶ Pathophysiology

Causes include multi-infarct dementia, Pick's disease, normal pressure hydrocephalus, Creutzfeldt–Jakob disease, and Alzheimer's disease, which is a diagnosis of exclusion.

▶ Diagnosis and Treatment

- Mainly supportive care for the patient and caregivers.
- Control medical comorbidities.
- Antidepressants, antipsychotics, and anxiolytics used as indicated.
- See Chapter 11, section X.

C. Amnestic Disorders

Memory impairment due to medical condition without other significant cognitive impairments. Korsakoff syndrome (thiamine deficiency), head trauma, seizures, CNS tumors, cerebrovascular disease, hypoglycemia, hypoxia, multiple sclerosis (MS), sedative–hypnotics, alcohol. Dissociative disorders have more selective memory deficits associated with stressful life events.

D. Neuropsychiatric Disorders Associated with HIV Infection

▶ Description

At least 50% with HIV infection have clinical neuropsychiatric complications; in 10% are initial event. HIV encephalopathy associated with subcortical dementia; syndrome of psychomotor slowing and impairment, forgetfulness, poor concentration, impaired problem solving and visuospatial skills, apathy, depression. CNS infection, tumor usually accompanied by headache, photophobia, focal signs, clouded consciousness. May need neuropsychological testing, lumbar puncture, neuroimaging. Dementia due to HIV is poor prognostic sign. Other psychiatric complications include delirium with acute mania or psychosis; anxiety; depression; adjustment disorder; substance abuse; increased suicide risk.

▶ Treatment Steps

1. Primary prevention: safe sex practices, avoid needle sharing.
2. Pre- and post-HIV test counseling.
3. Symptomatic treatment with individual, group, couples therapy, peer support.
4. Pharmacotherapy for specific disorder; stimulants sometimes used for HIV encephalopathy with apathy, depression. Use low doses of psychotropics, watch for drug interactions and side effects especially with antipsychotics.

▶ cram facts

PSYCHIATRIC SYNDROMES DUE TO HIV, ITS COMPLICATIONS, OR ITS TREATMENT

- HIV-associated dementia (HAD)
- Minor cognitive motor disorder (MCMD)
- CNS infections (toxoplasmosis, cytomegalovirus [CMV], herpes simplex virus [HSV] encephalitis, cryptococcal meningitis, tuberculosis)
- Progressive multifocal leukoencephalopathy (PML)
- Hypoxia due to lung infections
- CNS lymphoma
- Kaposi's sarcoma
- Mood, anxiety, and psychotic disorders
- Neuropsychiatric effects of HIV medications

III. SUBSTANCE-RELATED DISORDERS

A. Overview

► Epidemiology and Social Impact

Greater than 15% lifetime prevalence, 6% point prevalence in U.S. population. Impaired work and school performance, accidents, absenteeism, family conflict and violence, violent crime, theft, prostitution, medical and mental disorders. Social cost $67 billion annually.

► Prevention (Primary, Secondary)

Education, counseling of high-risk youth in culturally sensitive manner; increase minimum drinking age, price of cigarettes and alcohol, driving under the influence (DUI) enforcement; ban vending machines; improve early case identification and referral in primary care and emergency settings; improve accessability of treatment.

► Comorbidity

Often coexists with other substance-related, mood, anxiety, personality, pain, schizophrenic, attention deficit disorders. Intravenous drug use (IVDU) and crack use associated with HIV transmission, cellulitis, endocarditis. Chronic alcoholism associated with multiple system degenerative diseases.

► Pathophysiology

Cultural, psychological, genetic contributions. All substances enhance brain reward mechanisms involving opioid, amine, and γ-aminobutyric acid (GABA) systems. Use reinforced by relief of withdrawal symptoms. Environmental learning important.

► Diagnosis

History, drug screen, blood alcohol level detect recent use.

► Definitions

Abuse—Recurrent, maladaptive pattern of use during 12-month period despite physical hazard or legal, social, or occupational problems.

Dependence—Psychological (craving) or physical (tolerance, withdrawal); loss of control over use; preoccupation with obtaining and using substance; continued use despite adverse social, occupational, health consequences. Frequent denial, minimization.

Intoxication—Maladaptive behavior associated with recent ingestion. All substances can cause intoxication.

Withdrawal—Substance-specific syndrome following decreased use or cessation of regular use. Associated with alcohol, sedative hypnotics, amphetamines, cocaine, opiods, nicotine.

Tolerance—Increasing amounts of ingested drug necessary to produce same degree of intoxication.

Other Substance-Induced Disorders—Delirium, dementia, amnestic, psychotic, anxiety, mood, sexual, sleep disorders possible with various substances.

B. Alcohol

1. Dependence, Intoxication, Withdrawal

► Description/Diagnosis

Facilitates action of GABA receptor, inhibits *N*-methyl-D-aspartate (NMDA) glutamate receptor; also effects serotonin transmission.

► cram facts

SIGNS AND SYMPTOMS OF SUBSTANCE INTOXICATION AND WITHDRAWAL

Substance Category	Intoxication	Withdrawal
CNS depressants: alcohol, sedatives, hypnotics, anxiolytics	Disinhibition, slurred speech, drowsiness, ataxia, confusion, blackouts **Overdose:** respiratory depression, coma, death; barbiturates have low therapeutic index	Autonomic hyperactivity, anxiety, malaise, headache, nausea, vomiting, fever, mydriasis, seizures, delusions, hallucinations, delirium, death; can be life threatening
CNS stimulants: amphetamine, cocaine, other sympathomimetics	Euphoria, alertness, increased energy, loquaciousness, anorexia, insomnia, mydriasis, autonomic hyperactivity **Overdose:** agitation, aggression, fever, chills, arrhythmias, seizures, sudden cardiac death, cerebrovascular accident; paranoid psychosis, hallucinosis, delirium	Fatigue, insomnia or hypersomnia, anxiety, dysphoria, vivid dreams, agitation, drug craving; not life threatening (unless suicidal)
Opioids	Euphoria, analgesia, drowsiness, hypoactivity, miosis, anorexia, constipation, pruritus, nausea, vomiting, ataxia **Overdose:** hypotension, bradycardia, CNS and respiratory depression, pulmonary edema, seizures, coma	Flulike syndrome, tearing, dilated pupils, restlessness, yawning, sweating, piloerection, anxiety, tachycardia, hypertension, craving

---

Early *dependence:* injuries, accidents, gastritis, diarrhea, absenteeism, blackouts, irritability, insomnia; screen with CAGE (attempts to **C**ut down, **A**nnoyance of criticism of drinking, **G**uilt, morning **E**ye opener). May have elevated γ-glutamyl transpeptidase (GGT), mean corpuscular volume (MCV), aspartate transaminase (AST), alanine transaminase (ALT). Later: nutritional deficiencies, hepatitis, cirrhosis, gastrointestinal (GI) bleeding, pancreatitis, heart disease, hypertension, palmar erythema, gynecomastia, testicular atrophy, peripheral neuropathy, GI cancers, neuropsychiatric disorders.

Intoxication—Disinhibition, emotional lability, impaired judgment, incoordination, slurred speech, ataxia, coma, blackouts; accidents, violent acts, suicide, head injuries. Blood alcohol levels for nontolerant person:
- 100–150 mg/dL: incoordination, irritability (legal intoxication)
- 150–250 mg/dL: slurred speech, ataxia
- > 250 mg/dL: unconsciousness
- Blood alcohol level > 150 mg/dL without intoxication evidence of tolerance.

Withdrawal—Tremulousness, agitation, irritability, autonomic hyperactivity, nausea and vomiting, fever, seizures; delirium tremens (onset of delirium, vivid auditory, visual, tactile hallucinations, paranoid delusions 2–3 days past cessation of long-term, heavy use in medically compromised patients).

▶ Treatment Steps

1. *Intoxication*—treat supportively, evaluate for subdural infection, other substances.

2. *Withdrawal* (detoxification)—vital signs, electrolytes, glucose, magnesium, thiamine, vitamin B_{12}, folate, toxicology. Hydration—give thiamine *before* giving IV glucose to avoid precipitating acute thiamine deficiency and Wernicke's encephalopathy. Benzodiazepine taper adjusted to control symptoms; carbamazepine also used. Reduce stimulation, seclusion/restraint as necessary. Diagnose and treat underlying medical problems.

3. *Dependence*—detoxification as necessary. Confrontation of denial. Diagnose and treat persisting comorbid psychiatric disorders. Inpatient, residential, outpatient rehabilitation aimed at abstinence with 12-step, individual, group, family therapies. Maintenance of abstinence with Alcoholics Anonymous or similar group, halfway house; disulfiram (Antabuse—causes toxic reaction with ingestion of alcohol), opiate antagonist naltrexone (Revia—eliminates "high" from drinking, used with some highly motivated patients); SSRIs may promote abstinence.

2. Related Disorders

a. Alcohol hallucinosis

Vivid persistent hallucinations shortly after cessation *without delirium*. Rarely chronic. Treat with benzodiazepines, IV fluids, nutrition. High-potency antipsychotics if chronic.

b. Alcohol-induced persisting dementia

Follows prolonged and heavy ingestion. Impairment of memory and other cognitive deficits.

c. Alcohol encephalopathy **(Wernicke's encephalopathy)**

Abrupt onset of truncal ataxia, confusion, ophthalmoplegia (nystagmus, lateral rectus palsy) due to thiamine deficiency. Give thiamine before giving IV glucose (which utilizes thiamine for glucose metabolism).

d. Alcohol-induced persisting dementia **(Korsakoff syndrome)**

Severe, persistent retrograde and anterograde amnesia, confabulation, apathy, polyneuritis resulting from thiamine deficiency, following Wernicke's encephalopathy.

e. **Fetal alcohol syndrome**

In utero exposure to alcohol leading to microcephaly, growth retardation, craniofacial malformations, limb and heart defects, mental retardation, emotional and attentional problems.

C. Opioids (Opium, Morphine, Diacetylmorphine [Heroin], Methadone, Codeine, Meperidine, Pentazocine, Others)

▶ Description/Diagnosis

Heroin injected IV, subcutaneous ("skin popping"), snorted; opium smoked; pharmaceuticals ingested. Agonists at μ, κ, δ CNS opioid receptors.

Dependence—Highly addictive, rapid tolerance, weight loss, needle tracks, hyposexuality, amenorrhea, constipation, multiple medical problems including HIV infection, subacute bacterial endocarditis (SBE), cellulitis, criminal involvement, suicide, accidents.

Intoxication—Euphoria, analgesia, hypoactivity, anorexia, drowsiness, nausea and vomiting, constipation, pupillary constriction, hypotension, bradycardia.

Overdose—CNS and respiratory depression, pinpoint pupils, pulmonary edema, seizures, coma, death.

Withdrawal—Uncomfortable but not life threatening. Flulike syndrome of rhinorrhea, myalgias, nausea, vomiting, diarrhea; lacrimation, dilated pupils, restlessness, yawning, sweating, insomnia, piloerection, anxiety, tachycardia, hypertension, craving.

► Treatment Steps
1. *Overdose*—IV naloxone q 5 min, in certain cases can be used as a continuous IV infusion; support vital functions; observe up to 3 days; diagnose polysubstance overdose.
2. *Detoxification/Dependence*—abstinence through methadone titration, gradual taper or buprenorphine (agonist–antagonist); or symptomatic treatment of withdrawal with clonidine (reduces sympathetic output, observe for hypotension), antiemetics, analgesics. Pentazocine (Talwin) withdrawn with pentazocine. Naltrexone after detox for highly motivated patients; methadone maintenance for long-term addicts reduces social and medical problems; therapeutic communities, Narcotics Anonymous, supportive psychotherapy. Treat comorbid psychiatric disorders (antisocial personality disorder, depression, posttraumatic stress disorder [PTSD]) in 80%.

D. Stimulants (Amphetamine, Methamphetamine, Cocaine, Crack Cocaine, Other Sympathomimetics)

► Description/Diagnosis
Ingested, injected IV, snorted, smoked (crack). Highly addictive. Amphetamine longer acting, release of presynaptic norepinephrine and dopamine; cocaine blocks reuptake of norepinephrine, dopamine, 5-hydroxytryptamine (5-HT); both directly stimulate brain reward–pleasure centers.

Dependence—Rapid development of tolerance. Severe financial, social, health losses; weight loss, sexually transmitted disease (STD) risk through IVDU, prostitution, depression, irritability, sexual dysfunction, memory impairment, paranoid psychosis (psychotic disorder).

Intoxication—Euphoria, alertness, increased energy, anxiety, talkativeness, psychomotor agitation, impaired judgment, sexual arousal, anorexia, insomnia, pupillary dilatation, hypertension, tachycardia; may progress to hyperpyrexia, nausea and vomiting, visual or tactile hallucinations ("cocaine bugs"), paranoia, sudden cardiac death; delirium may develop rapidly, lasting 1–6 hours with olfactory or tactile hallucinations; may lead to seizures, death.

Withdrawal—"Crash," not medically dangerous; fatigue, insomnia/hypersomnia, anxiety, dysphoria, suicidal ideation, craving.

► Treatment Steps

1. *Intoxication*—Treated symptomatically (e.g., antiarrhythmic agents for arrhythmias, benzodiazepines for severe agitation, antipsychotics for psychosis); acidify urine.
2. *Withdrawal*—Treat supportively, observe for suicidality.
3. *Dependence*—Confront denial, drug rehabilitation program, Narcotics Anonymous, behavioral therapy for relapse prevention, supportive, individual, group therapies; dopamine agonists (e.g., amantadine) and desipramine sometimes used for cocaine cravings. Diagnose and treat comorbid psychiatric disorders (e.g., persistent depression, ADHD).

E. Sedatives, Hypnotics, and Anxiolytics (Benzodiazepines, Barbiturates, Methaqualone, Chloral Hydrate, Zolpidem, Others)

► Description/Diagnosis

Ingested, often in combination with other substances; rarely injected IV. Activate GABA-A receptor complex.

Dependence—Produces tolerance to sedative and euphoriant effects, fatigue, psychomotor impairment, amnesia, depression, headaches, GI disturbances.

Intoxication—Slurred speech, drowsiness, incoordination, ataxia, impaired attention and memory, disinhibition. Flumetrazepam ("roofies") associated with date rape.

Overdose—Barbiturates have low therapeutic index, frequently used in suicide; benzodiazepines have high therapeutic index but may be lethal in combination with other CNS sedatives. Respiratory depression, coma, death.

Withdrawal—Mild withdrawal syndrome of anxiety, insomnia, anorexia, dizziness common. Severe withdrawal syndrome is a medical emergency, associated with nausea, vomiting, malaise, autonomic hyperactivity, photophobia, tremor, hyperreflexia, hyperthermia, insomnia, delirium, seizures, death. Shorter-acting drugs cause most severe symptoms.

► Treatment Steps

1. *Overdose*—Gastric lavage, charcoal; maintain airway and blood pressure. Treat supportively. Flumazenil (benzodiazepine antagonist) does not reverse respiratory inhibition from benzodiazepines.
2. *Withdrawal*—Pentobarbital challenge test to determine usual daily dosage, substitute equivalent phenobarbital dose, taper 10%/day. Benzodiazepines may be substituted by long-acting agent (diazepam, clonazepam) and gradually withdrawn.
3. *Prevention*—Benzodiazepines generally safely prescribed but should not be prescribed for persons with a history of drug or alcohol abuse/dependence. Barbiturate dependency often iatrogenic.

F. Caffeine

Found in **coffee, tea, colas, chocolate, over-the-counter (OTC) stimulants, cold preparations.** Adenosine receptor antagonist.

Intoxication—Restlessness, insomnia, flushing, GI disturbance, anxiety, diuresis with intake > 250 mg/day (2 cups brewed coffee);

agitation, muscle twitching, cardiac arrhythmia, inexhaustibility with intake > 1 g/day.

Withdrawal—Headache, fatigue lasting 4–5 days.

G. Nicotine

► Description
Acetylcholine (nicotinic) agonist.

Dependence—Develops rapidly. Strongly conditioned. Associated with pulmonary, cardiac, peripheral vascular, neoplastic diseases.

Withdrawal—Craving, irritability, anxiety, weight gain, difficulty concentrating, headache; may last several weeks. Depression develops in some.

► Treatment Steps
Obtain commitment to stop on specific date. Education, counseling, smoking cessation groups; nicotine replacement sprays, gums, patches for moderate to severe addiction; continued smoking can cause cardiac death. Bupropion may enhance success rate and may be used in combination with nicotine replacement.

H. Inhalants (Glues, Solvents, Volatile Cleaners, Gasoline, Nitrates, Aromatic Hydrocarbons)

► Description

Intoxication—Light-headedness, euphoria, disinhibition, belligerence, apathy, impaired judgment, hallucinations, body distortions, slurred speech, accidents, injuries; progressing to ataxia, confusion, nystagmus, delirium, coma.

Chronic Use—Associated with weight loss, fatigue, breathing problems, facial rash, halitosis, dementia, irritability, emotional lability, hepatic and renal damage, cardiovascular and pulmonary symptoms, muscle damage, bone marrow suppression, peripheral neuropathy.

Withdrawal—Rare; sleep disturbance, irritability, jitteriness, sweating, nausea, vomiting, psychotic symptoms.

► Treatment Steps
1. Supportive medical care.
2. Young adolescents require substance abuse education, evaluation for conduct disorder.
3. Older users often debilitated and require substantial psychosocial and medical interventions.

I. Phencyclidine (PCP, Angel Dust)

► Description
An atypical hallucinogen. Smoked, snorted, eaten, injected. NMDA glutamate receptor antagonist.

Intoxication—Euphoria, unpredictability, paranoia, assaultiveness, belligerence, impulsiveness, psychomotor agitation, catatonia; vertical and horizontal nystagmus, hypertension, chest pain, renal failure, ataxia, dysarthria, diaphoresis, hyperacusis, hyperreflexia, myoclonic jerks, muscle rigidity, seizures, respiratory depression, coma. **Pupils normal size.** Elevated creatine phosphokinase (CPK), ALT, blood urea nitrogen (BUN), creatinine, myoglobinuria.

Chronic Use—May develop chronic psychosis, mood disorder, delirium, long-term neuropsychologic damage.

► Treatment Steps
Isolate in nonstimulating environment. May need physical restraint. Acidify urine to increase clearance of drug. Treat hypertension. Use benzodiazepines, antipsychotics symptomatically.

J. Hallucinogens (Lysergic Acid Diethylamide [LSD], Dimethyltryptamine [DMT], Psilocybin, Mescaline, MDMA [Ecstasy], Others)

► Description
Serotonin agonists. Eaten, sucked from paper, smoked.

Hallucinogen Hallucinosis—Intoxication produces wakeful hallucinosis, sympathomimetic effects, including pupillary dilatation, tachycardia, diaphoresis; perceptual changes, emotional intensity and lability; may be associated with anxiety or depression, ideas of reference, delusions, paranoid ideation, derealization, depersonalization, illusions, hallucinations, panic reactions ("bad trip").

Posthallucinogen Perception Disorder—A distressing, persistent reexperiencing of the same perceptual symptoms experienced while intoxicated ("flashback") with intact reality testing.

► Treatment Steps
1. "Bad trip" treated with reassurance, low stimulation.
2. Benzodiazepines, antipsychotics if symptoms severe.
3. Posthallucinogen perception disorder treated with benzodiazepine acutely or antipsychotic if persistent.

K. Cannabinoids (Marijuana, Hashish, Bhang, Ganja, Purified Tetrahydrocannabinol [THC])

Usually smoked, also eaten. Stimulates cannabinoid receptor. Urine drug screen positive up to 4 weeks past heavy use.

Intoxication—Euphoria or dysphoria, heightened sensation, time distortion, increased humorousness, increased appetite, impaired judgment, dry mouth, tachycardia, conjunctival injection; may produce suspiciousness, anxiety, depersonalization, incoordination; rarely, persecutory delusions, hallucinations. Pupils normal size.

Chronic Use—Apathetic, amotivational syndrome controversial; memory impairment. Bronchitis; decreased chance of pregnancy.

L. Anabolic Steroids

Ingested, intramuscular injection. Initially produces sense of wellbeing. **Chronic use** causes depression, psychosis, mania, acne, hepatic damage, infection from needle sharing, cerebrovascular accidents (CVAs), testicular atrophy and feminization in males, masculinization in females.

IV. SCHIZOPHRENIA AND OTHER PSYCHOTIC DISORDERS

▶ Definitions

1. *Hallucinations:* disturbed **sensory perceptions** occurring without external stimulation. Can occur in all sensory modalities, including auditory, visual, tactile, gustatory, olfactory.
2. *Delusions:* fixed, false **beliefs** (content of thought) based on incorrect inference about perception or experience, maintained despite evidence or overwhelming sentiment to the contrary. Common types include bizarre (e.g., loss of control over mind or body), grandiose, referential, nihilistic, persecutory, somatic, being controlled.
3. *Formal thought disorder:* disorganized speech, including incoherence, derailment, tangentiality, illogicality, neologisms.
4. *Psychosis:* impairment in ability to judge boundary between real and unreal. Symptoms include prominent hallucinations, delusions, bizarre or grossly disorganized behavior and speech.

A. Schizophrenia

▶ Description

Presence of two or more psychotic symptoms: delusions, hallucinations, disorganized speech, disorganized or catatonic behavior, negative symptoms (e.g., inappropriate or flat affect, poverty of speech, lack of motivation, anhedonia). Decreased occupational, interpersonal, self-care functioning. Duration of at least 6 months. May have premorbid schizotypal features, soft neurologic signs, motor abnormalities. Onset typically late teens to mid-twenties. Variable course, stable or deteriorating. Increased risk of medical illness, sudden death, suicide (10%), poverty, violence, victimization, substance disorders. Better prognosis with acute onset, later onset, good premorbid social/occupational history, positive symptoms, presence of mood symptoms, early and continued treatment, medication compliance, female gender, absence of structural brain abnormalities. Families with high levels of criticism and hostility ("expressed emotion") yield higher relapse rates.

▶ Pathophysiology

Biologic vulnerability triggered by stress. (Polygenic) genetic and environmental contributions, including possible perinatal infection and other insults. Dopamine hypothesis: symptoms associated with altered dopaminergic activity in mesocortical and mesolimbic tracts (typical antipsychotic medications block dopamine-D2 receptors). Newer antipsychotics affect serotonin 5-HT_{2A} receptors, others. Negative symptoms associated with enlargment of cerebral ventricles, cortical atrophy. Hypofrontality on functional neuroimaging. Stable neuropsychological deficits predict social/vocational outcome. Delusions, hallucinations have cultural component.

▶ Diagnosis

No pathognomonic signs or studies; rule out general medical etiology (substance intoxication/withdrawal, temporal lobe epilepsy, medication effects, CNS infection, trauma, tumor, endocrine and metabolic disorders). Rule out psychotic, affective, delusional personality disorders. Features pointing to a general medical etiology include older age, rapid onset of new symptoms, visual or olfactory hallucinations, neurologic symptoms, fluctuations of consciousness, clouded sensorium, cognitive impairment, constructional apraxia, catatonic features, abnormal physical exam.

▶ Treatment Steps

1. May require hospitalization for protection of self or others, stabilization.
2. Medication compliance and psychosocial treatments **independently** contribute to prevention of relapse.
3. Antipsychotic medication (typical or newer atypical neuroleptics).
4. Lithium, anticonvulsants, benzodiazepines, antidepressants, electroconvulsive therapy (ECT), may benefit some.
5. Psychosocial treatments, including patient and family education, family support/therapy, social skills training, vocational rehabilitation.
6. May need structured residential or treatment programs.

B. Delusional (Paranoid) Disorder

▶ Description

Persistent, nonbizarre, well-systematized delusion. Age of onset and psychosocial functioning variable. Types include:

- **Erotomanic**—one is loved by a famous other.
- **Grandiose**—one possesses great talent.
- **Jealous**—conviction that spouse/lover is unfaithful.
- **Persecutory**—one is conspired against. Most common type.
- **Somatic**—one has a physical abnormality (e.g., odor).

▶ Pathophysiology

Predisposed by immigration, deafness, severe stress.

▶ Diagnosis

No pathognomonic signs, tests. Rule out early dementias, CNS tumor, endocrine, metabolic disorders, stimulant abuse, basal ganglia trauma. Schizophrenia associated with more bizarre psychotic symptoms, prominent hallucinations, thought disorder, deteriorating course. Paranoid personality disorder has no true delusions.

▶ Treatment Steps

1. Course is variable. Hospitalization for inability to control suicidal or homicidal impulses, danger associated with delusions.
2. Supportive psychotherapy.
3. Antipsychotic medication for delusions. Antidepressants for depression.

C. Schizophreniform Disorder

▶ Description

Identical to schizophrenia but duration < 6 months. Good prognosis associated with acute onset, confusion and disorientation, full affect, good premorbid functioning.

▶ Treatment Steps

Antipsychotic medication at least 6 months.

D. Brief Psychotic Disorder

▶ Description

Sudden onset of psychotic symptoms, with emotional turmoil and confusion, often following obvious stressor, duration < 1 month.

Prognostic factors as in schizophreniform disorder. Suicide risk. Usual return to premorbid functioning. Predisposed to by personality disorder, PTSD.

► Diagnosis

Rule out schizophreniform and mood disorders, general medical etiology, factitious disorder, malingering, substance-related.

► Treatment Steps
1. Hospitalization as needed.
2. Antipsychotic or antianxiety agent.
3. Psychotherapy when stabilized.

E. Schizoaffective Disorder

► Description

Concurrent features of schizophrenia and depression or mania, with delusions or hallucinations without affective syndrome for at least 2 weeks. Subtype defined by mood syndrome (bipolar type with mania, depressed type with depression).

► Treatment Steps
1. Hospitalization, medical workup as with schizophrenia.
2. Bipolar type (manic or mixed episode): lithium and antipsychotic agent; latter may be reduced or discontinued with stabilization. Valproate, carbamazepine, ECT, clozapine also used.
3. Depressive type: antipsychotic with or without antidepressant; lithium, ECT also used.

F. Shared Psychotic Disorder

► Description

Delusion (usually persecutory) develops in context of submissive, dependent, isolated relationship with person with established delusion. Suicide/homicide pacts.

► Treatment Steps
1. Separate the two people.
2. Antipsychotic medication as needed.

V. MOOD DISORDERS

A. Definitions

1. Mania

Distinct period of elevated, expansive, or irritable mood with grandiosity, decreased need for sleep, talkativeness or pressured speech, racing thoughts, distractability, increased activity/agitation, impulsivity (excessive spending, gambling, promiscuity), which causes marked impairment or hospitalization. Lasts at least 1 week.

2. Hypomania

Same symptoms as mania, with less severity and impairment, lasting at least 4 days.

3. Major Depression

Sustained depressed mood or loss of interest/pleasure (anhedonia) with appetite/weight change, insomnia/hypersomnia, fatigue, psychomotor agitation/retardation, low self-esteem/guilt, trouble concentrating, thoughts of death or suicide for at least 2 weeks.

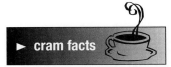
► cram facts

MNEMONIC FOR MAJOR DEPRESSION

SIG E CAPS

Sustained, distinct depressed mood × 2 weeks plus at least four of the following:

Sleep (increased or decreased)

Interest (loss of interest or pleasure)

Guilt (worthlessness)

Energy (decreased)

Concentration (decreased)

Appetite (increased or decreased)

Psychomotor change (retardation or agitation)

Suicidality (active or passive)

B. Unipolar Major Depression

▶ Description

See above. No history of mania/hypomania. Diurnal variation is common, with symptoms worse in A.M. Also associated with somatic symptoms (GI, genitourinary [GU], back pain, headache), tearfulness, obsessive rumination, anxiety. Children and adolescents may have behavioral problems, irritability, somatic complaints, failure to gain weight. Elderly may present with cognitive complaints (pseudodementia). Depressed patients more likely to die from cardiac disease, cancer, pulmonary disease, hip fractures. Over 50% suffer recurrence. Lifetime suicide risk 15%.

▶ Pathophysiology

Dysregulation of CNS neurotransmitter activity and neuroendocrine dysregulation, especially in hypothalamic–pituitary–adrenal (HPA) axis. Decreased serotonergic activity associated with violence, suicide. Antidepressants increase available monoamines at nerve terminals, alter receptor sensitivity and density. Genetic component, especially with severe, recurrent illness. Pathology of limbic system, basal ganglia, and hypothalamus. Sleep EEG shows delayed sleep onset, decreased rapid eye movement (REM) latency, increased first REM period length. Late-onset may have subcortical cerebrovascular disease. Early parental loss, psychiatric or medical illness, substance abuse predisposes; 25% identify precipitant, often loss.

▶ Diagnosis

Rule out other mood disorders. Rule out thyroid and adrenal disease, medications (steroids, diuretics, progestins, oral contraceptives, nonsteroidal anti-inflammatory drugs [NSAIDs], antivirals, antihypertensives, benzodiazepines, others), substance use/withdrawal, CNS disease (Parkinson's, MS, dementia, tumor), pancreatic and other malignancies, anemia, systemic infection, sleep apnea, lupus, uncontrolled diabetes, normal bereavement. Tests based on neuroendocrine dysregulation (dexamethasone suppression test, thyrotropin-releasing hormone stimulation test); sleep EEG generally not specific/sensitive enough or too expensive for routine clinical use. Over 50% have recurrence.

▶ Treatment Steps

1. Ensure safety—hospitalize for suicide risk.
2. Antidepressant medications (SSRIs generally first choice); if par-

▶ **differential diagnosis**

DEPRESSION	VS.	BEREAVEMENT
Mood pervasive, unremitting		Mood fluctuates
Pervasive low self-esteem, worthlessness		Self-reproach regarding deceased
May be suicidal		Usually not suicidal
May have sustained psychotic symptoms		May transiently hear voice or see image of deceased
Does not improve without treatment; average episode 6–9 months		Symptoms improve with time; severe symptoms usually gone by 2–6 months
Social withdrawal		Often welcomes social support

tially effective, may augment with lithium, another antidepressant, thyroid hormone. Continue treatment for 6–12 months if first episode. Antidepressants take 4–6 weeks for effect. Long-term maintenance treatment for recurrent illness.

3. ECT may be used for treatment-resistant or psychotic depression, rapid response, in the pregnant, elderly, or medically ill, or with previous good response.

4. Psychotherapy (i.e., cognitive, interpersonal, psychodynamic, couples) may be effective alone in mild depression. Combined therapy and medication most effective treatment.

5. Antipsychotics plus antidepressant or ECT for psychotic depression.

6. Phototherapy may help with seasonal pattern.

7. Diagnose and treat comorbid psychopathology (anxiety disorders, substance use, personality disorders, ADHD).

C. Bipolar Disorders

▶ Description

One or more manic episodes (see above) usually accompanied by one or more major depressive episodes. Bipolar depressions may have hypersomnia, severe lethargy. High suicide risk and rates of substance abuse. May become aggressive when manic. Classified as follows:

1. Type I—history of full-blown mania and major depression.
2. Type II—history of hypomania and major depression.
3. Rapid cycling—four or more mood episodes per year.
4. Mixed—full symptoms of both mania and depression intermixed or alternating rapidly for at least 1 week. Often psychotic. High suicide risk.

▶ Pathophysiology

Strong genetic diathesis; heterogeneous dysregulation of biogenic amine systems. One theory implicates kindling, repeated subthreshold stimulation of neuron-generating action potential in temporal lobes. Cycles occur more frequently over time. Initial episode may be stress related.

▶ differential diagnosis

PSYCHOTIC MANIA OR DEPRESSION	VS.	SCHIZOPHRENIA
Premorbid adjustment good		Premorbid adjustment poor in ≥ 50%
Family history of affective disorder		Family history affective disorder much less likely
Personality and functioning usually preserved between episodes		Chronic, often deteriorating course
Prior mood episodes		No prior mood episodes
Mood disturbance always present and begins before onset of psychosis		Psychosis usually precedes any mood symptoms
Psychotic features usually reflect underlying mood disturbance (e.g., somatic delusions in depression, grandiose delusions in mania)		Psychotic features often bizarre, persecutory, nihilistic

► Diagnosis

Rule out hyperthyroidism, medications (steroids, antidepressants, stimulants, sympathomimetics, others), substance intoxication/withdrawal, neurologic disorders (e.g., head injury, MS, seizure disorder), other psychiatric disorders (e.g., schizophrenia, personality disorders).

► Treatment Steps

1. Assess risk of suicide, dangerous poor judgment, assaultiveness, acute medical problems.
2. Acute mania—mood stabilizer: lithium generally effective in bipolar I, anticonvulsants (valproate, carbamazepine) may be more effective with rapid cycling or mixed types. Benzodiazepine or neuroleptic for acute symptom control. ECT also effective.
3. Acute depression—mood stabilizer with or without antidepressant if necessary (risk of precipitating mania); antipsychotic may be necessary for psychotic symptoms.
4. Maintenance therapy—mood stabilizers alone or in combination. Warranted after second episode or first in adolescents.
5. Psychotherapy useful for adjustment problems, education, prevention of relapse.

D. Cyclothymia

Chronic disturbance of at least 2 years' duration. Numerous hypomanic episodes and numerous depressive episodes of insufficient severity to qualify for mania or major depression. May respond to lithium, anticonvulsants, psychotherapy.

E. Dysthymia

► Description

Chronic disturbance of at least 2 years' duration. Depressed mood not of severity of major depression. Psychotherapy, antidepressants. Possibly exercise.

VI. ANXIETY DISORDERS

A. Panic Disorder

► Description

Recurrent discrete periods of intense anxiety (minutes to hours) that are initially unexpected. Dyspnea, paresthesias, chest pain, dizziness, palpitations, sweating, nausea, fears of going crazy or dying. Often associated with agoraphobia, fear of being in a place from which escape is difficult, such as outside the home alone, in a crowd, traveling on public transportation, driving on a bridge. Phobic avoidance of situations associated with attacks. Onset mid- to late twenties with chronic, relapsing course. First presentation usually to emergency rooms, primary care physicians.

► Pathophysiology

Genetic contribution. Disturbances in locus ceruleus (norepinephrine), serotonin, and GABA neurotransmission. Substances that induce panic include CO_2, lactate, isoproterenol. Initial episode often stress related. Frequent childhood history of anxiety disorder, some with history of childhood sexual/physical abuse.

► **Diagnosis**

Rule out hypoglycemia, pheochromocytoma, hyperthyroidism, hyperparathyroidism, adrenal dysfunction, autoimmune disorders, arrhythmias, cardiomyopathy, seizure disorder, pulmonary insufficiency, anemia, CNS diseases, B_{12} deficiency, caffeinism, sedative or alcohol withdrawal, hallucinogen or stimulant abuse, medication related. **Cued** (situationally bound) panic attacks may occur with other psychiatric disorders—phobias, OCD, PTSD. Mitral valve prolapse associated finding in 20–50%, but generally not clinically significant.

► **Treatment Steps**

1. Emergency management: reassurance, benzodiazepine.
2. Rule out acute medical event: myocardial infarction, pulmonary embolus, substance withdrawal, CNS insult, hypoglycemia, electrolyte abnormalities.
3. Antidepressants first line; high-potency benzodiazepines (e.g., clonazepam) work faster in severe cases. Buspirone alone ineffective.
4. Cognitive-behavior therapies effective for agoraphobia, relapse prevention in some. Combined therapy (medication + behavioral therapy) probably most effective.
5. Diagnose and treat comorbid anxiety disorders, depression (> 50%), suicidality, substance abuse, personality disorders, somatization, coronary artery disease.
6. Reduce or eliminate caffeine.

B. Obsessive–Compulsive Disorder

► **Description**

Recurrent intrusive images, impulses, thoughts (obsessions), and perseverative, ritualistic behaviors (compulsions) that produce anxiety if resisted. In most cases, experienced as senseless product of own mind (versus delusion). Typical obsessions involve contamination, sin, aggression, loss of control, order, doubt; common compulsions include washing, checking, counting. Onset childhood through early adulthood. Twenty-five percent have obsessions only. Course chronic.

► **Pathophysiology**

Genetic contribution, also genetically linked to Tourette syndrome. PET shows hypermetabolism in prefrontal cortex and caudate nuclei. Psychobiologic probes suggest abnormality in serotonin system. Autoimmunity to streptococcal infection in some childhood cases.

► **Diagnosis**

"Compulsive" behaviors such as eating, gambling, shopping give pleasure and are impulse-control disorders; performance of true compulsions reduces anxiety. May have chapped hands due to excessive washing. Rule out temporal lobe epilepsy, postencephalitic states, Tourette syndrome, MS, basal ganglia lesions, postconcussion syndrome, Sydenham's chorea. Obsessive–compulsive personality disorder lacks true obsessions/compulsions, lacks anxiety, not experienced as ego-alien.

► **Treatment Steps**

1. Serotonergic antidepressants (i.e., SSRIs, clomipramine).
2. Behavioral therapies (exposure plus response prevention).

3. Diagnose and treat comorbid suicidal risk, depression, substance abuse, Tourette syndrome, anorexia nervosa, schizotypal features, impulse-control disorders.

C. Specific Phobia

▶ Description

Irrational, excessive fear and avoidance of object or situation (other than fear of panic or social situation) (e.g., snakes, heights, blood).

▶ Treatment Steps

Behavioral and cognitive therapies (systematic desensitization).

D. Social Phobia

▶ Description

Fear of embarrassment, scrutiny of others; specific (e.g., eating in public, public speaking) or generalized. Onset adolescence, chronic course.

▶ Treatment Steps

1. Cognitive and behavioral psychotherapies.
2. β-Blockers for performance anxiety.
3. Antidepressants (not tricyclics), high-potency benzodiazapines.

E. Posttraumatic Stress Disorder

▶ Description

Exposure to markedly stressful event causing terror and helplessness (e.g., combat, rape, sexual abuse, torture, natural disaster). Symptoms from three categories: **reexperiencing** (recollections, nightmares, play in children); **emotional numbing** (avoidance, amnesia, restricted affect); **autonomic arousal** (insomnia, irritability). Comorbid depression, anxiety, dissociation, substance abuse, suicide attempts common.

▶ Treatment Steps

1. Hospitalize for acute suicide, violence risk.
2. Cognitive-behavioral and exposure therapies.
3. Antidepressants may be helpful.

F. Acute Stress Disorder

▶ Description

Symptoms of dissociation (numbing, detachment, derealization, depersonalization) experienced during/following extreme trauma; followed by reexperiencing, avoidance, and arousal symptoms as in PTSD. If symptoms present after 4 weeks, diagnose PTSD.

▶ Treatment Steps

1. Psychotherapy.
2. Mild sedation as indicated.

G. Generalized Anxiety Disorder

▶ Description

Unrealistic, persistent, excessive anxiety and worry unrelated to another psychiatric disorder for at least 6 months. Muscle tension, restlessness, fatiguability, difficulty concentrating, irritability, sleep disturbance. Other somatic complaints common. High comorbidity with depression. Medical conditions associated with anxiety listed under panic disorder.

► Treatment Steps
1. Psychotherapy.
2. Antidepressants, especially with comorbid depression. Buspirone does **not** cause sedation, psychomotor impairment, risk of tolerance or abuse. Benzodiazepines give more immediate relief.

H. Anxiety Disorder Due to a General Medical Condition

A wide range of medical disorders can produce symptoms of anxiety disorders, most frequently panic disorder, generalized anxiety disorder, and OCD. Specific medical disorders to consider are listed under each anxiety disorder. Suspect medical etiology with onset age > 35–40, presence of medical illness, atypical symptoms, or focal neurologic signs. Treat primary medical disorder; may require independent treatment of anxiety disorder if symptoms persist.

VII. SOMATOFORM DISORDERS

Physical symptoms not fully explained by a medical condition, severe enough to cause distress and impairment; unlike factitious disorders and malingering, the symptoms of somatoform disorders are **not intentionally produced** but are **strongly linked to psychological factors. In psychological factors affecting a medical condition, a known medical condition is present and develops or is exacerbated by psychological factors.**

A. Somatization Disorder

► Description

Recurrent, multiple, unfeigned somatic complaints not fully explained by physical disorder, for which medical attention sought. Often vague and dramatic presentation. Frequently includes chronic pain; GI, cardiopulmonary, neurologic symptoms; menstrual complaints, sexual problems. Onset before 30. Child sexual abuse predisposes. Comorbid alcohol, analgesic, sedative abuse; depression (> 80%), anxiety (> 25%), personality disorders. Chronic, fluctuating course. Rare in males. Genetic predisposition. Rule out disorders that present with vague, multiple, confusing symptoms. Conversion disorder presents with only pseudoneurologic symptoms.

► Treatment Steps
1. Regularly scheduled visits with primary care physician.
2. Tests, consultations only with evidence of illness.
3. Avoid opiates, benzodiazepines.
4. Antidepressants if indicated.
5. Psychiatric referral.

B. Conversion Disorder

Involuntary, psychogenic alteration of physical functioning, not limited to pain or sexual disturbance. Limited to neurologic symptoms (e.g., paralysis, blindness, mutism, pseudoseizures). Complete medical and neurologic evaluation to rule out confusing neurologic or medical disorders (e.g., MS, HIV encephalopathy, lupus) (25–50% eventually receive nonpsychiatric diagnosis). Comorbid personality disorders, substance abuse, depression, anxiety, previous neurologic or medical disorder. Resolution usually spontaneous. Hypnosis, anxiolytics, psychotherapy, amobarbital interview are all used.

► **cram facts**

SOMATOFORM AND RELATED DISORDERS

1. Somatoform Disorders
   • Symptoms are not intentionally produced
   • Symptoms not fully explained by medical condition
   • Symptoms linked to psychological factors
      a. Somatization disorder: Multiple somatic complaints
      b. Conversion disorder: Neurologic symptoms
      c. Pain disorder
      d. Hypochondriasis: Fear of specific disease
      e. Body dysmorphic disorder: Preoccupation with defect in appearance
2. Factitious Disorder
   Intentional production of symptoms for unconscious psychological reasons
3. Malingering
   Intentional production of symptoms for recognizable gain
4. Psychological Factors Affecting a Medical Condition
   Known medical condition develops/is exacerbated by psychological factors

---

C. Pain Disorder

Preoccupation with pain in absence of adequate physical findings or pathophysiologic mechanism to account for intensity or disabling psychosocial sequelae. "Invalid role" frequent. Comorbid analgesic, substance abuse, depression, anxiety, invalidism, inactivity, isolation. Rule out psychogenic disorders with known pathophysiologic mechanisms (e.g., tension headaches) (diagnosed as psychologic factors affecting medical condition). Rule out reflex sympathetic dystrophy. Treatment team with "gatekeeper"; cognitive and behavioral therapies including behavioral modification, biofeedback, relaxation; NSAIDs, antidepressants for pain.

D. Hypochondriasis

Preoccupation with fear of having a specific, serious disease, despite medical reassurance to the contrary. Not of delusional intensity. Duration at least 6 months. Comorbid depression, anxiety, dependence. Symptoms must not be due to panic attacks or part of OCD. Manage with regular medical visits, avoiding costly workups. Psychiatric referral.

E. Body Dysmorphic Disorder (Dysmorphophobia)

Preoccupation with imagined or slight defect in appearance; may or may not be of delusional intensity; causing marked distress/impairment (not including anorexia nervosa). May seek repeated cosmetic surgery. Comorbid depression, delusional disorder, social phobia, OCD, suicide risk. Psychotherapy, SSRI.

VIII. FACTITIOUS DISORDERS AND MALINGERING

A. Factitious Disorder (Munchausen Syndrome)

Intentional (but often compulsive) production or feigning of physical or psychological symptoms, presumably for unconscious psychological reasons (e.g., need to assume sick role). Comorbid severe personality disorders, substance abuse. Extensive medical knowledge—medical occupation, history of illness. Symptoms induced by parent in child, known as Munchausen's by proxy. Psychiatric consultation, confrontation sometimes helpful.

B. Malingering

Intentional production of physical or psychological symptoms for **obvious recognizable external incentive** (e.g., to avoid military service, evade prison, obtain drugs). Does not imply psychiatric disorder. Discrepancy with objective findings, uncooperative, vague.

IX. DISSOCIATIVE DISORDERS

Alteration in normally integrative functions of identity, memory, or consciousness.

A. Dissociative Identity Disorder

▶ Description

Two or more distinct personalities which recurrently take control of person's behavior and may or may not be aware of each other. Each personality may have its own set of memories, physiologic characteristics, sex, age, race. May have lapses of time, be told of behaviors of which they have no memories, or hear voices (pseudohallucinations) leading to misdiagnosis of schizophrenia. Severe sexual and psychological abuse in childhood. Ninety percent females. High comorbidity with borderline personality, somatization, depressive disorders.

▶ Treatment Steps
Intensive psychotherapy.

B. Amnestic Disorders

1. Psychogenic Fugue

Sudden, unexpected travel away from home with confusion about identity or assumption of new identity and amnesia for previous identity. Unaware of loss of identity. Lasts hours to months. Follows severe stress, personal rejection, loss.

2. Psychogenic Amnesia

▶ Description

Sudden inability to recall important personal information of a traumatic or stressful nature. Aware of loss.

▶ Treatment Steps
1. Rule out medical/neurologic etiology such as temporal lobe epilepsy, substance-induced amnesia, CNS tumor, closed head trauma, dementia, malingering.
2. Recovery generally rapid and spontaneous.
3. Hypnosis, amobarbital (Amytal) interview may assist in recovery of memories, differentiation from medical etiologies.
4. Psychotherapy.

C. Depersonalization Disorder

Persistent or recurrent feeling of detachment from one's body or self. May be accompanied by derealization, sense of detachment from, unreality of outside world. Mild forms common. Reality testing intact. May be precipitated by stressor, substance intoxication (alcohol, hallucinogen, marijuana). Course chronic. Rule out temporal lobe epilepsy, CNS tumor, encephalitis, migraine. SSRI may help.

X. SEXUAL AND GENDER IDENTITY DISORDERS

A. Sexual Dysfunctions

▶ **Description**

Disorders of all phases of sexual response cycle (Desire → Arousal → Orgasm → Resolution). Etiology can be medical, substance related, psychogenic, or combination.

a. **Sexual desire disorders**
   (1) Hypoactive sexual desire disorder—deficient or absent sexual fantasies or desire. Desire commonly decreased by major illness or surgery, especially those affecting body image.
   (2) Sexual aversion disorder—revulsion to and avoidance of sexual contact.

b. **Sexual arousal disorders**
   (1) Female sexual arousal disorder—inadequate subjective excitement and lubrication/swelling. Lack of lubrication may be related to hormonal patterns, medications.
   (2) **Male erectile disorder (impotence)**—inability to attain or maintain erection to complete sexual activity or lack of subjective excitement. Increases with age. From 20–50% are substance related or are due to medical illness or medication (see below). Spontaneous erections, morning erections, erections with masturbation indicate psychogenic etiology. Sensate focus techniques.

c. **Orgasmic disorders**
   (1) **Male and female orgasmic disorders**—persistent or recurrent delay or absence of orgasm following sexual excitement. Directed masturbation, sensate focus.
   (2) **Premature ejaculation**—persistent ejaculation with minimal stimulation before or shortly after penetration. Affects 30% of male population. Responds to behavioral techniques (squeeze technique).

d. **Sexual pain disorders**
   (1) **Dyspareunia**—genital pain before, during, or after intercourse. Most common in women, expecially with history of sexual trauma. Rule out pelvic pathology (e.g., vaginitis, endometriosis, cervicitis, postmenopausal thinning of vaginal mucosa).
   (2) **Vaginismus**—involuntary spasm of musculature of vagina which interferes with coitus. Sexual trauma common cause.

▶ **Pathophysiology**

Psychological etiologies include ignorance and misinformation; unconscious guilt, anger, anxiety; performance anxiety and fear of rejection; lack of communication between spouses; conditioned responses (e.g., fear of discovery in parental home leading to premature ejaculation).

▶ **Diagnosis**

Rule out medical and substance-induced etiologies (see Cram Facts).

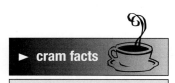

▶ **cram facts**

MEDICAL CAUSES OF SEXUAL DYSFUNCTION

- Diabetes
- Vascular disease
- Multiple sclerosis
- Trauma injury (spinal cord injury)
- Complication of prostate surgery
- Antihypertensives
- Antidepressants
- Anticholinergics
- Abuse of alcohol or illicit drugs

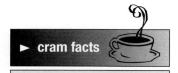

▶ **cram facts**

LAB WORKUP FOR ERECTILE DYSFUNCTION

- Glucose (rule out diabetes)
- Liver function tests (LFTs)
- Thyroid-stimulating hormone (TSH)
- Follicle-stimulating hormone (FSH) and luteinizing hormone (LH)
- Prolactin
- Testosterone

▶ **Treatment Steps**

1. Rule out medical and substance-induced causes and other psychiatric diagnoses.
2. Education, specific behavioral therapies, couples therapy, individual therapy.
3. Somatic therapies include medication (e.g., SSRI for premature ejaculation); external vacuum devices, alprostadil injections, sildenafil citrate, surgery (see Clinical Pearl).

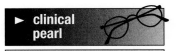

▶ **clinical pearl**

Do not use any of the phosphodiesterase 5 inhibitors with any form of nitroglycerin (Viagra [sildenafil], Cialis [tadalafil], Levitra [vardenafil]).

B. Paraphilias

▶ **Description**

Recurrent and intense sexual arousal in response to unusual fantasies or objects, of at least 6 months' duration. Patient has acted on or is distressed by the urges. Types include:

- Exhibitionism—exposure of one's genitals to strangers; rare in females.
- Fetishism—use of nonliving objects (e.g., undergarments); rare in females.
- Frotteurism—rubbing nonconsenting person.
- Pedophilia—prepubescent child; most common paraphilia.
- Sexual masochism—acts of being beaten, humiliated, bound, made to suffer.
- Sexual sadism—psychological or physical suffering of victim; rare in females.
- Transvestic fetishism—cross-dressing.
- Voyeurism—observing unsuspecting persons.

▶ **Treatment Steps**

1. Rule out schizophrenia, other brain diseases.
2. Insight-oriented psychotherapy, behavior therapy.
3. Antiandrogens (e.g., medroxyprogesterone acetate) sometimes used with dangerous hypersexuality.

C. Gender Identity Disorder

▶ **Description**

Distress about his/her assigned sex, desire to be or insisting one is opposite sex. May occur in children, adolescents, or adults. Few children carry diagnosis into adulthood. Often isolated, ostracized, depressed, may become suicidal. Attracted to either sex.

▶ **Treatment Steps**

1. Individual and family therapy with children.
2. Hormones, sex-reassignment surgery for selected adult "transsexuals" who have lived successfully as other gender.
3. Treat comorbid anxiety, depression.

XI. EATING DISORDERS

A. Anorexia Nervosa

▶ **Description**

Refusal to maintain minimal normal body weight (< 85%), intense fear of gaining weight, distorted body image, 95% female, **amenorrhea, potentially fatal.**

► Pathophysiology

Genetic component; possible hypothalamic disturbance; psychological resistance to demands of adolescence; cultural preoccupation with slimness in developed societies. Stress, dieting often precipitate.

► Diagnosis

Rule out weight loss due to depression, substance use, psychosis, acquired immune deficiency syndrome (AIDS), cancer, GI disorders (generally no body image disturbance, amenorrhea). Leukopenia, anemia, electrolyte abnormalities, dehydration, decreased thryoid function, sinus bradycardia.

► Treatment Steps

1. Hospitalize for dehydration, starvation, hypotension, electrolyte problems, hypothermia, suicide risk.
2. Treatment contract for weight gain.
3. Individual/cognitive behavioral/family therapy often used.
4. Antidepressants if depressed (avoid bupropion due to seizure risk).

B. Bulimia Nervosa

► Description

Recurrent binge eating, lack of control over eating, and compensatory behavior to prevent weight gain, including self-induced vomiting, laxatives/diuretics, strict dieting/vigorous exercise, overconcern with body shape. Usually normal weight. Purging and nonpurging types.

► Pathophysiology

Genetic component; decreased CNS serotonin, norepinephrine activity. Onset often during dieting. Family history of mood and substance disorders, obesity.

► Diagnosis

Dental erosion, caries, parotid enlargement, calloused fingers, metabolic alkalosis in 50%, dehydration, weakness, lethargy, GI problems, cardiac arrhythmias; comorbid anorexia, depression, personality disorders, stealing, substance abuse.

► Treatment Steps

1. Electrocardiogram (ECG), electrolytes, amylase, liver function tests.
2. Hospitalize for suicide risk, electrolyte imbalance, esophageal/gastric rupture.
3. Psychotherapy, nutritional counseling; SSRIs reduce binging. Do not prescribe bupropion due to risk of seizures. Monitor weight.

XII. SLEEP DISORDERS

A. Primary Sleep Disorders

1. Dyssomnias

► Description

Disturbance in the amount, quality, and timing of sleep.

a. **Primary insomnia**

Disturbance in initiating, maintaining, or feeling rested after sleep. Somatic tension/anxiety, conditioned response. Rule out psychiatric (one-third to one-half), general medical, or substance-induced cause. Sleep log, interview bed partner regarding awakenings, snoring, leg jerks. **Sleep hygiene treatment:**

- Regularize sleep hours.
- Use of bed **only** for sex or sleep.
- If not asleep in 30 minutes, leave bed and return only when drowsy.
- No napping.
- Regular exercise, but not immediately prior to bedtime.
- Reduce or eliminate alcohol, caffeine, sedative–hypnotics, cigarettes.
- Relaxation exercises may help.

Sedative–hypnotics (benzodiazepines, zolpidem) appropriate for short-term relief; long-term benefit unpredictable. OTC sleep aids contain antihistamines, anticholinergics—limited effectiveness and may lead to anticholinergic toxicity.

b. **Primary Hypersomnia**

Prolonged sleep, excessive daytime sleepiness, napping. Rule out medical, psychiatric etiologies, narcolepsy, sleep apnea; naps, stimulants.

c. **Narcolepsy**

► Description

Daytime drowsiness, irresistible sleep attacks; at times in combination with hypnagogic/hypnopompic hallucinations, sleep paralysis, cataplexy (loss of muscle control with strong emotions). Risk of accidents. Onset in adolescence, chronic course.

► Pathophysiology

Abnormality of REM-inhibiting mechanisms. May have genetic component. Associated with human lymphocyte antigen (HLA)-DR2.

► Diagnosis

Diagnose with careful history; polysomnographic sleep study shows REM at sleep onset.

► Treatment Steps

Short daytime naps; stimulants for sleep attacks; TCAs used for cataplexy, sleep paralysis. Family, employer education.

d. **Breathing-Related Sleep Disorder (Sleep Apnea)**

► Description

Episodes of breathing cessation during sleep. Obstructive (occlusion of upper airway during sleep, most common), central (reduced nocturnal respiratory drive), mixed types. Obesity predisposes. Accompanied by snoring, gasping, body movements, morning headaches, daytime sleepiness, memory impairment, inattention, anxiety, depression, hypertension, arrhythmias.

► Diagnosis

Rule out hypothyroidism. Overnight polysomnography (sleep study).

► Treatment Steps

1. Weight reduction.
2. Surgical removal of excess airway tissue as indicated.
3. Nasal continuous positive airway pressure (CPAP) for obstructive type.

4. Avoid sedatives, alcohol.

5. Protriptyline for central type.

e. Circadian Rhythm Sleep Disorder

Mismatch between environmental demands and person's sleep–wake pattern (e.g., shift work, jet lag, delayed sleep phase). Avoid shift work when possible. Avoid alcohol; low-dose hypnotics; bright-light therapy, melatonin.

f. Dyssomnia Not Otherwise Specified

(1) Periodic limb movements. Frequent, repetitive, low-amplitude limb jerks, leading to frequent awakenings, daytime sleepiness. Often occurs with restless legs syndrome. Most prevalent in elderly. Benzodiazepines, L-dopa, quinine.

(2) **Restless legs syndrome**—agonizing, deep creeping sensations in leg or arm muscles relieved by moving, massage. Peak incidence in middle age. Benzodiazepines, L-dopa, quinine, carbamazepine, others.

2. Parasomnias

▶ Description

Abnormal events that occur during sleep. The event is the focus, not daytime sleepiness. Relatively common in children. In adults, psychiatric evaluation indicated.

a. Nightmare disorder

Repeated awakenings, detailed recall. Usually during REM sleep. Rule out sedative withdrawal, SSRI use, depression, PTSD. TCAs, benzodiazepines.

b. Sleep terror disorder (pavor nocturnus)

Awaken with panicky scream, intense anxiety, tachycardia from stage 3 to 4 sleep. May not fully awaken and be relatively unresponsive to efforts of others to comfort, with morning amnesia. Comorbid sleepwalking disorder. Familial. Rule out temporal lobe epilepsy; mood, anxiety disorders in adults.

c. Sleepwalking disorder

Unresponsive during episode with morning amnesia. High-amplitude slow waves in stage 3 to 4 sleep. Protect from accidental injury (e.g., door and window latches). In adults, rule out psychopathology. Sleep hygiene, benzodiazepines, TCAs may help.

B. Sleep Disorders Related to Another Mental or Substance-Related Disorder

▶ Description

Depression and alcoholism most common causes of sleep disturbance.

- Depression: variable sleep continuity disturbance, delayed onset, shortened REM latency, increased REM density and duration.
- Mania: decreased sleep with decreased need for sleep.
- Panic disorder: difficulty falling and staying asleep; panic attacks during stage 2 or 3.
- Posttraumatic stress disorder: insomnia, disturbing dreams.
- Psychosis: variability in sleep continuity.
- Alcohol abuse, dependence: acutely induces sleep with wakefulness, anxiety dreams; with chronic use sleep is fragmented; abstinence acutely causes insomnia, nightmares.

- Dementia: disrupted sleep continuity, polyphasic sleep–wake schedule.
- Delirium: agitation, combativeness, wandering, confusion, fragmented sleep.

XIII. IMPULSE-CONTROL DISORDERS

Failure to resist an impulse to perform an act that is harmful to the person or others, with increasing tension before committing the act, and experience of pleasure at the time of the act. The act is ego syntonic. Subsequent guilt may or may not follow. Course usually chronic. May be attempts to master painful affects. CNS serotonin dysregulation strongly implicated in impulsivity; soft neurologic signs, nonspecific abnormal EEG. Comorbid mental retardation, head trauma, epilepsy. Rule out other psychiatric disorder which may share features (e.g., antisocial personality disorder, mania, ADHD, substance-related disorders).

A. Intermittent Explosive Disorder

▶ Description

Discreet episodes of loss of control of aggressive impulses grossly out of proportion to precipitant, resulting in serious assault or destruction of property. Frequently poor recall for episode. Not otherwise aggressive.

▶ Treatment Steps

Combined psychotherapy and medication. Lithium, anticonvulsants, SSRIs. **Benzodiazepines may cause disinhibition.**

B. Kleptomania

Failure to resist impulses to steal unneccessary or trivial items. Insight-oriented or behavioral psychotherapy, SSRIs.

C. Pathologic Gambling

Maladaptive gambling behavior, including preoccupation and loss of control. Treatment includes psychotherapy, Gamblers Anonymous (GA), SSRIs.

D. Pyromania

Deliberate fire setting and fascination with fire. Onset usually childhood. Behavioral therapy.

E. Trichotillomania

Recurrent pulling out of one's own hair that results in noticeable hair loss. Usually surreptitious. Childhood or adolescent onset. Psychotherapy, SSRI.

XIV. ADJUSTMENT DISORDERS

▶ Description

Maladaptive, excessive emotional and behavioral responses that occur within 3 months of a stressor that is **within range of normal experience** (unlike PTSD), such as school problem, marital discord, job loss, illness. Significant impairment in social or occupational functioning. Classified by predominant symptoms: depression, anxiety, mixed emotional features, disturbance of conduct, mixed disturbance of conduct and emotions. Adolescents frequently have behavioral symptoms, whereas adults often have mood, anxiety symptoms. Does not persist more than 6 months after stressor is terminated. Not diagnosed in presence of Axis I disorder, uncomplicated bereavement, or exacerbation of Axis II (personality) disorder.

► Pathophysiology

Greater vulnerability with history of serious medical illness, disability, parental loss during childhood.

► Treatment Steps

1. Evaluate suicide risk, risk of medical noncompliance.
2. Psychotherapy, antianxiety, antidepressant medication sometimes helpful.
3. Stress reduction through social support exercise, relaxation, cognitive reframing, attention to health habits.

XV. PERSONALITY DISORDERS (AXIS II)

► Description

Persistent, inflexible, maladaptive patterns of thinking, feeling, and behaving causing dysfunction or subjective distress. Onset late adolescence.

A. Odd/Eccentric Cluster

1. Paranoid Personality Disorder

Interprets actions of others as malicious, demeaning, or threatening. Hypervigilant, hypersensitive to criticism. Not psychotic.

2. Schizoid Personality Disorder

Isolated, indifference to social relationships, restricted range of emotional experience.

3. Schizotypal Personality Disorder

Peculiarities of ideation, appearance, behavior. Deficit in interpersonal relatedness, constricted affect, excessive social anxiety. May respond to low-dose antipsychotics.

B. Dramatic/Emotional Cluster

1. Antisocial Personality Disorder

Pattern of exploitative, socially irresponsible, destructive, impulsive behavior with no remorse; substance abuse, precocious sexual activity, violent. Childhood history of conduct disorder essential for diagnosis. Aggressivity may respond to SSRI, anticonvulsants. Treat comorbid substance abuse, anxiety, depression.

2. Borderline Personality Disorder

Instability of self-image, identity, relationships, and mood. Chronic feelings of emptiness, intense personal attachments, impulsivity, inappropriate anger, suicide gestures, substance abuse and other self–destructive behavior common. Frequent histories of childhood abuse. Long-term psychotherapy; SSRI or carbamazepine helpful for mood stability, decreasing impulsivity; low-dose antipsychotic may help for psychotic symptoms, severe cognitive distortions. Avoid benzodiazepines. Treat comorbid disorders.

3. Histrionic Personality Disorder

Excessive but shallow and labile emotionality and attention seeking. Need for praise, reassurance.

4. Narcissistic Personality Disorder

Grandiose, exploitative, entitled, rageful if humiliated, lacking in empathy.

C. Anxious/Inhibited Cluster

1. Obsessive–Compulsive Personality Disorder

Perfectionist, inflexible; preoccupied with rules; ambivalent, controlling, stingy, constricted affect, driven.

2. Dependent Personality Disorder

Submissive, passive, clingy behavior; lets others make important decisions; easily hurt, preoccupied with abandonment. Chronic physical illness predisposing factor.

3. Avoidant Personality Disorder

▶ **Description**

Fearful of rejection, timid, inhibited but **desirous of relationships** (versus schizoid personality disorder); frequent comorbid anxiety disorders (e.g., social phobia, generalized anxiety disorder).

▶ **Pathophysiology of Personality Disorders**

Genetic contribution in antisocial personality disorder, schizotypal, paranoid; childhood sexual/physical abuse in many borderlines, antisocials, avoidants; nonspecific neurologic abnormalities; decreased CNS serotonin associated with impulsivity, aggression; schizotypals genetically, biologically related to schizophrenia.

▶ **Treatment Steps**

1. Rule out medical/psychiatric causes of acute personality change.
2. Evaluate risk of suicide, aggression, especially with substance intoxication; hospitalize for protection of self/others.
3. Diagnose and treat comorbid Axis I disorders; depression, anxiety, psychosis, substance use, ADHD, somatization.
4. Cognitive–behavioral, interpersonal, psychodynamic, behavioral, family, group therapies all utilized depending on specific disorder and patient.

XVI. BIOLOGIC THERAPIES

A. Antipsychotic Medication (Neuroleptics)

▶ **Description**

Classes—Low potency (e.g., thioridazine, chlorpromazine); **high potency** (e.g., haloperidol, fluphenazine); **atypical** (e.g., clozapine, risperidone, olanzapine, quetiapine, ziprasidone). Haloperidol and fluphenazine can be given as long as long-acting IM preparation.

Indications—Acute schizophrenia and other schizophrenias—acute psychotic disorders (e.g., amphetamine-induced psychosis); chronic schizophrenia; psychosis in context of major depression or mania; Tourette syndrome (Haldol); acute agitation, aggression or psychosis in delirium, dementia. Low-dose antipsychotics may be helpful in some personality disorders.

Mechanism of Action—Postsynaptic blockade of mesolimbic dopamine-D2 receptors. Atypical antipsychotics also block 5-HT$_2$ receptors, others.

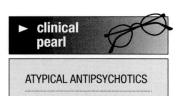

▶ **clinical pearl**

ATYPICAL ANTIPSYCHOTICS

- Good for negative symptoms of schizophrenia.
- Fewer extrapyramidal side effects than traditional antipsychotics.

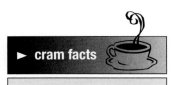

► cram facts

OLANZAPINE (ZYPREXA)

- Weight gain is a common side effect.
- Hyperglycemia and diabetes are also associated with olanzapine and may limit the use of the drug.

Pharmacokinetics—Marked interindividual differences in blood levels.

Side Effects—EPS greater for high-potency drugs; anticholinergic/hypotension/sedation/cardiac effects greater for low-potency drugs. Acute dystonic reactions, pseudo-parkinsonism treated with anticholinergic agents, e.g., benztropine (Cogentin). Tardive dyskinesia (abnormal involuntary movement scale [AIMS] exam to evaluate symptoms every 6 months). Atypical antipsychotics cause less EPS, tardive dyskinesia; clozapine causes agranulocytosis in 1%, requiring weekly CBC; also anticholinergic, seizures, weight gain, sialorrhea. All antipsychotics (possibly excepting molindone) cause weight gain, sedation, side effects, lower seizure threshold.

Toxicity—Neuroleptic malignant syndrome (NMS), idiosyncratic reaction with rapid development of rigidity, hyperpyrexia, autonomic instability, delirium, confusion, mutism, myoglobinuria with CPK elevation. Supportive care, dantrolene, bromocriptine.

B. Mood Stabilizers

1. Lithium

► Description

Indications—Acute mania, acute depression, and maintenance treatment of bipolar disorder; cyclothymic disorder; schizoaffective disorder; segmentation of antidepressants in major depression; intermittent explosive disorder, mental retardation with aggressiveness or self-mutilation. Lithium may have antisuicidal effect independent of its antidepressant effect. **Never discontinue lithium abruptly.**

Mechanism of Action—Uncertain.

Pharmacokinetics—Rapid absorption. Monitor 12-hour blood levels, therapeutic range 0.8–1.2 mEq/L. **Narrow margin of safety.** Lower doses in elderly.

Side Effects—Tremor, GI distress, weight gain, polyuria, mental dulling, ECG changes, dermatologic reactions, peripheral edema, hypothyroidism, goiter. Low risk of fetal cardiac anomaly if used during first trimester. Prelithium workup includes thyroid function tests, BUN, creatinine, urinalysis; ECG if age > 40.

Toxicity—Due to overdose, sodium depletion, drugs that increase levels (NSAIDs, diuretics, metronidazole): nausea, vomiting, diarrhea, renal failure, neuromuscular irritability, ataxia, coarse tremor, confusion, delirium, hallucinations, seizures, stupor, coma. **Lithium levels > 3.0 is medical emergency.** IV saline or hemodialysis, supportive treatment.

2. Anticonvulsants (Carbamazepine, Valproate)

Indications—Acute mania, maintenance treatment of bipolar disorder, schizoaffective disorder, intermittent explosive disorder. Anticonvulsants may be more effective than lithium in treatment of rapid cycling or mixed bipolar disorders. Lamotrigine, gabapentin, topiramate also used.

Mechanism of Action—Uncertain; may prevent kindling (repetitive subthreshold electrical or chemical stimuli producing autonomous epileptic focus).

Pharmacokinetics—Valproate serum levels 50–150; inhibits metabolism of many drugs oxidized in the liver, thereby increasing their serum levels. Carbamazepine serum levels 6–12; induces hepatic metabolism of many drugs including valproate, antidepressants, haloperidol, benzodiazepines, thereby decreasing their levels. Induces own metabolism, requiring dosage adjustments.

Side Effects—Valproate: GI distress, sedation, tremor, weight gain, benign transaminase elevation, thrombocytopenia, alopecia, ataxia, mild cognitive impairment; rare hemorrhagic pancreatitis, hepatitis may cause major malformations in pregnancy. Carbamazepine: sedation, dizziness, ataxia, GI distress, clumsiness, benign elevation of liver enzymes, leukopenia, cognitive disturbances; exacerbation of cardiac conduction delays; rare blood dyscrasias, hepatitis. Teratogenic in pregnancy. Get CBC, liver and renal function tests prior to treatment. Instruct patient taking carbamazepine to report fever, sore throat, weakness, petechiae, bruising, bleeding.

Toxicity—Valproate: severe neurologic symptoms. Hemodialysis. Carbamazepine: atrioventricular (AV) block, stupor, coma, neurologic symptoms. Supportive management.

C. Antidepressants

Indications—Major depression, bipolar depression, depression prophylaxis, atypical depression (SSRIs, monoamine oxidase inhibitors [MAOIs]), dysthymic disorder, panic disorder, generalized anxiety disorder, social phobia (MAOIs, SSRIs), PTSD, bulimia, obsessive–compulsive disorder (SSRIs and clompiramine), impulse control disorders, chronic pain (TCAs), ADHD, others.

Mechanism of Action—Uncertain. All antidepressants increase availability of CNS monamines, primarily norepinephrine and serotonin, with subsequent changes in neuroreceptors and other neuronal adaptations. Full response takes 4–6 weeks, longer for OCD.

1. Tricyclic Antidepressants

Examples—Amitriptyline (Elavil), imipramine (Tofranil), doxepin (Sinequan), nortriptyline (Pamelor).

Pharmacokinetics—Marked interindividual differences in blood levels. Nortriptyline has therapeutic window above which response declines. SSRIs, others increase serum levels of TCAs.

Side Effects—Anticholinergic including dryness, blurred vision, urinary hesitancy, constipation, ileus, tachycardia, memory disturbance; watch for additive toxicity. Sedation, orthostasis, falls in the elderly, weight gain, impotence, seizures. Slowed cardiac conduction (quinidine-like effect)—avoid use in patients with prolonged QT interval, bifascicular or left bundle branch block, or status post myocardial infarction. Obtain pretreatment ECG if age > 40 or history of cardiac disease.

Toxicity—High, doses of > 1 g toxic, often fatal due to arrhythmias, seizures, hypotension. CNS depressant effects potentiated by alcohol, sedative–hypnotics. Supportive care.

2. Monoamine Oxidase Inhibitors

Examples—Phenelzine (Nardil), tranylcypromine (Parnate).

Pharmacokinetics—Rapidly absorbed. Inhibition of > 85% platelet MAO in blood sample is a measure of effective dose.

Side Effects—Requires tyramine-free diet (i.e., no cheese, liver, red wine, aged meats, others). Anticholinergic (as above), headache, orthostasis, insomnia, sedation, weight gain, sexual dysfunction (impotence, anorgasmia).

Toxicity—**Hyperadrenergic crisis** due to MAO inhibition in gut with inability to metabolize pressors in medications (sympathomimetics, stimulants) or food (tyramine), results in sudden severe headache, hypertension, mydriasis, diaphoresis, cardiac arrhythmias; treat with nifedipine (Procardia) orally or phentolamine IV. **Serotonin syndrome** (diarrhea, nausea, headache, altered consciousness, tremor, neuromuscular irritability, hyperthermia, hypertension, tachycardia, seizures, coma, death) with serotonergic agents (e.g., SSRIs, buspirone, clomipramine); also with **meperidine,** dextromethorphan. Similar symptoms in overdose. Treat supportively. **Stop MAOIs at least 2 weeks before starting TCAs, SSRIs.**

3. Selective Serotonin Reuptake Inhibitors

Examples—Fluoxetine (Prozac), fluvoxamine (Luvox), paroxetine (Paxil), sertraline (Zoloft).

Pharmacokinetics—Inhibition of hepatic microsomal oxidative enzymes, increasing serum levels of many drugs, including TCAs, others.

Side Effects—Jitteriness, headache, nausea, diarrhea, anxiety, **sexual dysfunction,** insomnia, apathy, sedation. **No** or few anticholinergic, antihistaminic effects (e.g., orthostasic changes, seizures, cardiotoxic effects). Safety and side effect profile make them first choice agents especially in elderly. Relatively safe in overdose. Discontinue fluoxetine at least 5 weeks before starting MAOI.

4. Others

Bupropion (Wellbutrin)—Weak reuptake blocking effects on serotonin and nonrepinephrine. Affects reuptake of dopamine. Stimulating. Agitation, restlessness, insomnia. Also used in ADHD. Ineffective against panic. Contraindicated in bulimia, seizure disorders due to higher risk of seizures. **Does not cause sexual dysfunction, cardiotoxicity, weight gain, significant drug interactions.**

Venlafaxine (Effexor)—Inhibits uptake of both norepinephrine and 5-HT (like TCAs) but lacks anticholinergic and antihistaminic side effects. Side effects similar to SSRIs. May cause persistent increased diastolic blood pressure. Stimulating. Effective in depression, generalized anxiety disorder, possibly pain.

Trazodone (Desyrel)—Serotonergic. May be less effective than other antidepressants. Often used as hypnotic. Nausea, sedation, orthostasis, mental clouding. Rarely, cardiac arrhythmia, priapism.

Nefazodone (Serzone)—Inhibits serotonin reuptake, also blocks postsynaptic serotonin receptors. Headache, dry mouth, nausea, constipation, sedation. Less jitteriness, sexual dysfunction than SSRIs.

Mirtazapine (Remeron)—Effects on α-adrenergic and serotonin systems. **Highly sedating,** moderately anticholinergic, significant weight gain.

► clinical pearl

Bupropion (marketed as Zyban) is used to help smoking cessation.

D. Antianxiety Medications

1. Benzodiazepines

Examples—Diazepam (Valium), lorazepam (Ativan), alprazolam (Xanax), clonazepam (Klonopin), temazepam (Restoril). Rapidity of onset, potency and half-life differentiate individual use.

Indications—Generalized anxiety disorder; agitation; panic disorder (potent agents, e.g., clonazepam, alprazolam), social phobia, alcohol withdrawal; adjustment disorders, situational anxiety, primary insomnia, mania and acute psychosis (short-term treatment); also anticonvulsant, muscle relaxant.

Mechanism of Action—Upregulate GABA transmission.

Pharmacokinetics—Well absorbed. Lorazepam effective intramuscularly. Use lorazepam, oxazepam in elderly or with liver disease. Absorption interfered with by food, antacids.

Side Effects—Sedation, impaired anterograde memory, impaired motor coordination, depression, CNS/respiratory depression. May have rebound anxiety, nightmares with shorter-acting agents (e.g., triazolam). Relatively safe in overdose unless in combination with other CNS depressants. Risk of dependence greatest with high-potency, short-acting agents (e.g., alprazolam, lorazepam). Avoid prescribing with history of substance abuse/dependence, aggression (risk of disinhibition). Pharmacologic dependence is not the same as addiction.

Withdrawal—Anxiety, insomnia, tremor, headache, tachycardia, GI discomfort, diaphoresis, delirium, seizures. Most severe with high-potency, short-acting agents (e.g., alprazolam); longer duration of use, higher dose, abrupt withdrawal.

2. Buspirone (Buspar)

Pharmacologically unrelated to benzodiazepines. No abuse/dependence. Onset of action is weeks. 5-HT$_1$ receptor agonist.

Indications—Generalized anxiety disorder, augmentation of antidepressants. Ineffective for panic disorder.

Side Effects—Dizziness, nausea, headache, restlessness. **No** withdrawal symptoms, sedation, CNS depression, or psychomotor impairment.

E. Electroconvulsive Therapy

Involves administration of electrical impulse (usually brief pulse) to brain to generate generalized electrical seizure by unilateral (nondominant hemisphere) or bilateral placement of electrodes. Seizures that last 30–90 seconds are effective. Rapid onset of action makes it preferred in acute situations (e.g., intense suicidality, delirious mania).

Indications—Severe major depression, especially with psychotic features (may be treatment of choice), in elderly (more sensitive to side effects of antidepressants), in pregnancy, with previous good response; unresponsive mania; acute suicide risk; acute schizophrenia; catatonia; severe obsessive–compulsive disorder.

Side Effects—Retrograde and anterograde memory impairment with bilateral administration, transient confusion, headache, muscle aches, anesthetic complications, tardive seizures.

Contraindications—No absolute contraindications. Due to increased blood pressure during procedure, increased intracranial pressure (brain tumor), recent myocardial infarction, recent or evolving stroke, leaking aneurysms represent significant risk. Other risk factors include cervical spine fractures, severe osteoarthritis, cardiac arrhythmias. Obtain complete history and physical, ECG, LFTs; EEG, spine films if indicated.

XVII. SUICIDE, VIOLENCE, LEGAL ISSUES

A. Suicide

1. Demographic Risk Factors
Psychiatric disorder; male sex; Caucasian; peak incidence 20–24; also high in elderly; single, divorced, or widowed; poor health; social isolation; unemployed, drop in economic status. Ninth leading cause of death in the United States.

2. Individual Risk Factors

► Description
Recent losses, hopelessness, rage, turmoil, insomnia, physical illness, chronic pain, previous attempt, family history of suicide, expressed intent, thoroughness of plan, lack of future plans (e.g., giving away possessions), possession of means (e.g., firearm), psychiatric diagnosis (alcohol/substance dependence, major depression, bipolar depression or mixed states, schizophrenia [especially command hallucinations to suicide], personality disorders, conduct disorder, anxiety disorders).

► Treatment Steps
1. **Ask about suicidal thoughts, intent, plan; 80%** give warnings of intent.
2. Assess risk and develop safety plan.
3. Hospitalize for severe psychiatric symptoms, lack of social support, substance use, plan with possession of means, history of impulsivity, inability to contract for safety plan.

B. Violence

1. Risk Factors

► Description
Recent violent acts, verbal/physical threats, carrying weapons, progressive agitation, **alcohol/drug intoxication or withdrawal,** paranoid features, command violent auditory hallucinations, **brain disease** (dementia, trauma, epilepsy, mental retardation, infection, tumor), mania, antisocial personality, impulse dyscontrol, massive panic; young males, lower socioeconomic status, few social supports.

► Treatment Steps
1. **Ensure safety of self, staff, patient.**
2. Assess and treat underlying cause; rule out acute brain disease.
3. Antipsychotic (e.g., haloperidol) and benzodiazepine (e.g., lorazepam) can be given PO, IM, or IV for paranoid delusions, command hallucinations, acute agitation. Do not give benzodiazepines with head injury.

4. Restraints as needed.
5. Hospitalization as needed.

2. Family Violence

a. **Child Abuse**—see Section I.I.

b. **Partner Abuse**

▶ Description

Risk factors include pregnancy, younger age, social isolation, child abuse in home. History may be incompatable with injury. Repetitive injuries to head, face, neck, breasts, abdomen. Depression, PTSD, somatic complaints, substance abuse, suicide attempts. Present in > 20% of women seeking medical care. Routine inquiry in privacy makes diagnosis. Barriers to leaving abusive situation include shock and denial, self-blame, helplessness, presence of children, financial dependency, lack of job skills, fear of retaliation.

▶ Treatment Steps

1. Treat and document injuries.
2. Evaluate suicide potential.
3. Ensure confidentiality and safety of victim and children—risk of severe abuse increases when abused partner decides to leave.
4. Assess resources, continued risk (threats, extent of previous injury, presence of weapons, stalking, substance abuse).
5. Referrals for social, legal, psychiatric, medical resources.

c. **Elder Abuse**

▶ Description

Abuser generally relative/caretaker; victim may fear disclosure due to dependency. Family stress. History of violence, previous injuries, physical deterioration: brusing, head injury, burns, decubiti, contractures, dehydration, lacerations, diarrhea, impaction, malnutrition, urine burns, signs of neglect, sexual assault, PTSD symptoms.

▶ Treatment Steps

1. Interview privately.
2. Document and treat injuries.
3. Social service evaluation of living situation.
4. Mandatory reporting in most states.

C. Legal Issues

1. Informed Consent

Requires that patient be informed about treatment, alternative treatments, potential risks and benefits; patient must understand and freely and knowingly give consent. Exception: emergencies (i.e., patient in imminent physical danger).

2. Confidentiality

Hippocratic oath and law bind physician to secrecy. Exceptions: contagious disease, child/elder abuse, suicide, gun and knife wounds; duty to protect (Tarasoff rule) requires psychotherapist to warn potential victims of patient's expressed intent to harm if threat realistic (e.g., if patient not currently hospitalized).

3. Involuntary Commitment

Laws vary according to state. Typically requires risk or action of self-harm, danger to others, or grave disability due to mental illness.

BIBLIOGRAPHY

American Psychiatric Association. *Diagnostic and Statistical Manual of Mental Disorders,* 4th ed. Text Revision. Washington, DC: American Psychiatric Association, 2000.

Andreasen AC, Black DW. *Introductory Textbook of Psychiatry,* 3rd ed. Washington, DC: American Psychiatric Press, 2001.

Hyman SE, Arana GW, Rosenbaum JF. *Handbook of Psychiatric Drug Therapy,* 5th ed. Boston, MA: Little, Brown & Co., 2005.

Kaplan HI, Sadock BJ. *Synopsis of Psychiatry,* 9th ed. Baltimore: Williams & Wilkins, 2002.

Pulmonary Medicine | 16

I. HEALTH AND HEALTH MAINTENANCE

A. Respiratory Tract Infection

▶ Description

Epidemiology—**Pneumonia: More common in alcoholics, elderly, patients with chronic lung disease, chronic disease** (cancer, diabetes, immunocompromise, etc.). Pneumonia is either community acquired or hospital acquired (hospital acquired, defined as pneumonia ≥ 48 hours after admission). **Bronchitis** may be bacterial or viral, and in adults is often from smoking (chronic bronchitis). Source of infection may be **aspiration, inhalation,** or **hematologic/contiguous spread. Sinusitis has to be included within respiratory tract infection. It can be chronic as well as acute and can be seen in outpatient as well as inpatient population.**

Impact—Vast number of people affected, time lost from work, cost of prescription and over-the-counter (OTC) cough/cold preparations, and mortality.

Prevention—Vaccination where indicated (children: diphtheria, pertussis; susceptible adults: influenza, pneumococcal), and education (including hygiene, smoking cessation, etc.).

Prevention of Complications in Human Immunodeficiency Virus (HIV)/ Acquired Immune Deficiency Syndrome (AIDS) Patients—Antiretroviral tharapy may reduce infection incidence. Trimethoprim–sulfamethoxazole for *Pneumocystis carinii* prophylaxis (aerosolized pentamidine if patient is allergic to sulfa drugs), isoniazid for reactive purified protein derivative (PPD) patients, hygiene, patient education.

B. Chronic Bronchitis, Emphysema, Larynx and Lung Carcinoma

▶ Description

Epidemiology—In **chronic bronchitis, emphysema, lung and larynx carcinoma,** smoking is the major cause. **Most common lung tumor type: adenocarcinoma. Most head/neck cancer is squamous cell,** and **alcohol is an additional risk factor.** There is an increased risk of metachronous/synchronous head and neck cancers.

Impact—Vast morbidity/mortality and cost.

Prevention—Patient education, including smoking cessation and reduction in alcohol and environmental risks (nickel, arsenic, asbestos, radiation, etc.).

C. Tuberculosis

▶ Description

Epidemiology—**Most often due to *Mycobacterium tuberculosis.* Marked impact in underdeveloped areas,** immunocompromised hosts (HIV+, cancer), and **airborne transmission by prolonged close exposure.**

Prevention of active disease in patients with evidence of tubercular infection (e.g., positive PPD) is now called "Treatment of latent TB infection" (LTBI).

INH 10 mg/kg/day (up to a maximum of 300 mg/day) for 9 months is the recommended therapy for LTBI.

D. Occupational and Environmental Pulmonary Disease and Asthma

► Description

Epidemiology—Exposure to occupational and environmental toxins results in a wide range of pulmonary disorders (acute, firefighters smoke inhalation, or over many years, asbestosis-induced mesothelioma, berylliosis, and coal miner's disease). Risk factors for occupational asthma includes atopy (allergic rhinitis, eczema), smoking, and genetic factors. Occupational factors include type and intensity of offending agent (organic versus inorganic, high or low molecular weight, etc.).

Prevention—**Avoid exposure to offending agent,** including toxin/dust control, adequate ventilation, and mask/respirator protection, can also consider premedication depending on clinical scenario.

E. Postoperative Pulmonary Complications

► Description

Epidemiology—Complications include **atelectasis** (most common), **respiratory failure,** pneumonia/aspiration, and **hypoxemia.**

Risk Factors—Chronic obstructive pulmonary disease (COPD), **obesity, smoking,** arteriosclerotic cardiovascular disease (ASCVD), congestive heart failure (CHF), upper abdominal surgery, age > 70.

Preoperative Assessment—History and physical examination for everyone; pulmonary function testing and/or arterial blood gas (ABG) in selected high-risk cases.

Prevention—Chest physical therapy (CPT), incentive spirometry (IS), deep breathing, early mobilization, and the use of perioperative nebulizer treatments with albuterol and/or ipratropium bromide (Atrovent).

F. Newborn Respiratory Distress Syndrome

See also Chapter 14, section IV.

► Description

Epidemiology—**Lack of surfactant** resulting in atelectasis.

Other risk factors—Maternal diabetes, cesarean section delivery, male sex.

Prevention—**Avoid prematurity; betamethasone** given 48–72 hours before delivery in fetuses < 32 weeks, treatment with exogenous surfactant, check lecithin/sphingomyelin (L/S) ratio (over 2:1 is okay).

G. Pulmonary Aspiration

► Description

Prevent aspiration in high-risk patients (elderly, neurologic disorders, intubation/tracheostomy/sedated patients). **Prevent and mini-**

mize symptoms with H_2 antagonists, elevate head of bed, safe feeding tube flow rates, cricoid pressure during intubation, preoperative and postoperative fasting.

II. MECHANISMS OF DISEASE, DIAGNOSIS, AND TREATMENT

A. Nose, Sinus, Pharynx, Larynx, and Trachea

1. Common Cold

▶ Symptoms/Diagnosis
Rhinitis, sneezing, headache, malaise, and cough. Clinical diagnosis.

▶ Pathology/Treatment
Rhinovirus commonly, many others possible (adenovirus, respiratory syncytial virus [RSV], influenza, etc.). Supportive treatment.

2. Pharyngitis

▶ Symptoms
Fever, dry/sore throat, headache, and cough.

▶ Diagnosis/Treatment
See Cram Facts.

▶ Treatment Steps
Supportive if viral.

3. Tonsillitis

▶ Symptoms/Diagnosis
Sore throat, halitosis, high fever. Diagnose clinically, throat culture.

▶ Pathology
Group A, β-hemolytic strep is **common;** other bacterial/viral agents possible.

▶ Treatment Steps
Antibiotics as per culture report, symptomatic measures.

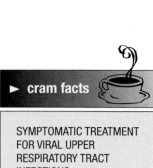

▶ cram facts

SYMPTOMATIC TREATMENT FOR VIRAL UPPER RESPIRATORY TRACT INFECTIONS

- Keep well hydrated.
- Acetaminophen/nonsteroidal anti-inflammatory drugs (NSAIDs) for fever, pain.
- Warm salt water gargles for pharyngitis/laryngitis.
- Pseudoephedrine or phenlylephrine for nasal congestion.
- Guiafenesin for chest congestion.
- Avoid aspirin in children.

▶ cram facts

PHARYNGITIS AND "STREP THROAT"

- Although viruses can be a common cause of pharyngitis, it is important to rule out bacterial infection, most commonly with group A *Streptococcus* (*S. pyogenes*). If present, it must be treated to prevent complications.
- Clues to the presence of *S. pyogenes* include cervical lymphadenopathy, fever, pharyngeal and tonsillar exudates, and the absence of cough. However, rapid strep testing or routine throat culture are still used to diagnose *S. pyogenes.*
- Treatment is given to prevent complications (peritonsillar or retropharyngeal abscess, meningitis, endocarditis, acute rheumatic fever, and glomerulonephritis).
- Antibiotics include penicillin and erythromycin.
- If viral etiology, supportive care only.

4. Peritonsillar Abscess

▶ Symptoms

Dysphagia, fever, pain, trismus (hard to open mouth).

▶ Diagnosis

History and physical exam (uvula displaced by peritonsillar mass/swelling), culture of aspirate. May be a complication of untreated strep throat.

▶ Treatment Steps
1. **Surgical drainage.**
2. **Antibiotics.**

5. Thrush

▶ Description

Moniliasis.

▶ Symptoms

White patch in mouth; **removable.** Dysphagia may be present if thrush is in posterior oropharynx and/or the esohagus.

▶ Diagnosis

History and physical (bleeding surface after scraping plaque off), fungal culture, potassium hydroxide (KOH) prep.

▶ Pathology

Excess *Candida* (*C. albicans* usually). Much more common in immunocompromised adults and infants.

▶ Treatment Steps

Antifungal (nystatin, fluconazole, etc.).

6. Sinusitis

▶ Symptoms

Facial pain/pressure, fever, headache, referred pain (teeth).

▶ Diagnosis

History and physical (sinus tender to percussion, purulent rhinitis, decreased transillumination), x-ray and computed tomography (CT) scan, culture from sinus.

▶ Pathology

Streptococcus and *Haemophilus influenzae* common; **maxillary most common.**

▶ Treatment Steps
1. **Antibiotics.**
2. **Decongestants** (pseudoephedrine, phenylephrine).
3. Drainage with decongestants. Also use nasal saline spray.
4. Irrigation.

7. Allergic Rhinitis

▶ Symptoms

Sneezing, itchy/watery eyes, nose blocked and/or runny.

▶ Diagnosis

History and physical (blue, boggy turbinates), allergy testing, nasal smear for eosinophils.

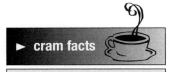

▶ cram facts

SIGN OR SYMPTOM: EPISTAXIS

Think of: **Common things first**—nose picking!; coagulopathies (or anticoagulation); other trauma besides nose manipulation; severe hypertension; dry mucosa; iatrogenic (e.g., nasogastric tube placement); arteriovenous malformations less frequently but need to think of it; Goodpasture's, Wegener's, and others less frequent such as ectopic pregnancy, etc.

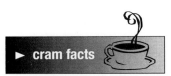

▶ cram facts

Only maxillary and ethmoid sinuses are present in children. Ethmoid sinusitis more frequent in children. Cavernous sinus thrombosis: sinusitis complication (facial edema, meningitis, ophthalmoplegia).

▶ cram facts

Vasomotor rhinitis: rhinitis and nasal vascular congestion, nonallergic, etiology unknown.

► **Treatment Steps**
1. Anti-inflammatory drugs (nasal corticosteroids, cromolyn sodium).
2. Antihistamines and/or decongestants.
3. Allergy shots in patients with severe recurrent disease not controlled on above treatment.

8. **Nasal Polyps**

► **Description/Symptoms**
Swollen mucosa/submucosa polypoid tissue. Nasal obstructive symptoms.

► **Diagnosis**
History and physical examination (polyp: smooth, blue, wet appearance).

► **Pathology**
Associated with allergic rhinitis, cystic fibrosis, and asthma with aspirin intolerance (asthma triad).

► **Treatment Steps**
Medical or surgical.

9. **Croup**

9–1. Acute Laryngotracheobronchitis (Croup)

► **Description**
An acute viral illness seen in young children.

► **Symptoms**
Cold symptoms at onset, then **barking cough, slight fever, inspiratory/expiratory stridor.**

► **Diagnosis**
History and physical examination, chest/lateral neck x-ray (see Fig. 16–1).

► **Treatment Steps**
1. **Humidification of air.**
2. **Racemic epinephrine.**
3. Oxygen.
4. Steroids.
5. Supportive care (see Table 16–1).

9–2. Epiglottitis

► **Description/Symptoms**
Dangerous airway-compromising infection. Presents with **high fever, respiratory obstruction, dyspnea, drooling, dysphagia,** barking cough, **inspiratory** stridor.

► **Diagnosis**
History and physical, **cherry-red epiglottis, lateral neck x-ray,** blood culture.

► **Pathology**
Children ages 2–7, **usually *H. influenzae* type b, supraglottic.** Incidence of *H. influenzae* is decreasing since most children are immunized.

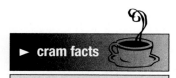

► **cram facts**

In adults, part of triad resulting in asthma.
Childhood nasal polyps: rule out cystic fibrosis.

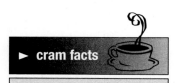

► **cram facts**

SIGN OR SYMPTOM: WHEEZING

Think of: **All that wheezes is not asthma!** Asthma, congestive heart failure (CHF), airway hyperactivity (postinfectious), foreign object (especially in children), pseudoasthma (vocal cord dysfunction), and a few others that are not as common.

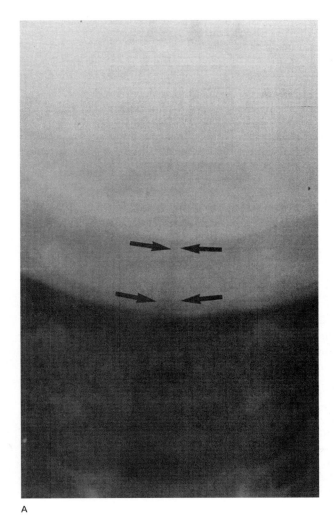

A

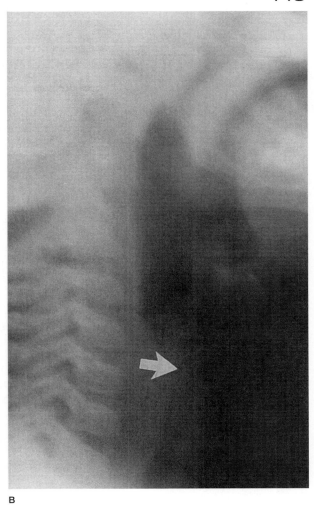

B

Figure 16–1. Croup (laryngotracheobronchitis [LTB]). **A:** Posteroanterior view of the upper airway shows the so-called "steeple" sign, the tapered narrowing of the immediate subglottic airway (arrows). **B:** Lateral view of the upper airway shows good delineation of the supraglottic anatomy. The subglottic trachea is hazy and poorly defined (arrow) because of the inflammatory edema that has obliterated the sharp undersurface of the vocal cords and extends down the trachea in a diminishing manner.

16-1

CONSIDERATIONS FOR THERAPY FOR ACUTE LARYNGOTRACHEOBRONCHITIS

Outpatient	Hospital
Humidified air	Humidified air (if tolerated) and oxygen[a]
Oral hydration	Racemic epinephrine or L-epinephrine[b]
Fever control	Decadron (0.6 mg/kg intramuscularly given once)
Plan for physician follow-up visit after phone communication	Fever control
Decadron (outpatient use may be appropriate if there is adequate follow-up care)	Hydration
	Antiviral drugs for influenza A virus or respiratory syncytial virus

[a] Based on pulse oximetry readings of PaO_2 < 95% in room air.

[b] Nebulized treatment: 0.2 mL (for 5–10 kg body weight), 0.5 mL (11–15 kg), 0.7 mL (16–20 kg), and 1.0 mL (≥ 21 kg) in 3.5 mL normal saline solution. L-epinephrine is given in one-half the dose of racemic epinephrine.

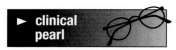

EPIGLOTTITIS

On lateral neck x-ray, look for "thumb sign."

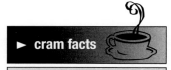

- *Epiglottitis*—examine epiglottis only with cardiorespiratory support team available, as examination may provoke laryngospasm/complete airway loss/cardiac arrest!
- *Spasmodic croup*— children 1–3, night onset, lasts few hours, usually viral, **no fever.**

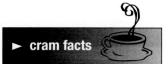

SIGN OR SYMPTOM: COUGH

Causes of acute cough (< 3 weeks' duration) are viral or bacterial upper repiratory tract infections (e.g., common cold, acute bacterial sinusitis), allergic rhinitis, and environmental irritants. Most common causes of chronic cough (> 3 weeks' duration) are postnasal drip, asthma, gastroesophageal reflux disease, chronic bronchitis, bronchiectasis, and drugs like angiotensin-converting enzyme inhibitors.

▶ Treatment Steps
1. **Antibiotics** (cefuroxime [Zinacef]), or other third-generation cephalosporin.
2. Treat nonimmunized household contacts (usually with rifampin).

10. Pertussis (Whooping Cough)

▶ Symptoms
Three stages of illness: **Catarrhal stage** (coryza, 1–2 weeks), **paroxysmal stage** (coughing and inspiratory whoop, 2–4 weeks), **convalescent stage** weeks later.

▶ Diagnosis
History and physical exam, nasopharyngeal culture, leukocytosis. The cough in pertussis is distinctive. Patients often have paroxysms of cough. Patients make the posttussive "whooping" sound about 50% of the time. Coughing spells are often followed by posttussive emesis.

▶ Pathology
Bordetella pertussis; infants under 2 years.

▶ Treatment Steps
1. **Erythromycin** will help in catarrhal stage.
2. Otherwise, **supportive care.**
3. Treat household contacts.

11. Nasopharyngeal Carcinoma
See Chapter 6, section VII.D.

12. Carcinoma of the Larnyx
See Chapter 6, section VII.D.

13. Chronic Laryngitis

▶ Symptoms
Persisting hoarseness; recurrent acute laryngitis episodes.

▶ Diagnosis
History and physical examination, laryngoscopy.

▶ Pathology
Chronic irritation (smoking, overuse of voice, reflux).

▶ Treatment Steps
1. Voice rest.
2. Speech therapy.
3. Steroids.
4. Treatment for reflux disease.

14. Larynx and Pharynx Trauma

▶ Symptoms/Diagnosis
Stridor, hoarseness, subcutaneous emphysema. Laryngoscopy for direct visualization.

▶ Pathology
Injuries include thyroid cartilage fracture, contusions, arytenoid dislocation.

▶ Treatment Steps
1. **Do not intubate.**
2. Observation if stable.
3. Tracheotomy if airway obstruction.

15. Tracheoesophageal Fistula
See Chapter 14, section VIII.B.

B. Pulmonary Infections

1. Acute Bronchitis

▶ **Description/Symptoms**
Large airway inflammation/infection, causing productive cough, fever, mild shortness of breath. Often due to a viral infection. More likely bacterial in smokers/patients with COPD.

▶ **Diagnosis**
History and physical, chest x-ray (CXR) should be clear, sputum culture. (Presence of an infiltrate would lead to a diagnosis of pneumonia rather than bronchitis.)

▶ **Treatment Steps**
1. Antibiotics (if underlying COPD, Gram stain and culture of sputum are unnecessary and often misleading, because normal respiratory tract flora are often seen).
2. Otherwise supportive (hydration, expectorants, bronchodilators).

▶ **cram facts**

ARTERIAL BLOOD GASES/ACID–BASE DISORDERS

Use this as a Q.I.G. (Quick Interpretation Guidelines):
• Easy access for close approximation.
• Will help you figure out acute respiratory disorders and from there you will be able to accurately calculate CHRONIC and/or FIXED disorders.
• When using this table, there is a diagonal correlation (as shown); change will be approximately 1:0.1 (remember the formula for accuracy).
• Check:
  • pH   Alk. ↑ or Ac. ↓
  • Paco$_2$ Alk. ↓ or Ac. ↑
  • Look at HCO$_3$ and calculate (when indicated)
  • Pao$_2$ Hypoxia ↓ or NL ↑
• Remember:

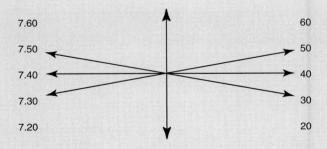

Ex. 7.40/40—Nl
7.50/30—Resp. Alk.
7.30/50—Resp. Ac.

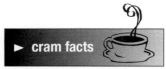

SIGN OR SYMPTOM: HEMOPTYSIS

Think of: First need to figure out if it is true hemoptysis or if it is epistaxis or hematemesis. The most common causes of hemoptysis are bronchitis/bronchiectasis and carcinoma. One-third of the cases are due to unknown causes. Other less common causes are arteriovenous malformations, foreign bodies, mitrial stenosis, trauma, infections (like tuberculosis, aspergilloma), pulmonary embolism, and vasculitis/autoimmune diseases (Wegener's granulomatosis, systemic lupus erythematosus (SLE), Goodpasture's syndrome).

2. Bronchiolitis

▶ Description
Lower respiratory tract infection, with **small airway inflammation/ obstruction.**

▶ Symptoms/Diagnosis
Tachypnea, wheezing, fever, and **cough.** Diagnose clinically. Chest x-ray may show overinflation.

▶ Pathology
Viral (RSV common); affecting **infants younger than 2 (not exclusive of pediatric patients), also seen (rarely) in adults.**

▶ Treatment Steps
1. Ribavirin for RSV.
2. **Oxygen.**
3. Fluids.

3. Pneumonia

3–1. General Facts

▶ Description
Infection of the lower respiratory tract caused by a variety of different pathogens (bacterial, viral, fungal).

▶ Symptoms
Typically, bacterial pneumonia is characterized by fever, cough productive of purulent sputum, and difficulty breathing. Exam often reveals signs of consolidation (rhonchi). CXR often shows an infiltrate. Other symptoms may (or may not) exist based on the infectious organism causing the pneumonia.

▶ Diagnosis
Initial treatment should start based on the history and physical, keeping in mind the patient's medical history and what type of pneumonia is most likely in that particular patient (see Cram Facts).

▶ Treatment Steps
Guided by the specific etiology.

▶ cram facts

SCENARIOS FOR PNEUMONIA

- A young, otherwise healthy adult may have an atypical pneumonia due to *Mycoplasma pneumoniae.*
- An elderly patient with COPD likely has a bacterial pneumonia, or, if in the winter, possible infection with influenza.
- An AIDS patient with a low CD4 count and subacute illness may have *Pneumocystis carinii* pneumonia (PCP).
- A patient whose mentation is altered (e.g., postop from anesthesia or other sedatives) or who has swallowing dysfunction from a stroke may have aspiration pneumonia.

3-2. Influenza and Pneumonia

▶ Description

Influenza is an acute respiratory infection caused by an RNA virus. Common types of the virus are types A and B. Typically, the strain of influenza varies from year to year, and vaccines are developed trying to anticipate the specific strains.

▶ Symptoms

Influenza most commonly presents with the acute onset of malaise, myalgias, fever, chills, cough, and sore throat. In certain patients, pneumonia can develop. The pneumonia may be caused by the influenza itself, a secondary bacterial pneumonia, or a mixed picture.

▶ Diagnosis

Throat or nasal swabs can confirm the presence of influenza (and specific type, A or B). CXR can reveal infiltrates/pneumonia.

▶ Treatment Steps

1. Rest/fluids/symptomatic treatment with analgesics/antipyretics.
2. If the infection is discovered within the first 48 hours, treatment can begin with oseltamivir (Tamiflu) given for 5 days. This medication can also be given after close contact with an infected individual as prophylaxis. Amantadine can be used for prophylaxis and treatment of influenza A infections only.
3. Antibiotics often needed if pneumonia develops.

3-3. Atypical Pneumonia

▶ Description/Symptoms

In contrast to a "typical" bacterial pneumonia, atypical pneumonia often presents with a subacute onset, nonproductive cough, multiple extrapulmonary symptoms (headache, sore throat, gastrointestinal [GI] complaints), and minimal findings on exam. However, the x-ray often shows a diffuse or patchy, often bilateral infiltrate.

▶ Diagnosis

Based on clinical picture and patient risk factors. Sputum culture may help with identifying specific pathogen.

▶ Pathology

Classically due to *Mycoplasma pneumoniae* or *Chlamydia pneumoniae* and seen in young, otherwise healthy patients. Other, much less common organisms include *Chlamydia psittaci, Coxiella burnetii,* and *Francisella tularensis.*

▶ Treatment Steps

Based on suspected pathogen. Antibiotics must cover these "atypical" pathogens. Antibiotics include erythromycin, doxycycline, azithromycin, clarithromycin, levofloxacin, and tetracycline.

3-4. Legionella

▶ Description/Symptoms

Pneumonia caused by the aerobic, gram-negative bacillus *Legionella* species (*Legionella pneumophila* in 80–90% of cases). Risk factors include smoking, elderly, and immunosuppressed patients.

▶ Diagnosis

A few aspects of the illness should raise suspicion for *Legionella.* These include headache, diarrhea, high fever, lack of organisms on sputum Gram stain despite multiple neutrophils, hyponatremia, abnormal liver function tests (LFTs), and failure to respond to typical antibiotic therapy (β-lactam drugs).

Special lab testing can be done for *Legionella*, which includes direct fluorescent antibody (DFA) staining of sputum, *Legionella* urine antigen testing, and serologies.

► Treatment Steps

Medications include those antibiotics active against "atypical" organisms (erythromycin, doxycycline, azithromycin, clarithromycin, levofloxacin, and tetracycline).

3–5. Pneumococcal Pneumonia

► Description/Symptoms

Presentation is consistent with typical bacterial pneumonia (see section II.B.3–1). Complications can include pleural effusion (transudative or empyema), meningitis.

► Diagnosis

Clinical picture. Gram stain shows gram-positive diplococci (Fig. 16–2).

► Treatment Steps

Most β-lactam antibiotics and fluoroquinolones are effective. Prevention with vaccination (see Table 16–2).

3–6. Staphylococcal Pneumonia

► Description/Symptoms

S. aureus is a rare cause of pneumonia. It is more common in infancy/early childhood or debilitated patients. The course is rapidly progressive with a relatively high mortality. After a short prodrome, patients have acute respiratory distress.

► Diagnosis

Clinical setting, and organism seen on Gram stain and culture (Fig. 16–2).

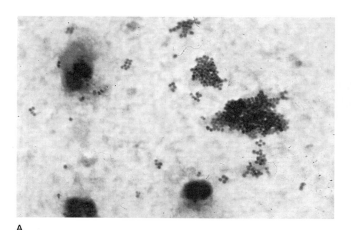
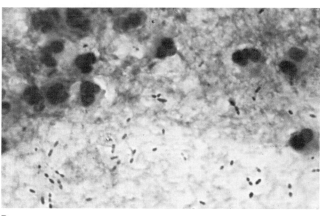

Figure 16–2. A: Gram-stained smear of pus containing *Staphylococcus aureus*. **B:** Gram-stained smear of sputum containing *Streptococcus pneumoniae*. (Photographs courtesy of Joseph M. Campos.)

16-2

VACCINATIONS

PNEUMOCOCCAL POLYSACCHARIDE VACCINE (PPV)

PPV protects against 23 serotypes of pneumococcus. According to Centers for Disease Control and Prevention (CDC) guidelines, vaccine is indicated for:

- All adults 65 years of age or older
- Patients > 2 years old with a chronic health condition (e.g., cardiopulmonary disease, diabetes, cirrhosis, alcoholism)
- Patients > 2 years old with immunosuppression from various causes (renal failure, HIV/AIDS, certain cancers, long-term steroids/radiation or chemotherapy)
- Patients postsplenectomy (surgical or nonfunctional spleen, e.g., patients with sickle cell anemia)

INFLUENZA

The 2004–2005 influenza season saw a "scare" with a nationwide shortage of influenza vaccine. Ordinarily, vaccine is offered annually to all individuals. Due to the shortage, highest-risk groups were vaccinated first, including:

- Children aged 6–23 months
- Adults aged ≥ 65
- Women who are pregnant during influenza season
- Patients aged 2–64 with underlying chronic medical conditions
- Residents of nursing homes and other long-term care facilities
- Health care workers with direct patient contact
- Children aged 2–18 years on chronic aspirin
- Caregivers and household contacts of children aged < 6 months

▶ **Treatment Steps**

Aggressive supportive therapy. Vancomycin may be needed initially until the sensitivity of the organism is known. Vancomycin can be changed to an alternative antibiotic if the isolate is not methicillin-resistant *S. aureus* (MRSA).

3–7. Pneumocystis carinii *Pneumonia (PCP)*

▶ **Description**

Pneumocystis carinii is a ubiquitous unicellular eukaryote, and differing opinions exist as to whether it is classified as a protozoan or fungus. It is the most common opportunistic respiratory infection in patients infected with HIV, and can cause disease in other immunocompromised populations. PCP is an AIDS-defining illness.

▶ **Symptoms**

Classically, patients have a subacute illness (lasting usually a few weeks) consisting of dry cough, fever, malaise, fever, weight loss, and dyspnea. Patients are very commonly hypoxemic.

▶ **Diagnosis**

CXR classically shows diffuse bilateral infiltrates (see Fig. 16–3). May be hard to diagnose in a patient with no prior diagnosis of HIV and who may not fully disclose all risk factors. In a patient who has never had PCP before, it is better to isolate the organism (which may require bronchoscopy and bronchoalveolar lavage).

▶ **Treatment Steps**

Trimethoprim–sulfamethoxazole (Bactrim) is the standard of care. In patients with severe allergy, other options include pentamidine, dapsone, and atovaquone. The use of steroids (prednisone) is somewhat controversial. It is thought that steroid treatment decreases inflammation produced by the organism. It is usually reserved only for patients with HIV/AIDS who are hypoxemic.

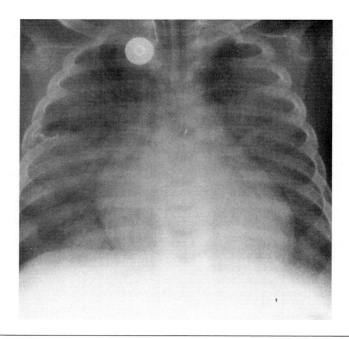

Figure 16–3. Chest radiograph of *Pneumocystis carinii pneumonia* (PCP) in a 6-month-old infant seropositive for HIV infection who developed severe tachypnea, dry cough, and progressive respiratory distress. The frontal chest radiograph shows the diffuse "ground glass-like" air space (alveolar) infiltration of the lungs typical of PCP. Sutures in the right lung are from a previous lung biopsy.

3–8. Aspiration Pneumonia

▶ Description/Symptoms

Pneumonia occurring when food or gastric aspirate enters the lung. Common scenarios include patients with stroke and dysphagia, and patients with altered sensorium (delirium, sedation).

▶ Diagnosis

Clinical scenario. CXR classically shows right middle or lower lobe infiltrate.

▶ Treatment Steps

Antibiotics used to cover gram-positive and anaerobic infections, including clindamycin and amoxicillin/clavulanate (Augmentin).

3–9. Other Causes of Pneumonia

- *Pseudomonas aeruginosa* (and other gram-negative pathogens) uncommonly cause pneumonia. *Pseudomonas* is regarded as a cause of nosocomial pneumonia. Suspect in patients recently or frequently hospitalized or patients who live in nursing homes. Antipseudomonal antibiotics include piperacillin/tazobactam, ceftazidime, and most aminoglycosides. *P. aeruginosa* is a common pathogen in patients with cystic fibrosis.
- *Francisella tularensis* is a gram-negative bacteria relatively uncommon in the United States. However, three states (Arkansas, Oklahoma, and Missouri) account for more than 50% of all cases in the United States. Pulmonary tularemia has a high mortality rate.
- *Coxiella burnetii* is the organism causing Q fever. Cattle, sheep, and goats are the reservoirs for the organisms and farmers and veterinarians are at highest risk. Doxycycline is the treatment of choice.
- *Chlamydia psittaci* is an obligate intracellular parasite that causes psittacosis. This diagnosis should be considered in patients with

community-acquired pneumonia who have had exposure to birds. Doxycycline is the treatment of choice.

4. Tuberculosis

► Description
Mycobacterial infection due to *Mycobacterium tuberculosis;* pulmonary, genitourinary (GU), GI, bone, and meningitis may present. More common in HIV/AIDS patients, homeless persons.

► Symptoms
Asymptomatic, or **weight loss, night sweats, cough,** malaise, and hemoptysis.

► Diagnosis
History and physical, CXR, sputum **culture** and polymerase chain reaction (PCR) testing and smear for **acid-fast bacilli,** skin test, tissue/body fluid exam for *M. tuberculosis.* (See Fig. 16–4.)

► Treatment Steps
1. **Start four drugs (isoniazid [INH] 300 mg daily plus rifampin 600 mg daily, pyrazinamide (PZA), and ethambutol) until culture sensitivities arrive.**
2. **Narrow treatment according to sensitivities to complete 6 months of treatment.**
3. **In HIV, follow strict culture sensitivities. Always monitor liver enzymes and tailor drug therapy to individual case.**
4. **Other treatment modalities include DOT (direct observe therapy) for the poor compliance patient.**

5. Histoplasmosis

► Description
Most patients who are exposed to this soil mold (*Histoplasma capsulatum*) are asymptomatic. Patients who develop clinical manifestations are often immunocompromised.

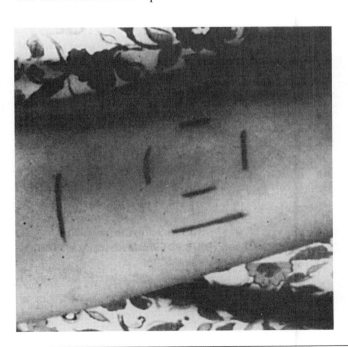

Figure 16–4. A positive Mantoux reaction, which consists of an inner zone of induration and an outer zone of edema and erythema. (From *Pediatric Infectious Diseases Principles and Practice,* Appleton & Lange, 1995.)

► cram facts

TUBERCULOSIS (TB)

Old disease in new times. Etiology *M. tuberculosis.* Pathologically will see caseating granulomas. Transmission by aerolized droplets. Therefore, overcrowded areas, poor ventilation, health care workers, immunosuppression, and many others are risk factors. There are four commonly known types of infection: primary TB, miliary TB, dormant TB (leading to reactivation TB), and extrapulmonary manifestations of TB.

- Symptoms: Fatigue, weight loss, night sweats, fevers, productive cough.
- Diagnosis: History and physical, sputum sample (identify *M. tuberculosis* bacilli on acid-fast stain and culture). CXR, PCR, positive PPD.
- Treatment: Most commonly use INH, rifampin, pyrazinamide, ethambutol, streptomycin (important to correlate with specific sensitivies and population group for choices of combination of 3–4 drugs and duration).
- Prevention: Screening individuals via skin testing (PPD) and initiating treatment if skin test is positive.

> ► **cram facts**
>
> *Renal TB*—sterile pyuria.
> - *INH*—side effects include neuropathy from pyridoxine loss, and hepatitis.
> - *Positive TB skin test (PPD) in person with history of bacillus Calmette–Guérin (BCG) vaccine does not necessarily indicate infection. CXR needed.*

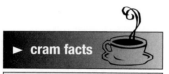

> ► **cram facts**
>
> Progressive disseminated histoplasmosis: associated with AIDS, do blood/bone marrow culture and treat with amphotericin B.

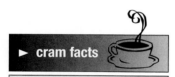

> ► **cram facts**
>
> COCCIDIOIDOMYCOSIS
>
> Diabetics and blacks tend toward progressive infection.

► **Symptoms**

Asymptomatic, or **nonproductive cough, myalgia,** fever, chest pain, mild flulike presentation.

► **Diagnosis**

History and physical, CXR (Fig. 16–5), serologic testing; in some cases, might need lung biopsy (see Fig. 16–6).

► **Pathology**

Histoplasma is a soil mold. **Bird/bat droppings in soil grow spores, which are inhaled.** The endemic areas for *H. capsulatum* include most of the midwestern and south central United States (the Ohio, Missouri, and Mississippi River valleys).

► **Treatment Steps**

1. **In mild case no treatment indicated.**
2. **If more ill, then ketoconazole 400 mg/day,** or amphotericin B.

6. **Coccidioidomycosis**

► **Description**

Infection with *Coccidioides immitis;* common Southwest U.S. mold.

► **Symptoms**

Asymptomatic or flulike presentation, arthralgia, erythema nodosum/multiforme rash. Can be difficult to differentiate from other respiratory infections.

► **Diagnosis**

History and physical, serologic testing. Travel or residence in an endemic area is important. CXR is nonspecific.

► **Treatment Steps**

1. **If mild, no treatment or possibly oral fluconazole.**
2. **If severe, give amphotericin B.**

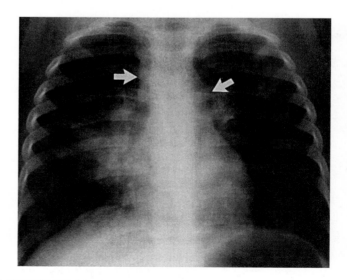

Figure 16–5. Histoplasmosis. Frontal chest radiograph taken during the acute phase shows a perihilar infiltrate on the right extending into the right middle lobe as well as bilateral hilar and paratracheal adenopathy (arrows). (From *Pediatric Infectious Diseases Principles and Practice,* Appleton & Lange, 1995.)

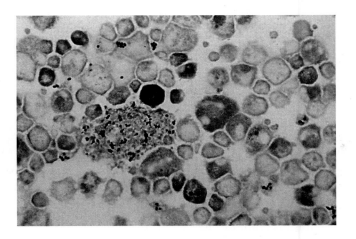

Figure 16–6. *Histoplasma* in the cytoplasm of a macrophage detected by Grocott staining of bronchoalveolar lavage.

7. Cryptococcosis

► Description
Infection with *Cryptococcus neoformans,* an encapsulated yeast. Two principal sites of infection are lungs and central nervous system (CNS), causing meningitis.

► Symptoms
Fever, cough, and dissemination in immunocompromised patients. Clinical picture can vary from minimal symptoms to acute respiratory distress syndrome (ARDS).

► Diagnosis
Fungal culture, CXR.

► Pathology
C. neoformans infection; in **soil and pigeon droppings. Risk factors** include **AIDS and corticosteroid use.**

► Treatment Steps
Amphotericin B plus flucytosine for severe pulmonary disease.

8. Lung Abscess

► Symptoms
Purulent/putrid sputum, cough, chest pain, fever.

► Diagnosis
History and physical, **CXR (cavities and air–fluid level),** bronchoscopy/culture, CT scan, lung biopsy.

► Pathology
Anaerobic bacteria most often (bacteroides, peptostreptococcus). **Risk factors: poor dentition and aspiration** (CNS disease, overdose, alcoholism, etc.).

► Treatment Steps
1. Antibiotics **penicillin G, 2 million units IV every 4 hours.**
2. Clindamycin 600 mg every 6 hours.
3. Surgical drainage rarely.

C. Obstructive Airway Disease

General information: Using pulmonary function tests (PFTs), pulmonary diseases can be classified as having either a restrictive or obstructive pattern (although in certain cases a mixed picture exists) (see Table 16–3).

1. Chronic Obstructive Pulmonary Disease (COPD)—General

COPD in general refers to three disease processes: chronic bronchitis (CB), emphysema, and asthma. (However, other diseases can cause obstructive lung disease, including bronchiectasis, cystic fibrosis, and allergic bronchopulmonary aspergillosis [ABPA].)

► Symptoms

Symptoms common to COPD, regardless of CB or emphysema, include worsening dyspnea and progressive decrease in exercise tolerance. (Other symptoms are more specific to each disorder; see below.)

► Diagnosis

In general, diagnosis is made based on the clinical scenario. Technically, the diagnosis should be made with PFTs but often, prior to PFTs, the diagnosis is made clinically and empiric treatment is started.

► Treatment Steps

From a medication standpoint, the two conditions are treated fairly similarly.

1. Inhaled medications:
   - Anticholinergics: Ipratroprium bromide (Atrovent) usually four times per day. Tiotropium (Spiriva) is newer and used once a day.
   - Ipratroprium or tiotropium is usually administered with a short-acting β-agonist (albuterol).
   - Long-acting β-agonist (salmeterol) used twice a day.
   - Corticosteroids (fluticasone, beclomethasone).

16-3

PULMONARY FUNCTION TESTS (PFTs)

DEFINITIONS
- FEV_1: Amount of air exhaled in the first second of forced exhalation
- FVC: Forced vital capacity (total volume of air exhaled from full lungs)
- DLCO: Diffusion capacity, gives information on gas exchange at the level of the alveoli
- TLC: Total lung capacity (volume of air in full lungs)
- RV: Residual volume (volume of air left in lungs after full expiration)

DESCRIPTION
- There are many subtleties to interpretation of PFTs. However, these are some high-yield facts.

OBSTRUCTIVE
- FEV_1 and FVC are both depressed.
- Ratio of FEV_1 to FVC is depressed.
- In emphysema, DLCO is depressed.
- FEV_1 can determine severity of disease. FEV_1 that is 60–70% of normal may be moderate chronic obstructive pulmonary disease (COPD), while FEV_1 < 50% of normal is severe COPD.

RESTRICTIVE
- FEV_1 and FVC are both depressed, *but*
  - Ratio of FEV_1 to FVC is normal.
  - TLC is reduced.

► cram facts

SLEEP-DISORDERED BREATHING

Background

Abnormal ventilation in sleep is found by the presence of apneic and/or hypoxic events. Most commonly recognized sleep disordered breathing: obstructive sleep apnea (OSA), central sleep apena, and mixed events. There are other disorders of clinical importance but less frequently seen, such as primary alveolar hypoventilation and obesity hypoventilation syndrome.

Etiology

Not certain in all cases, but in OSA there is a true obstruction of the airway, usually at the level of the posterior pharynx.

Symptoms

Snoring, morning headaches, difficulty concentrating and decreased memory capability, obesity, daytime hypersomnolence, dry mouth in A.M., sensation of choking or gasping for air in the middle of the night, peripheral edema. Pauses in breathing while asleep.

Diagnosis

History and physical. Polysomnography, overnight continuous pulse oximetry (helps, but not diagnostic).

Treatment

1. Continuous positive airway pressure (CPAP).
2. Oral appliances.
3. Surgical intervention.
4. Weight reduction.
5. BiPAP in severe cases.
6. Tracheostomy.

- In an acute exacerbation, albuterol with atrovent is often given as a nebulized solution.
2. Theophylline is used in some patients but has multiple toxicities.
3. Acute exacerbations are treated with empiric antibiotics, which should provide broad-spectrum coverage (against pneumococcus, *H. influenzae, Legionella* species, and gram-negative enterics). Azithromycin, levofloxacin, and trimethoprim–sulfamethoxazole have all been used.
4. Concerns with hospitalization: ABGs can assess hypoxemia as well as retention of carbon dioxide (hypercapnia). Oxygen should be administered for hypoxemia. If initial treatment for the acute exacerbation does not improve hypercapnia, other methods may be needed (such as bilevel positive airway pressure [BiPAP] or intubation with mechanical ventilation).

2. COPD—Chronic Bronchitis

► Description/Symptoms

Classically, patients are referred to as "blue bloaters" and have productive cough and recurrent pulmonary infections. With further progression, respiratory and cardiac failure develop (cor pulmonale) with edema and weight gain.

► Diagnosis/Treatment

See above (section II.C.1).

3. COPD—Emphysema

▶ **Description/Symptoms**

Patients are referred to as "pink puffers" and have a long history of progressive dyspnea. Cough is not a predominant symptom; it presents late in the illness and is usually nonproductive. Patients are eventually cachexic, with a barrel chest. They often adopt the tripod position to facilitate breathing. Chest can be hyperresonant with distant heart sounds.

▶ **Diagnosis/Treatment**

See above (section II.C.1).

4. α₁-Antitrypsin Deficiency

▶ **Description**

A genetic defect resulting in depressed levels of α_1-antitrypsin. The primary result is panacinar emphysema occurring at a young age. Hepatic cirrhosis can also develop.

▶ **Symptoms**

Symptoms of emphysema at early age (or in nonsmoker).

▶ **Diagnosis**

Clinical scenario. Can check serum levels of α_1-antitrypsin. **CXR (basal bullae, not only found at the bases),** high-resolution CT scan of chest, and PFTs.

▶ **Pathology**

Excess elastase (without α_1-antitrypsin to inactivate it), results in lung damage.

▶ **Treatment Steps**

1. Make sure patient quits smoking.
2. Treatment for emphysema (see above, section II.C.3).
3. Replacement therapy with purified human α_1-antitrypsin.
4. Lung volume reduction surgery is sometimes done, as is lung transplantation.

5. Asthma

See Chapter 7, section II.B.2.

6. Bronchiectasis

▶ **Description**

Bronchial infection/inflammation, resulting in **bronchi dilation.**

▶ **Symptoms**

Productive purulent cough, weight loss, hemoptysis, clubbing.

▶ **Diagnosis**

History and physical. Bronchography was the traditional technique for diagnosing bronchiectasis, but is no longer recommended. High-resolution CT scan of the chest is the diagnostic test of choice.

▶ **Treatment Steps**

1. Chest physical therapy.
2. Antibiotics.
3. Bronchodilators.
4. Surgery.

7. Allergic Bronchopulmonary Aspergillosis (ABPA)

► **Description**

ABPA is a hypersensitivity reaction to *Aspergillus* fungus; most commonly seen in patients with asthma and cystic fibrosis.

► **Symptoms**

Wheezing, central bronchiectasis, productive cough.

► **Diagnosis**

See Cram Facts.

► **Treatment Steps**

Prednisone. New studies suggest some role of antifungals (itraconazole) in selected patients with this disease.

8. Cystic Fibrosis (CF)

► **Description**

Autosomal recessive genetic disorder of exocrine gland function involving multiple organ systems. Pulmonary involvement exists in 90% of patients surviving the neonatal period. Pancreatic exocrine gland dysfunction also occurs.

► **Symptoms**

Steatorrhea, cough, sputum production, diabetes.

► **Diagnosis**

Clinical scenario, **sweat chloride test** (> 60 mEq/L of sweat chloride is diagnostic of CF).

► **Treatment Steps**

Multidisciplinary approach:
1. **Chest physical therapy.**
2. Antibiotics.
3. Inhaled Dornase alfa (recombinant human DNAse—cleaves extracellular DNA and thus decreases the viscosity of sputum).
4. Double lung transplantation (end-stage lung disease).

D. Atelectasis

► **Description/Symptoms**

Lung collapse (segment or lobe). Patients have shortness of breath, hypoxia, fever.

► **Diagnosis**

History and physical, CXR.

► **Pathology**

Bronchi obstruction (frequently mucus/secretions plug). **Most frequent postop pulmonary problem.** Risk factors include COPD/smoking, obesity, age > 70, and upper abdominal/thoracic surgery.

► **Treatment Steps**

1. Incentive spirometry.
2. Deep breathing exercises.
3. OOB (out of bed).
4. Chest physical therapy.
5. Continuous positive airway pressure (CPAP).
6. Bronchoscopy (if atelectasis is severe).

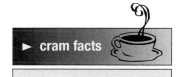

► **cram facts**

DIAGNOSIS OF ABPA

If six of seven criteria are met, almost 100% have ABPA:
- History of asthma
- Peripheral eosinophilia
- Pulmonary infiltrates
- Positive skin test to *Aspergillus*
- High serum immunoglobulin E (IgE)
- Positive IgE and IgG for *Aspergillus*
- Central bronchiectasis

► **cram facts**

If azoospermia noted, or *Pseudomonas aeruginosa* in sputum, think cystic fibrosis.

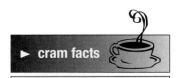

► **cram facts**

Mendelson syndrome: gastric aspiration, often postop, may cause ARDS. Most risky time for aspiration during surgery is during anesthetic induction.

E. Pneumothorax and Hemothorax

1. Pneumothorax
See Chapter 8, section II.E.

2. Hemothorax

► **Description**
Blood in pleural space, usually caused by trauma or as a postprocedural complication.

► **Symptoms**
Dyspnea; if massive, shock.

► **Diagnosis**
History and physical, **decubitus film (can detect decrease in hematocrit if severe enough), true blood will clot unlike other bloody effusions.**

► **Treatment Steps**
1. *Very small*—observe.
2. *All others*—**chest tube** (32–40 French with 20 cm water suction).
3. **Possible thoracotomy** (for continued bleeding > 200 mL/hour).

F. Pneumoconiosis

1. Asbestosis

► **Description**
An interstitial lung disorder caused by long-term exposure to asbestos.

► **Symptoms**
Asymptomatic, or exertional dyspnea, cough.

► **Diagnosis**
History and physical, CXR (pleural thickening/plaques, effusion, and opacities), pulmonary function testing (restrictive disease), lung biopsy.

► **Pathology**
Histologic hallmark—ferruginous bodies. Asbestosis may lead to **mesothelioma and lung cancer. Additional risk if patient smokes.**

► **Treatment Steps**
1. **None.**
2. Stop smoking.

2. Silicosis

► **Description**
Silica-induced fibrosing lung disease; with increased risk of mycobacterial infections and lung cancer.

► **Symptoms**
Asymptomatic or **exertional dyspnea and cough.**

► **Diagnosis**
History and physical, CXR (**upper lobe nodules** and **eggshell hilar node calcification**).

► **Pathology**
Found with sandblasters/miners; TB and bacteria may coexist with silicosis. Silicosis may be **acute, chronic,** or **accelerated** in type.

► **cram facts**

Prevention: in areas of known possible asbestos exposure (removal sites, industrial pipe maintenance, etc.), body suits and respirator masks (EPA [Environmental Protection Agency] approved) required as other government-regulated measurements are to be followed.

► Treatment Steps
1. No specific treatment.
2. Annual screening for mycobacterial disease.

3. **Sarcoidosis**

► Description
Multisystem granulomatous disorder, commonly with pulmonary involvement.

► Symptoms
Asymptomatic, or **fever, dyspnea, skin/eye/CNS/cardiac symptoms** (erythema nodosum, iritis, arrhythmia, nerve palsy).

► Diagnosis
History and physical, CXR **(bilateral enlarged hilar adenopathy), biopsy,** elevated angiotensin-converting enzyme, possibly elevated calcium, skin test anergy. Pulmonary function test. (See Cram Facts.)

► Pathology
Etiology unknown; more common in blacks.

► Treatment Steps
Corticosteroids. Cutaneous sarcoid: chloroquine (Plaquenil).

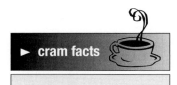

G. Respiratory Failure

1. **Newborn Respiratory Distress (Hyaline Membrane Disease)**

► Symptoms
Respiratory distress (cyanosis, grunting, tachypnea).

► Diagnosis
History and physical, CXR **(air bronchograms** and fine reticular pattern).

► Pathology
Deficient surfactant, and high lung surface tension.

► Treatment Steps
1. **Oxygen.**
2. Mechanical ventilation.
3. **CPAP.**

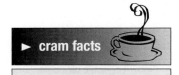

2. **Acute Respiratory Distress Syndrome (ARDS)**

► Description
Acute lung damage syndrome, from **increased pulmonary (alveolar) permeability.**

► Symptoms
Dyspnea, tachypnea, tachycardia.

► Diagnosis
See Cram Facts.

► Pathology
Etiology includes **infection, aspiration, shock, drugs,** and multiple other conditions.

► Treatment Steps
1. **Supportive.**
2. Treat underlying etiology.

► cram facts

DIAGNOSIS OF ACUTE LUNG INJURY AND ARDS
(as defined by the 1994 American European Consensus conference)

ACUTE LUNG INJURY

- Arterial hypoxemia (Pao_2/Fio_2 ratio, ≤ 300)
- Pulmonary artery wedge pressure ≤ 18 mm Hg or no clinical evidence of left atrial hypertension, and
- Bilateral infiltrates consistent with pulmonary edema on frontal CXR (infiltrates can be mild)

ARDS

- Same criteria as acute lung injury, but more severe hypoxemia (Pao_2/Fio_2, ≤ 200)

Fio_2 = fraction of inspired oxygen.

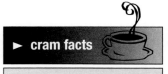

► cram facts

Hypoxemia—depressed Po_2
Hypercapnia—elevated Pco_2

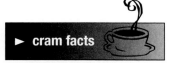

► cram facts

PULMONARY EMBOLISM

- Etiology: may vary. Venous stasis, venous thrombosis, hypercoagulable states (e.g., SLE, malignancies), protein C and S deficiency, oral contraceptives, antithrombin III deficiency, and others.
- Symptoms: sudden onset dyspnea, pleuritic chest pain, hemoptysis, palpitations, syncope, split S2 sound.
- Diagnosis: history and physical, CXR, ventilation–perfusion scan, electrocardiogram (S1, Q3, T [V] 1–3), venous ultrasound of legs, pulmonary angiography, and arterial blood gas (respiratory alkalosis with or without significant hypoxia but increased A-a gradient).
- Treatment: anticoagulation, O_2, thrombolitics, embolectomy, filter.

3. "Lung protective ventilation" with low tidal volumes (6 mL/kg ideal body weight).
4. **Positive end-expiratory pressure (PEEP).**

3. **Acute and Chronic Respiratory Failure**

► Symptoms
Dyspnea, hypoxemia (headache, confusion, tachycardia, shock).

► Diagnosis
History and physical, **arterial blood gas (hypoxemia/hypercapnia).** PFTs are useful in chronic respiratory disease but are not useful in the acute setting.

► Pathology
Etiology includes ARDS, pulmonary edema, drugs, and neuromuscular conditions. **Reduced Po_2 etiology: impaired diffusion, ventilation–perfusion mismatch, hypoventilation, right–left shunt, and reduced inspired Po_2.**

► Treatment Steps
1. **Control airway.**
2. **Oxygen.**
3. Improving ventilation by limiting sedation/discontinuing sedative medications.
4. More often ventilation assistance is needed with either noninasive ventilation (CPAP or BiPAP) or invasive ventilation (intubation with ventilator).

H. Pulmonary Vascular Disorders

1. **Pulmonary Embolism (PE)**

► Description
Pulmonary thrombus, via the right side of the heart, from the venous system.

► Symptoms
Chest pain, cough, hemoptysis, tachycardia/tachypnea, **or nonspecific** symptoms (apprehension).

► Diagnosis

History (sudden onset!) and physical (fever, rales, or normal), arterial **blood gas (increase A-a gradient), lung scan** (ventilation–perfusion), CXR, electrocardiogram (ECG) with sinus tachycardia and/or S1, Q3, T3, pulmonary angiography (gold standard), search for deep vein thrombosis (DVT) in lower extremities.

► Pathology

Mostly from deep leg vein thrombi and pelvic venous system (less frequent etiology).

► Treatment Steps

1. **Anticoagulation** (heparin, then Coumadin).
2. Thrombolytic medication (use with massive PE and hypotension).
3. **If cannot use anticoagulation, vena caval filter. Prevention** important for high-risk groups (orthopedic surgery, pelvic/abdominal surgery associated with malignancy, surgery with history of DVT or PE).
4. Embolectomy (use in nonresponding shock case).
5. In pregnancy where Coumadin is contraindicated, need to use heparin subcutaneously until term is reached (keeping therapeutic partial thromboplastin time [PTT]).

   Anticoagulation: heparin 5,000–10,000 U (80 U/kg) **bolus IV, then 1,000 U/hour (18 U/kg/hour IV), PTT (1.5–2 times control), duration 5–10 days. After 96 hours, start Coumadin (to maintain INR > 2.0).** Continue Coumadin 3 months.

   Monitor platelet count: **heparin-induced thrombocytopenia.**

2. Pulmonary Hypertension

► Description

Elevated pulmonary artery pressure.

► Symptoms

Chest pain, dyspnea, lethargy, syncope, and occasional hemoptysis.

► Diagnosis

History and physical **(shortened second heart sound split and louder P2, weak peripheral pulse/cold hands),** ECG (right heart-strain pattern), CXR, polycythemia. Increase pulmonary artery pressures (PAP), pulmonary capillary wedge pressure (PCWP) is usually normal (increased PCWP in pulmonary hypertension from cardiac causes). Pulmonary function tests show normal lung volumes with low diffusion capacity.

► Etiology

Major etiology is **hypoxia,** but may also be from obstruction, shunts, or unknown etiology (primary pulmonary hypertension).

► Treatment Steps

1. **Oxygen.**
2. **Vasodilators.**
3. Anticoagulation.
4. Calcium channel blockers.
5. Prostaglandins.

3. Cor Pulmonale

See also Chapter 1, section II.D.

► Description

Right ventricular hypertrophy (RVH) secondary to pulmonary disease.

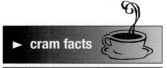

► cram facts

SIGN OR SYMPTOM: ARRHYTHMIAS

Think of: Important to define if they are atrial or ventricular in origin. Think of cardiac ischemia, thyroid disease, medication-induced stress, drugs, post–myocardial infarction (MI) pulmonary embolism, mitral valve prolapse, panic attacks; other less frequent but you need to be aware of: Wolff–Parkinson–White, multifocal atrial tachycardia (MAT), and prolonged QT, just to mention a few.

► **Symptoms**
Dyspnea, weight gain, wheezing.

► **Diagnosis**
History and physical (cyanosis, edema, ascites, clubbing), ECG (RVH), CXR (**large pulmonary artery** [main and left/right descending, and RVH]), echocardiogram.

► **Treatment Steps**
1. **Oxygen.**
2. Bronchodilators.
3. Diuretics.
4. Treat right heart failure.

4. **Pulmonary Edema**

► **Symptoms**
Dyspnea, diaphoresis, anxiety, wheezing, tachycardia, cyanosis.

► **Diagnosis**
See Cram Facts.

► **Treatment Steps**
1. Oxygen.
2. Diuretics.
3. Morphine sulfate.
4. Venodilators.
5. Dopamine if hypotensive.

5. **Vasculitis**

5–1. Goodpasture's Syndrome

► **Description**
An autoimmune disorder characterized by antiglomerular basement membrane antibodies (anti-GBM), causing diffuse pulmonary hemorrhage and glomerulonephritis. (See also Chapter 7.)

► **Symptoms**
Hemoptysis, glomerulonephritis, anemia, chills/fever/chest pain.

► **Diagnosis**
Clinical scenario, **anti–GBM antibodies,** renal biopsy.

► **Treatment Steps**
1. **Prednisone.**
2. **Cyclophosphamide.**
3. **Plasmapheresis.**

5–2. Wegener's Granulomatosis

► **Description**
Necrotizing upper and lower pulmonary granulomatous vasculitis with glomerulonephritis.

► **Symptoms**
Cough, dyspnea, lethargy, conjunctivitis, glomerulonephritis, fever, purulent sinusitis.

► **Diagnosis**
Clinical scenario, lung or renal biopsy.

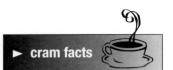

► **cram facts**

PULMONARY EDEMA/CHF

- **Symptoms:** Dyspnea, DOE (dyspnea on exertion), orthopnea, paroxysmal nocturnal dyspnea (PND)
- **Signs:** Peripheral edema; rales/crackles; jugular venous distention (JVD); sometimes pink, frothy sputum
- **CXR:** Bilateral infiltrates or "cephalization," Kerley B lines
- **Echocardiogram:** Useful in documenting depressed ejection fraction and valvular disease

► **clinical pearl**

Antineutrophil cytoplasmic antibody (c-ANCA) is associated with Wegener's granulomatosis. Perinuclear antineutrophil cytoplasmic antibody (p-ANCA) is associated with polyarteritis nodosa.

▶ differential diagnosis

PLEURAL EFFUSIONS

How to classify them?: Need to have one or more of the following Lights' Criteria parameters to be an exudative effusion:

1. Pleural protein to serum protein ratio > 0.5.
2. Pleural LDH to serum LDH > 0.6.
3. Pleural LDH > ⅔ upper serum LDH.

Criteria suggesting need for aggressive treatment of pleural effusion:

1. Pleural LDH > 1,000.
2. Pleural pH < 7.2.
3. Bacteria present on pleural fluid stain.

- **Transudates:** CHF, pulmonary emboli, nephrotic syndrome, ascites, myxedema, peritoneal dialysis, severe atelectasis, and superior vena cava syndrome.
- **Exudates:** empyema, parapneumonic effusions, malignancies, TB, Meigs' syndrome, pancreatic disease, sarcoidosis, connective tissue disease, Dressler syndrome, postpericardiomy syndrome, chylothorax, infections (viral, fungal), asbestosis, uremia.
- **Others:** hemothorax, esophageal rupture.

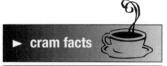

▶ cram facts

Pleurodynia—epidemic infection **in young people, coxsackie B virus,** supportive treatment.

▶ cram facts

1. **Transudate**—pleural fluid protein divided by serum protein under 0.5 and pleural lactic dehydrogenase (LDH) divided by serum LDH under 0.6. Noted in CHF, and **renal/liver** disease.
2. **Exudate**—protein and LDH numbers **above** the transudate values. Empyema or complicated parapneumonic effusions (LDH > 1,000 or pH of fluid < 7.20 and/or decrease glucose concentration). Noted in **infections, malignancy, and trauma.**

▶ Treatment Steps
1. **Cyclophosphamide.**
2. **Corticosteroids.**

Attention: There are other types of vasculitis but these are the most frequently asked in test questions. Be aware of the others.

I. Pleural Disorders

1. Pleurisy

▶ Description/Symptoms
Pleural inflammation, causing **inspiratory pain** (usually unilateral, and of rapid onset), **dyspnea.** Clinical diagnosis.

▶ Treatment Steps
1. Indomethacin.
2. Intercostal nerve block.

2. Pleural Effusion

▶ Symptoms
May be asymptomatic or present as per primary etiology, also **dyspnea, pleuritic chest pain.**

▶ Diagnosis
History and physical, CXR (lateral decubitus film), pleural fluid exam. (See Differential Diagnosis and Cram Facts.)

▶ Pathology
Increased capillary permeability or hydrostatic pressure, or decreased lymph drainage or oncotic pressure.

▶ Treatment Steps
Treat primary etiology.

J. Pulmonary Neoplasm—Primary and Metastatic Tumors

See Chapter 6, section VII.D.

III. PRINCIPLES OF MANAGEMENT

A. Intubation, Tracheostomy, and Assisted Ventilation

▶ Description

1. *Intubation*—endotracheal tube: via oral or nasal route, with position confirmed by x-ray and auscultation (where available, also can use CO_2 detector for airway as an aid to confirm position). Nasal tube is more difficult to suction through than oral tube (and has increased infection risk after 5 days). Endotracheal intubation may be maintained without time limit (in prolonged intubations or recurrent intubations watch for tracheostenosis, also watch for increased balloon pressures and tracheal trauma). If long-term ventilation is needed, tracheostomy is considered.

2. *Tracheostomy*—easier to suction through than oral tube. More comfortable to patients for prolonged/extended periods of time. Air must be humidified. As all tubes, bypass normal nose/upper airway humidification. Same precautions as above.

3. *Assisted ventilation*—decision to intubate is clinical in nature. Clinical signs to look for: paradoxical respirations, increased JVD, pulsus paradoxicus, and increased lethargy or severe confusion. ABG is also very useful in documenting the severity of hypoxemia or hypercapnia.

   (a) *Initial settings:* FIO_2, 100%; tidal volume, 10 mL/kg; assisted control (A/C) or intermittent mandatory ventilation (IMV), 10–14 breaths/min (always need to correlate with clinical scenario).

   (b) **Most common modes of mechanical ventilation use**—IMV: delivers set respiratory rate per minute with set tidal volume with each of those breaths. In between machine breaths, patient can generate his/her own breaths with tidal volume determined by patient's effort, allowing for patient's own muscles to be exercised.

   (c) *A/C*—patient receives set rate per minute with set volumes with each breath. Any extra breaths generated by the patient, in addition to the ones already set, will be assisted (the machine will complete/supplement each breath [volume]) for patient.

B. Massive Hemoptysis

▶ Description
Blood flow of 200–600 mL into the pulmonary system within 24 hours.

▶ Symptoms
Hemoptysis, hypoxia, dyspnea, lethargy, wheezing.

▶ Diagnosis
History and physical exam, CXR and lab, bronchoscopy.

▶ Pathology
Bronchiectasis, TB, vasculitis, fungal cavitations, abscess, and coagulopathies most commonly.

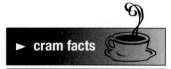

▶ **cram facts**

PEEP added to A/C or IMV to produce constant positive ventilation pressure; most useful for pulmonary edema, ARDS, or other conditions in which oxygenation is poor, with settings of 3–20 cm water.

- *Complications of PEEP*—reduced cardiac output and pneumothorax.
- *Ventilator problem*— disconnect patient from machine, and ventilate by bag. Hard to ventilate: suction patient, and rule out pneumothorax, tube position problem, or obstruction. Treat as indicated.

▶ Treatment Steps
1. Oxygen.
2. Fluids.
3. Bronchoscopy.
4. Correct coagulopathy.
5. A-gram embolization.
6. Surgery.

BIBLIOGRAPHY

Adams GL. *Fundamentals of Otolaryngology,* 6th ed. Philadelphia: W.B. Saunders, 1997.

Bass JB, et al. Treatment and Tuberculosis Infection in Adults and Children. *Am Rev Resp Dis,* May 1994; 1359–1374.

Baum GL. *Textbook of Pulmonary Diseases,* Vols. 1 & 2, 6th ed. Boston: Little, Brown & Co., 1998.

Civetta JM. *Critical Care.* Philadelphia: J.B. Lippincott, 1992.

Dosman JA. *The Medical Clinics of North America, Obstructive Lung Disease,* Vol. 74. Philadelphia: W.B. Saunders, May 1990.

Freundlich IM. *A Radiologic Approach to Diseases of the Chest,* 2nd ed. Baltimore: Williams & Wilkins, 1997.

George RB. *Chest Medicine, Essentials of Pulmonary and Critical Care Medicine,* 5th ed. Baltimore: Williams & Wilkins, 2005.

Guenter CA. *Pulmonary Medicine,* 2nd ed. Philadelphia: J.B. Lippincott, 1982.

Light RW. *Pleural Diseases,* 3rd ed. Philadelphia: Lea & Febiger, 1995.

Middleton E. *Allergy Principles and Practices,* Vols. I & II, 3rd ed. St. Louis: Mosby, 1988.

Muller NL, et al. *Fraser and Pare's Diagnosis of Diseases of the Chest,* Vols. I–III. Philadelphia: W.B. Saunders, 1999.

Murray JF. *Textbook of Respiratory Medicine,* 3rd ed. Philadelphia: W.B. Saunders, 2001.

Pennington JE. *Respiratory Infections: Diagnosis and Management.* New York: Raven Press, 1988.

Pinsky MR. *Pathophysiologic Foundations of Critical Care.* Baltimore: Williams & Wilkins, 1993.

Renal System and Urology

I. HEALTH AND HEALTH MAINTENANCE

A. Urinary Tract Infection

Epidemiology—More frequent in females (except in neonates), and increases with age.

Impact—Recurrent infections and renal damage.

Risk Factors—Obstructive uropathy (calculus, stricture/valves), vesicoureteral reflux, diabetes mellitus, sexual activity, and pregnancy.

Prevention—Patient education, for both prevention/hygiene, early intervention/treatment, and prophylactic antibiotics where indicated.

B. Toxic Nephropathy

Epidemiology—Common causes include **analgesics, penicillin/sulfa, phenytoin sodium (Dilantin), cimetidine (Tagamet), heavy metals,** and **aminoglycosides.** Noted in chronic pain patients with continued analgesic use.

Impact—Papillary necrosis/renal failure.

Risk Factors—Compounds listed, occupational/environmental exposure to toxins, and both calcium disorders (sarcoid, multiple myeloma, etc.) and antineoplastic agents.

Prevention—Patient education and early intervention/diagnosis (discontinue the offending agent). Special consideration is given to the elderly in whom reduced renal function may contribute to elevated serum toxin levels and earlier toxicity.

C. Renal Failure/Disease Prevention

Prevention of acute renal failure and of urinary tract disease secondary to formation of calculi and/or obstruction. Where **absorptive hypercalciuria** is noted, **reduced-calcium diet, ion-exchange resin (sodium cellulose), hydration,** and **orthophosphates.** For **renal hypercalciuria** use **thiazides.** For **hyperuricosuria** use **allopurinol.** For **struvite/chronic infection** stones, use **repeat cultures/antibiotics.** For **hypercystinuria, alkalinize the urine.** For **obstructions,** treat/remove obstruction when indicated.

D. Limiting Renal Disease Progression

Control underlying disorder (hypertension, diabetes mellitus, etc.). Dietary measures include protein/potassium/phosphorus restriction for chronic renal failure. Limit extra dietary magnesium, treat acidosis, and supply additional calcium when required.

II. MECHANISMS OF DISEASE AND DIAGNOSIS

A. Male Reproductive System Disorders

1. Prostatitis

▶ Symptoms
Dysuria, chills/fever, low back pain, perineal pain, frequency.

► Diagnosis

History and physical, **large (boggy if chronic) tender prostate gland.**
Avoid prostate massage (bacteremia risk).

► Pathology

Escherichia coli **(usually aerobic gram-negative rods).** *Chlamydia,* nonspecific inflammation.

► Treatment Steps

1. Antibiotics (e.g., fluoroquinolones, tetracycline), often treated for up to 6 weeks.
2. Nonsteroidal anti-inflammatory drugs (NSAIDs).
3. Sitz baths.

2. Epididymitis

► Symptoms

Tender, enlarged testicle and/or epididymis; fever; scrotal thickening.

► Diagnosis

History and physical, **scrotum** may be **red/tender.** Pyuria, epididymis tender. Urethra/urine culture and Gram stain (if patient is having discharge).

► Pathology

Organisms include *Neisseria gonorrhoeae, E. coli,* and *Chlamydia.*

► Treatment Steps

1. Tetracycline, fluoroquinolones, or antibiotic as per culture.
2. NSAIDs.
3. Scrotal support.

3. Orchitis (Testicular Inflammation)

► Symptoms

Fever, testicular size increase, scrotal pain, and erythema.

► Diagnosis

History and physical, rule out mumps or torsion, usually no urethral symptoms/discharge.

► Treatment Steps

1. Antibiotic (if bacterial).
2. NSAIDs.
3. Scrotal support.
4. Warm soaks.

4. Urethritis

► Symptoms/Diagnosis

Urethral discharge, dysuria. Urethral culture and Gram stain (to rule out sexually transmitted diseases and other infection).

► Pathology

Sexual transmission common. Gonococcal and nongonococcal urethritis (*Chlamydia, Trichomonas,* herpes simplex).

► Treatment Steps

Antibiotics tailored to the specific etiology.

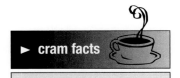

► cram facts

Orchitis may be associated with mumps, tuberculosis, or other infections.

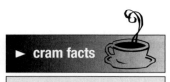

cram facts

TREATMENT OPTIONS
FOR GONORRHEA

- Cefixime (Suprax) 400 mg PO × 1
- Ceftriaxone (Rocephin) 400 mg PO × 1
- Ciprofloxacin 500 mg PO × 1
- Ofloxacin 400 mg PO × 1

Note: Gonorrhea and chlamydia are usually treated as if they coexist.

cram facts

Testicular torsion is a urologic emergency! If not diagnosed and treated promptly, infarction and loss of testicle may occur.

5. **Sexually Transmitted Diseases (STDs)**
See also Chapter 13.

5–1. Gonorrhea

▶ Symptoms
Caused by infection with *N. gonorrhoeae*. **Dysuria, urethritis/discharge (thick yellow).** Less commonly can cause pharyngitis.

▶ Diagnosis
History and physical, culture/Gram stain **(gram-negative intracellular diplococci).**

▶ Treatment Steps
See Cram Facts.

5–2. Syphilis
See also Chapter 9, section I.C.4.

▶ Description
STD caused by the spirochete *Treponema pallidum*. Four stages: primary, secondary, latent, and tertiary.

▶ Symptoms
Penile painless lesion: chancre (primary syphilis).

▶ Diagnosis
Serologic test for syphilis (rapid plasma reagin [RPR], Venereal Disease Research Laboratory [VDRL]) and fluorescent treponemal antibody absorption (FTA-ABS) studies.

▶ Treatment Steps
Benzathine penicillin G, 2.4 million U IM (if allergic to penicillin, give doxycycline). For primary disease, one injection. (See also Chapter 9, section I.C.4.)

5–3. Chlamydia

▶ Symptoms
Dysuria, frequency, or asymptomatic. Possible abnormal vaginal discharge. Often coinfection with gonorrhea. Caused by infection with *Chlamydia trachomatis*.

▶ Diagnosis
Urethral culture/Gram stain, *Chlamydia* culture.

▶ Treatment Steps
1. Doxycycline 100 mg twice daily for 1 week (not safe in pregnancy).
2. Azithromycin 1 g PO.
3. Metronidazole 2 g PO.

6. **Testicular Torsion**

▶ Description
Testicular rotation and loss of blood supply. **Most common cause of scrotal swelling in children.**

▶ Symptoms
Testicular pain/swelling, vomiting and/or abdominal pain. May have initially only abdominal pain; check scrotum!

▶ **Diagnosis**

History and physical, pain unchanged or worse with testicular elevation. Urine negative, and affected testicle may be elevated in position.

▶ **Pathology**

Abnormal tunica vaginalis attachment allowing room for testicular
twisting ("bell-clapper deformity").

▶ **Treatment Steps**

Surgery (within 4–6 hours, if possible).

7. Cryptorchidism (Undescended Testicle)

▶ **Symptoms**

None. Pick up on exam only (50% of premature males have undescended testicle).

▶ **Diagnosis**

History and physical. Rule out retractile testis (hyperactive cremaster
muscle pull). In adults, consider computed tomography (CT).

▶ **Pathology**

Failure of testes to descend normally. Exact cause not defined.

▶ **Treatment Steps**

1. Surgery by age 1 **(orchiopexy).**
2. Hormones have been tried (human chorionic gonadotropin
   [hCG]).

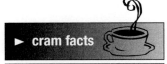

CRYPTORCHIDISM

- Undescended testicle
  has an increased risk of
  developing cancer.
- Risk is not reduced with
  orchiopexy.

8. Neoplasm of the Testis—Seminoma

See Chapter 6, section VII.F.11–2.

9. Prostate Neoplasm—Benign Prostatic Hyperplasia (BPH)

▶ **Description**

Enlargement of the prostate gland due to glandular and/or stromal
hyperplasia. Exceedingly common in men as they age.

▶ **Symptoms**

Obstruction (hesitancy, dribbling, reduced stream force), and urgency, nocturia, frequency. Some cases of BPH can cause near total
obstruction of urinary flow and result in renal failure.

▶ **Diagnosis**

History and physical. Ultrasound, urodynamics, cystoscopy.

▶ **Pathology**

Hyperplasia or increased tone of bladder neck/prostatic urethra, increasing incidence with age.

▶ **Treatment Steps**

1. Watchful waiting.
2. α-Blocker (prazosin, terazosin, doxazosin [Cardura], tamsulosin
   [Flomax]).
3. Bulk reducers (finasteride [Proscar]), 5α-reductase inhibitor. Inhibits conversion of testosteron to dihydrotestosterone.
4. Surgical reduction (transurethral prostatectomy [TURP]).

SCROTAL MASS

- Testicular tumor
- Hydrocele
- Varicocele
- Epididymal cyst
- Testicular torsion
- Epididymal orchitis
- Hernia
- Inguinal cord tumor
- Hematoma

10. Prostate Cancer

See Chapter 6, section VII.G.4.

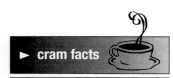

► cram facts

HYPOSPADIAS

- Commonly associated with other conditions such as inguinal hernias and cryptorchidism (undescended testes).
- The penis is more likely to have chordee, which is ventral shortening and curvature.

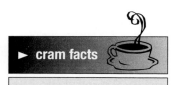

► cram facts

Most common etiology of ambiguous genitalia, adrenal hyperplasia (check for Y chromosome).

► cram facts

SIGN OR SYMPTOM: HEMATURIA

Think of: Kidney stones, cystitis, menstrual cycle, anticoagulation/coagulopathy, bladder cancer, trauma, Foley catheter manipulation, infections (common as well as uncommon, such as *Schistosoma haematobium)*, renal failure (in some ways).

11. Penile Disorders—Hypospadias

► **Description**
Most frequent urologic anomaly, with meatus below penis tip.

► **Symptoms**
None. May be associated with **chordee (ventral penile curve).**

► **Pathology**
Urethral ridges do not fuse, possibly hereditary.

► **Treatment Steps**
Surgical if meatus too proximal. Look for associated anomalies.

12. Hydrocele and Varicocele

► **Description**

Hydrocele—Fluid around testis (in tunica vaginalis layers).

Varicocele—Pampiniform plexus vein dilation.

► **Symptoms**
Nontender scrotal mass.

► **Diagnosis**
Transillumination, history and physical, ultrasound. Varicocele may be absent when supine, increase if straining/standing (Valsalva).

► **Pathology**

Hydrocele—**Patent processus vaginalis.**

Varicocele—Inefficient pampiniform valves.

► **Treatment Steps**
1. Observation.
2. Surgical if not resolving on own, or if resulting in infertility (varicocele), or symptoms (pressure).

13. Urethral Stricture

► **Symptoms**
May be **asymptomatic,** prostatitis, obstruction (abnormal stream angle/spraying, or narrow stream), cystitis.

► **Diagnosis**
Cystourethrogram, history and physical, flow studies, culture, cystoscopy.

► **Pathology**
May have history of **gonorrhea,** trauma, or other infections causing fibrotic narrowing of the urethra.

► **Treatment Steps**
1. Optical internal urethrotomy.
2. Primary resection.
3. Dilation.

B. Bladder/Collecting System Disorders

1. Cystitis

► **Description**
Cystitis is bladder infection. (See Cram Facts.)

► **Symptoms/Diagnosis**

Cystitis presents as dysuria, frequency, nocturia, urgency. Urine dip, urinalysis, and culture used in certain cases.

► **Pathology**

Cystitis usually from *E. coli.*

► **Treatment Steps**

1. Antibiotics.
2. Intravenous pyelogram (IVP), cystoscopy for recurrent/persistent cases.

2. Carcinoma of the Bladder

See Chapter 6.

3. Nephrolithiasis

► **Description**

Calculi (stones) in the urinary tract.

► **Symptoms**

Severe pain, nausea/vomiting, flank pain, hematuria. **Caliceal,** may be asymptomatic; **proximal ureter,** severe intermittent flank pain, colic; **distal ureter**/ureterovesicle junction, radiating pain, bladder irritation, groin pain.

► **Diagnosis**

History and physical, IVP, urine analysis. **Uric acid stones not visible on plain x-ray** (see Fig. 17–1).

► **Treatment Steps**

1. Prevention of further episodes: hydration and medical evaluation.
2. Symptomatic stones: small stones (5 mm) supportive measures and spontaneous passage (6 weeks). Larger or completely obstructive stones: upper tract—extracorporeal lithotripsy, lower tract—ureteroscopy.

4. Ureteral Reflux

► **Description**

Reflux of urine into ureter with voiding.

► **Symptoms**

Infection/pyelonephritis, kidney damage/uremia.

► **Diagnosis**

History and physical, urine analysis and culture, IVP, **voiding cystourethrography.**

► **Pathology**

Short intramural ureter.

► **Treatment Steps**

1. Medical (watch and wait, antibiotics).
2. Surgical (ureteral reimplantation).

5. Neurogenic Bladder

► **Symptoms**

Voiding dysfunction. Failure to empty urine; failure to store urine.

► **cram facts**

- *Dysuria* may be symptom of cystitis, or urethral syndrome in females.
- *Pyuria* is leukocytes in urine, but **not necessarily infection** (pyuria and negative culture: rule out tuberculosis).
- *Hematuria* may be sign of infection, cancer, found in runners, renal disease. Always abnormal in males; IVP and cystocope to rule out tumor.
- *Casts* suggest **renal disease** (leukocyte, pyelonephritis; red blood cell [RBC] casts, glomerulitis).

► **cram facts**

NEPHROLITHIASIS

- Pain is often excruciating.
- Requires aggressive hydration and pain medications.
- Urinalysis will often show microscopic hematuria.
- Calcium-containing stones are seen on x-ray.
- CT scanning is now used to visualize calculi.

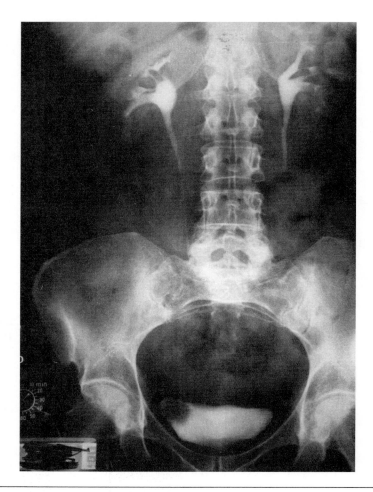

Figure 17–1. Abdominal plain film demonstrating radiopaque staghorn calculus.

► Diagnosis

History and physical, urodynamic testing (cystometrogram [CMG], flowmeter, etc.).

► Pathology

Sensory, motor, uninhibited, reflex, and **autonomous.**

Sensory—No sensation of full bladder, diabetics, herniated disk.

Motor—Sensation okay, but cannot initiate contraction, disk, polio, tumor.

Uninhibited—No control, brain/central nervous system (CNS) lesion or disease.

Reflex Spinal Cord Injury, Autonomous—No connection from bladder to brain, spinal trauma.

► Treatment Steps

Failure to empty:

1. Clean intermittent catheterization.
2. Sphincterotomy.

Failure to store:

1. Anticholinergics.
2. Collagen injections.
3. Bladder sling or artificial sphincter.

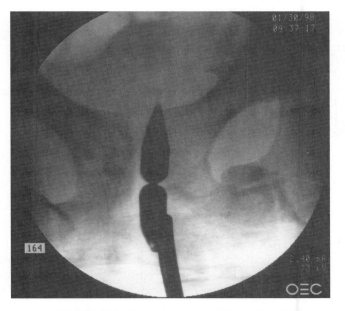

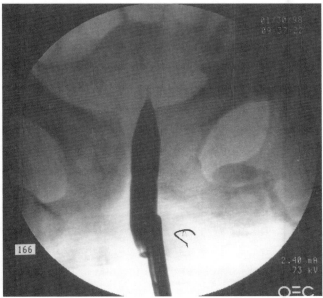

Figure 17–3. Bulbar urethral stricture before and after balloon dilatation.

► Treatment Steps

Antibiotics (IV cephalosporin and aminoglycoside). If recurrent/chronic infection, rule out organic disease and coexisting medical conditions.

2. Glomerulonephritis

► Description

Kidney inflammation with glomeruli as area of disorder.

► Symptoms

Hematuria, proteinuria, reduced glomerular filtration rate (GFR) resulting in **hypertension, edema.**

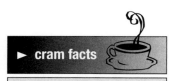

► Diagnosis

History and physical, urine analysis and culture, serologic studies to attempt to define cause.

► Pathology

Inflammation/immune deposits resulting in glomerular injury. (See Cram Facts.)

► Treatment Steps

Varies according to etiology.
1. Acute—diuresis, bed rest, antihypertensives.
2. Rapid progression—steroids, cytotoxics, plasmapheresis.

3. Minimal Change Disease (MCD)

► Description/Treatment

MCD refers to a pathologic lesion of the glomerulus. It is the most common cause of nephrotic syndrome in children and is usually very responsive to steroids (prednisone), with a good prognosis. It is less responsive to steroids and has a slightly worse prognosis in adults.

► Pathology

Under light microscopy, the glomerulus is basically normal. Immunohistochemistry is also unremarkable. However, changes are seen on electron microscopy: retraction of the epithelial foot processes, sometimes referred to as fusion of the foot processes.

4. Immunoglobulin A (IgA) Nephropathy

► Description

Berger's disease (a variety of Henoch–Schönlein purpura).

► Symptoms

Gross hematuria after viral infection, fever, proteinuria, dysuria.

► Diagnosis

History and physical, possible elevated serum IgA, **biopsy.**

► Pathology

Immune deposits of IgA on glomeruli.

► Treatment Steps

None.

5. Diabetic Nephropathy

► Description

This is a clinical syndrome associated with diabetes, proteinuria, and, if uncontrolled, progressive renal failure. Patients are symptomatic as renal failure develops. It is the leading cause of chronic renal failure.

► Pathology

Microvascular glomerular damage (thickening of the glomerular basement membrane) and **Kimmelstiel–Wilson lesions (nodular deposits in glomeruli).**

► Treatment Steps

See Cram Facts.

6. Nephrotic Syndrome

See Chapter 19.

TREATMENT OF DIABETIC NEPHROPATHY

- **Prevention is of the utmost importance.**
- Excellent diabetic control (goal: hemoglobin $A_{1C} < 7.0$).
- Excellent blood pressure control (< 120/80).
- Routine screening of urine for microalbuminuria (a small but abnormal degree of albumin in the urine, 30–300 mg/day).
- Treatment of microalbuminuria with angiotensin-converting enzyme (ACE) inhibitors or angiotensin receptor blockers.
- Early follow-up with a nephrologist is prudent.
- If renal insufficiency progresses to failure, counseling and preparation should begin for hemodialysis and/or renal transplant.

7. Proteinuria

See Chapter 19.

8. Interstitial Nephropathy

► **Symptoms**

Polyuria, nocturia, acute renal failure, fever, rash, joint pain.

► **Diagnosis**

History and physical, eosinophilia, renal biopsy.

► **Pathology**

Wide variety of infections, toxins (heavy metals), calcium disorders, drugs, and systemic disorders as etiologic agents.

► **Treatment Steps**

1. Remove offending agent.
2. Treat primary disease.

9. Renal Failure

9–1. Acute

► **Description**

A decline in renal function over a short period of time (hours to days). (See Cram Facts.)

► **Symptoms**

Vary based on cause of the renal failure. Important to assess a decline in urine output, change in the quality of the urine flow or color, dysuria, hematuria, increase in abdominal size. Look for signs of volume status: skin turgor, peripheral edema.

► **Diagnosis**

Assess for symptoms as above. Ask about any new medications that have been started. Routine labs include chemistries (specifically for potassium, CO_2, BUN, creatinine, magnesium, phosphate, calcium). Also, urinalysis, urine electrolytes (particularly urine sodium and creatinine). Routine CBC, liver function tests (LFTs), electrocardiogram (ECG), and chest x-ray (CXR). Other studies (e.g., KUB [kidneys, ureters, bladder] or CT scan to rule out nephrolithiasis) are done as indicated.

► **Pathology**

See Table 17–1.

17-1

ACUTE RENAL FAILURE

Because there are so many different etiologies of renal failure, it is common to try and decide which of the following three basic pathways is most likely to be related to the renal disease:

PRERENAL

Conditions in which there is decreased flow to the kidney. Commonly includes volume depletion (from gastrointestinal bleed, overdiuresis, severe dehydration). Also includes relative intravascular volume depletion and reduced renal blood flow (i.e., congestive heart failure, cirrhosis).

INTRINSIC RENAL

Conditions affecting the kidney directly. Includes the glomerulonephridites, acute tubular necrosis, rhabdomyolysis, multiple myeloma, interstitial nephritis, and amyloidosis.

POSTRENAL

Obstruction of flow existing somewhere in the urinary tract. In men, common cause is BPH. Also extrinsic compression by pelvic mass, kidney stones. One rule of thumb is when a patient is seen initially, a Foley catheter should be placed. This will help to see if there is distal obstruction. Additionally, a renal ultrasound should be done to rule out hydronephrosis.

▶ **Treatment Steps**

Varies according to the etiology. Some guidelines:

1. Prerenal: Improving renal blood flow may be accomplished with iv hydration, stopping ACE inhibitors, and in certain cases using vasopressors (dopamine).
2. Intrinsic renal: Varies according to etiology.
3. Postrenal: Foley catheter can be curative if obstruction caused by BPH. Removal of kidney stone, or ureteral or urethral stent if there are stenoses causing a blockage.
4. In all cases, meticulous attention paid to urine output and management of electrolyte imbalances (hyperklemia). Also, remove all potentially nephrotoxic medications (NSAIDs, ACE inhibitors) and adjust the doses of necessary medications according the creatinine clearance.
5. Dialysis is used in certain cases (see Cram Facts).

9–2. Chronic

▶ **Description**

Long-term renal function reduction.

▶ **Symptoms**

May have reduced urine output, **lethargy, hypertension, myopathy, pruritus,** pericarditis, **anemia.**

▶ **Diagnosis**

See Renal Failure (Acute).

▶ **Pathology**

Etiology in numerous disorders.

▶ **Treatment Steps**

1. Diet control.
2. Balance electrolytes.
3. Treat anemia, osteodystrophy.
4. Dialysis.

10. Renal Osteodystrophy

▶ **Description**

Skeletal abnormality secondary to chronic renal failure. Diagnose with typical x-ray findings.

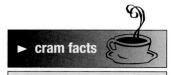

▶ **cram facts**

Most common skeletal lesion in chronic renal failure (CRF): **osteitis fibrosa. Lack of erythropoietin results in CRF anemia. Serum phosphate is elevated with reduced GFR** (e.g., chronic renal failure).

Total serum calcium is reduced in CRF.

► Symptoms

Children—growth retardation, rickets.

Adults—may be asymptomatic, or **bone pain, proximal muscle weakness.**

► Pathology

Subperiosteal bone resorption. Results in **osteitis fibrosa** and **osteomalacia.**

► Treatment Steps

Control serum calcium/phosphorus (phosphate binders), parathyroidectomy. **Drug of choice for hypocalcemia/secondary hyperparathyroidism is vitamin D.**

11. Papillary Necrosis

► Description

Kidney papilla necrosis.

► Symptoms

Hematuria, fever, flank pain, renal failure.

► Diagnosis

History and physical, IVP, urine analysis, and culture.

► Pathology

Ischemic, usually associated infection. Chronic disease, toxins, obstructions. Often seen in patients with sickle cell disease. May be a complication of pyelonephritis.

► Treatment Steps

1. Treat primary etiology (infection, etc.).
2. Remove mechanical obstruction.

12. Hypertensive Renal Disease

12–1. *Preeclampsia/Pregnancy-Induced Hypertension*

See Chapter 13.

12–2. *Eclampsia*

See Chapter 13.

13. Renovascular Hypertension

► Description

Stenosis of the renal arteries can cause systemic hypertension.

► Symptoms

Hypertension, may be **rapid onset at any age, difficult to control, childhood** or **older adult onset.**

► Diagnosis

History and physical (epigastric bruit), IVP, renal/digital subtraction angiography (DSA), renal vein renin ratio > 1.5.

► Treatment Steps

1. Medication (captopril).
2. Surgical (including angioplasty).

14. Nephrosclerosis

► Description

A clinical syndrome involving long-standing hypertension, hyperten-

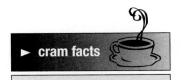

► cram facts

RENAL ARTERY STENOSIS

- In a young female, suspect fibromuscular dysplasia, often amenable to stenting.
- In older patients, suspect atherosclerosis as the cause.

sive retropathy, hypertrophy of the left ventricle, minimal proteinuria, and progressive renal insufficiency/failure.

► **Symptoms**
Often asymptomatic. Over time, signs and symptoms of renal disease develop. Clinical diagnosis. Renal failure, proteinuria, hematuria, small kidneys, or no symptoms.

► **Treatment Steps**
Control blood pressure and renal disease.

15. Lupus Nephritis

► **Description**
Lupus may present as interstitial nephritis or glomerulonephritis.

► **Symptoms**
Hematuria, proteinuria, hypertension, edema, red cell/hyaline casts.

► **Diagnosis**
History and physical, urine analysis, lupus symptoms (rash, fever, weight loss, joint symptoms, etc.), serologic testing (antinuclear antibodies [ANA], anti-DS-DNA, etc.), renal biopsy.

► **Pathology**
Interstitial fibrosis and inflammation. Includes several histologic types **(minimal, mesangial, focal, diffuse, and membranous).**

► **Treatment Steps**
Prednisone, cyclophosphamide, azathioprine. Close follow-up by nephrologist and rheumatologist.

16. Inherited Disorders—Polycystic Kidney Disease

► **Description**
Hereditary cystic kidney disorder.

► **Symptoms**
Hematuria, flank pain, hypertension, pyelonephritis, uremia.

► **Diagnosis**
History and physical (enlarged kidney), IVP, **ultrasound. Child: bilateral flank mass.**

► **Pathology**

Adult Polycystic Kidney Disease—autosomal dominant, cysts.

Infantile Polycystic Disease—autosomal recessive, collecting duct dilation.

► **Treatment Steps**
1. Blood pressure control.
2. Dialysis.
3. Renal transplant.

17. Neoplasms—Wilms' Tumor
See Chapter 6, section VII.G.2.

18. Renal Cell Carcinoma
See Chapter 6, section VII.G.1.

► **cram facts**

Cysts also in liver and pancreas. Positive association of polycystic kidney disease and intracranial aneurysms.

D. Electrolyte and Acid–Base Disorders

1. Hyponatremia

▶ **Description**
Sodium < 130 mEq/L.

▶ **Symptoms**
Confusion, vomiting, coma, nausea, lethargy.

▶ **Pathology**
Excess salt loss (diuretic use), water retention (renal/cardiac failure, syndrome of inappropriate antidiuretic hormone [SIADH]). (See also Chapter 3.)

▶ **Treatment Steps**
Salt loss—give saline.
Water excess—restrict water.

2. Hypernatremia

▶ **Description**
Elevated sodium, > 145 mEq/L.

▶ **Symptoms**
Thirst, hypotension, oliguria, hyperpnea, coma.

▶ **Pathology**
Excess water loss, impaired thirst, and solute loss (diabetic ketoacidosis).

▶ **Treatment Steps**
Replace free water slowly. **If sodium is corrected too rapidly, cerebral edema can result. This can be fatal.**

3. Hypokalemia

▶ **Description**
Potassium < 3.5 mEq/L.

▶ **Symptoms**
Arrhythmia, muscle weakness/cramps, rhabdomyolysis.

▶ **Diagnosis**
History and physical, serum electrolytes, ECG (smaller/wider T wave, U wave, atrioventricular [AV] block).

▶ **Pathology**
Etiology **in gastrointestinal (GI) and urinary loss, decreased intake** (uncommon), **shift into cells** (delirium tremens, hypothermia, increased insulin as in hyperglycemia therapy).

▶ **Treatment Steps**
1. Oral potassium replacement.
2. IV replacement **under** 20 mEq/hour.

4. Hyperkalemia

▶ **Description**
Potassium > 5 mEq/L.

▶ **Symptoms**
Diarrhea, weakness.

▶ **clinical pearl**

SODIUM DISORDERS

- Both hypo- and hypernatremia need to be managed very carefully.
- Too rapid correction of hypernatremia can cause brain edema.
- Too rapid correction of hyponatremia can cause central pontine myelinosis (CPM). In CPM, central nervous system sequelae can vary, but the most devastating is known as "locked in syndrome," in which the patient has paralysis of the limbs and lower cranial nerves, but vertical eye movements, blinking, and alertness remain intact.

▶ **cram facts**

HYPONATREMIA

- **Diuretics:** Generally mild, worsened by free water intake, loss of K+, volume depletion, usually thiazide diuretics.
- **SIADH:** Nonphysiologic release of antidiuretic hormone. Impaired water but normal Na+ excretion. Multiple etiologies: drugs, neuropsychiatric, pulmonary, postsurgical state. Raise serum Na+ at appropriate rate and treat underlying cause.
- **Edematous states:** Renal failure, cardiac failure, cirrhosis. Requires specific therapeutic approaches.

► differential diagnosis

HYPOKALEMIA

- Thiazide and loop diuretics
- Low dietary intake
- Vomiting or other GI loss
- Potassium-free IV fluids
- Mineralocorticoid excess
- Penicillin derivatives
- Periodic paralysis— hypokalemic form

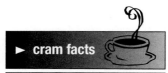

► cram facts

Periodic paralysis: low, normal, or high potassium, muscle weakness.

► clinical pearl

HYPERKALEMIA WITH ECG CHANGES

Acute treatment includes:
1. Calcium IV to stabilize the cardiac myocyte membrane.
2. Insulin and glucose to facilitate potassium exchange into the cells.
3. Sodium bicarb used in certain situations.
4. Kayexalate must also be given to facilitate removal of potassium from the body.

► **Diagnosis**
History and physical, serum electrolytes, ECG (wide QRS, peaked T).

► **Pathology**
Reduced renal excretion, excess intake, adrenocortical insufficiency.

► **Treatment Steps**
1. Stop potassium.
2. Exchange resin (sodium polystyrene sulfonate [Kayexalate]).
3. Insulin/50% glucose.
4. Dialysis in certain cases.

5. Volume Depletion

► **Symptoms**
Thirst, dehydration (sunken eyes, reduced skin turgor, etc.), **coma.**

► **Diagnosis**
History and physical, **increased serum sodium, BUN,** and **osmolality.**

► **Pathology**
Excessive water loss, reduced intake, or "third spacing."

► **Treatment Steps**
1. Slow replacement of free water.
2. Replace sodium as needed.

6. Volume Excess

► **Description**
Free water excess.

► **Symptoms**
Weakness, nausea, seizure, coma.

► **Diagnosis**
History and physical, electrolytes (low sodium, BUN).

► **Pathology**
SIADH, renal failure, congestive heart failure (CHF).

► **Treatment Steps**
Restrict free water. Subcategory: water intoxication—psychiatric component, restrict fluids.

7. Alkalosis

7–1. Metabolic

► **Description**
Elevated pH and elevated carbon dioxide.

► **Symptoms**
May have symptoms of hypokalemia, lethargy, tetany, volume depletion.

► **Diagnosis**
History and physical, **elevated anion gap,** blood gas **(elevated pH** and **serum bicarbonate).**

► **Pathology**
Reduced acid or gain of bicarbonate. Often caused or worsened by volume depletion, diuretics.

► Treatment Steps
Correct electrolyte abnormality and primary cause.

7–2. Respiratory

► **Description**
Elevated pH with low carbon dioxide, caused by hyperventilation.

► **Symptoms**
Syncope, tetany, anxiety, perioral paresthesias.

► **Treatment Steps**
See Cram Facts.

8. Acidosis

8–1. Metabolic

► **Description**
Reduced blood pH and bicarbonate. Separate into elevated or nonelevated anion gap. Anion gap = sodium – (bicarb + chloride).

► **Symptoms**
Thirst, lethargy, coma, dehydration, and primary disease symptoms.

► **Diagnosis**
History and physical, arterial blood gas. Evaluation of individual disorders.

► **Pathology**

Elevated Anion Gap—Diabetic ketoacidosis, lactic acidosis, starvation, methanol/salicylate/ethylene glycol ingestion.

Normal Anion Gap—Diarrhea, renal tubular acidosis.

► **Treatment Steps**
Correct primary etiology. **Lactic acidosis: acidosis associated with shock and metabolic disorders, significant mortality.**

8–2. Respiratory

► **Description**
Reduced pH and elevated P_{CO_2}. Often occurs in respiratory failure, commonly in patients with underlying chronic obstructive pulmonary disease (COPD).

► **Symptoms**
Lethargy, disorientation, coma, headache, anxiety.

► **Diagnosis**
History and physical, arterial blood gas (hypercapnia).

► **Pathology**
Inadequate ventilation.

► **Treatment Steps**
This is a medical emergency, and ventilation needs to be improved in order to lower the P_{CO_2} level. Treatment of the underlying condition is warranted; however, mechanical ventilation is often needed. In certain scenarios, "noninvasive" ventilation can be used (continuous positive airway pressure [CPAP] or bilevel positive airway pressure [BiPAP]) via face mask, but often intubation with mechanical ventilation is needed.

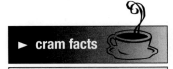

► cram facts

RESPIRATORY ALKALOSIS

Patient is breathing rapidly. Etiology could be as simple as anxiety or as serious as pulmonary embolism. Look for underlying cause and treat appropriately.

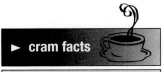

► cram facts

RENAL TUBULAR ACIDOSIS

• **Distal:** Primary, inherited, drugs, nephrocalcinosis, idiopathic hypercalciuria, hypervitaminosis D, hyperthyroidism, multiple myeloma, hyperparathyroidism.
• **Proximal:** Primary, Wilson's disease, heavy metals, carbonic anhydrase inhibitors, scleroderma, tetracycline, amyloid, nephrotic syndrome, acute hepatitis.

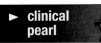

► clinical pearl

ANION GAP METABOLIC ACIDOSIS

Commonly used mnemonic is **MUDPILES:**
Methanol
Uremia
DKA
Paraldehyde (very rare cause)
Iron or Isoniazid ingestion
Lactic acidosis (which itself has many causes)
Ethanol, ethylene glycol
Salicylates

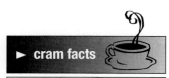

► cram facts

HYPERCALCEMIA

- The most common etiology in the outpatient setting is primary hyperparathyroidism (see Chapter 3)
- The most common etiology in the inpatient setting is malignancy.
- If asymptomatic, investigate etiology and follow calcium levels.
- If symptomatic, inpatient treatment:
  - Initially, aggressive hydration with normal saline, followed by diuresis with loop diuretics (furosemide), not thiazides.
  - Bisphosphonates are very effective. Pamidronate (Aredia) is given as a one-time intravenous dose.

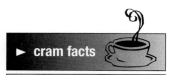

► cram facts

HYPOCALCEMIA AND NEONATES

Rule out DiGeorge anomaly, a rare but serious condition (see Chapter 7).

9. **Hypomagnesemia**

   ► Symptoms
   Tetany, lethargy, delirium, CNS irritability, muscle cramps. ECG findings are nonspecific but can include ST depression, loss of voltage, PR prolongation, and widened QRS.

   ► Pathology
   Etiology includes **alcoholism, malnutrition, diabetic ketoacidosis, diuretics.**

   ► Treatment Steps
   Replace magnesium (IV or IM).

10. **Hypercalcemia**

    ► Description
    Serum calcium > 10.2 mg/dL.

    ► Symptoms
    Renal failure, **nausea/vomiting,** confusion, ECG (short QT, long PR).

    ► Pathology
    Etiology includes **sarcoidosis, cancer, milk-alkali, hyperthyroid/hyperparathyroidism.**

    ► Treatment Steps
    See Cram Facts.

11. **Hypocalcemia**

    ► Description
    Low serum calcium (< 8.4 mg/dL).

    ► Symptoms
    Tetany, Chvostek's sign, Trousseau's sign, perioral paresthesia, muscle cramps.

    ► Pathology
    Etiology includes **renal failure, vitamin D deficiency, hypoparathyroidism, malabsorption.**

    ► Treatment Steps
    1. Control etiology.
    2. Administer calcium and vitamin D.

E. Kidney and Urinary System Trauma

► Description
Renal injury, minor (contusion, cut, hematoma), and **major** (deeper cut/rupture, pedicle injury). **Ureteral injury:** most often surgical mishap, external cause most often gunshot.

► Symptoms
Pain, shock, flank ecchymosis.

Injury to Upper Urinary Tract—Hematuria.

Injury to Posterior Urethra—Blood at meatus, distended bladder, voiding difficulty.

Ureter Ligation—Presents as **pain, nausea/vomiting, fever postop.**

► Diagnosis

History and physical, IVP, CT, **angiography,** KUB. Evaluate urethra with retrograde study. **If blood at meatus: do not catheterize. Do retrograde cystography to evaluate bladder.**

► Pathology

Renal—Blunt, by auto accident most common.

Pedicle Injury—Left renal vein most often injured, usually penetrating injury.

Ureter—Often surgical injury, **hysterectomy commonly.**

► Treatment Steps

Kidney—Penetrating, surgical exploration; blunt, medical, or surgical.

Bladder—Contusion, catheter; **rupture,** surgery.

Ureter—Surgical (may need stent, anastomosis, bladder reimplantation, depending on injury).

Urethra—Partial rupture, suprapubic cystotomy; complete rupture, drainage, and suprapubic cystotomy.

F. Kidney Transplant Rejection

► Description

Allograft rejection. **Acute type most common.**

► Symptoms

Lethargy, edema, oliguria, fever. Elevated blood pressure, diminishing renal function and proteinuria may indicate **chronic graft rejection.**

► Diagnosis

History and physical, renal scan, renal biopsy.

► Pathology

Immunologic host reaction, where **activated helper T cells** and **macrophages damage donor tissue.**

► Treatment Steps

Rejection types: Hyperacute (immediate, no treatment, nephrectomy), acute accelerated (after several days, no treatment, nephrectomy), acute (after 1–3 weeks, immunosuppression), chronic (no treatment). Rule out muscular or obstructive pathology.

G. Hepatorenal Syndrome

► Description

Cirrhosis and renal failure.

► Symptoms

Cirrhosis (jaundice, ascites, etc.), renal failure (azotemia, oliguria).

► Diagnosis

History and physical, clinical picture (oliguria and severe liver disease), **no urine sediment. Low wedge pressure may suggest prerenal azotemia,** not hepatorenal syndrome.

► Pathology

Cause unknown.

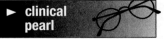

► clinical pearl

CALCIUM

- Do not forget to correct the calcium level when the albumin is abnormal.
- Corrected calcium = 0.8 times (normal albumin – measured albumin) + reported calcium. *Example:* Normal albumin is 4 mg/dL, measured albumin is 1.5 mg/dL, calcium is 9.0 mg/dL.
- Corrected calcium = 0.8 × (4 – 1.5) + 9.0, which is 11.0 mg/dL. *Note:* If ionized calcium is measured, no correction is needed.

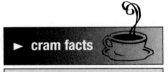

► cram facts

HEPATORENAL SYNDROME

- The kidneys retain the ability to function normally.
- If a patient with hepatorenal syndrome restores hepatic function (or gets a liver transplant), the kidneys can again function normally.

► **Treatment Steps**

Treat etiology if possible, dialysis(?), fluids to rule out hypovolemia.

BIBLIOGRAPHY

Cahill, J., *Updates in Emergency Medicine.* New York: Kluwer Academic/Plenum Publishers, 2003.

Resnick MI. *Critical Decisions in Urology,* 2nd ed. Hamilton, Ontario: B.C. Decker, 2004.

Rose BD. *Clinical Physiology of Acid–Base and Electrolyte Disorders,* 5th ed. New York: McGraw-Hill, 2000.

Walsh PC, Retik AB, Vaughan ED Jr., Wein AJ. *Campbell's Urology,* 8th ed. Philadelphia: W.B. Saunders, 2002.

Surgical Principles

I. ESOPHAGUS

A. Achalasia

▶ Description

Motility disorder characterized by a triad of: primary esophageal aperistalsis and atony; megaesophagus; failure of lower esophageal sphincter (LES) relaxation. The LES fails to relax with swallowing. Circular muscle of the LES is thickened. Auerbach's plexus absent.

▶ Symptoms

Dysphagia (often with liquids), regurgitation of undigested food and aspiration while recumbent, minimal pain.

▶ Diagnosis

Esophagram—Marked dilation above constricted distal esophagus. Abnormal peristalsis.

Endoscopy—Excludes an esophageal stricture whether benign or malignant.

Esophageal Manometry—Uncoordinated peristalsis, primary peristalsis absent, gastroesophageal (GE) sphincter has above-normal resting pressure and does not relax with swallowing.

Complications of untreated achalasia: megaesophagus, increased risk of squamous cell carcinoma.

▶ Treatment Steps

1. Pneumatic dilatation.
2. Botulinum toxin injected in LES.
3. Longitudinal esophageal myotomy (open or laparoscopic) is surgical procedure of choice. Usually, antireflux procedure (e.g., Nissen or Toupet fundoplication) added to myotomy.

B. Hiatal Hernia and Reflux Esophagitis

1. Sliding Hiatal Hernia

▶ Description

Esophagogastric junction and proximal stomach displaced into mediastinum. Ninety-five percent of hiatal hernias are sliding. Symptoms caused by accompanying esophageal reflux. There is no true hernia sac.

▶ Symptoms

Most hiatal hernias are asymptomatic. Symptoms of gastroesophageal reflux disease (GERD) can occur, including retrosternal burning pain especially lying supine, lifting, or straining; regurgitation of bitter fluid; nocturnal cough, recurrent pneumonia from aspiration; dysphagia. Bleeding rare.

▶ Diagnosis

Chest x-ray (CXR): Air–fluid level in mediastinum. GE reflux may be evident on esophagram. Esophagoscopy to rule out other lesions and document esophagitis. Distal esophagus pH monitoring most sensitive test.

▶ Treatment Steps

1. No treatment if asymptomatic.
2. Treat GERD symmptoms medically (see Chapter 4).

3. Surgical antireflux procedures—Nissen fundoplication, Hill repair, Belsey fundoplication.

2. Paraesophageal Hiatal Hernia

▶ **Description**
Esophageal junction in normal anatomic position. Stomach herniates through hiatus usually to left of esophagus. May strangulate or volvulize leading to rapid death (20–30%).

▶ **Symptoms**
Fullness after meals, epigastric postprandial pain (69%), bowel sounds in chest, early postprandial vomiting (50%), breathlessness while eating. Chronic blood loss in up to one-third of patients due to recurrent bleeding from the gastric mucosa.

▶ **Diagnosis**
CXR: air–fluid level in mediastinum. Esophagram establishes the diagnosis. Esophagoscopy to rule out Barrett's esophagus.

▶ **Treatment Steps**
Because of high rate of complications, all paraesophageal hiatal hernias should be surgically repaired (abdominal and/or thoracic approach) with or without an accompanying antireflux procedure. Good to excellent surgical results in 80–90% of patients.

C. Esophageal Cancer

▶ **Description**
Squamous carcinoma most common cell type: distal third (30%), middle third (50%), upper third (20%). Spreads by lymphatics, vascular invasion, and direct extension. Adenocarcinoma 5–10% of primary carcinomas of esophagus. Frequency of adenocarcinoma has increased and currently accounts for > 50% all esophageal tumors. Extraesophageal extension present in high percentage of patients at time of diagnosis. Highly aggressive. Five-year survival rate only 3% when lymph nodes are involved.

▶ **Symptoms**
Progressive dysphagia, odynophagia, chest pain, weight loss.

▶ **Diagnosis**

Esophagram—Irregular mass narrowing lumen of esophagus, minimal proximal dilatation.

Esophagoscopy—Biopsy for tissue diagnosis, tumor length. Rule out gastric involvement.

Bronchoscopy—For upper- and middle-third lesions to rule out tracheobronchial involvement.

Computed tomographic (CT) scan and endoscopic ultrasonography (EUS) helps with staging. Other imaging studies used for staging are: magnetic resonance imaging (MRI), positron-emission tomography (PET), and video-assisted thoracoscopic surgery (VATS).

▶ **Treatment Steps**
1. Surgery; only 30% resectable. Esophagectomy (transhiatal blunt esophagectomy or Ivor Lewis procedure), total or partial, depending on tumor location and size. Stomach or the left-sided

colon are used to reestablish gastrointestinal (GI) tract continuity. Resection may also provide palliation in low-risk patients.

2. Radiation therapy preoperative may shrink tumor mass allowing resection. Combined with chemotherapy may be effective adjuvant therapy. However, no definitive survival advantage to either chemo- or radiation therapy has been demonstrated.

3. Endoscopic laser therapy used to establish esophageal patency in unresectable obstructing tumors.

D. Esophageal Perforation

1. Instrumental Perforation Causes

The most common cause of esophageal perforation is iatrogenic disruption, which includes endoscopy, dilation, paraesophageal surgery, Sengstaken–Blakemore (SB) tube, intubation, sclerotherapy.

▶ **Description**

Susceptible at areas of narrowing: cricopharyngeal area, midportion near aortic arch and mainstem bronchi, diaphragmatic hiatus.

▶ **Symptoms**

Dysphagia, pain, fever, neck tenderness and crepitus (with cervical perforations), chest pain, dyspnea, shock, mediastinal air (Hamman's sign).

▶ **Diagnosis**

X-rays: soft tissue air, mediastinal air (takes 1 hour to be seen), pleural effusion, pneumothorax, mediastinal widening. Esophagram shows site of perforation (usually into left pleural cavity).

▶ **Treatment Steps**

1. Antibiotics for all patients.
2. Observation for those patients with small localized perforation with minimal symptoms and no sepsis.
3. Surgical repair required in almost all cases.
   a. Early diagnosis (< 24 hours)—primary repair.
   b. Late diagnosis—primary reinforced repair, drainage alone (cervical perforation), esophageal exclusion and diversion, or esophagectomy (if underlying significant esophageal pathology, e.g., cancer is present).

▶ **Criteria for Nonoperative Therapy**

Contained mediastinal leak, free drainage back into esophagus, minimal symptoms, no sign of sepsis. Surgical repair possible within 24 hours of perforation. After 24 hours, resection combined with diverting procedures may be necessary ("spit fistula").

2. Spontaneous Perforation

▶ **Description**

Postemetic transmural perforation usually following an alcoholic binge (Boerhaave syndrome). Patients generally present with mediastinitis. Posterior, distal esophagus most usual site. Fifty percent with concomitant GERD.

▶ **Symptoms**

Sudden, severe pain in lower chest and upper abdomen; shock; rigid abdomen.

► Differential Diagnosis

Pancreatitis, myocardial infarction, perforated peptic ulcer, dissecting aortic aneurysm.

► Diagnosis/Treatment

Same as instrumental perforation.

II. STOMACH AND DUODENUM

A. Peptic Ulcer Disease (PUD)

1. Duodenal Ulcer

► Description

Associated with acid hypersecretion. Increased number of parietal cells. Peak incidence between the ages of 20 and 60. Typically, periods of remission and exacerbation. Ninety-five percent occur in duodenal bulb (posterior wall within 2 cm of the pylorus). Risk factors include: *Helicobactor pylori* (almost 100%), tobacco use, nonsteroidal anti-inflammatory drugs (NSAIDs), and Zollinger–Ellison syndrome.

► Symptoms

Epigastric pain, pain relieved by food and/or antacids, nocturnal awakenings, nausea, vomiting, and anorexia. Approximately one-third are asymptomatic.

► Diagnosis

Endoscopy is 95% accurate and is diagnostic procedure of choice. Upper GI series 75–80% accurate, showing an ulcer crater or scarring of the duodenal bulb. The saline load test can be used to determine gastric outlet obstruction.

► Treatment Steps

Medical—See Chapter 4.

Surgical—Indications for surgery are hemorrhage, perforation (Fig. 18–1), obstruction, and intractability.

Surgical procedures:
1. Perforated duodenal ulcer—vagotomy and pyloroplasty, vagotomy and antrectomy, highly selective vagotomy (laparoscopic or open), omentopexy (Graham patch) with vagotomy.
2. Bleeding duodenal ulcer—oversew the bleeder with pyloroplasty and truncal vagotomy.
3. Obstructing duodenal ulcer—truncal vagotomy with gastrojejunostomy.

2. Gastric Ulcer

► Description

Appear later in life. Peak incidence in fifth decade. More common in men. Usually no acid hypersecretion. Cause factor is mucosal injury or defect in "mucosal defense" that renders mucosa susceptible to gastric acid. Majority occur on lesser curve of stomach. Malignant potential (10%). Ninety percent have *H. pylori*.

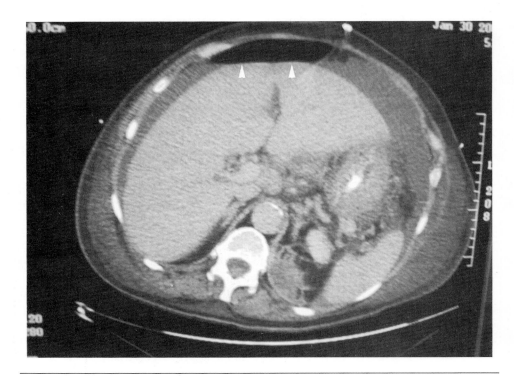

Figure 18–1. Abdominal CT scan showing free air (arrows) in the peritoneal cavity, consistent with a perforated viscus.

► Types
1. Ulcer located at incisura angularis on the lesser curvature (low acid output, associated with blood group A).
2. Ulcers located in stomach and duodenum (high acid output, associated with blood group O).
3. Ulcer located in pylorus or prepyloric area (high acid output, associated with blood group O).
4. Ulcer located high in stomach (juxtacardia, low acid output).
5. Ulcer located anywhere in stomach (associated with NSAIDs).

► Symptoms
Similar to duodenal ulcer. Pain localizes to left of midline, mostly postprandial.

► Diagnosis
Upper GI series can localize (90% sensitive). Endoscopy (97% sensitive) important. Must biopsy ulcer 8–12 times to rule out malignancy.

► Treatment Steps
1. Principles of medical treatment are similar to those of treatment of duodenal ulcer. (See Chapter 4.)
2. Because recurrence rate is higher after medical therapy, surgical therapy should be considered earlier. Procedure of choice is antrectomy with Billroth I anastomosis. No vagotomy with type I gastric ulcers.
   - Type 1: distal gastrectomy (use Billroth I).
   - Types 2, 3: antrectomy with truncal vagotomy.
   - Type 4: extended distal gastrectomy or 90% near total gastrectomy with Roux-en-Y esophagogastrojejunostomy.

B. Gastric Carcinoma

▶ Description

Adenocarcinoma is the most common (95%); classified into ulcerating (25%), polypoid (25%), superficial spreading (15%, best prognosis), linnitus plastica or "leather bottle" (10%), and advanced (35%). Risk factors include: dietary (nitrosamines, smoked/salted or pickled foodstuffs), tobacco use, alcohol, and environmental factors. Almost all have *H. pylori*. Adenomatous polyps and atypical gastritis are premalignant lesions. Most have adenocarcinoma and are located in the antrum. Cancer at the gastroesophageal junction is associated with Barrett's esophagus and GERD. Major factors influencing survival are level of spread through gastric wall and lymph node involvement. Seventy-five percent have metastasis at the time of diagnosis. Age range: 50–70 years; male-to-female ratio is 2:1.

▶ Symptoms

- Early—vague, nondescript symptoms.
- Late—indigestion, postprandial fullness, eructation, loss of appetite, heartburn, vomiting. Pain pattern is similar to peptic ulcer disease.

▶ Diagnosis

Barium Meal Upper GI Series (Double Contrast)—polypoid mass, ulcer crater not extending outside boundary of gastric wall, nondistensible stomach.

Endoscopy—With biopsy, 90% accurate. Endoscopic ultrasound may be of value in determining depth of tumor and presence of enlarged lymph nodes.

CT Scan—Evaluation of metastatic spread.

▶ Treatment Steps

1. Radical subtotal gastrectomy for cure, distal lesions.
2. Radical total gastrectomy for proximal lesions. Half of those operated on are resectable.
3. Chemotherapy reserved for unresectable or recurrent disease (no impact on survival).
4. Gastrojejunostomy for palliative bypass in unresectable disease.
5. Radiotherapy to control pain and bleeding in unresectable cases.

III. SMALL INTESTINE

A. Obstruction

▶ Description

Can be classified into:

- Simple—no vascular compromise.
- Strangulating—vascular obstruction.
- Paralytic ileus—impairment of muscle function, closed-loop blockage at two points.

Can be caused by adhesions (70%), hernia (8%), tumor (9%), inflammatory disease (4%), volvulus, or intussusception.

▶ **differential diagnosis**

SMALL BOWEL OBSTRUCTION

- Adhesions
- Malignancy
- External hernia
- Volvulus
- Crohn's disease
- Intra-abdominal abscess
- Intussusception
- Radiation stricture
- Foreign body
- Gallstone ileus

► Symptoms

Crampy abdominal pain, vomiting, obstipation, distention, failure to pass flatus.

► Diagnosis

High-pitched bowel sounds on physical examination. Peritoneal signs signify peritonitis secondary to strangulation and/or perforation. X-ray: distended small-bowel loops in stepladder pattern, air–fluid levels. Small bowel follow-through and CT scan may delineate the point of obstruction.

► Treatment Steps

1. Nonsurgical management for partial small bowel obstruction (SBO), which includes replacing electrolyte losses, intravenous fluids, nothing by mouth (NPO), and often nasogastric tube decompression.
2. Consider trial of long-tube decompression. Uncommonly used secondary to risk of perforation or intussusception.
3. Complete SBO—surgery as needed.
4. Operative therapy: exploratory laparotomy with lysis of adhesions and small bowel resection if indicated.
5. Septrafilms (hyaluronic acid) can be used to reduce adhesions (by 50%).

► Results

Morbidity—30% (60% with strangulated bowel, 20% with neoplasia, 20% with adhesion and hernia).

B. Neoplasms

► Description

Jejunum and ileum, 5% of all tumors of GI tract. Benign are more common. Most are asymptomatic; 10% become symptomatic.

Benign Tumors—Leiomyomas (18–20%), lipomas (15%), neurofibromas (10%), adenomas (15%), polyps (15%), hemangiomas (13%), fibromas (10%).

Malignant Tumors—Adenocarcinomas (30–50%), lymphomas (15%), leiomyosarcomas (20%), carcinoids (30–50%). Less than 5% metastatic tumors (melanoma, gastric carcinoma).

► Symptoms

Bleeding and obstruction. Weight loss in nearly all malignant tumors. Carcinoid syndrome (flushing, pain, diarrhea, bronchoconstriction, valvular disease) from release of vasoactive substances from metastatic carcinoid tumors.

► Diagnosis

Often made at time of laparotomy. Bowel obstruction with no previous surgery is suspicious for neoplasm. Small-bowel series (enteroclysis is most sensitive). Endoscopy (procedure of choice with duodenal neoplasms). Arteriography (useful with vascular neoplasms: hemangiomas). CT/MRI may complement staging. Biochemical analysis of urine samples (5-hydroxyindoleacetic acid in carcinoid tumors).

► Treatment Steps

1. Wide resection.
2. Bypass for palliation.

C. Radiation Injury

▶ Description

Pathogenesis involves progressive obliterative vasculitis. May be diagnosed many years remote from time of radiation therapy.

▶ Symptoms

Obstruction due to stricture, bleeding from ulcerated mucosa, necrosis with perforation, fistula formation, abscess formation.

▶ Treatment Steps

1. Avoid surgery if possible. (Total parenteral nutrition [TPN] used with severe symptomatic disease, poor nutritional status.) Minimal dissection.
2. Resection or bypass with wide margins. May need to exteriorize if bowel viability is in question.

D. Meckel's Diverticulum

▶ Description

Congenital anomaly, persistent omphalomesenteric duct. A true diverticulum found on the antimesenteric border. Found in 2% of the population. Two feet from ileocecal valve; 2 inches long. May contain heterotopic tissue (pancreas, gastric mucosa, other types). Four percent symptomatic, usually in childhood.

▶ Symptoms

May mimic appendicitis if Meckel's diverticulitis is present. Bleeding (more common in children). Intestinal obstruction from intussusception (more common in adults).

▶ Diagnosis

X-ray and small-bowel series unreliable. Technetium scan will localize heterotopic gastric mucosa, if present (accuracy, 90%).

▶ Treatment Steps

1. Surgical resection (with GI bleeding, excise diverticulum with sufficient margin of ileum to encompass ulceration). The contralateral ileal wall is usually the source of the bleeding and therefore, a wedge resection is not appropriate.
2. Incidental finding at laparotomy: leave alone.

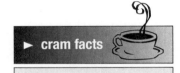

▶ **cram facts**

MECKEL'S DIVERTICULUM "RULE OF TWOS"

- 2% of population
- 2 feet from ileocecal valve
- 2 inches long
- 2 types of heterotopic tissue (pancreas, gastric mucosa)
- Shaped like a 2
- 2x more common in males
- 2% symptomatic

E. Crohn's Disease

▶ Description

Chronic inflammatory disease of the GI tract. There are three types: inflammatory, fibrostenotic, and fistulizing. Unknown cause. Peak age of onset is between second and fourth decades. Transmural involvement of bowel wall, noncaseating granulomas, aphthous ulcers, malignant potential, extraintestinal manifestations are common. Obstruction and perforation with abscess and fistula formation. Skip lesions. Seventy percent progress to operation for complications of the disease. Anal manifestations of the disease are common.

▶ Symptoms

Crampy abdominal pain, diarrhea, nausea and vomiting, fear of eating, weight loss.

▶ Diagnosis

Physical Examination—Abdominal mass right lower quadrant. Check for other sites of disease (e.g., perianal area for fistula).

Endoscopy—Reddened mucosa, skip lesions. Biopsy.

Small Bowel Series—String sign, fistulas. Thickened bowel wall.

▶ Treatment Steps

Medical Therapy—Antibiotics, steroids, sulfasalazine, 5-aminosali-cyclic acid (ASA), immunosuppressive agents (6-mercapto-purine, azathioprine), bowel rest, central hyperalimentation.

Surgical Therapy—(Use eventually required in 75%). Indications: failure of medical therapy or complications of the disease. Surgery: excision, bypass, stricturoplasty. Contraindications to stricturoplasty are fistula, open perforation, abscess, associated inflammatory mass.

Recurrence—(40% within 5 years, 60% within 10 years, 75% within 15 years). The major problem in surgical treatment.

IV. COLON, RECTUM, ANUS

A. Carcinoma of the Colon and Rectum

▶ Description

Second most common malignancy. Pathogenesis unclear. Likely environmental influence. Diets high in fat, low in fiber: higher incidence. Other risk factors (25%): first-degree relatives, inherited genetic syndrome, prior colorectal cancer or adenomatous polyp, inflammatory bowel disease, hereditary nonpolyposis colorectal cancer (HNPCC) or Lynch syndrome, familial polyposis coli. Seventy-five percent have no specific risk factors. The sigmoid colon in the most common primary site and the liver, the most common site of metastasis. Screening: digital examination, stool for occult blood, sigmoidoscopy, colonoscopy.

▶ Symptoms

Right-Sided Lesions—Dull abdominal pain, occult bleeding.

Left-Sided Lesions—Change in bowel habits, visible blood, change in stool caliber.

Rectal Lesions—Tenesmus, incomplete evacuation, blood-streaked stool.

▶ Diagnosis

Digital examination, barium enema, colonoscopy, CT scan, endorectal ultrasound, liver function tests, CXR. Carcinoembryonic antigen level (provides a baseline level for future comparison). Screen 50 years or older annually for fecal occult blood and every 5 years with flexible sigmoidoscopy, or colonoscopy every 10 years.

▶ Treatment Steps

Operative excision with adequate margins. Rectal carcinoma: level of resection depends on location of tumor. Lesions < 8 cm from anal verge may need abdominoperineal resection; > 8 cm, low anterior resection. Adjuvant therapy in colorectal cancer: (1) for stage 2 and 3 rectal cancer, 5-fluorouracil (5-FU) and postoperative radiation therapy; (2) no role for radiation therapy in colon cancer. Additional chemotherapy is appropriate for stage 3 and 4 colon cancer.

B. Diverticular Disease

1. Diverticulosis

▶ **Description**

Colonic outpouching from bowel wall. Males and females equal incidence. Sixty-five percent of population by age 85. Bleeding occurs in 15%. Hemorrhage arises in right colon in 70–90%. Seventy percent stop bleeding spontaneously; 30% have recurrent bleeding.

▶ **Symptoms**

Blood per rectum, minimal pain.

▶ **Diagnosis**

Endoscopy, bleeding scan, arteriography.

▶ **Treatment Steps (Lower GI Bleed or Diverticulosis)**

1. Selective infusion of vasopressin or rarely angioembolization.
2. Segmental colonic resection if bleeding site is localized.
3. Subtotal colectomy if bleeding not localized.

2. Diverticulitis

▶ **Description**

Inflammation of diverticulae. Limited to sigmoid colon in 90%. Inflammation is usually contained by pericolic fat and mesentery.

▶ **Symptoms**

Left lower quadrant (LLQ) pain, anorexia, nausea and vomiting, fever, abdominal mass.

▶ **Diagnosis**

Clinical presentation, CT scan. Barium enema and colonoscopy only after acute inflammation lessened (usually > 1 week following acute episode).

▶ **Treatment Steps**

1. Bowel rest, antibiotics, intravenous fluids, analgesia.
2. If there is an abscess, CT-guided drainage.
3. Elective surgical resection in young, diabetic, immunocompromised, or one prior episode of diverticulitis. Surgical resection when inflammation has subsided (approximately 8 weeks following recent attack).
4. Operations for diverticular disease:

   One-Stage Procedure—Resection and primary anastomosis.

   Two-Stage Procedure—Hartman operation (sigmoid resection, and decending colostomy, mucous fistula or leaving a rectal stump as a "Hartman's pouch"). Operating room sigmoid resection, primary anastomosis, and proximal diverting colostomy.

   Three-Stage Procedure—Colostomy and drainage. Subsequent resection as a second procedure. Subsequent takedown of colostomy and primary ananstomosis. This series of procedures is uncommonly done secondary to prolonged hospital stay, increased morbidity and mortality.

C. Ulcerative Colitis

▶ **Description**

Mucosal inflammation, crypt abscesses, mucosa sloughs, colon becomes shortened. Two peaks in incidence: second and sixth decades.

► cram facts

ULCERATIVE COLITIS VS. CROHN'S DISEASE OF THE COLON

	Ulcerative Colitis	Crohn's Disease
Rectum	Involved	Spared in 25%
Colon	Begins in rectum with proximal spread	Neocolonic pattern frequent
Ileum	Rarely involved	Commonly involved as "skip lesions"
Mucosal involvement	Circumferential	Patchy, segmental

Can involve rectum alone or entire colon. Malignant potential increases with time (2–5% at 10 years, then 1% 1 year thereafter). Extraintestinal manifestations (arthralgias, ankylosing spondylitis, sclerosing cholangitis, and liver dysfunction, uveitis, nephrolithiasis).

► Symptoms

Bloody diarrhea, fever, crampy abdominal pain, tenesmus, urgency, incontinence.

► Diagnosis

Endoscopy—Friable, erythematous mucosa.

Barium Enema—Loss of haustral markings, stricture, stovepipe colon.

► Treatment Steps

Medical—Intravenous fluids, NPO, steroid enemas, correct electrolyte abnormalities, sulfasalazine.

Surgery—Reserved for treatment of complications (hemorrhage, perforation, toxic megacolon, carcinoma, intractability).

Total proctocolectomy with ileostomy. Proctocolectomy with ileoanal anastomosis (ileal J pouch).

D. Hemorrhoids

► Description

Internal hemorrhoids above dentate line. External below dentate line. Location of internal hemorrhoids: right anterior, right posterior, left lateral. Causes: Hereditary, straining, portal hypertension, and pregnancy.

► Symptoms

Bleeding, pruritus ani, pain (secondary to thrombosis).

► Diagnosis

Physical examination, anoscopy.

► Treatment Steps

1. Medical symptomatic relief (high-fiber diet, stool softeners, bulk agents [psyllium]).
2. Rubber band ligation. Contraindication to banding—presence of foreign material (e.g., breast or penile implant, or pacemaker).
3. Surgical excision. Indication for surgical hemorrhoidectomy—

stage 4 hemorrhoids that fail conservative therapy. Contraindication to surgical hemorrhoidectomy—inflammatory bowel disease, suspicion of neoplasm.

4. Anal dilatation. Uncommonly done secondary to incontinence issue.

E. Anal Fissure

▶ **Description**

Superficial linear ulceration in the posterior midline. Sentinel pile (skin tag), seen in chronic fissures. Ulceration occurs in the squamous epithelium; therefore, very painful. Straining at stool. Constipation. Condition is cyclic. Secondary anal fissures occur secondary to inflammatory bowel disease, malignancy, acquired immune deficiency syndrome (AIDS), syphilis, tuberculosis.

▶ **Symptoms**

Exquisite pain, painful defecation, blood on toilet paper.

▶ **Diagnosis**

Sentinel pile, painful digital examination, endoscopy when acute episode resolved.

▶ **Treatment Steps**

1. Acute fissure is treated nonsurgically. Chronic fissure is treated operatively with consideration for biopsy.
2. Local cleansing agents.
3. Sitz baths.
4. Topical ointments.
5. Stool softeners.
6. Anal dilatation.
7. Lateral internal sphincterotomy (open or closed).

V. APPENDIX—APPENDICITIS

▶ **Description**

Appendix: variable location in relation to the cecum. Teniae converge on appendix. Closed-loop obstruction of lumen, vascular congestion, serosal inflammation, perforation.

▶ **Symptoms**

Pain, anorexia, vomiting, diarrhea, cutaneous hyperesthesia, guarding and rebound at McBurney's point, Rovsing's sign, psoas sign, obturator sign, Blumberg's sign.

▶ **Diagnosis**

Physical examination. Fecalith in right lower quadrant (RLQ) is diagnostic, altered right psoas shadow. Leukocytosis (may be absent). Ultrasound and CT scan useful in equivocal cases. However, use clinical judgment. If appendicitis is still clinically suspected despite negative lab or radiologic workup, seek surgical opinion.

▶ **Treatment Steps**

1. Intravenous fluids and antibiotic therapy.
2. Appendectomy (open or laparoscopic). Normal appendix is removed as an incidental finding of malrotation or if an exploration is done for possible appendicitis (to avoid future confusion over the diagnosis).

VI. GALLBLADDER

A. Acute Cholecystitis

▶ Description

Bacterial or chemical inflammation of the gallbladder. Cystic duct obstruction and altered bile chemistry are two conditions necessary to cause acute cholecystitis. Occurs in the 4th to 8th decade. Incidence higher in females. Obstruction of the cystic duct. Bacteria in 50–75% (*Escherichia coli, Klebsiella, Enterobacter*).

▶ Symptoms

Right upper quadrant (RUQ) or epigastric pain. Pain radiates to tip of scapula. Nausea and vomiting.

▶ Diagnosis

Physical examination: Murphy's sign. Mild jaundice. Ultrasound is the most sensitive and specific diagnostic test to detect stones and surrounding inflammation, and can provide other anatomic information in the hepatobiliary system. Hepatoiminodiacetic acid (HIDA) scan 90% accurate (normal HIDA, gallbladder fills in 30 minutes).

▶ Treatment Steps

Antibiotics. Cholecystectomy, delayed or immediate. Percutaneous cholecystostomy in poor-risk patients. Not to be performed in the presence of gallbladder gangrene or perforation (Fig. 18–2). **Variant forms:** empyema of gallbladder, gangrene, acalculous cholecystitis.

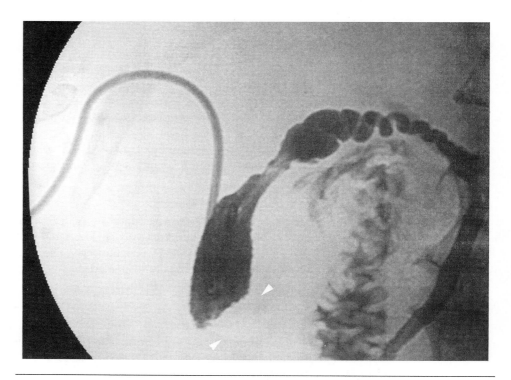

Figure 18–2. Cholecystotomy tube cholangiogram showing a somewhat decompressed gallbladder filled with gallstones. The arrows point to the portion of the gallbladder containing stones. This patient had calculus cholecystitis in the setting of severe hemodynamic instability and was too sick for an open cholecystectomy.

B. Chronic Cholecystitis

▶ **Description**

Repeated attacks of acute cholecystitis. Stones almost always present.

▶ **Signs and Symptoms**

Pain in RUQ and epigastric pain. May radiate to tip of scapula. Nausea and vomiting. Attacks often follow large meals.

▶ **Diagnosis**

Physical examination. Ultrasound to identify stones. Oral cholecystography if symptoms are typical but ultrasound negative. Endoscopic retrograde cholangiopancreatography (ERCP) to identify cholesterol crystals if other tests negative and symptoms persist.

▶ **Treatment Steps**

Laparoscopic cholecystectomy for routine management. An open cholecystectomy is indicated in cases of cirrhosis, bleeding disorders, pregnancy, gallbladder cancer, and severe cardiopulmonary disorders.

C. Cholangitis

▶ **Description**

Infection in the biliary tree. Bacteria (commonly *E. coli*, *Klebsiella*, *Enterococcus*), obstruction, increased pressure. Most commonly associated with choledocholithiasis.

▶ **Symptoms**

Fever and chills, jaundice, biliary colic (Charcot's triad). Severe: additional hypotension and mental confusion (Reynolds' pentad).

▶ **Diagnosis**

Clinical presentation. RUQ tenderness. Elevated white blood cell count, bilirubin, and alkaline phosphatase. Ultrasound of RUQ to document gallstones. CT scan to rule out periampullary malignancies or liver abscesses.

▶ **Treatment Steps**

Antibiotics. Triple antibiotics if severe (60% of cases with multiple organisms). Endoscopic sphincterotomy with stone extraction. Exploratory laparotomy, cholecystectomy with common bile duct exploration and T-tube drainage.

D. Gallstone Ileus

▶ **Description**

Antecedent cholecystointestinal or choledochointestinal fistula. Gallstone obstructs at intestinal narrowing (usually in distal ileum). Occurs more likely in the elderly (70s) and is four times more common in women. Less commonly Bouveret's syndrome (stone enters and obstructs the duodenum). Gallbladder carcinoma occurs in 15% of those with gallstone ileus.

▶ **Symptoms**

Pain in RUQ. Distention. Nausea. Vomiting. Colicky abdominal pain.

▶ **Diagnosis**

Air in biliary tree (pneumobilia) occurs in 40%. Dilated small-bowel loops. Opaque stone in the intestinal tract (15–20%). Nonopaque stone in intestinal tract identified by ultrasound.

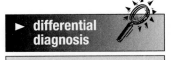

▶ **differential diagnosis**

BILIARY OBSTRUCTION

- Gallstones
- Benign strictures
- Malignant strictures
- Pancreatitis
- Extrinsic compression
- Obstructed biliary stents

▶ Treatment Steps

1. Fluid resuscitation, correction of electrolyte abnomalities, naso-gastric decompression, antibiotic prophylaxis.
2. Exploratory laparotomy, enterotomy proximal to the impacted stone with removal of the stone. Repair of biliary–enteric fistula.
3. Cholecystectomy if medically stable.

E. Gallbladder Carcinoma

▶ Description

Most common malignancy of biliary tract. Association with gall-stones (95%, particularly larger ones), porcelain gallbladder (calci-fied wall, should have cholecystectomy even if asymptomatic), biliary adenoma, biliary infection with *Salmonella*. Adenocarcinoma in 82%. More common in females. One to two percent undergo cholecystec-tomy. Tends to be diagnosed in advanced stage. Seventy percent have liver metastases at the time of diagnosis.

▶ Symptoms

Nonspecific. Pain. Weight loss. Jaundice. Anorexia. RUQ mass.

▶ Diagnosis

Advanced disease: CT scan. Curable, localized disease found at time of cholecystectomy.

▶ Treatment Steps

If tumor localized to mucosa and submucosa, cholecystectomy. Serosal or lymph node involvement: cholecystectomy with node re-section and hepatic wedge resection. If N2 nodes (peripancreatic, duodenal, portal, celiac, or superior mesenteric artery [SMA]) are present, do not proced with resection. **Results:** overall 5-year survival rate, 2–5%.

VII. LIVER

A. Hepatocellular Carcinoma

▶ Description

More common in Africa and Asia. Risk factors include: cirrhosis, hepatitis B, hemochromatosis, schistosomiasis, aflatoxin, and α_1-antitrypsin deficiency. Eighty percent of primary liver tumors. Very often presents in advanced stage.

▶ Symptoms

Pain, distention, weight loss, fatigue, anorexia, fever, jaundice, as-cites.

▶ Diagnosis

The tumor marker, α-fetoprotein (AFP) is elevated (although fibro-lamellar type seen in younger patients, it is not associated with AFP elevation). CT scan with or without percutaneous biopsy. Arteriogra-phy. **Intraoperative ultrasound.**

▶ Treatment Steps

1. Only 25% are resectable (5-year survival rate: 18–36%). Can re-move up to 80% of liver.
2. Transplantation.
3. Palliation: intra-arterial chemotherapy, hepatic artery ligation.
4. Cryoablation developing as alternative to resection.

B. Pyogenic Liver Abscess

▶ **Description**

Follows an acute abdominal infection. Routes: portal system, ascension from the biliary tree, hepatic artery, direct extension, trauma. Untreated, 100% mortality rate; treated, 20% mortality rate. Right lobe more common. Solitary or multiple. Bacteria: *E. coli, Klebsiella,* enterococcus, bacteroides. May rupture into adjacent peritoneal, pericardial, or thoracic cavities.

▶ **Symptoms**

Fever, malaise, chills, anorexia, weight loss, abdominal pain, RUQ tenderness, jaundice, hepatomegaly.

▶ **Diagnosis**

Leukocytosis (very high); CXR: atelectasis, pneumonia, effusion (all right-sided), CT scan, ultrasound, arteriography.

▶ **Treatment Steps**

1. Eliminate abscess and underlying cause.
2. Percutaneous drainage if single.
3. Operative drainage if multiple or multilocated abscess.
4. Long-term antibiotics, especially for multiple small hepatic abscesses.

C. Amebic Liver Abscess

▶ **Description**

Prevalence higher in tropical zones, travelers to tropical countries. More common in males, peak incidence fourth decade. Spread by fecal–oral route of *E. histolytica.* Typically reaches the liver by way of the portal vein from intestinal amebiasis. Only 5% of people infected with amebiasis develop liver abscess. Ninety percent in right lobe. May grow to large size. History to separate from hydatid cyst. Amebic abscess fluid looks like anchovy paste.

▶ **Symptoms**

Recent diarrheal syndrome in minority. Similar to pyogenic abscess.

▶ **Diagnosis**

Serum antibody for *E. histolytica* (indirect hemagglutinin test). Only one-third have positive amebic stool cultures.

▶ **Treatment Steps**

1. Metronidazole 750 mg by mouth, three times a day for 10 days.
2. Operative treatment reserved for rupture.
3. Percutanous drainage may be considered. In cases of abscess refractory to Flagyl, large left liver lobe abscess, bacterial contamination (10–15%). There is danger of anaphylaxis from spillage with open drainage of cyst.

VIII. PORTAL HYPERTENSION/ESOPHAGEAL VARICEAL BLEEDING

▶ **Description**

Present when portal venous pressure exceeds 15 mm Hg. Collaterals between portal and systemic venous circulations lead to splenic varices, hemorrhoids, and esophageal varices. Commonly associated with cirrhosis (United States) and schistosomiasis (worldwide).

► Symptoms

Ascites. Hepatic encephalopathy, hypersplenism, hemorrhoids, caput medusa, esophageal variceal bleed. Stigmata of cirrhosis: spider angiomata, palmar erythema, testicular atrophy, gynecomastia, hepatomegaly. Jaundice.

► Diagnosis

Liver function tests, liver biopsy, hepatitis profile, endoscopy if bleeding.

► Treatment Steps

Acute variceal bleed (50% mortality):

1. Injection sclerotherapy by way of esophagogastroduodenoscopy (EGD); 90% initial success.
2. Vasopressin infusion or octreotide (somatostatin) infusion.
3. Balloon tamponade (Sengstaken–Blakemore tube).
4. Transjugular intrahepatic portosystemic shunt (TIPS).
5. Emergency portosystemic shunt.

Shunt procedures:

1. End-to-side and side-to-side shunts are nonselective and are associated with encephalopathy.
2. Selective shunts (e.g., distal splenorenal Warren shunt) is associated with cirrhosis.

Prophylactic treatment: β-blocker (propranolol) long-term prophylactic medication in portal hypertension (HTN) to prevent esophageal varices from bleeding.

IX. PANCREAS

A. Acute Pancreatitis

► Description

Inflammation from escape of active pancreatic enzymes. Eighty percent due to alcohol and biliary disease (predominantly gallstones). Trauma, hyperlipidemia, hypercalcemia, pancreas divisum. Also caused by scorpion, *Ascaris,* or *Clonorchis sinensis*. Drugs causing pancreatitis: azithioprine, furosemide, Tylenol/flagyl/Zantac, erythromycin/tetracycline. Ninety percent mild cases; 10% life-threatening.

► Symptoms

Epigastric and back pain, fever, tachycardia, hypotension, nausea, vomiting, epigastric tenderness, flank ecchymosis (Grey–Turner's sign), periumbilical ecchymosis (Cullen's sign).

► Diagnosis

Serum amylase and lipase, hypocalcemia, hyperbilirubinemia, leukocytosis, CT scan (dynamic angio-CT also measures amount of pancreatic necrosis). CT-guided fine-needle aspiration (FNA) differentiates infected compared to sterile pancreatic necrosis. Upper gastrointestinal (UGI) series, sentinal loop on plain film abdomen, ultrasound of biliary tree.

► Treatment Steps

1. Bowel rest, NPO, intravenous fluids, analgesia, nasogastric tube, antibiotics. Antibiotics especially if pancreatic necrosis is present.

2. TPN for prolonged cases.

3. ERCP and endoscopic sphincterotomy to treat gallstone pancreatitis.

4. Surgery: correct biliary disease (e.g., cholecystectomy for gallstone pancreatitis); reserved for complications of pancreatitis (abscess, ascites, hemorrhagic, pseudocyst). Pancreatic debridement and open packing/closed lavage for pancreatic necrosis; 50% develop infection and mostly with gram-negative rod bacteria.

B. Chronic Pancreatitis

▶ Description

Recurrent abdominal pain of pancreatic origin. Irreversible damage. Exocrine and endocrine insufficiency. **Most often alcohol related (70%).** Ten-year survival rate only 43%.

▶ Symptoms

Epigastric and back pain, anorexia and weight loss, pancreatic insufficiency with malabsorption, steatorrhea, possibly diabetes.

▶ Diagnosis

Clinical findings:

Plain Films—Pancreatic calcifications.

CT Scan—Calcifications, size of pancreas.

ERCP—Identify ductal abnormalities ("chain of lakes").

SMA and Celiac Arteriogram—Pseudo-aneurysm with or without splenic/portal vein thrombosis.

▶ cram facts

RANSON'S CRITERIA (PREDICTING THE SEVERITY OF ACUTE PANCREATITIS)		
On Admission		
W	WBC	> 16,000/mm³
A	Age	> 55 yr
G	Glucose	> 200 mg/dL
A	AST	> 250 IU/dL
L	LDH	> 350 IU/L
At 48 Hours		
B	Base deficit	> 4 mEq/L
E	Estimated fluid gain	> 6 L
C	Calcium	< 8 mg/dL
H	Hct fall	> 10%
U	Urea rise	> 5 mg/dL
P	Pao₂	< 60 mm Hg

AST, aspartate transaminase; LDH, lactic dehydrogenase; WBC, white blood count.

Mortality rate in acute pancreatitis closely related to the number of positive Ranson signs (1% if up to 2 signs, 15% if 3–4, 40% if 5–6, and 100% if 7–8 signs present).

Note: Amylase is not part of the Ranson's criteria.

► Treatment Steps
1. Analgesia, correct exocrine and endocrine function.
2. Surgery: indications: intractable abdominal pain, local complications, main duct stenosis, pancreas divisum, rule out malignancy. Ampullary procedures; transduodenal sphincteroplasty.
3. Ductal drainage procedures: side-to-side pancreaticojejunostomy (Puestow procedure).

C. Pancreatic Carcinoma

► Description
Ninety percent duct cell adenocarcinoma (remainder are cystadenoma and acinar cell carcinoma); 65% arise in pancreatic head. Present in advanced stage. Fifth leading cancer-related death. Other risk factors include advanced age, smoking, diabetes, alcohol abuse, exposure to benzidine, naphthylamine, and partial gastrectomy.

► Symptoms
Jaundice, weight loss, abdominal pain, pain in epigastrium and back, palpable gallbladder (Courvoisier's sign).

► Diagnosis
Liver function tests (LFTs) reflect ductal obstruction. Elevated carcinoembryonic antigen (CEA), CA 19–9, occult blood in stool. CT scan to evaluate size of tumor and relation to surrounding structures (Fig. 18–3), ERCP or percutaneous transhepatic cholangiography, arteriography (define anatomy/resectability), percutaneous biopsy. Prognostic factors in pancreatic carcinoma include lymph node status, margin involvement, vascular invasion, and need for blood transfusion.

► Treatment Steps
Resection for cure, if possible: pancreaticoduodenectomy. Five-year survival rate, 15–35%. Bypass for palliation: choledochojejunostomy,

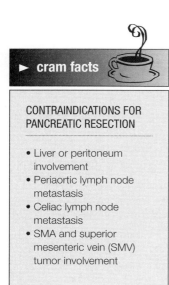

► **cram facts**

CONTRAINDICATIONS FOR
PANCREATIC RESECTION

- Liver or peritoneum involvement
- Periaortic lymph node metastasis
- Celiac lymph node metastasis
- SMA and superior mesenteric vein (SMV) tumor involvement

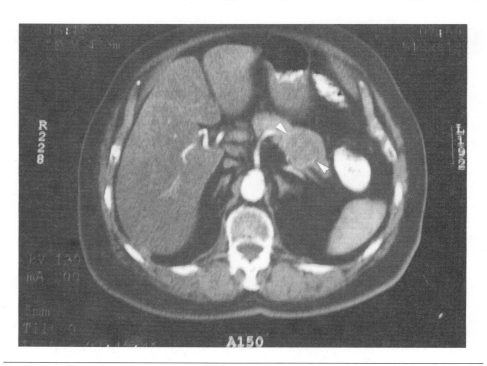

Figure 18–3. Abdominal CT scan showing an oval-shaped distal pancreatic mass (arrows). This patient will be managed with a distal pancreatectomy and possible adjuvant therapy depending on the stage of the tumor.

gastrojejunostomy. Adjuvant chemo- and radiation therapy improve survival.

D. Endocrine Tumors of the Pancreas

1. Insulinoma

Most common. β-cell origin. Equal distribution throughout the pancreas. Eighty percent solitary benign; 10% malignant. Whipple's triad. Fasting hypoglycemia (insulin:glucose ratio > 0.3). Elevated C-peptide and proinsulin. Preoperative localization: CT scan localizes tumors > 1 cm. Arteriography. Intraoperative ultrasound used in localization. Resection is curative for large lesions, and enucleation also adequate for small lesions. Debulk for palliation. Medical therapy: diazoxide.

2. Gastrinoma

Second most common. Hypergastrinemia and PUD (especially in unusual locations). Zollinger–Ellison syndrome. Elevated fasting gastrin and secretin stimulation test. Fifty percent malignant. Resection for cure. Preoperative localization. Explore if localization attempts fail. Eighty percent of lesions found in the gastrinoma triangle (boundaries are: cystic–common bile duct, second to third part of duodenum, and neck–body junction of the pancreas). Somatostatin and high-dose omeprazole for treatment.

3. Glucagonoma

From α cells. Mainly in the body and the tail of the pancreas. Elevated plasmin glucagon is diagnostic. Hyperglycemia. Majority are malignant. Necrolytic migratory erythema. Present in advanced stage. Resect for cure. Debulk for relief of symptoms.

4. VIPoma (Vasoactive Intestinal Polypeptide Tumors) or WDHA Syndrome (Watery Diarrhea, Hypokalemia, Achlorhydria, or Verner–Morrison Syndrome)

Fifty percent have metastasis at presentation, and treatment is subtotal pancreatectomy if no tumor found in the presence of the syndrome.

X. SPLEEN

A. Trauma

▶ Description

Most commonly injured organ in blunt trauma. Associated with left chest rib fractures.

▶ Symptoms

Nonspecific abdominal pain. Left upper quadrant (LUQ) pain. Pain referred to left shoulder (Kehr's sign).

▶ Diagnosis

Clinical suspicion (e.g., multiple left-sided rib fractures). Gross blood on diagnostic peritoneal lavage. Focused abdominal sonography for trauma (FAST) is frequently the first study done on a trauma patient with a suspected splenic injury. CT scan findings in stable patients.

► Treatment Steps

Splenectomy. Splenic salvage in appropriate cases. Nonoperative therapy in children. Vaccinate the splenectomy patient against *Haemophilus influenzae* B, pneumococcus, and meningococcus (encapsulated organism).

B. Immune Thrombocytopenic Purpura

► Description

Persistently low platelet count. Antiplatelet factor (circulating immunoglobulin G [IgG]) directed against a platelet antigen. Majority are young women. Childhood cases typically occur after a viral illness under age 6. Also associated with human immunodefieciency virus (HIV).

► Symptoms

Spontaneous bleeding. Spleen normal size or small.

► Diagnosis

Thrombocytopenia, bone marrow aspirate megakaryocytes.

► Treatment Steps

1. Steroids, response in 3–7 days. Complete remission with steroids is rare.
2. IV gamma globulin (1–2 g/kg), plasmapheresis.
3. Elective splenectomy, when refractory to medical management (75% of cases), i.e., persistent thrombocytopenia (platelets < 80,000) or recurrence after tapering or discontinuation of steroids.
4. Emergent splenectomy with central nervous system (CNS) bleeding.
5. Laparoscopic splenectomy is an option.

C. Hodgkin's Disease

► Description

Malignant lymphoma; Reed–Sternberg cells; asymptomatic lymphadenopathy: cervical (70%), axillary, inguinal. Four pathologic subtypes: lymphocyte predominance (best prognosis), nodular sclerosis (most common), mixed cellularity, lymphocyte depletion (worst prognosis). Metastasize in predictable patterns (spread via lymphatics).

► Symptoms

Asymptomatic lymphadenopathy, night sweats, weight loss, pruritus, malaise.

► Diagnosis

Hematologic tests, bone marrow aspirate, LFTs, CT scan abdomen and chest, CXR, lymph node biopsy, lymphangiogram. Staging laparotomy: splenectomy, liver biopsy (bilateral), lymph node sampling, oophoropexy. Bilateral bone marrow biopsy from the iliac crest. In women of childbearing years, fix ovary to the pelvic wall or behind uterus to protect it from radiation.

► Treatment Steps

1. Radiation (all stages).
2. Chemotherapy (stage III A or above).
3. Staging laparotomy: when result may change therapy. It is controversial and mainly for stages I and II. Improved imaging and liberal use of chemotherapy has made staging laparotomy less common.

D. Non-Hodgkin's Lymphoma (NHL)

Clinical course and natural history more diverse than Hodgkin's. Usually older patients are more common than with Hodgkin's disease. Pattern of spread is variable; two grades: high-grade (diffuse) or low-grade (nodular). Two-thirds have asymptomatic lymphadenopathy. Onset may be in extranodal site (e.g., gastric non-Hodgkin's lymphoma). May appear as asymptomatic splenomegaly. Constitutional symptoms commonly present. Chemotherapy and radiation therapy. It is spread via the bloodstream and can present as a superior vena cava (SVC) syndrome, acute spinal cord compression syndrome, central obstruction or meningeal involvement. Indications for splenectomy in NHL are hypersplenism, pancytopenia, symptomatic splenomegaly, and recurrent splenic infarcts.

E. Postsplenectomy Sepsis

► Description

Risk highest for splenectomy for thalassemia and reticuloendothelial (RE) diseases like Hodgkin's, lowest for trauma and idiopathic thrombocytopenic purpura (ITP). Risk may be as high as 1% per year. Risk greatest for children younger than 4 years, and within 2 years of splenectomy. Fifty percent mortality rate.

► Symptoms

Preceded by upper respiratory infection (URI). Followed by nausea, vomiting, headache, confusion, shock, coma, death within 24 hours.

► Diagnosis

Clinical suspicion. Blood cultures positive for *Streptococcus pneumoniae* in 50%. Encapsulated organisms predominate (pneumococci, *H. influenzae*).

► Treatment Steps

1. Broad-spectrum antibiotics.
2. Supportive care.
3. Prophylaxis: Pneumovax, prophylactic antibiotics.

XI. ARTERIAL DISEASE

A. Arterial Embolism

► Description

Heart is the source of arterial emboli in 90% (see Cram Facts). Left atrial myxoma (histology of its embolus is diagnostic). Symptoms are acute in onset and occur at bifurcations (femoral bifurcation most common).

► Symptoms

Pulselessness, pain, pallor, paresthesias, paralysis, and poikilothermia.

► Diagnosis

Physical examination, duplex scan, arteriography.

► Treatment Steps

1. Heparinization.
2. Consider thrombolytic therapy (tPA).
3. Embolectomy (does not treat the embolus but prevents further emboli or propagation of thrombosis) can restore flow to tissues.

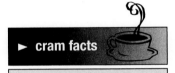

► cram facts

CARDIAC SOURCES OF EMBOLI

- Left ventricular thrombus (post-MI patients)
- Left atrium clot (atrial fibrillation)
- Valvular disease (prosthetic valve, endocarditis, rheumatic heart disease) with or without right-to-left cardiac shunt
- Left atrial myxoma (primary cardiac tumor, no risk factors)

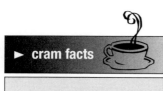

► cram facts

ATHEROSCLEROSIS RISK FACTORS

• Cigarette smoking
• Diabetes
• Hypertension
• Hyperlipidemia
• Genetics

B. Aortoiliac Occlusive Disease

► Description

Arteriosclerosis involves arteries singly or in combination. Slow progression of occlusive disease allows for collateral formation.

► Symptoms

Claudication, rest pain, tissue loss. Leriche syndrome: buttock claudication, impotence, diminished femoral pulses, bruit, thrill, elevation pallor, dependent rubor.

► Diagnosis

History and physical. Noninvasive tests: ankle–brachial index (Fig. 18–4), pulse volume recording, duplex scan, arteriography.

► Treatment Steps

Medical—Control risk factors, control hypertension, lower cholesterol, stop smoking, cilastozol (Pletal), exercise program.

Surgical—Bypass, endarterectomy, angioplasty with or without stent (consider patient's comorbid factors and location and extent of the lesion in deciding for stent or open procedure).

C. Abdominal Aortic Aneurysm

► Description

Typically involve infrarenal aorta, but may extend above renals. Most are fusiform. More degenerative than atherosclerosis. More common in males. (See Fig. 18–5.)

► Symptoms

Intact aneurysms are asymptomatic. Expanding or leaking causes back pain and abdominal pain. Pulsatile abdominal mass.

► Diagnosis

Physical examination, calcific outline on plain x-ray, ultrasound, CT scan (Fig. 18–6), arteriography.

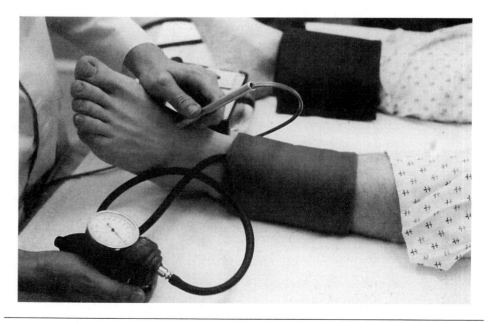

Figure 18–4. Measurement of ankle–brachial index. Doppler instrument identifies the dorsal pedal artery.

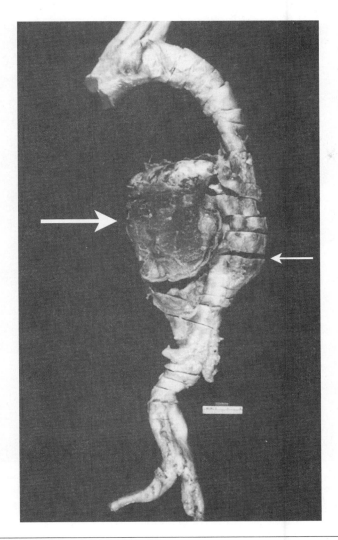

Figure 18–5. Entire lenth of aorta from acending aortic segment to iliac bifurcation obtained at necropsy. Note the dilatation of an abdominal aortic aneurysm (small arrow) which has ruptured to cause a large adjacent hematoma (large arrow). Scale in centimeters.

▶ Treatment Steps
1. Asymptomatic less than 5 cm: observe.
2. Greater than 5 cm: Elective aneurysmectomy with aortobifemoral graft or tube graft.
3. Endovascular repair (stent grafts) undergoing clinical trials. Endovascular abdominal aortic aneurysm (AAA) repair has more limitations based on anatomic issues.

D. Femoropopliteal Occlusive Disease

▶ Description
Arteries involved singly or in combination.

▶ Symptoms
Claudication, rest pain, tissue loss.

▶ Diagnosis
Physical examination, noninvasive tests, arteriography.

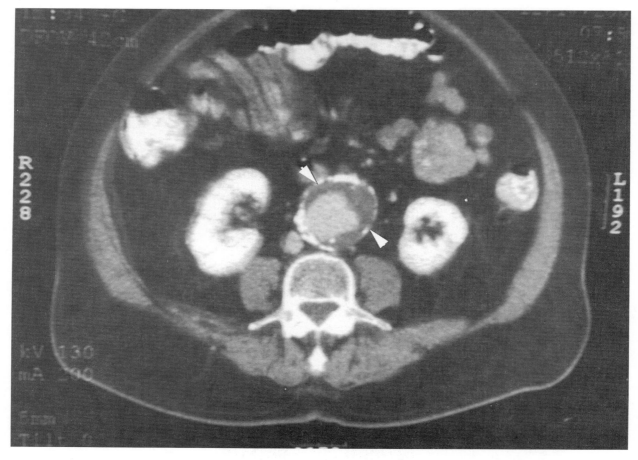

Figure 18–6. Abdominal CT scan with intravenous contrast showing an abdominal aortic aneurysm (arrows). Note the white inner lumen surrounded by a darker mural thrombus and an outer white ring of calcification around the aneurysm.

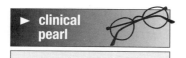

► **clinical pearl**

Cilastozol (Platal) should not be used in patients with heart failure.

► Treatment Steps
1. Control risk factors, cilastozol (Pletal), pentoxifylline (Trental), exercise programs.
2. Surgery for disabling claudication, rest pain, or tissue loss.

E. Cerebrovascular Disease

► Description
Lesions of the extracranial cerebral vessels. Decreased cerebral perfusion from occlusive lesions, thrombosis, or embolization. Majority due to thromboembolic etiologies.

► Symptoms
Transient ischemic attacks (amaurosis fugax), stroke, vertebral–basilar insufficiency (ataxia, vertigo, diplopia), diminished pulses, bruits.

► Diagnosis
Duplex scan, arteriography (Fig. 18–7). Angiogram can be done as an intervention, but CT or magnetic resonance angiography is possible without the risks of an invasive procedure.

► Treatment Steps
1. Medical therapy. Antiplatelet agents (aspirin, persantine, ticlopide).

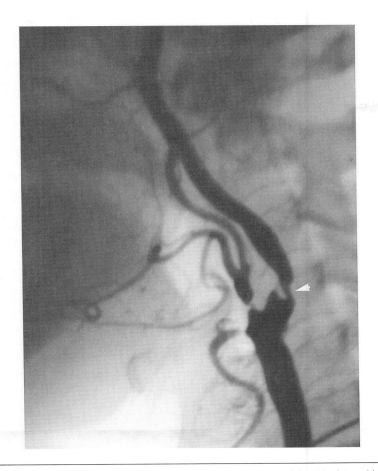

Figure 18–7. Carotid angiogram showing a high-grade stenosis of the origin of the internal (arrow) as well as the external carotid artery.

2. Endarterectomy.
3. Carotid balloon angioplasty with stenting undergoing clinical trials.

XII. VENOUS DISEASE

A. Deep Vein Thrombosis (DVT)

▶ **Description**
Those at risk: elderly, bedridden, hip replacement and other orthopedic procedures, pelvic and abdominal procedures, trauma, malignancy, and estrogen therapy. Virchow's triad: stasis, intimal damage, hypercoagulability.

▶ **Symptoms**
Asymptomatic in 50%, swelling, tenderness, Homan's sign (calf pain with dorsiflexion of foot). *Phlegmasia alba dolens:* milk leg. *Phlegmasia cerulea dolens:* venous gangrene.

▶ **Diagnosis**
Duplex scan, venography, impedance plethysmography, fibrinogen scan (best study for calf DVT).

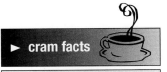

▶ **cram facts**

MEDICATIONS FOR DVT

- Unfractionated heparin (maintain partial thromboplastin time 1.5 × control)

or

- Low-molecular-weight heparin (once or twice daily subcutaneous injection)

and

- Warfarin (Coumadin) orally for long-term treatment

► Prophylactic Measures
1. Early ambulation postoperatively.
2. Low-dose subcutaneous heparin or enoxaparin/low-molecular-weight heparin.
3. Elastic compression stocking or intermittent pneumatic compression device.

► Treatment Steps
1. Bed rest (for iliofemoral DVT or extensive clot burden).
2. Thrombolytic therapy with iliofemoral DVT.
3. Gradient compressive hose.
4. Inferior vena cava (IVC) filter if failure of anticoagulation or contraindications or complications from anticoagulation.
5. Venous thrombectomy (and fasciotomies for compartment syndrome in cases of severe compromise). Very uncommon.

B. Varicose Veins

► Description
Dilated, tortuous veins in the leg.

Primary—Normal deep system.

Secondary—Diseased deep system.

► Symptoms
Dull ache, feeling of leg heaviness relieved by elevation. Dilated veins along anatomic distribution of greater and lesser saphenous veins. May be accompanied by signs of chronic deep venous disease.

► Diagnosis
Clinical examination, Trendelenburg test, duplex scan, Perthes' test.

► Treatment Steps
1. Support hose.
2. Sclerotherapy.
3. Ligation and stripping.

C. Superficial Thrombophlebitis

► Description
Inflammation and thrombosis of vein, pain, swelling, warmth. Treat with hot compresses, leg elevation, analgesics, excision of vein if purulent, systemic anticoagulation if process extends to deep venous system, or ascending superficial thigh. Mondor disease is superficial thrombophlebitis of the thoracoepigastric veins of the anterior chest wall or breast. Migratory thrombophlebitis is associated with pancreatic carcinoma.

D. Pulmonary Embolus
See Chapter 16.

XIII. HERNIA

A. Indirect Hernia

► Description
Fifty percent of all hernias. Congenital defect. Patent processus vaginalis. Lateral to inferior epigastric vessels. Chronic intra-abdominal pressure elevation. Rule out colon disease, prostate (strain to void), or pulmonary (chronic cough).

► **Symptoms**

Pain, groin mass.

► **Diagnosis**

Physical examination. Reducible or irreducible; incarcerated or strangulated.

► **Treatment Steps**

1. High ligation of sac. Close defect in transversalis fascia.
2. Laparoscopic hernia repair also an option.
3. If incarcerated or strangulated, open abdomen (midline incision).

B. Direct Hernia

► **Description**

Weakness in the inguinal floor (Hesselbach's triangle). Most common in elderly or young heavy lifters.

► **Treatment Steps**

1. Cooper's ligament repair.
2. Mesh repair (open versus laparoscopic) also an option.

XIV. WOUND INFECTIONS

► **Description**

Usually caused by break in sterile technique, carrier in operating room, ruptured viscus, large wound inoculum. Local factors: devitalized tissue, foreign body, hematoma, seroma. Systemic risk factors: age, steroids, immunosuppression, diabetes, obesity, length of operation, and blood transfusion.

► **Symptoms**

Fever, pain, erythema, drainage, swelling.

► **Diagnosis**

Physical examination, cultures.

► **Treatment Steps**

1. Drainage.
2. Debridement.
3. Antibiotics.

XV. THYROID

A. Hyperthyroidism

► **Description**

Increased levels of thyroid hormone. Loss of normal feedback. Graves' disease, autoimmune. Thyroid-stimulating immunoglobulins in 90% with Graves' disease.

► **Symptoms**

Heat intolerance, sweating, insomnia, muscle weakness, weight loss, nervousness, irritability, staring appearance, fine hair or alopecia, exophthalmos, vitiligo, onycholysis.

► **Diagnosis**

T_4 and T_3 levels high. Thyroid-stimulating hormone (TSH) is low. Elevated radioactive iodine uptake.

► Treatment Steps
1. Antithyroid drugs—propylthiouracil or tapazole, radioiodine (^{131}I).
2. Subtotal thyroidectomy.

B. Nontoxic Nodular Goiter

► Description
Compensatory response to decreased production of thyroid hormone, inadequate intake of iodine, medications that impair hormone production, enzyme deficiency.

► Symptoms
Compression of neck structures, cough, fullness in neck, neck mass.

► Diagnosis
Exam, ultrasound of thyroid gland. Increased TSH. Decreased levels of thyroid hormone.

► Treatment Steps
1. Thyroid hormone replacement.
2. Surgery reserved for compressive symptoms, cosmesis, threat of malignancy.

C. Thyroid Carcinoma

► Description
Low overall mortality. Favorable prognosis for most cell types. Papillary, 60–70%. Follicular, 15–20%. Medullary. Anaplastic aggressive. Previous neck irradiation. Best prognosis is papillary.

► Signs & Symptoms
Solitary neck mass most common. Lymphadenopathy.

► Diagnosis
Thyroid function tests, thyroid scan, ultrasound, fine-needle aspiration, neck exploration.

► Treatment Steps
1. Surgery: thyroid lobectomy and isthmusectomy, subtotal thyroidectomy, total thyroidectomy. Procedure depends on cell type and size of tumor.
2. Postoperative thyroid suppression.
3. Radioactive iodine for metastatic disease.

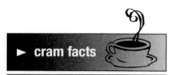

► cram facts

RISK FACTORS FOR
THYROID CARCINOMA

- Extremes of age
- Rapid growth
- Local invasion
  (hoarseness and fixation)
- External radiation
- Cold hypofunctional
  nodule + family history
  (medullary and papillary)

XVI. PARATHYROID—PRIMARY HYPERPARATHYROIDISM

► Description
Increase in serum parathyroid hormone. Single or multiple parathyroid adenomas or hyperplasia.

► Signs and Symptoms
Weakness, anorexia, nausea, constipation, renal colic, renal stones, osteoporosis, osteitis fibrosa cystica, subperiosteal resorption, pancreatitis, gallstones, depression, anxiety.

► Diagnosis
Increased serum calcium, decreased serum phosphate. Increased serum parathyroid hormone: carboxyterminal fragment longer half-life, biologically inactive. Chloride-to-phosphate ratio > 33. Localiza-

tion: CT scan, venous catheterization, and sampling. Thallium-technetium subtraction scan.

▶ Treatment Steps
1. Surgery: One enlarged gland, remove.
2. Generalized hyperplasia: Remove 3.5 glands or total parathyroidectomy with reimplantation.

XVII. ADRENAL

A. Primary Hyperaldosteronism

▶ Description
Excess aldosterone secretion. No adrenocorticotropic hormone (ACTH) regulation. One percent of all cases of hypertension. More common in women. Adenoma in 75%, hyperplasia in 25%. The most common adrenal tumor is incidental. Surgical resection for any functional tumor or any adreanal tumor ≥ 5 cm.

▶ Symptoms
Hypertension, headache, weakness, polydipsia, edema.

▶ Diagnosis
Elevated serum aldosterone levels, decreased serum renin level. Hypernatremia, hypokalemia, hypochloremia, alkalosis. Localization: CT scan, MRI, venous catheterization, and sampling.

▶ Treatment Steps

Adenoma—Surgical removal, adrenalectomy.

Hyperplasia—Medical therapy, spironolactone.

B. Hypercortisolism

▶ Description

Cushing's Disease—Pituitary ACTH excess usually from a pituitary adenoma that leads to adrenal hyperplasia.

Cushing Syndrome—If due to an adrenal source of cortisol, low ACTH. More common in women, young age. Seventy-five percent of adrenal tumors are benign, 98% unilateral.

▶ Symptoms
Change in menstrual cycle, virilization, weight gain, lassitude, muscle weakness, psychiatric disturbance, hypertension, edema, purple striae, buffalo hump.

▶ Diagnosis
Plasma cortisol levels, low-dose dexamethasone suppression test, urinary-free cortisol excretion, ACTH assay, high-dose dexamethasone suppression test, metapyrone test, CT scan.

▶ Treatment Steps

Cushing's Disease—Transsphenoidal hypophysectomy.

Cushing Syndrome (if caused by adrenal neoplasm)—Adrenalectomy.

C. Pheochromocytoma

▶ Description
Catecholamine-producing tumors for amine precursor uptake and decarboxylation (APUD) cells. Neural crest origin. Adrenal medulla

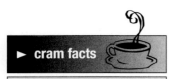
or sympathetic system. Of all patients with hypertension, 0.1%. Malignant, 10%; bilateral, 10%; in adrenal or periadrenal area, 90%.

► Symptoms

Sustained or paroxysmal hypertension, perspiration, pallor, flushing, palpitation, trembling, weakness, anxiety.

► Diagnosis

Urine for catecholamine metabolites: Vanillylmandelic acid (VMA), normetanephrine, metanephrine. Urinary-free epinephrine and norepinephrine. Localization: metaiodobenzylguanidine (MIBG) scan, CT scan.

► Treatment Steps

1. Surgery: Preparation with α-blocking agent phenoxybenzamine, followed by β blockade (propranolol hydrochloride [Inderal]).
2. Adrenalectomy with careful intraoperative monitoring.

XVIII. LUNG

A. Lung Cancer

► Description

Peak incidence 50–70 years. Cigarette smoking, exposure to asbestos, other toxic agents. Cell types: squamous (40–70%), adeno-

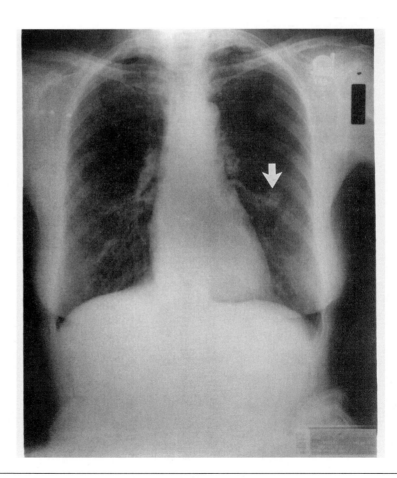

Figure 18–8. Posterior–anterior (PA) chest film showing left lung carcinoma (arrow).

carcinoma (15%), bronchoalveolar (5%), undifferentiated (20–30%). Most common malignancy in males.

▶ Symptoms
Cough, dyspnea, chest or shoulder pain, hoarseness, weight loss, clubbing, hemoptysis. May be asymptomatic.

▶ Diagnosis
CXR (Fig. 18–8), sputum cytology, CT scan, bronchoscopy, transpleural needle biopsy, mediastinoscopy, open-lung biopsy.

▶ Treatment Steps
1. Thoracotomy with wedge resection.
2. Lobectomy.
3. Pneumonectomy.
4. Radiation.
5. Chemotherapy.

B. Lung Abscess

See Chapter 16.

C. Pneumothorax

See Chapter 16.

XIX. BREAST

A. Breast Cancer

▶ Description
Most common cancer in females; can occur in males. Risk factors: previous cancer, heredity, early menarche, late menopause. Ductal or lobular accounts for 85%; spreads by lymphatic and hematogenous routes.

▶ Symptoms
Painless lump, nipple discharge, erythema, asymmetry, nipple inversion, bone pain, weight loss. Edema of overlying skin (peau d'orange); hard, irregular, fixed mass in advanced cases.

▶ Diagnosis
Liver function tests may be elevated in advanced cases, hypercalcemia with bone metastasis, CXR, CT scan of abdomen, mammography (Fig. 18–9), breast biopsy, fine-needle aspiration.

▶ Treatment Steps
1. Breast conservation: lumpectomy with axillary dissection, radiation therapy; stage I and stage II.
2. Mastectomy.
3. Adjuvant chemotherapy (cylophosphamide, methotrexate, 5-FU). Antiestrogen therapy (tamoxifen).

Note: Equivalent survival with modified radical mastectomy (MRM) versus lumpectomy, axillary node dissection, and radiation.

B. Mammary Dysplasia

▶ Description
Incidence peaks age 35–40. Most common breast complaint. Common cause of breast mass. Atypical hyperplasia premalignant.

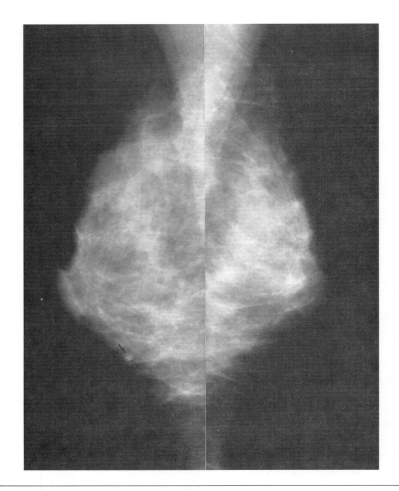

Figure 18–9. Bilateral mammogram dominant fibroglandular material (white) with little accompanying fat (black on mammography). Small focus of microcalcifications (arrows).

► Symptoms
Breast pain varying with menstrual cycle. Breast masses may appear in cyclic manner. Tender mass; thickened, nodular areas.

► Diagnosis
Physical examination, mammography.

► Treatment Steps
1. Biopsy dominant masses to rule out carcinoma.
2. Avoid caffeine.
3. Danazol in severe cases.
4. Simple mastectomy with breast reconstruction in severe cases.

C. Fibroadenoma

► Description
Common cause of breast mass in young women, peak age to 25. May grow to large size. Unusual to find cancer invading fibroadenoma.

► Symptoms
Asymptomatic mass, found incidentally. Firm, freely movable.

► Diagnosis
Physical examination, needle biopsy.

► Treatment Steps
1. Observation.
2. Excisional biopsy.

D. Intraductal Papilloma

► Description
Benign; may degenerate if allowed to enlarge. Grows within ducts. Nipple discharge, bloody.

► Symptoms
Nipple discharge. May be too small to feel on physical examination.

► Diagnosis
Physical examination. Note area of discharge on nipple and areolar palpation.

► Treatment Steps
Excision.

E. Breast Abscess

► Description
Most associated with lactation.

► Signs and Symptoms
Fever, erythema, tender mass.

► Diagnosis
Physical examination.

► Treatment Steps
1. Antibiotics.
2. Operative drainage.
3. Biopsy wall of abscess and skin to rule out inflammatory carcinoma.

XX. SKIN AND SOFT TISSUE

A. Melanoma

► Description
Increasing incidence (1/75, eighth most common cancer in the world), ultraviolet irradiation. Genetic predisposition: fair skin, blonde hair, blue eyes higher risk. Majority originate de novo 10–50% from preexisting nevi. Ninety percent in skin, rest in eye, anus, viscera. Distant metastasis occur in lungs and liver. Four types: lentigo maligna, superficial spreading, acral lentiginous, nodular. Prognosis depends on level of invasion, thickness, and ulceration.

► Symptoms
Change in existing nevus: bleeding, ulceration, irregular border, size change.

► Diagnosis
Biopsy: full thickness. Breslow thickness best prognosis factor.

► Treatment Steps
1. Wide local excision.
2. Amputation.
3. Lymph node dissection.

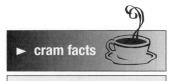

► cram facts

RISK FACTORS FOR MELANOMA

- Sun exposure
- Dyplastic nevus syndrome
- Xeroderma pigmentosum
- Family history of other skin cancer (nonmelanoma)
- High socioeconomic status
- Family history of melanoma

4. Isolated limb perfusion.
5. Immunotherapy.

B. Soft Tissue Sarcomas

▶ Description

Uncommon. One percent of malignant tumors. Liposarcomas, malignant fibrous histiocytomas, leiomyosarcomas, fibrosarcomas, rhabdomyosarcomas are most common. Hematogenous spread to lung. The most common site is the extremities. Adult: most common types are malignant fibrous histiocytoma and liposarcoma. Children: most common types are rhabdomyosarcoma and fibrosarcoma. Stewart–Treves syndrome—angiosarcoma in edematous extremity post modified radical mastectomy for breast cancer.

▶ Symptoms

Painless mass, enlarging. May become painful and interfere with function. Most often in lower extremities.

▶ Diagnosis

Biopsy along longitudinal axis of extremity (do not cross fascial compartments). CT scan or MRI of area. CXR.

▶ Treatment Steps

1. Surgical resection: avoid simple enucleation.
2. Irradiation, surgery, and chemotherapy in combination (limb sparing).

BIBLIOGRAPHY

Cameron J. *Current Surgical Therapy,* 8th ed. Philadelphia: Mosby, 2004.
Emery, SE. *Surgery of the Cervical Spine.* Philadelphia: W.B. Saunders, 2003.
Hardy JD. *Textbook of Surgery.* Philadelphia: J.B. Lippincott, 1988.
Sabiston D. *Textbook of Surgery,* 17th ed. Philadelphia: W.B. Saunders, 2001.
Schwartz ST. *Principles of Surgery,* 8th ed. New York: McGraw-Hill, 2004.

Symptoms, Signs, and Ill-Defined Conditions

19

I. CARDIORESPIRATORY SYSTEM AND CHEST

A. Cough

▶ **Description**

Protective respiratory reflex, induced by stimulation of respiratory tree receptors.

▶ **Symptoms**

Cough. May be productive or nonproductive (dry).

▶ **Diagnosis**

History and physical, chest x-ray (CXR), pulmonary function testing (PFTs), sputum analysis (culture and cytology), upper gastrointestinal (UGI) (rule out reflux/aspiration), empiric trial of PPI (proton pump inhibitor) for reflux.

▶ **Pathology**

See Cram Facts below.

▶ **Treatment Steps**

As per individual condition.

B. Hemoptysis

▶ **Description**

Bloody sputum production.

▶ **Symptoms**

Ranges from sputum tinged with blood to expectoration of frank blood. May see shortness of breath.

▶ **Diagnosis**

History and physical, **CXR, bronchoscopy,** computed tomographic (CT) scan of chest, pulmonary angiography, labs (prothrombin time [PT], partial thromboplastin time [PTT], complete blood count [CBC]).

▶ **cram facts**

PARANEOPLASTIC SYNDROMES IN LUNG CANCER

- **Metabolic and endocrine:** Cushing's syndrome, syndrome of inappropriate antidiuretic hormone (SIADH), hypercalcemia, gynecomastia
- **Cutaneous:** Ancathosis nigricans, erythema gyratum
- **Cardiovascular:** Thrombophlebitis, marantic endocarditis
- **Hematologic:** Anemia, disseminated intravascular coagulation (DIC), eosinophilia, thrombocytosis
- **Neuromuscular:** Dermatomyositis, Eaton–Lambert syndrome, myasthenia gravis, peripheral neuropathy
- **Others:** Clubbing

▶ **clinical pearl**

HISTORY

- Timing of cough
- Current or past tobacco smoke
- Occupational exposures
- Productive or nonproductive
- Blood tinged

▶ **cram facts**

COUGH

One of the most challenging diagnostic and treatment dilemmas encountered in clinical practice. Although an innocent symptom, it can be very annoying and a significant manifestation of a bigger and more severe problem. To figure out any medical problem, go to the basics: pathology and physiology of the normal and the ill (etiology). Therefore, explore the different alternatives: a reflex, an inflammatory process, irritation/hypersensitivity, manifestation of other airway problem between others.

- **Diagnosis:** History and physical, CXR, PFTs, esophageal pH probes, fiberoptic flexible bronchoscopy, and other studies as indicated.
- **Differential Diagnosis:** Asthma, foreign body, congestive heart failure (CHF), chronic aspiration, pneumonia, sinusitis, severe gastroesophageal reflux disease (GERD), malignancies, angiotensin-converting enzyme (ACE) inhibitor related, other pulmonary diseases.
- **Treatment:** Will vary depending on the insulting factor (etiology). Could be as simple as bronchodilators and/or H_2 blockers, or as complex as bronchoscopy for foreign body retrieval.

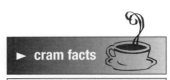

► **cram facts**

Cough complications: syncope, rib fractures. Asthma may present with cough only, without wheezing.

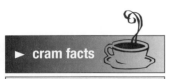

► **cram facts**

X-RAYS

Look carefully at x-rays, and remember: CXR—look for heart size, infiltrates, and their locations and for volume loss, masses, diaphragms (positions), hardware (endotracheal tube, nasogastric tube). Look for pneumothorax and free air under the diaphragm. KUB (kidney/urinary tract/bladder)—look for gas patterns, stones, and REMEMBER: the rule of 20/80% (20% of gallstones are seen on KUB and 80% of kidney stones are seen on KUB).

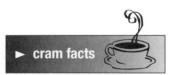

► **cram facts**

Posterior pack blocks sphenopalatine artery (anterior bleeding from ethmoid arteries).
   Most frequent bleeding site: Kiesselbach's area.

► Pathology

A result of **carcinoma, bronchitis,** tuberculosis (TB), pulmonary embolism, coagulation disorder, Goodpasture's syndrome, mycetomas, **bronchiectasis,** hemosiderosis, Wegener's disease, and mitral stenosis.

► Treatment Steps

1. Supportive.
2. Control cough (codeine).
3. Intubation.
4. Tamponade or thoracotomy for massive hemorrhage/tumor.

C. Epistaxis

► Symptoms

Nasal bleeding (slight or brisk), hypertension.

   Anterior Bleed—Often one side only.

   Posterior Bleed—Both sides, coughing/choking on blood.

► Diagnosis

History and physical examination.

► Pathology

Anterior (**Kiesselbach's** or Little's plexus bleeding, trauma, low humidity), or **posterior** sites. Additional etiologies: hypertension, nasal foreign body, tumor, vascular abnormalities/arteriosclerosis, leukemia, bleeding disorders, and infection.

► Treatment Steps

Anterior:
1. Pressure/packing.
2. **Cautery.**

Posterior:
1. **Posterior pack/balloon.**
2. Artery ligation.

D. Dyspnea

► Description

Air hunger.

► Symptoms

Subjective complaint of **uncomfortable shortness of breath, of more than expected severity for activity level.**

► Diagnosis

History and physical, cardiac and pulmonary evaluation as guided by the history. **Note the patient's vital signs.** Pulse, blood pressure, pulse ox. CBC, SMA-12, electrocardiogram (ECG), CXR, arterial blood gas (ABG), 2-dimensional (2-D) echo, ventilation/perfusion (V/Q) scan, cardiac enzymes (creatine kinase [CK], CK-MB, troponin), PFTs, stress test.

► Pathology

Most frequently pulmonary or cardiac disease, of acute or chronic nature. Deconditioning and psychogenic factors may be present.

► Treatment Steps

Treat primary problem.

E. Chest Pain

► Symptoms
Chest pain. May be pleuritic (pleurisy), exacerbated by chest wall palpation (costochondritis) or exercise (angina), or episodic (spasm?) and atypical (other disorders).

► Diagnosis
History and physical, cardiac workup (ECG, 2-D echocardiogram, stress testing, arteriography), CXR. Other studies may include V/Q scan, high-resolution CT scan of chest, ultrasound of aorta, and gastrointestinal (GI) workup.

► Pathology
Rule out **angina pectoris:** ischemic cardiac pain. Other etiologies include pleurisy, pericarditis, costochondral disease, GERD, esophageal spasm, neuritis, pulmonary embolism, aortic aneurysm, pulmonary hypertension, valvular disorders, and others.

► Treatment Steps
Treat as per specific etiology.

F. Palpitations

► Description
Subjective sensation of additional/irregular or strong heartbeats, or chest discomfort related to cardiac rhythm.

► Symptoms
As described. Depending on etiology, may also experience chest pain, anxiety, light-headedness, or syncope.

► Diagnosis
History and physical, ECG (see Figs. 19–1 and 19–2), 2-D echocardiogram, Holter monitor, CBC, thyroid-stimulating hormone (TSH).

► Pathology
Sensation of abnormal beats (palpitations) may reflect significant cardiac pathology or be of no importance whatsoever.

► **cram facts**

SHORTNESS OF BREATH

This is a large differential diagnosis. By system:

Pulmonary
Asthma, pulmonary embolism, chronic obstructive pulmonary disease (COPD) exacerbation, acute bronchitis, pneumonia, aspiration, airway obstruction (due to foreign body or tumor), pleural effusion, cor pulmonale.

Cardiac
Angina, myocardial infarction (MI), CHF, pericarditis, cardiomyopathy, arrhythmia.

Other
Anemia (acute or severe and chronic), metabolic disorders (metabolic acidosis due to diabetic ketoacidosis [DKA]), end-stage liver disease with ascites, pregnancy, acute intoxications, panic attacks.

► **cram facts**

- *Orthopnea*—supine dyspnea
- *Platypnea*—upright dyspnea
- *Hyperpnea*—increase minute volume

Figure 19–1. A patient with palpitations due to atrial flutter.

532

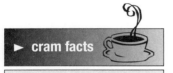

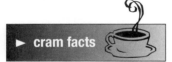

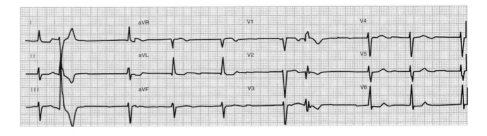

Figure 19–2. A patient with palpitations due to PVCs (premature ventricular contractions).

► Treatment Steps
As per individual condition.

G. Cyanosis

► **Description**
Blue color of mucous membranes and/or skin and nail beds. Clubbing (see Section II.C).

► **Symptoms**
As described. May be associated with other symptoms depending on specific disorder.

► **Diagnosis**
History and physical, cardiopulmonary evaluation (ABG/ECG/echo/CXR/cath/PFTs). **Newborn with cyanosis:** oxygen (100%) will improve hypoxemia with pulmonary disorders, but have negligible effect with intracardiac shunt lesions.

► **Pathology**
Reduced arterial oxygen concentration from central (cardiac shunt or pulmonary pathology), or peripheral (vasoconstriction) mechanisms.

► **Treatment Steps**
As per individual condition.

H. Hypoxemia

► **Description**
Inadequate blood oxygen.

► **Symptoms**
Lethargy, mental status change, arrhythmia, headache, palpitations, impaired judgment.

► **Diagnosis**
History and physical (cyanosis, tachycardia, etc.), cardiopulmonary evaluation, ABGs, response to oxygen, A-a gradient (see the following), and **hemoglobin. Most specific physical sign of hypoxemia: cyanosis.**

► **Pathology**
Etiologies include **V/Q mismatch, right-to-left shunt, diffusion abnormality, alveolar hypoventilation,** and **reduced inspiratory oxygen content.**

► **Treatment Steps**
As per condition, but **oxygen** is critical.

I. Shock

▶ Description
Inadequate tissue perfusion.

▶ Symptoms
Hypotension, tachypnea, tachycardia, mental confusion, cyanosis.

▶ Diagnosis
History and physical (weak pulse, reduced urinary output, fever, poor skin color, etc.). Other procedures as indicated (blood cultures, hemodynamic monitoring, etc.).

▶ Pathology
Primary etiology includes **cardiogenic** and **hypovolemic** disorders. Other sources include trauma and sepsis.

▶ Treatment Steps
1. Cardiopulmonary resuscitation (CPR) (including ventilatory support, cardiac monitoring, acid–base management, and fluids/vasopressors).
2. Treatment of primary disorder.

J. Respiratory Failure

▶ Description
Inadequate oxygen or carbon dioxide exchange.

▶ Symptoms
Tachypnea, tachycardia, mental confusion, cyanosis, wheezing/dyspnea.

▶ **cram facts**

WEDGE HEMODYNAMICS

Watch those hemodynamics—don't blow them off; they are trying to tell you something (e.g., high CO/low SVR suggests sepsis; low CO/high SVR/high wedge pressure suggests cardiogenic shock; equalization of pressures suggests tamponade; high wedge, your patient could be wet; low wedge, your patient might be intravascularly depleted; high RA/high PAP with pad-wedge > 5 suggests pulmonary hypertension).
CO = cardiac output
SVR = systemic vascular resistance
PAP = pulmonary artery pressure

▶ **cram facts**

COMMON ADRENAL CORTEX AND MEDULLA PROBLEMS

- **Adrenal crisis:** weakness, abdominal pain, fever, confusion, nausea and vomiting, dehydration, hypotension, can see skin pigmentation, high K and low NA and elevated adrenocorticotropic hormone (ACTH). Patients may look like they're in septic shock. Treat with hydrocortisone and fluids.
- **Addison's disease:** weakness, abdominal pain, diarrhea, nausea and vomiting, anorexia, amenorrhea, increased pigmentation in nipples and creases, sparse axillary hair, hypotension, low sodium, High potassium and calcium, neutropenia, eosinophilia, high ACTH. Treat with replacement therapy, glucocorticoids, and mineralocorticoids.
- **Cushing syndrome:** purple striae, central obesity, muscle wasting, thin skin, hirsutism, hypertension, hyperglycemia, low potassium, free urinary cortisol, and high serum cortisol. Treat with resection of tumor.
- **Hirsutism:** menstrual problems, acne, virilization, high serum testosterone. Treat with antiandrogens.
- **Hyperaldosteronism:** weakness, hypertension, polyuria and polydipsia, low potassium, high serum and urine aldosterone, low serum renin level. Treat with surgery if indicated, spironolactone, antihypertensives.
- **Pheocromocytoma:** sudden onset of headaches, palpitations, hypertension, diaphoresis, abdominal and thoracic pain, nausea and vomiting, weakness, visual disturbances, anxiety, tremors, elevated urinary catecholamines and metabolites. Treat with surgical removal of tumor and treatment of hypertension.

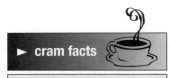

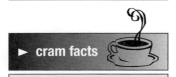

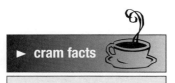

► Diagnosis

History and physical, **most important test is ABGs;** clinical findings of respiratory failure, and CXR may all be helpful. Note vitals—pulse, blood pressure, pulse ox, temperature.

► Pathology

Hypercarbia ($PaCO_2 > 50$) and/or hypoxemia ($PaO_2 < 60$).

► Treatment Steps

1. **Oxygen** (with or without intubation and mechanical ventilation).
2. Treatment of primary problem (drug overdose, infection, trauma, etc.).

II. SKIN

A. Edema

► Description

Increased tissue fluid, swelling of affected area.

► Diagnosis

History and physical, evaluation of cardiac, renal, hepatic, and vascular systems. Commonly CBC, SMA-12, urinalysis (UA), CXR, 2-D echo, lower extremity Dopplers, possible stress test.

► Pathology

Interstitial fluid excess. "Third spacing" due to low oncotic pressure: cirrhosis, nephrotic syndrome. Also venous insufficiency, obstruction to venous flow by tumor or DVT (deep vein thrombosis), CHF, medications (calcium channel blockers, rofecoxib, thiazolidinediones).

► Treatment Steps

1. Treat primary condition.
2. Reduce salt and fluids.
3. Diuretics (cardiac causes).

B. Jaundice

► Description

Yellow skin and **mucous membranes,** secondary to elevated bilirubin levels.

► Symptoms

Yellow skin/mucosa, may have **dark urine, pruritus,** light-colored stools, and symptoms of individual etiologic disorder.

► Diagnosis

History and physical (look for subungual jaundice and scleral icterus as well as skin discoloration), CBC with smear, lactic dehydrogenase (LDH), liver function tests (LFTs), ultrasound or CT scan of liver/abdomen, HIDA (hepatoiminodiacetic acid) scan, ERCP (endoscopic retrograde cholangiopancreatography), liver biopsy.

► Pathology

Unconjugated—Etiology includes excess bilirubin production (hemolytic disorders), or **faulty liver conjugation or uptake** (genetic disorders).

Conjugated—Reduced liver production (hepatic disease of various types, including inflammation, infection, and obstruction).

► Treatment Steps
Treat primary condition.

C. Clubbing

► Description
Distal phalanx nail deformity.

► Symptoms
Loss of nail plate-to-finger angle (convex nails), with fingernail thickness greater than distal interphalangeal (DIP) joint thickness.

► Diagnosis
Physical examination.

► Pathology
Common to many cardiopulmonary disorders (bronchiectasis, pulmonary hypertension, atrial septal defect, lung cancer, cystic fibrosis, cyanotic congenital heart disease, etc.), possibly secondary to hypoxemia. May also be familial.

► Treatment Steps
Treat primary condition.

D. Pruritus

► Symptoms
Sensation of itching (via skin nerve-ending stimulation).

► Diagnosis
History and physical, routine lab studies, and evaluation for any underlying disease as indicated.

► Pathology
May relate to local factors (dry skin, allergy), medications, or systemic pathology (uremia, malignancy, endocrine/thyroid disease, liver disease).

► Treatment Steps
1. Symptomatic treatment.
2. Corticosteroids topical/oral.
3. Antihistamines.

► **clinical pearl**

PRURITUS

• Young female—not pregnant, think PBC (primary biliary cirrhosis). Check LFTs (elevated alk phos).
• Young female—pregnant, possible cholestasis of pregnancy.
• Irtractable pruritus, poor living conditions, think scabies. Check for burrows in hand.

► **clinical pearl**

History and physical is of utmost importance. Obtain the 7 dimensions of a symptom (PPQRST). Things to ask:

Quality of pain—Crampy, dull, knife-like, sharp, intermittent (colicky)

Region—Diffuse or localized to a certain quadrant? Does it radiate?

Severity—"On a scale of 1 to 10" how bad is the pain, how has it interfered with daily life?

Timing—How long has it been present? What were you doing when it started? Speed of onset?

Palliation/Provocation—Is the pain better or worse with eating? Position? Defecating?

Also important—What other symptoms are occuring? Fever, nausea, vomiting, diarrhea, hematemesis, hematochezia, constipation, decreased oral intake, urinary symptoms, vaginal discharge, travel history, sexual history.

► **cram facts**

• *Dubin–Johnson syndrome*—genetic, conjugated jaundice disease, elevated urine coproporphyrin type 1 rather than type 3.
• *Gilbert syndrome*—genetic, most frequent unconjugated disorder, glucuronyl transferase deficiency.
• *Neonatal jaundice*—most frequent type is physiologic (no treatment needed); **high prolonged bilirubinemia may cause kernicterus (brain damage),** aggressive therapy required as per current literature/tables.
• *Carotenemia*—"jaundice," normal bilirubin, excess carrot ingestion.
• *Obstructive jaundice*—serum glutamic-oxaloacetic transaminase (SGOT) < 300, and **alkaline phosphatase** three times normal.
• *Drugs causing jaundice*—griseofulvin, erythromycin estolate, oxacillin, and **chloramphenicol**.

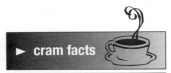

► **cram facts**

Peritonitis patients remain still. Viscus perforation causes severe pain.

- *Referred pain*—hepatic to right shoulder; uterine to back
- *Obstruction*—bowel sounds high-pitched, distention, pain
- *Cervical motion tenderness*—rule out pelvic inflammatory disease (PID)
- *Vomiting blood*—lesion above ligament of Treitz
- *Grey–Turner's sign*—flank ecchymosis
- *Cullen's sign*—periumbilical ecchymosis

III. DIGESTIVE SYSTEM AND ABDOMEN

A. Abdominal Pain

► **Description/Symptoms**
Pain in the abdominopelvic region (may include signs of peritonitis, referred pain, abdominal rigidity, etc.).

► **Diagnosis**
History and physical (see Cram Facts). CBC, SMA-12, amylase, lipase, UA, obstruction series, ECG, possibly CT scan of abdomen and pelvis, ultrasound, intravenous pyelography (IVP), bimanual pelvic exam with cultures.

► **Pathology**
Wide etiology including both acute and chronic events, and both abdominal and referred pain (cardiac) (see Fig. 19–3).

► **Treatment Steps**
As per individual condition.

B. Infantile Colic

► **Description**
Prolonged infant crying/abdominal pain.

► **Symptoms**
Crying episodes, with clenched fists and **legs pulled up.**

► **Diagnosis**
Clinical.

► **Pathology**
Uncertain, but most often resolves by 12 weeks of age.

► **Treatment Steps**
1. Reduce infant stress.
2. Increase parent relaxation/supportive care for parents.
3. Hot water bottle for infant.
4. Simethicone drops (Mylicon).
5. Burping.

C. Hepatomegaly (Enlarged Liver)

► **Symptoms**
Asymptomatic, or abdominal mass, right upper quadrant or shoulder pain.

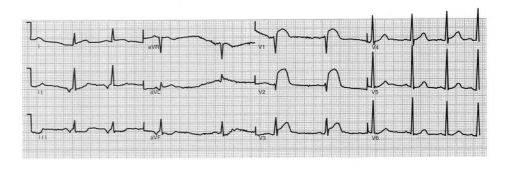

Figure 19–3. Patient with an MI actually presenting as abdominal pain.

▶ Diagnosis

History and physical—may lead you to possible etiology (see Clinical Pearl). Based on clinical scenario: LFTs, CBC, LDH, hepatitis serologies (hepatitis A, B, C), ferritin, ultrasound, CT scan abdomen.

▶ Pathology

Numerous possible etiologies.

▶ Treatment Steps

Treat primary condition.

D. Splenomegaly

▶ Symptoms

Asymptomatic or abdominal mass, left upper quadrant or shoulder pain.

▶ Diagnosis

History and physical, ultrasound, CT, and radioisotope scan.

▶ Pathology

Numerous possible etiologies (hemolytic anemia, portal hypertension and hepatocellular disease, mononucleosis, sarcoid, leukemia/lymphoma, storage disorders, idiopathic).

▶ Treatment Steps

Treat primary condition.

E. Ascites

▶ Description

Excess peritoneal fluid.

▶ Symptoms

Enlarging abdomen. May also have nausea, abdominal pain, edema, weight gain, and dyspnea.

▶ Diagnosis

History and physical—on history, ask about prior liver disease or cirrhosis (see Clinical Pearl). On physical exam, look for fluid wave, shifting dullness, bulging flanks. Ultrasound is helpful; paracentesis is essential to determine the cause of ascites.

    Paracentesis: It is essential to ask for cell count with differential, cytology, and albumin. Calculate the SAAG (serum ascites:albumin gradient. SAAG > 1.1 is consistent with ascites due to cirrhosis.

▶ Pathology

    Exudate—Protein > 3 g/100 mL (**TB, cancer,** and others).

    Transudate—Cirrhosis and CHF.

▶ Treatment Steps

As per individual condition. For **cirrhosis: restrict salt, diuretics** (furosemide, aldactone), **Le Veen shunt.**

F. Dysphagia

▶ Description

Difficulty swallowing.

▶ **clinical pearl**

HEPATOMEGALY—HISTORY

- Medications—Ask about use of over-the-counter medications, particularly those containing acetaminophen. Can cause "accidental" acetaminophen toxicity, epecially with alcohol use. Also hepatotoxicity reported with certain herbs.
- Travel and sexual history—for exposure to hepatitis A, B.
- Prior inhalational or intravenous drug use, blood transfusion prior to 1993, tatoos with questionable needle antiseptic techniques, hemophiliacs—exposure to hepatitis C.
- Diabetes, obesity—NASH (non-alcoholic steatohepatitis, sometimes called fatty liver).
- Prior diagnosis of cirrhosis or chronic hepatitis—hepatocellular carcinoma.
- Prior diagnosis of other malignancy—possible liver metastases.
- Family history of cirrhosis—hemochromatosis, Wilson's disease, α_1-antitrypsin deficiency.

▶ **clinical pearl**

HEPATOSPLENOMEGALY

Enlarged liver and spleen are often seen together (hepatosplenomegaly). Cirrhosis of any etiology as well as a portal vein thrombosis (Budd–Chiari) can cause portal hypertension.

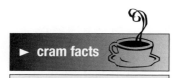

▶ **cram facts**

- *Felty syndrome*—splenomegaly, rheumatoid arthritis, and **granulocytopenia**
- *Gaucher's disease*—excess cerebroside, splenomegaly

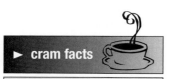

▶ **cram facts**

- *Most frequent cause of ascites*—cirrhosis
- *Treatment for ascites fluid removal*—paracentesis
- *Meig syndrome*—ovarian tumor, transudative ascites
- *Spontaneous bacterial peritonitis*—ascites complication with fever, elevated number of ascitic polymorphonuclear cells (> 250/μL), **pain**, organism on Gram stain.

▶ Symptoms
Difficulty swallowing, weight loss, regurgitation.

▶ Diagnosis
History and physical, barium swallow or UGI series, **endoscopy.**

▶ Pathology
Esophageal constriction may be due to **tumor, achalasia, stricture, esophageal ring** (Schatzki's ring may cause intermittent dysphagia), or **neuromuscular disorders.**

▶ Treatment Steps
As per individual condition.

G. Nausea and Vomiting

▶ Symptoms
Nausea, possibly followed by tachycardia, hypersalivation, and vomiting.

▶ Diagnosis
History and physical, x-ray studies (obstruction series), lab studies, endoscopy.

▶ Pathology

Gastrointestinal	Appendicitis, ileus, small bowel obstruction, gastric or duodenal ulcer, pancreatitis
Metabolic	Pregnancy, uremia, DKA
Psychogenic	Bulemia
Oncologic	Chemotherapeutic agents
CNS	Vertigo (Ménière's and acute labyrinthitis), neoplasm, migraine headache
Endocrine	Gastroparesis (commonly due to diabetes)
Cardiac	MI

▶ Treatment Steps
1. Treat primary condition.
2. Antiemetics include scopolamine, meclizine, and corticosteroids.

H. Diarrhea

▶ Description
Acute or chronic diarrheal illness (**increased stool weight per 24 hours**).

▶ Symptoms
Diarrhea (mild or severe), dehydration, fever if infectious.

▶ Diagnosis
History and physical, stool studies (fecal white blood count [WBC], ova and parasites, *Clostridium difficile* antigen and toxin), CBC, SMA-12, amylase, lipase, stool electrolytes (sodium and potassium), stool osmolarity.

▶ Pathology
Physiology includes **secretory, osmotic, impaired motility,** and **absorptive disorders.** Etiology includes **infection, medications,** and **in-**

flammatory bowel disease. Effect of fasting on diarrhea types—secretory, no effect; osmotic, diarrhea stops.

▶ Treatment Steps
1. Rehydration.
2. Treat primary condition (amebiasis/giardiasis: metronidazole; pseudomembranous colitis: metronidazole).
3. Antidiarrheals (if infection is absent).

I. Fecal Incontinence

▶ Description/Symptoms
Inability to maintain stool continence. Termed *encopresis* in children.

▶ Pathology
Anal sphincter disorder (idiopathic, postsurgical, trauma, Crohn's, etc.). May also relate to impaction, diabetes, and neuromuscular disease.

▶ Treatment Steps
1. Anal sphincter exercises (consult physician).
2. Biofeedback.
3. Medication.

J. Anorexia Nervosa
See also Chapter 15.

▶ Description
Weight loss disorder.

▶ Symptoms
Weight loss, depression, amenorrhea, distorted self-image.

▶ Diagnosis
History and physical examination, lab studies (SMA-12, CBC) examination of nails and teeth. Rule out GI disease: GI studies (UGI, endoscopy, barium enema [BE], etc.).

▶ Pathology
Typically in adolescent females, with unknown etiology (though family and social situations/pressures play a role).

▶ Treatment Steps
1. Psychiatric/psychological care.
2. Medication (cyproheptadine, chlorpromazine).

K. Failure to Thrive in Infancy

▶ Symptoms
Insufficient weight gain or growth, lethargy, emotional/behavioral disorders.

▶ Diagnosis
History and physical, laboratory, and other studies as indicated.

▶ Pathology
Etiology most often includes psychological disorders and deprivation/abuse.

▶ **cram facts**

- *Odynophagia*—painful swallowing. Most common cause is infection (candida, herpes simplex virus, cytomegalovirus)
- *Chalasia*—lower esophageal sphincter (LES) **does not close**
- *Achalasia*—pressure of LES elevated, with poor esophageal peristalsis
- *Barrett's esophagitis*— **esophageal columnar epithelium** (instead of squamous epithelium), **secondary to reflux,** with **tricture and adenocarcinoma** as potential **complications**
- *Globus hystericus*— **psychogenic, continuous "lump in throat" feeling,** may improve after swallowing
- *Plummer–Vinson syndrome*—**esophageal web** and **iron deficiency anemia**

▶ **differential diagnosis**

HEMATEMESIS

- Gastritis
- Peptic ulcer disease
- Esophageal varices
- Malignancy
- Mallory–Weiss tear
- Aortojejunal fistula

HEMATOCHEZIA

- Upper GI bleed
- Angiodysplasia
- Hemorrhoids
- Malignancy
- Colitis (not always)
- Certain infectious diarrheas
- Diverticulitis

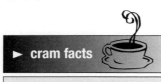

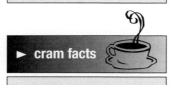

► Treatment Steps
1. Treat any coexisting medical disorder.
2. Family counseling.
3. Social service intervention.
4. Possible child foster placement.

IV. NERVOUS SYSTEM AND SPECIAL SENSES

A. Headache

► Description
Head pain.

► Symptoms

Migraine—**Throbbing, unilateral, nausea/vomiting,** photophobia, phonophobia.

Cluster—**Periorbital, severe pain, unilateral autonomic signs.**

Tension—**Bilateral, neck muscles tight, tight band feeling.**

Acute Central Nervous System (CNS)—**Acute-onset severe headache, neurologic signs.**

► Diagnosis
History and physical examination, lab testing (glucose, CBC), x-ray head/sinuses, electroencephalogram (EEG), CT/magnetic resonance imaging (MRI) studies, lumbar puncture (LP).

► Pathology
May include **migraine, cluster, tension, CNS disease, exertional,** and others (carbon monoxide, nitrites, temporal arteritis, temporomandibular joint [TMJ], etc.), as a result of inflammation or alteration of pain-sensitive CNS structures.

► Treatment Steps
As per individual condition.

B. Delirium

► Description
Alteration of consciousness.

► Symptoms
Confusion, memory difficulty, disorientation, agitation, perception disturbance.

► Diagnosis
History and physical examination, lab studies CBC, SMA-12, B_{12}, folate, rapid plasma reagin (RPR), TSH, urine drug screen, possibly LP, CT of head, EEG.

► Pathology
Etiology includes **infection, medication, metabolic disease, cardiac disease, sleep deprivation,** and CNS **disease.** Most frequent in elderly hospital patients, and resulting from complex and multiple factors.

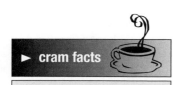

► Treatment Steps

1. Diagnose and treat the primary condition.
2. Provide orientation for the patient.
3. Nursing support.
4. Discontinue unnecessary medications and avoid anticholinergic and sedative–hypnotic medications.
5. Allow sleep (intensive care unit [ICU] psychosis).
6. Avoid restraints.
7. Medication if necessary, i.e., if patient is very agitated or psychotic (low-dose haloperidol [Haldol], antipsychotics [risperidol]).

C. Coma

► Description

State of **unconsciousness,** and unresponsiveness, resulting from metabolic, CNS pathology, and other causes.

► Symptoms

Unresponsiveness.

► Diagnosis

History and physical examination, EEG, CT, laboratory studies (SMA-12, CBC, drug screen, PT, PTT, ABGs, thyroid functions), **LP.**

► Pathology

Only two causes: extensive bilateral cerebral disorder or brain stem disorder.

► Treatment Steps

1. Cardiopulmonary resuscitation.
2. **Dextrose** (50 mL of 50% given IV).
3. **Naloxone.**
4. **Thiamine** (100 mg IV).
5. Correct metabolic abnormalities.
6. Treatment as per individual condition.

D. Convulsions

► Description

Seizure, and/or uncontrolled contraction of muscles.

► Symptoms

As described for following seizure disorders:

Grand Mal—Tonic–clonic, incontinence, postictal lethargy.

Petit Mal—Staring/absence spells, patient possibly unaware.

Partial—Simple (consciousness not lost), or complex (possible unconsciousness). Both may have sensory and/or motor signs.

► Diagnosis

History and physical examination, EEG, CT/MRI, laboratory studies, including blood cultures and toxicology screening.

► Pathology

Convulsions—Wide etiology (epilepsy, poisoning, infection, heatstroke, etc.).

Seizures—Generalized or partial (focal). Wide variety of CNS causes (trauma, metabolic, drugs/drug withdrawal, congenital disease, etc.).

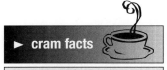

► cram facts

- **Pupils reactive and small**—narcotics, metabolic, and pontine pathology
- **Pupils fixed and dilated**—anoxia, and scopolamine overdose (OD)
- **Pupils face hemiparesis side**—pontine lesion
- **Pupils face strong side**—unilateral cerebral hemisphere lesion
- **Other antidotes**—benzodiazepines (give flumazenil)

► clinical pearl

SLEEP HYGEINE

Helpful for all patients with insomnia:
Avoid alcohol
Avoid caffeine after midday
Avoid exercising late at night
Avoid naps
Keep consistent bedtimes and awake times

OTHER SLEEP DISORDERS

1. Obstructive sleep apnea— clues: obesity, snoring at night, witnessed apnea when sleeping. Diagnose with polysomnography (sleep study). First-line treatment continuous positive airway pressure (CPAP).
2. Restless legs—motor restlessness of legs. Can disrupt sleep. Can be associated with iron deficiency anemia, peripheral neurophathy. Treat with amitriptyline, gabapentin.
3. Narcolepsy—severe daytime hypersomnolence also diagnosed with sleep study. Treat with stimulants.
4. Depression—screen through history.

► cram facts

Average sleep time: consists of 25% REM (rapid eye movement, dreaming) stages, and **the rest is non-REM.** Duration of REM sleep: five nightly episodes of **10–30 minutes** each.

► Treatment Steps
1. Neurologic workup.
2. Medication (see Chapter 11).

E. Insomnia

► **Symptoms**
Inability to sleep, disrupted sleep, or perceived poor sleep quality.

► **Diagnosis**
Clinical, psychological evaluation, routine laboratory studies, sleep studies, EEG.

► **Pathology**
May result from medication, depression, anxiety, and/or alcohol use. Also may be a primary sleep disorder (see Cram Facts).

► **Treatment Steps**
1. Treat coexisting medical disorders.
2. Psychological evaluation.
3. Progressive relaxation/biofeedback.
4. Sleep hygiene.

F. Syncope

► **Description**
Fainting.

► **Symptoms**
Sudden loss of consciousness.

> *Vasovagal*—May have diaphoresis, ringing in the ears, and blurry vision prior to fainting.
>
> *Orthostatic*—Postural-related symptoms.
>
> *Cardiac*—Possibly exercise induced.

► **Diagnosis**
History and physical, Holter monitor, ECG, EEG, and laboratory studies (rule out hypoglycemia and seizure disorders).

► **Pathology**
Reduced cerebral blood perfusion, via reduced cardiac output/venous return, or other disorders.

► **Treatment Steps**
Treat primary disorder.

G. Ataxia

► **Description**
Disorder of muscle coordination.

► **Symptoms**
Balance loss, may have limb, gait, or dysarthric ataxia.

► **Diagnosis**
History and physical, CT/MRI. MRI is superior to CT in imaging the cerebellum.

► **Pathology**
Cerebellar or brain stem pathology. Multiple disorders (drugs/alcohol, B_{12} deficiency, hypothyroidism, viral infection, etc.).

► **Treatment Steps**
Treat primary condition.

H. Weakness

► **Description**
Muscle and/or neurologic disease resulting in reduced muscle strength.

► **Symptoms**
Weakness (may include reduced deep tendon reflexes, and fasciculations). Try to distinguish muscle weakness from generalized fatigue.

► **Diagnosis**
History and physical, laboratory studies (CK, aldolase), CT/MRI, LP, electromyogram (EMG)/nerve conduction velocity (NCV), PFTs.

► **Pathology**
Neurologic (most often myasthenia gravis, Guillain–Barré syndrome), infectious, endocrine, psychological, and other conditions (botulism, medication, etc.).

► **Treatment Steps**
As per individual condition.

I. Dysphasia

► **Description**
Impaired speech and verbal comprehension. Aphasia—acquired disorder of language due to brain damage.

► **Symptoms**

Receptive (Posterior)—Difficulty with comprehension, speech remains fluent.

Expressive (Anterior)—Difficulty with expression, speech fluency disturbed.

► **Diagnosis**
History and physical/neurologic examination.

► **Pathology**
Brain pathology (cerebrovascular accident [CVA], trauma, infection), typically of **dominant temporal lobe.**

► **Treatment Steps**
1. Treat primary condition.
2. Speech therapy when stable.

J. Dyslexia

► **Description**
Reading disorder.

► **Symptoms**
Reading disorder without associated intellectual or visual disability.

► **Diagnosis**
History and physical, reading tests.

► **Pathology**
Cortical developmental disorder.

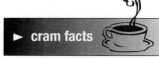

Valsalva induced: Micturition and cough syncope.

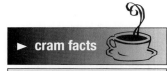

- **Midcerebellar disease**—wide stance, short steps.
- **Lateral cerebellar disease**—wide stance, swaying.
- **Hemiparesis**—weak arm, reduced arm motion, weak leg.
- **Parkinsonian gait**—short steps, diminished arm swing, stooped.
- **Senile gait**—slow, may appear similar to parkinsonian gait.
- **Dyskinetic gait**—involuntary jerking or dancelike movements.
- **Cerebral atrophy gait**—may have short steps, similar to parkinsonism.

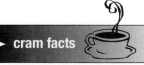

- **Proximal weakness**—often a myopathy, Guillain–Barré, nerve root lesion, and spinal muscular atrophy.
- **Distal weakness**—often a neuropathy.
- **Cranial/facial weakness**—myotonic dystrophy and neuromuscular junction disease.
- **Painful weakness**—polymyositis and myotonic dystrophy.
- **Weakness**—also consider multiple sclerosis (MS) and chronic fatigue syndrome.

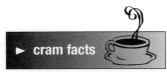

- **Broca's dysphasia**—nonfluent with good comprehension.
- **Wernicke's dysphasia**—fluent with poor comprehension.
- **Global dysphasia**—nonfluent, poor comprehension.
Cortical locations include speech (left motor cortex), and reading/writing (left angular gyrus).

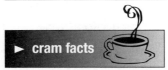

▶ cram facts

- **Ménière's disease**—endolymphatic hydrops, tinnitus, hearing loss, and episodic vertigo; give **diuretic** and reduce salt intake to treat.
- **Acoustic neuroma**—tinnitus, hearing loss, and chronic vertigo.
- **Vestibular neuronitis**—nausea/vomiting and vertigo with **normal hearing,** possibly viral etiology; treat with antihistamines and fluids.

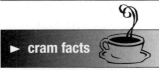

▶ cram facts

- *Oculomotor (third nerve) weakness*—rule out aneurysm and tumor with unreactive pupil. Muscle weakness with normally reactive pupil is less ominous (may be ischemic in elderly).
- *Trochlear (fourth nerve) weakness*—usually trauma induced; cannot look down on inward deviation (superior oblique).
- *Abducens (sixth nerve)*—cannot look outward, most often tumor.

▶ Treatment Steps
Tutoring.

K. Vertigo

▶ Description
Sensation of "the room spinning."

▶ Symptoms
Inappropriate perception of motion, often of abrupt onset (peripheral disease) with associated nausea and vomiting. May have nystagmus (peripheral disease, horizontal; central pathology vertigo, vertical nystagmus).

▶ Diagnosis
History and physical, CT/MRI, electronystagmography (ENG), brain stem auditory-evoked responses (BAER), and audiologic testing.

▶ Pathology
Vestibular disorder.

▶ Treatment Steps
1. Medication.
2. Attempt to fatigue response.
3. Surgery.

L. Diplopia

▶ Symptoms
Double vision; may demonstrate head tilt/compensation (head turns toward weak lateral rectus muscle with sixth nerve lesion).

▶ Diagnosis
History and physical examination, laboratory studies, CT/MRI.

▶ Pathology
Loss of eye muscle strength (neurologic disease, infection, tumor, and trauma).

▶ Treatment Steps
Treat individual condition.

V. URINARY SYSTEM

A. Dysuria

▶ Symptoms
Pain with urination, possibly associated with other urinary tract signs and symptoms (frequency, urgency).

▶ Diagnosis
History and physical, UA and culture, cystoscopy, x-rays (KUB, possibly renal ultrasound or spinal CT).

▶ Pathology
Urinary tract inflammation; suggestive of infection, though other etiologies possible (stone, foreign body, tumor, etc.).

▶ Treatment Steps
1. Treat primary disorder.
2. Antibiotics empirically or as per culture.

B. Pyuria

▶ Description
White blood cells in the urine.

▶ Symptoms
Asymptomatic, or symptoms of infection (urgency, frequency, nocturia, etc.). In a female, ask about vaginal discharge, sexual history.

▶ Diagnosis
Midstream UA, and culture, KUB (rule out stone and foreign body).

▶ Pathology
Urinary system inflammation (suggestive of infection), with **polymorphonuclear leukocytes in the urine.**

▶ Treatment Steps
1. Antibiotics as per culture.
2. Treatment of other coexisting disorders.

C. Glycosuria

▶ Description
Urine glucose.

▶ Symptoms
Often asymptomatic.

▶ Diagnosis
UA, dipstick tests (Clinitest, Testape).

▶ Pathology
Urinary glucose after renal threshold is exceeded (may indicate diabetes). Also noted with **renal glycosuria: normal serum glucose with disorder of glucose reabsorption** (congenital, drug/heavy metal induced, or associated with Fanconi syndrome).

▶ Treatment Steps
Blood glucose control.

D. Hematuria

▶ Description
Presence of red blood cells (RBCs) in urine (> 3–5 RBC per hpf).

▶ Symptoms
Microscopic hematuria is asymptomatic. If associated with kidney stones, may see flank pain and/or dysuria. If due to infections, may see symptoms of urinary tract infection (UTI) (dysuria, frequency, urgency). If severe glomerulonephritis (GN), may see signs of renal failure.

▶ Diagnosis
UA, microscopic analysis of urine looking for cells, casts, crystals. Urine culture, SMA-7.

▶ Pathology
Depending on etiology. Need to consider infection (simple UTI, hemorrhagic cystitis, pyelonephritis), nephrolithiasis, bladder or kidney malignancy, intrinsic kidney disease (nephritic or nephrotic GN).

▶ Treatment
Treat the underlying disorder.

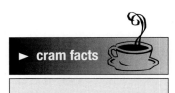

▶ cram facts

Diplopia in a young woman— think of MS (multiple sclerosis).

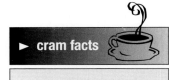

▶ cram facts

- *Sterile pyuria*—rule out renal TB.
- *Casts*—renal inflammation.
- Urine eosinophils— think drug-induced allergic interstitial nephritis?

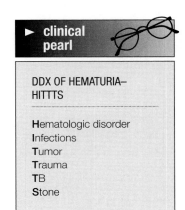

▶ clinical pearl

DDX OF HEMATURIA– HITTTS

Hematologic disorder
Infections
Tumor
Trauma
TB
Stone

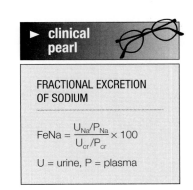

▶ clinical pearl

FRACTIONAL EXCRETION OF SODIUM

$$FeNa = \frac{U_{Na}/P_{Na}}{U_{cr}/P_{cr}} \times 100$$

U = urine, P = plasma

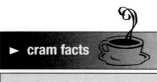

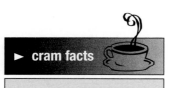

E. Azotemia

► **Description**

Elevated blood urea nitrogen (BUN) and creatinine.

► **Symptoms**

Multisystem abnormalities with renal failure (skeletal, metabolic, cardiovascular, hematologic, etc.). (See Chapter 17.)

► **Diagnosis**

History and physical, UA, urine soduim, urine creatinine, laboratory studies, SMA-12, magnesium, phosphorus, cystoscopy, Foley catheter insertion (may treat and define obstruction), renal ultrasound.

► **Pathology**

Renal failure may be **prerenal** (dehydration or decreased blood flow to kidneys), intrinsic renal disease, or **postrenal** (obstruction).

► **Treatment Steps**

Prerenal—Fluids.

Renal—Treat primary renal injury (e.g., stop offending medication; for rhabdomyolysis, give mannitol).

Postrenal—Remove obstruction.

F. Proteinuria

► **Description**

Elevated urinary protein, indicating renal parenchymal disease.

► **Symptoms**

Asymptomatic, unless severe (nephrotic syndrome—see below).

► **Diagnosis**

UA (dipstick method), followed by 24-hour urine protein study (> 400 mg/24 hr is abnormal).

► **Pathology**

A result of **abnormal proteins (Bence Jones), inadequate reabsorption, glomerular permeability disorder, or renal flow dysfunction.**

► **Treatment Steps**

Treat primary condition.

G. Nephrotic Syndrome

► **Description**

Syndrome involving glomerular dysfunction with massive loss of protein in the urine.

► **Symptoms**

Peripheral edema, ascites, occasionally anasarca, pleural effusion, periorbital edema. Also can see hypertension, hyperlipidemia, and hypercoagulability (renal vein thrombosis in particular).

► **Diagnosis**

History and physical, **24-hour urine protein collection (> 3.5 g/day proteinuria),** laboratory studies (**hypoalbuminemia,** hyperlipidemia), UA (**casts, oval fat bodies), renal biopsy.** Biopsy will delineate the type of GN present and see a secondary etiology.

► Pathology

Wide etiology. More common systematic causes include diabetes mellitus (DM), systemic lupus erythematosus (SLE), intravenous drug use, amyloidosis, hepatitis B, Hodgkin's disease, human immunodeficiency virus (HIV). Idiopathic nephrotic syndrome can also occur. The most common type in children is minimal change disease, in blacks focal segmental glomerulosclerosis, and whites membranous nephropathy.

► Treatment Steps

Treat underlying etiology if possible. Can use loop diuretics for edema, hydroxymethylglutaryl coenzyme A (HMG CoA) reductase inhibitors for hyperlipidemia, ACE inhibitors for proteinuria and blood pressure control, and anticoagulation if thrombosis is present.

H. Renal Colic

► Description

Ureteral spasm and pain, most commonly due to kidney stone.

► Symptoms

Flank or Testicle Pain—Upper ureter stone.

Flank/Abdomen Pain, Nausea/Vomiting—Pelvic brim–level stone.

Groin Pain—Distal ureter stone.

Dysuria/Urgency—Vesical stone.

Also chills, fever, muscle spasm, and signs of bladder irritation.

► Diagnosis

History and physical, x-ray (KUB, IVP), UA, ultrasound, CT scan.

► Pathology

Obstructive ureteral pain secondary to hyperperistalsis (etiology including infection, metabolic and renal disorders).

► Treatment Steps

1. Hydration and analgesia.
2. When stone will not pass, stone removal or lithotripsy.
3. Metabolic workup for the etiology of the stone.

I. Urinary Incontinence

► Description

Loss of urinary retention control.

► Symptoms

Atonic Bladder—Urinary retention and overflow incontinence.

Spastic Neuropathic Bladder—Incontinence.

Infection—Incontinence, symptoms of infection.

Stress Incontinence—Incontinence with exertion and straining.

► Diagnosis

History and physical, UA and culture, urodynamic evaluation (cystometry, uroflowmetry), and x-ray studies (excretory urography, CT, ultrasound, etc.).

► Pathology

Causes of incontinence: Neurologic, stress incontinence, outlet obstruction with overflow incontinence, inflammation, medications, trauma, dementia, and infectious etiology.

► Treatment Steps

As per individual condition (includes medication, surgery, catheterization, etc.).

J. Urinary Retention

► Description

Loss of ability to fully empty the bladder.

► Symptoms

Abdominal **pain, urgency** (without results), nocturia, bladder spasm.

► Diagnosis

History and physical, UA and culture, postvoid residual (after patient voids, insert catheter and record amount of residual urine) urodynamic evaluation, x-ray studies (retrograde urethrography), ultrasound, and obtain laboratory studies (BUN, creatinine, electrolytes, and glucose).

► Pathology

A result of medication (anticholinergics and sympathomimetics), obstruction (cancer, benign prostatic hypertrophy [BPH], stone, valves), or neurologic disease.

► Treatment Steps
1. Remove obstruction.
2. Dilate stricture.
3. Stop offending medication.

K. Oliguria

► Description

Reduced urine production.

► Symptoms

As described, **urine volume 100–400 mL/day,** may cause renal failure (lethargy, hypertension, hematuria, and/or proteinuria), increased BUN/creatinine.

► Diagnosis

History and physical, UA, laboratory studies (BUN, creatinine, calcium, electrolytes, ABGs, urinary osmolality/electrolytes, etc.).

► Pathology

Typically secondary to prerenal pathology (hypovolemia, CHF, burns, etc.), renal pathology (renal failure/disease), or obstruction.

► Treatment Steps

Always start with a fluid challenge. May need diuretics, dialysis.

VI. GENERAL

A. Fever of Unknown Origin

► Description

Fever > 101°F for more than 3 weeks or unexplained even after a 1-week hospital evaluation or three outpatient visits.

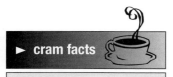

► cram facts

- Retention complications—hydronephrosis, renal failure.
- **Most frequent cause of retention in older men**—benign prostatic hypertrophy.
- **In child**—rule out posterior urethral valves (voiding cystourethrogram).

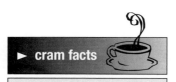

► cram facts

- **Anuria**—urinary output < 100 mL/day.
- **Prerenal oliguria**—urinary osmolality > 500, and urine sodium < 20.
- **Renal oliguria**—urinary osmolality < 350; urine sodium > 40.

► **Symptoms**

May be nonspecific (lethargy, hot/cold flashes, sweating), or symptoms associated with the primary disorder.

► **Diagnosis**

History and physical. Further testing as history and/or physical findings dictate (culture blood/urine/sputum/stool, chest/gallbladder x-rays, laboratory testing: CBC, heterophile, RPR, HIV, etc.), bone scan, CT scan of chest/abdomen, and others.

► **Pathology**

Fever induced by very wide variety of disorders (infection, fungal, medication, tumor, connective tissue, viral, psychogenic, metabolic disorders, etc.).

► **Treatment Steps**

Treat individual disorder.

B. Lymphadenopathy

► **Description**

Enlarged lymph nodes.

► **Symptoms**

Asymptomatic or local tenderness. May demonstrate signs/symptoms of associated disorder.

► **Diagnosis**

History and physical, laboratory studies as indicated (heterophile antibodies, HIV, blood culture, serologic testing, etc.), **biopsy** is diagnostic.

► **Pathology**

Infection (localized or widespread) or tumor (lymphoma or metastatic) can cause lymphadenopathy. Examples include disseminated HIV, mononucleosis, cat-scratch disease. Other etiologies include sarcoidosis, phenytoin sodium.

► **Treatment Steps**

Treat specific disorder.

► **differential diagnosis**

SWOLLEN JOINT (SYNOVIAL) FLUID

- **Hemorrhagic:** Trauma, Charcot joint, coagulation disorders, prosthesis, sickle cell disease
- **Inflammatory:** Rheumatoid arthritis (RA), Reiter syndrome, acute crystal synovitis, Crohn's disease, rheumatic fever, viral etiology, psoriatic disease
- **Noninflammatory:** Osteoarthritis, RA, SLE, scleroderma, aseptic necrosis
- **Purulent:** bacterial infections

BIBLIOGRAPHY

Green GB. *Washington Manual of Medical Therapeutics,* 31st ed. Philadelphia: Lippincott Williams & Wilkins. 1998.

Hurst JW. *Medicine for the Practicing Physician,* 3rd ed. Boston: Butterworth-Heinemann, 1992.

Kutty K. *Kochar's Concise Textbook of Medicine.* Philadelphia: J.B. Lippincott, 2003.

Pryse-Phillips WE. *Essential Neurology,* 4th ed. New York: Medical Examination Publishing Co., 1992.

Rakel RE. *Textbook of Family Practice,* 6th ed. Philadelphia: W.B. Saunders, 2001.

Tanagho EA. *Smith's General Urology,* 15th ed. Norwalk, CT: Appleton & Lange, 2000.

Weiner WJ. *Emergent and Urgent Neurology.* Philadelphia: J.B. Lippincott, 1992.

Woodley M. *Manual of Medical Therapeutics,* 27th ed. Boston: Little, Brown & Co., 1992.

Index